Current Cancer Biomarkers

Edited by

Farhadul Islam
Department of Biochemistry and Molecular Biology,
University of Rajshahi, Rajshahi, Bangladesh

Current Cancer Biomarkers

Editor: Farhadul Islam

ISBN (Online): 978-981-5079-36-4

ISBN (Print): 978-981-5079-37-1

ISBN (Paperback): 978-981-5079-38-8

First published in 2023.

Bentham Science Publishers Pte. Ltd.
80 Robinson Road #02-00
Singapore 068898
Singapore
Email: subscriptions@benthamscience.net

BENTHAM SCIENCE

CONTENTS

FOREWORD

CANCER is the leading cause of the world's death toll and has the greatest adverse economic impact from premature death and disability, ultimately causes of death worldwide. Its economic burden is 1.5 percent of the world's gross domestic product (GDP), around $900 billion excluding direct medical costs, which is 19 percent higher than heart disease. Thus, alleviating cancer will save millions of lives and billions of dollars.

The burden of cancer and economic impacts can be improved, if the disease is diagnosed with precancerous lesions or even early-stage of cancer. Also, the quality of life of patients could be improved by providing personalized treatment and counselling based on the prognosis of the disease. However, robust and effective markers for screening, diagnosis, prognosis and prediction are yet to be established.

The book 'Current Cancer Biomarkers' provides a comprehensive review, and details the clinical implications of currently useful and potential biomarkers for screening, diagnosis and management of patients with cancer. This book could help clinicians, medical students and researchers, at least to some extent, to collect scientific and clinical information on cancer biomarkers.

M. Khalilur Rahman Khan
Professor of Physics & Dean Faculty of Science
University of Rajshahi
Rajshahi-6205
Bangladesh

PREFACE

Cancer is the second leading cause of human mortality worldwide, and researches in the field are enormous to fight against the deadly disease. The huge research on cancer includes cancer biomarker development, diagnosis and detection method development, cellular & molecular characterization of cancers, target identification, therapy development, clinical management, and so on. Since the clinical outcome of patients with cancer largely depends on early and proper diagnosis of the disease, thus, significant efforts on cancer biomarker research are going based on cancer biomarkers for detection, diagnosis, prognosis, therapy response, molecular typing, classification and stratification of cancers. Therefore, this book, Current Cancer Biomarkers, provides a comprehensive review based on the current status of biomarkers for various types of cancer, which could give great potential in disseminating the knowledge and information to a broad range of readers.

This book starts with an introduction to the basic characteristics of cancer biomarkers, which are used for various cancer treatments, and the biomarkers are under development. The next major portion of the book highlights the potential and effective biomarkers such as genomic, epigenomic, transcriptomic, and proteomics, cellular and morphologic factors associated with cancer, indicating the occurrence of cancers. The other part of the book discusses novel technologies to detect and analyse potential cancer biomarkers in point-of-care applications.

This book provided an all-inclusive review and the most updated information based on different aspects of cancer markers in the clinical setting. We hope that the topics covered in this book are useful and enrich our understanding of the disease, which could help better manage patients with cancers.

I am thankful to all the Authors and the editorial staff from Bentham Science for their contribution and support.

Farhadul Islam
Department of Biochemistry and Molecular Biology
University of Rajshahi
Rajshahi
Bangladesh

List of Contributors

Afraa Mamoori	Department of Pathology and Forensic Medicine, School of Medicine, University of Babylon, Hillah, Iraq
Alfred King-yin Lam	Pathology Queensland, Gold Coast University Hospital, Gold Coast, Australia School of Medicine and Dentistry, Menzies Health Institute Queensland, Griffith University, Gold Coast, Australia
Amal Rabti	Sensors and Biosensors Group, Analytical Chemistry & Electrochemistry Lab. (LR99ES15), Faculty of Science, University of Tunis El Manar, Tunis El Manar, Tunisia
Amal Raouafi	Sensors and Biosensors Group, Analytical Chemistry & Electrochemistry Lab. (LR99ES15), Faculty of Science, University of Tunis El Manar, Tunis El Manar, Tunisia
Amira Ben Hassine	Sensors and Biosensors Group, Analytical Chemistry & Electrochemistry Lab. (LR99ES15), Faculty of Science, University of Tunis El Manar, Tunis El Manar, Tunisia
Asif Ahmed	Biotechnology and Genetic Engineering Discipline, Khulna University, Khulna 9208, Bangladesh
Chamath D. Ranaweera	National Cancer Institute of Sri Lanka, Maharagama, Sri Lanka Sunshine Coast Hospital and Health Service, QLD, Australia,
Dan H. V. Tran	Molecular and Cellular Pathology, School of Medicine and Dentistry, Griffith University, Gold Coast, Australia
Farhadul Islam	Department of Biochemistry and Molecular Biology, University of Rajshahi, Rajshahi-6205, Bangladesh
Md Abedul Haque	The University of Texas MD Anderson Cancer Center, Houston, Texas-77033, USA
Md Arifuzzaman	Institute of Tissue Banking and Biomaterial Research, Atomic Energy Research Establishment, Savar, Dhaka-1349, Bangladesh
Md Morsaline Billah	Biotechnology and Genetic Engineering Discipline, Khulna University, Khulna 9208, Bangladesh
Md Nazmul Islam	School of Health & Life Sciences, Teesside University, Middlesbrough TS1 3BA, United Kingdom National Horizons Centre, Teesside University, Darlington DH1 1HG, United Kingdom
Mostafa Kamal Masud	Australian Institute for Bioengineering and Nanotechnology (AIBN), The University of Queensland, Brisbane, QLD, 4072 Australia International Center for Materials Nanoarchitectonics (WPI-MANA), National Institute for Materials Science, Tsukuba, Ibaraki, 305-0044 Japan
Noureddine Raouafi	Sensors and Biosensors Group, Analytical Chemistry & Electrochemistry Lab. (LR99ES15), Faculty of Science, University of Tunis El Manar, Tunis El Manar, Tunisia
Plabon Kumar Das	Institute for Glycomics, Griffith University, Gold Coast, Australia

Riham Zayani	Sensors and Biosensors Group, Analytical Chemistry & Electrochemistry Lab. (LR99ES15), Faculty of Science, University of Tunis El Manar, Tunis El Manar, Tunisia
Sarath S. Joseph	Molecular and Cellular Pathology, School of Medicine and Dentistry, Griffith University, Gold Coast, Australia
Sharmin Aktar	Department of Biochemistry and Molecular Biology, Mawlana Bhashani Science and Technology University, Tangail-1902, Bangladesh School of Medicine and Dentistry, Griffith University, Gold Coast, QLD, Australia
Sujani M.K. Gamage	School of Medicine and Dentistry, Griffith University, Gold Coast, QLD, Australia, Faculty of Medicine, University of Peradeniya, Galaha Rd, 20400, Sri Lanka
Tracie T. Cheng	School of Medicine, Menzies Health Institute Queensland, Griffith University, Gold Coast, Australia
Vinod Gopalan	Molecular and Cellular Pathology, School of Medicine and Dentistry, Griffith University, Gold Coast, Australia

Part 1: Introduction and Clinically Used Biomarker

CHAPTER 1

Introduction: Current Status and Future Advances in Cancer Biomarkers

Farhadul Islam[1,*]

[1] *Department of Biochemistry and Molecular Biology, University of Rajshahi, Rajshahi-6205, Bangladesh*

Abstract: Cancer is a major health problem and a leading cause of morbidity and mortality worldwide. The cancer burden can be reduced significantly using reliable, robust, sensitive, accurate, validated and specific biomarkers for early diagnosis, better prognosis and prediction. Traditionally, a number of biomolecules exhibit the potential to be used as diagnostic, prognostic and predictive biomarkers roles, however, they failed to be used in point-of-care settings for routine analysis. Recent advancements in sequencing techniques and analytical methods facilitate the development of novel and effective cancer biomarkers (liquid biopsies) with the fidelity of clinical application. These biomarkers provide personalized "omics" based information on the pathological state, molecular nature and biological aggressiveness of individual patients. Nevertheless, standardized platforms and/or methods for these biomarkers are yet to be established. Thus, adopting a combination of classical and new cancer biomarkers would offer a better understanding of the disease, resulting in improved clinical outcomes for patients with cancer.

Keywords: Biomarkers, Cancer markers, Cancer management, Cancer burden, Cell-free DNA, Circulating tumour DNA, Circulating tumour cells, Classical cancer markers, Clinical application, Diagnostic markers, Drug toxicity, Liquid biopsy, Non-coding RNAs, Predictive markers, Prognostic markers, Personalized treatment, Precise medication, Tumour-derived exosomes, Tumor-derived extracellular vesicles.

INTRODUCTION

Cancer, a group of diseases, can affect any part of the body, involving uncontrolled growth and proliferation of cells caused by different factors, resulting in extreme molecular and cellular heterogeneity in different and even in a single cancer [1]. However, one defining feature of cancer is the rapid generation of abnormal cells that can grow beyond their usual boundaries and

* **Corresponding author Farhadul Islam:** Department of Biochemistry and Molecular Biology, University of Rajshahi, Rajshahi-6205, Bangladesh; E-mail: farhad_bio83@ru.ac.bd

have the potential of local invasion and distance metastasis- migrating to the other parts of the body. The latter, metastases, is the primary reason for cancer-related mortality in patients with cancers.

Cancer is a major health burden and a leading cause of death worldwide. In 2020, cancer accounted for about ten million deaths, with 19.3 million cases globally [2]. According to GLOBOCAN 2020, 1 in 5 people develop cancer during their lifetime, while 1 in 8 men and 1 in 11 women die from the disease globally [3]. The burden of cancer can be reduced (30 to 50%) by avoiding risk factors (*e.g.* tobacco and alcohol use, unhealthy diet, physical inactivity, air pollution, other non-communicable diseases *etc.*) and by using existing evidence-based prevention strategies. In addition, the cancer burden can also be reduced by early detection, proper care and appropriate treatment modalities [4]. Many cancers have a high chance of cure if diagnosed early in the disease.

Early detection and diagnosis of cancers, especially asymptomatic cases, are challenging and effective markers or methods yet to be established for point-o--care applications. Thus, there is an urgent need to develop effective biomarkers or panel of biomarkers (cancer biomarkers), which can diagnose patients with cancer at early stage with high specificity and sensitivity. Also, sensitive and specific biomarkers for stratification of stages, disease progression and therapy response could improve the clinical outcome of patients with various cancers. A biomarker or biological marker is a measurable indicator of biological condition and/or state using blood, urine, stool or soft tissues [5]. Measurement of a biomarker provides information on normal biological/cellular processes, pathogenic processes or pharmacologic responses to therapy. Thus, in principle, cancer or tumour biomarker is a biomolecule or part of biomolecules found in blood, urine, stool or body tissues, which elevated in the presence of cancer in biological samples. These biomarkers can be generated directly by a cancer cell or by a non-cancer cell in presence of cancer. Most of the cancer biomarkers can be categorized as tumour-specific antigens or tumour-associated antigens. They could be either (i) products of mutated oncogenes, (ii) products of tumour suppressor genes, (iii) products of other mutated genes, including (a) overexpressed or abnormally expressed cellular proteins or protein fragments, (b) tumour antigens produced by oncogenic viruses, (c) oncofetal antigens, (d) altered cell surface glycoproteins and glycolipids and (e) cell-type specific differentiation antigens, and (iv) altered or aberrant genetic and epigenetic make-up in cancer cells. Thus, a biomarker can be genetic materials, such as DNA, RNAs, including non-coding RNAs, or their products, *i.e.* proteins or peptides or even epigenetic changes, such as DNA-methylation. However, an ideal cancer biomarker should have the following criteria for effective use in clinical applications [6].

A. Produced in the presence of cancer (significantly elevated levels).

B. Associated with the cancer burden and provide sufficient lead time (length of time between the disease detection and its usual clinical presentation and diagnosis).

C. Significantly higher levels in blood, urine, stools or other biological samples in patients with cancer than in healthy individuals, especially at early or preclinical stages of patients.

D. Highly sensitive and specific for cancer types, preferably one type of cancer.

E. Easy, cost-effective, less labour intensive and able to measure in small quantities in point-of-care settings.

Classical Cancer Biomarker

A cancer biomarker can be used for screening, diagnosis, monitoring disease progression, therapy response and disease recurrence/relapse [7], therefore, giving the information of the disease status in particular patients, which in turn can facilitate the personalized cancer management in patients. Thus, cancer biomarkers can be classified into three broad categories, (i) diagnostic, (ii) prognostic and (iii) predictive biomarkers. However, a biomarker can be used for more than one clinical applications, thereby can fall into more than one of these groups.

Diagnostic Cancer Biomarkers

As mentioned earlier that early detection of cancer can significantly reduce the cancer burden, thereby alleviating economic and social costs associated with cancer. Early detection of cancer allows better response to the treatment, resulting in higher survival rates and less morbidity, along with the lower cost of management [8]. Therefore, a significant improvement can be made in patients with cancers by detecting them at earlier stages, especially at the asymptomatic stages and avoiding delays in proper care.

Early cancer detection can be carried out by screening of mass population using appropriate biomarker tests with the aim to identify individuals with findings indicative of specific cancer or pre-cancer at the asymptomatic phase. Identification of abnormalities during screening suggests further tests to diagnose the disease. The screening test must be inexpensive and safe enough to be used by mass populations and should be very highly sensitive and specific to avoid too many false positives in tested populations [9]. The screening programs for early detection are effective for some cancer types but not all cancer types. Also, the screening programs are far more complex and resource-intensive, requiring special equipment and resource personnel. The most widely used screening methods for early detection cancer are human papilloma virus (HPV), Papanicolaou (Pap) cytology and visual inspection with acetic acid (VIA) testing for cervical cancer, mammography screening for breast cancer. Also, human choriogonadotrophin can be used for germ cell tumours and gestational trophoblastic disease, α-fetoprotein can be used for hepatic and testicular carcinomas screening [9, 10]. However, an effective biomarker test for mass population screening and early cancer detection in clinical settings is yet to be established and poised a greatest challenge in cancer research and management.

On the contrary, a diagnostic cancer biomarker should narrow down the diagnosis and identify specific individual patients in clinical settings. Thus, a diagnostic biomarker test should be prescribed to individuals who have already developed symptoms of specific cancer types. However, there is no well-established biomarker test recommended in clinical practice for cancer diagnosis [6, 11]. Although, a number of well-known markers are widely used as a facilitator in the diagnosis and/or stratification of the cancers' pathological state. Since, there is no specific and recommended tumour biomarker for diagnosis, they should not be used for cancer diagnostic purposes, while they can be used to monitor or screen certain cancer types or certain cancer cases [12, 13]. Inappropriate and over-investigation would be the results of these biomarker tests if applied without understanding their utility in patient care.

Prognostic Cancer Biomarkers

Prognostic markers are biomarkers used to measure the progression of the disease using patients' biological samples. They are biomolecules, factors or biological characteristics that can be measured objectively and evaluated to predict the outcome of a disease or response to a therapeutic intervention among individuals with the same trait [14]. Thus, they provide information about the patient's overall outcome irrespective of therapeutic intervention.

The clinically useful prognostic biomarkers are used to stratify the patients into groups, thereby guiding them toward personalized medication. In cancer, the widely used traditional prognostic markers include tumour size, grade, lymph node metastasis, stage and distance metastasis. Larger tumour size, higher grade, advanced staging and presence of metastasis are associated with poor prognosis in patients with cancer [15]. In addition, cancer-specific prognostic markers also used in patient with various cancers. For example, estrogen, progesterone and HER2 levels are used as prognostic markers for patients with breast cancer [16].

Additionally, advances in molecular techniques in genomics, epigenetics and proteomics research, such as microarray, and deep or high throughput sequencing, have provided better opportunities to identify new biomarkers for cancer prognosis. These new generations of prognostic markers can be genetic (*i.e.,* DAN), epigenetic (*e.g.* methylation, non-coding RNAs), signalling pathways, proteins or protein fragments and metabolic molecules [17, 18]. The newly developed biomarkers can provide information that can facilitate the oncologist to guide personalised management of patients with cancer.

Predictive Cancer Biomarkers

Predictive biomarkers can be used to predict the likelihood benefit of specific therapy and optimize ideal treatment for clinical outcomes [19]. In oncology, predictive biomarkers assess the probable response of the tumour to the drug, thereby introducing a level of personalized treatment regimen in patients. Thus, an effective predictive biomarker could reduce the cost in considerable amounts as the therapy or drugs would be used only in patients likely get benefit from the treatment. However, till now, only a small number of biomarkers such as K-ras mutations, ER, PR and HER2/neu levels, BCR-ABL fusion protein, c-Kit mutations and EGFR1 mutations *etc*., have predictive clinical utility for patients with cancer [14, 20]. For example, BCR-ABL fusion protein and EGFR1 mutations are used as predictive biomarkers for patients with chronic myeloid leukaemia and non-small cell lung carcinomas, respectively in clinical care [14]. Also, predictive biomarkers (K-ras mutations) in metastatic colorectal cancer can evaluate and improve patients' survival rates [19]. In addition, a number of predictive biomarkers are gaining clinical acceptance as their objective measurements can give clinical response to the drug; patients only expressing the specific marker will response to the specific drug or will have higher degree of response while patients without the marker won't exhibit significant drug response [21]. Thus, in individual case by case scenario, predictive markers can differentiate the patients as responder from non-responder to guide the choice of anticancer therapy, resulting in sparing the patients from unnecessary toxicity and side effects of the regimen, thereby improving cancer care.

Future Cancer Biomarkers

The discovery and development of traditional cancer biomarkers could improve the survival rates and quality of life of patients, thereby having significant impacts on the better management of patients with cancers. However, research in the field of classical/traditional cancer biomarkers development is currently discouraging, as most of the newly identified cancer biomarkers are abandoned or fail clinical validation due to poorer analytical performance, resulting in no clinical utility in practical applications [22]. Nonetheless, the recent advancement of sequencing technologies, such as next-generation sequencing, high-throughput or deep sequencing *etc*., improved analytical platforms and/or methods to detect and analyse single cell or cells cluster allows to identify and develop new generation of cancer biomarkers, popularly known as "liquid biopsy", with the potential of clinical utility for patients with cancers [23]. These liquid biopsies have been receiving enormous attention in recent years as easy, rapid and non-invasive tools for cancer screening, diagnosis, prognosis and prediction of therapeutic intervention in cancer patients [24]. The potential candidate for effective liquid biopsies, includes but not limited to, circulating tumour cells (CTCs), metastatic-CTCs, circular tumour-DNA (ctDNA), cell free-DNA (cfDNA), non-coding RNAs (*e.g.* microRNA, long non-coding RNA, circular RNAs *etc.*), cancer epigenetics, tumour derived exosomes (TEX), tumour derive extracellular vesicles (TD-EVs) *etc*., exhibiting promising clinical utility in clinical applications.

CTCs are the disseminated cancer cells found in the peripheral blood in solid malignancies and their presence in blood and quantity associated with the prognosis of various cancers, including breast, colorectal, head and neck, lung, oesophageal, pancreatic, gastric *etc*., cancers [25]. In addition, molecular and functional characterization of CTCs provide personalized information about the patients, which in turn can dictate the diagnosis, prognosis and prediction of therapy. Profiling of CTCs can also have the potential to be used for predicting micrometastasis, monitoring progression and stratification of cancer [25]. However, analytical grade platforms and /or methodologies for the detection and characterization of CTCs yet to be established. Thus, standardised methods or technologies must be developed to detect and analyse CTCs for their clinical applications.

ctDNA is a tumour-derived DNA fragment found in the peripherals blood, originated only from tumour cells and CTCs. As ctDNA reflect the entire cancer genome, it has the potential of clinical utility as liquid biopsy by drawing blood at various time points to monitor disease progression [26]. Higher levels of ctDNA associated with larger tumour size and ctDNA harbour similar cancer-associated mutations in genomic DNA of patients with cancer, indicating that ctDNA can be used as a cancer detection, prognostic and treatment follow up biomarker [27, 28]. In addition, ctDNA can predict the presence of tumour recurrence by detecting minimal residual disease, whereas conventional imaging methods, such as CT, PET or MRI scan may unable to detect presence of disease after tumour resection. However, the clinical utility of ctDNA for primary cancer screening is limited by the sensitivity of the current technologies to detect low levels of ctDNA presence in patients with small tumours at early stages of the disease [27]. Therefore, clinical application of ctDNA is would be established by developing standardised methods for ctDNA processing and analysis along with the standardization of sample collection, downstream processing such as DNA extraction, amplification, quantification and validation must need to be established for routine analysis in clinical settings.

cfDNA is the freely circulating DNA fragments with a predominant 166bp length, found in the bloodstream, however, not necessarily of tumour origin [29]. The length of fragmentation is an indication of apoptotic fragmentation and altered cfDNA fragmentation is detected in cancer patients [29, 30]. As cfDNA is possibly derived from necrotic, apoptotic and living cells, their profiling and characterization of such epigenetic alterations have potential clinical applications for early detection, prognosis and prediction of therapy response [31].

Non-coding RNAs, including microRNAs (miRNAs), long non-coding RNAs (lncRNA), *etc*., are RNA molecules that do not translate into a specific protein, however, they regulate the expression and functionality of their targets, either at post-transcriptional or post-translational levels [32]. Since they regulate the expression of tumour suppressors and oncogenes, their alterations in cancer are associated with cancer initiation and disease progression [33]. A number of noncoding RNAs, such as miRNA-1, miRNA-34b, miRNA-miRNA-186, HOTAIR, GAS5, and SNORD50, *etc*., are associated with prognosis and diagnosis of various cancers [33 - 35]. Thus, profiling and validation of non-coding RNAs in cancer could have potential biomarkers implication for cancer diagnosis, prognosis and prediction of clinical outcome inpatients with cancer.

Exosomes are nanovesicles derived from all types of cells carrying information (*e.g*. mRNA, miRNA, circular RNA and proteins) originating from the parental cells. Tumour-derived exosomes (TEXs) carry endogenous cargos containing molecules that reflect the pathological status of cancer, thus, providing their potential to be used as novel non-invasive cancer diagnostics, prognostics and monitoring biomarkers [36, 37]. Also, tumour-derived extracellular vesicles (TD-EVs) can carry multiple cargoes containing DNA, RNAs, and proteins during distant metastasis. Paracrine signalling mediated by TD-EVs between adjacent cancer cells allows crosstalk, which in turn modulates the tumour microenvironment in favour of becoming a premetastatic niche [38]. Hence, TD-EVs could be a potential biomarker for cancer development and metastasis. Therefore, analysis of TD-EVs and TEXs derived genetic materials and proteomics have widespread potential use in cancer diagnosis and treatment. However, established and standardized methods for accurate and sensitive detection and isolation need to be develop for their clinical applications.

CONCLUDING REMARKS

The trial and error approach to cancer treatment and management is largely empirical, costly, and more frequently ineffective, resulting in poor clinical outcomes. The traditional 'one size fits all' strategy lead some patients (patients with aggressive tumour load) under treatment, whereas to other patients (patients with indolent disease) over treatments, thereby generating drug-associated toxicity. On the other hand, recent personalised or individualized strategies based on molecular and functional characterization of each cancer patient would provide precise information for the better management of each case. Personalized therapy provides the right drug to the right patient at the right time with the correct dose and schedule. This could provide an optimum clinical outcome for patients with cancer, however, without reliable, robust, validated, sensitive, specific and accurate cancer biomarkers, personalized precise medication would not be successful in practical applications.

CONSENT FOR PUBLICATION

Not applicable.

CONFLICT OF INTEREST

The author declares no conflict of interest, financial or otherwise.

ACKNKOWLEDGEMENT

The author is thankful to the University of Rajshahi for providing the technical support.

REFERENCES

[1] https://www.who.int/news-room/fact-sheets/detail/cancer

[2] Ferlay J, Ervik M, Lam F, *et al.* Global Cancer Observatory: Cancer Today. Lyon: International Agency for Research on Cancer 2020.https://gco.iarc.fr/today

[3] GLOBOCAN 2020: New global cancer data. https://www.uicc.org/news/globocan-2020-new-glo-al-cancer-data

[4] Early FC. https://www.cancer.org/healthy/find-cancer-early.html American Cancer Society.

[5] Hirsch MS, Watkins J. A comprehensive review of biomarker use in the gynecologic tract including differential diagnoses and diagnostic pitfalls. Adv Anat Pathol 2020; 27(3): 164-92. [http://dx.doi.org/10.1097/PAP.0000000000000238] [PMID: 31149908]

[6] Duffy MJ. Tumor markers in clinical practice: a review focusing on common solid cancers. Med Princ Pract 2013; 22(1): 4-11. [http://dx.doi.org/10.1159/000338393] [PMID: 22584792]

[7] Sawyers CL. The cancer biomarker problem. Nature 2008; 452(7187): 548-52. [http://dx.doi.org/10.1038/nature06913] [PMID: 18385728]

[8] Konforte D, Diamandis EP. Is early detection of cancer with circulating biomarkers feasible? Clin Chem 2013; 59(1): 35-7.
[http://dx.doi.org/10.1373/clinchem.2012.184903] [PMID: 22522223]

[9] Buchen L. Cancer: Missing the mark. Nature 2011; 471(7339): 428-32.
[http://dx.doi.org/10.1038/471428a] [PMID: 21430749]

[10] Diamandis EP. Cancer biomarkers: can we turn recent failures into success? J Natl Cancer Inst 2010; 102(19): 1462-7.
[http://dx.doi.org/10.1093/jnci/djq306] [PMID: 20705936]

[11] Pavlou MP, Diamandis EP, Blasutig IM. The long journey of cancer biomarkers from the bench to the clinic. Clin Chem 2013; 59(1): 147-57.
[http://dx.doi.org/10.1373/clinchem.2012.184614] [PMID: 23019307]

[12] Kilpatrick ES, Lind MJ. Appropriate requesting of serum tumour markers. BMJ 2009; 339(sep22 1): b3111.
[http://dx.doi.org/10.1136/bmj.b3111] [PMID: 19773324]

[13] Krishnan STM, Philipose Z, Rayman G. Lesson of the week: Hypothyroidism mimicking intra-abdominal malignancy. BMJ 2002; 325(7370): 946-7.
[http://dx.doi.org/10.1136/bmj.325.7370.946] [PMID: 12399347]

[14] Oldenhuis CNAM, Oosting SF, Gietema JA, de Vries EGE. Prognostic versus predictive value of biomarkers in oncology. Eur J Cancer 2008; 44(7): 946-53.
[http://dx.doi.org/10.1016/j.ejca.2008.03.006] [PMID: 18396036]

[15] Islam F, Gopalan V, Pillai S, Lu C, Kasem K, Lam AK. Promoter hypermethylation inactivate tumor suppressor *FAM134B* and is associated with poor prognosis in colorectal cancer. Genes Chromosomes Cancer 2018; 57(5): 240-51.
[http://dx.doi.org/10.1002/gcc.22525] [PMID: 29318692]

[16] Yeung C, Hilton J, Clemons M, *et al.* Estrogen, progesterone, and HER2/neu receptor discordance between primary and metastatic breast tumours—a review. Cancer Metastasis Rev 2016; 35(3): 427-37.
[http://dx.doi.org/10.1007/s10555-016-9631-3] [PMID: 27405651]

[17] Liu S, Wu M, Wang F. Research progress in prognostic factors and biomarkers of ovarian cancer. J Cancer 2021; 12(13): 3976-96.
[http://dx.doi.org/10.7150/jca.47695] [PMID: 34093804]

[18] Winder T, Lenz HJ. Molecular predictive and prognostic markers in colon cancer. Cancer Treat Rev 2010; 36(7): 550-6.
[http://dx.doi.org/10.1016/j.ctrv.2010.03.005] [PMID: 20363564]

[19] Ruiz-Bañobre J, Kandimalla R, Goel A. Predictive Biomarkers in Metastatic Colorectal Cancer: A Systematic Review. JCO Precision Oncology 2019; 3: 1-17.
[http://dx.doi.org/10.1200/PO.18.00260]

[20] Batis N, Brooks JM, Payne K, Sharma N, Nankivell P, Mehanna H. Lack of predictive tools for conventional and targeted cancer therapy: Barriers to biomarker development and clinical translation. Adv Drug Deliv Rev 2021; 176: 113854.
[http://dx.doi.org/10.1016/j.addr.2021.113854] [PMID: 34192550]

[21] La Thangue NB, Kerr DJ. Predictive biomarkers: a paradigm shift towards personalized cancer medicine. Nat Rev Clin Oncol 2011; 8(10): 587-96.
[http://dx.doi.org/10.1038/nrclinonc.2011.121] [PMID: 21862978]

[22] Diamandis EP. Present and future of cancer biomarkers. Clinical Chemistry and Laboratory Medicine (CCLM) 2014; 52(6): 791-4.
[http://dx.doi.org/10.1515/cclm-2014-0317] [PMID: 24803613]

[23] Watanabe K, Nakamura Y, Low SK. Clinical implementation and current advancement of blood liquid biopsy in cancer. J Hum Genet 2021; 66(9): 909-26.
[http://dx.doi.org/10.1038/s10038-021-00939-5] [PMID: 34088974]

[24] Freitas C, Sousa C, Machado F, *et al.* The role of liquid biopsy in early diagnosis of lung cancer. Front Oncol 2021; 11: 634316.
[http://dx.doi.org/10.3389/fonc.2021.634316] [PMID: 33937034]

[25] Chauhan A, Kaur R, Ghoshal S, Pal A. Exploration of circulating tumour cell (CTC) biology: A paradigm shift in liquid biopsy. Indian J Clin Biochem 2021; 36(2): 131-42.
[http://dx.doi.org/10.1007/s12291-020-00923-4] [PMID: 33867703]

[26] Wan JCM, Massie C, Garcia-Corbacho J, *et al.* Liquid biopsies come of age: towards implementation of circulating tumour DNA. Nat Rev Cancer 2017; 17(4): 223-38.
[http://dx.doi.org/10.1038/nrc.2017.7] [PMID: 28233803]

[27] Avanzini S, Kurtz DM, Chabon JJ, *et al.* A mathematical model of ctDNA shedding predicts tumor detection size. Sci Adv 2020; 6(50): eabc4308.
[http://dx.doi.org/10.1126/sciadv.abc4308] [PMID: 33310847]

[28] Yong E. Cancer biomarkers: Written in blood. Nature 2014; 511(7511): 524-6.
[http://dx.doi.org/10.1038/511524a] [PMID: 25079538]

[29] Mouliere F, Robert B, Arnau Peyrotte E, *et al.* High fragmentation characterizes tumour-derived circulating DNA. PLoS One 2011; 6(9): e23418.
[http://dx.doi.org/10.1371/journal.pone.0023418] [PMID: 21909401]

[30] Mouliere F, Chandrananda D, Piskorz AM, *et al.* Enhanced detection of circulating tumor DNA by fragment size analysis. Sci Transl Med 2018; 10(466): eaat4921.
[http://dx.doi.org/10.1126/scitranslmed.aat4921] [PMID: 30404863]

[31] Tran NH, Kisiel J, Roberts LR. Using cell-free DNA for HCC surveillance and prognosis. JHEP Reports 2021; 3(4): 100304.
[http://dx.doi.org/10.1016/j.jhepr.2021.100304] [PMID: 34136776]

[32] Das PK, Siddika MA, Asha SY, *et al.* MicroRNAs, a promising target for breast cancer stem cells. Mol Diagn Ther 2020; 24(1): 69-83.
[http://dx.doi.org/10.1007/s40291-019-00439-5] [PMID: 31758333]

[33] Das PK, Asha SY, Abe I, Islam F, Lam AK. Roles of non-coding RNAs on anaplastic thyroid carcinomas. Cancers (Basel) 2020; 12(11): 3159.
[http://dx.doi.org/10.3390/cancers12113159] [PMID: 33126409]

[34] Islam F, Gopalan V, Vider J, *et al.* MicroRNA-186-5p overexpression modulates colon cancer growth by repressing the expression of the FAM134B tumour inhibitor. Exp Cell Res 2017; 357(2): 260-70.
[http://dx.doi.org/10.1016/j.yexcr.2017.05.021] [PMID: 28549913]

[35] Islam F, Gopalan V, Law S, Tang JCO, Chan KW, Lam AKY. MiR-498 in esophageal squamous cell carcinoma: clinicopathological impacts and functional interactions. Hum Pathol 2017; 62: 141-51.
[http://dx.doi.org/10.1016/j.humpath.2017.01.014] [PMID: 28188753]

[36] Verdi J, Ketabchi N, Noorbakhsh N, *et al.* Development and clinical application of tumor-derived exosomes in patients with cancer. Curr Stem Cell Res Ther 2022; 17(1): 91-102.
[http://dx.doi.org/10.2174/1574888X16666210622123942] [PMID: 34161212]

[37] Luo R, Liu M, Yang Q, *et al.* Emerging diagnostic potential of tumor-derived exosomes. J Cancer 2021; 12(16): 5035-45.
[http://dx.doi.org/10.7150/jca.59391] [PMID: 34234872]

[38] Qiao F, Pan P, Yan J, *et al.* Role of tumor-derived extracellular vesicles in cancer progression and their clinical applications (Review). Int J Oncol 2019; 54(5): 1525-33.
[http://dx.doi.org/10.3892/ijo.2019.4745] [PMID: 30864674]

CHAPTER 2

Tumour Markers in Clinical Use

Sujani M. K. Gamage[1,2,*], **Chamath D. Ranaweera**[3,4], **Tracie T. Cheng**[1], **Sharmin Aktar**[1,5], **Vinod Gopalan**[1] and **Farhadul Islam**[6]

[1] *School of Medicine, Griffith University, Gold Coast, QLD, Australia*

[2] *Faculty of Medicine, University of Peradeniya, Galaha Rd, 20400, Sri Lanka*

[3] *National Cancer Institute of Sri Lanka, Maharagama, Sri Lanka*

[4] *Sunshine Coast Hospital and Health Service, QLD, Australia*

[5] *Department of Biochemistry and Molecular Biology, Mawlana Bhashani Science and Technology University, Tangail-1902, Bangladesh*

[6] *Department of Biochemistry and Molecular Biology, University of Rajshahi, Rajshahi-6205, Bangladesh*

Abstract: Despite ever-growing experimental evidence for the utility of a wide range of tumour markers, only a handful are understood to be useful in clinical applications. Tumour markers are useful for screening and diagnosis of cancers, prognostication, guiding treatment pathways and post-treatment surveillance studies. The tumour makers play a significant role in cancer care and the markers included in the current treatment guidelines will be discussed in detail in this chapter. The utility of the tumour markers in the management of colorectal, breast, thyroid, hepatobiliary, pancreatic, ovarian, testicular, neuroendocrine and prostate cancer are detailed herein to provide an update on the current use of tumour markers in the clinical settings.

Keywords: Alpha-fetoprotein (AFP), Breast cancer, Calcitonin cancer, Cancer treatment, Carcinoembryonic antigen (CEA), Chromogranin A, Colorectal cancer, Current guidelines in cancer care, CA 125, CA 19.9, Follow-up in cancer care, Hepatobiliary cancer, Neuroendocrine tumours, Ovarian cancer, Pancreatic cancer, Prostate cancer, Prostate-specific antigen (PSA), Screening, Surveillance, Testicular cancer, Thyroglobulin (Tg), Thyroid cancer, Tumour markers.

INTRODUCTION

Tumour marker is a substance (commonly a protein, enzyme or hormone) that is present or produced either by tumour cell or by other cells in the body due to the effects of cancer, which can be detectable in body fluids or tissue and provides

* **Corresponding author Sujani M. K. Gamage:** School of Medicine, Griffith University, Gold Coast, QLD, Australia; E-mail: s.kodagodagamage@griffith.edu.au

valuable information about the aggressiveness of cancer, potential treatment modalities as well as disease and treatment outcomes. Also, they can either be produced within the cancer cells or by the non-cancerous cells as a result of the metabolic alterations caused by cancer [1]. Genetic alterations are also being considered tumour markers, especially for screening purposes. Theoretically, an ideal tumour marker should have the following characteristics: (i) having a high degree of specificity to the particular tumour; (ii) possessing high sensitivity to rule out possible false positives; (iii) allowing a sufficient time frame (lead time) to alter the natural course of the disease; (iv) detectable levels being reliably correlated with the tumour burden, while closely reflecting tumour progression; (v) having a short half-life, permitting serial measurements and (vi) being affordable for patients. Unfortunately, such an ideal tumour marker does not exist, and the available markers have their advantages and limitations [2].

Tumour markers are particularly important in assessing treatment response and residual disease, surveillance and follow-up. Following treatment, normalization of tumour markers usually denotes adequate cancer resection/ treatment. Normalized tumour marker levels with radiological evidence of persistent disease may indicate that the tumour is non-viable. There may be a transient increase in tumour marker levels following effective treatment, secondary to cell lysis. Therefore, an increase in tumour marker levels on its own does not signify treatment failure. However, increasing tumour markers in a clinically deteriorating patient may indicate treatment failure or recurrence, warranting further work-up [3].

Though there are experimental evidence for the utility of a wide range of tumour markers for each cancer, only a handful are used in the actual clinical setting (Table **1**). Selected tumour markers, which are routinely used in the clinical setup and are important in the diagnosis and management of cancers, will be discussed in detail in this chapter.

Markers for Colorectal Cancer

Colorectal cancer (CRC) is the third most common cancer worldwide, affecting mostly the population in developed countries [4]. However, the prognosis of patients with CRC depends mainly on the cancer staging at the time of presentation. Tumour markers have particular importance in the diagnosis of disease and determination of prognosis of patients with CRC. Carcinoembryonic antigen (CEA) is the most used tumour marker in clinical practice for CRC. In addition, tissue polypeptide-specific antigen (TPS), carbohydrate antigen (CA 19.9), hematopoietic growth factors (HGF-s) and tumour-associated glycoprotein-72 (TAG-72) are promising as potential tumour markers in CRC [5, 6].

Macrophage-colony stimulating factor (M-CSF), granulocyte-macrophage-colony stimulating factor (GM-CSF), Cathepsin D, interleukin-3, interleukin-6 and enzymes, such as Alcohol Dehydrogenase and Lysosomal Exoglycosidases, are also recognised as potential CRC related tumour markers [7 - 10]. However, these are still not widely used in clinical practice. Since most cancer-related deaths are due to metastasis, investigations on circulating tumour cells (CTCs) will be promising with respect to gaining information on the prognosis and treatment response of patients with CRC [11 - 13]. Nevertheless, currently, only CEA is considered a reliable marker for CRC in clinical practice.

Diagnosis

CEA is an oncofetal antigen present in most epithelial tumours and is the most versatile and frequently used tumour marker in clinical settings [6]. Relative cost-effectiveness has warranted its use in routine clinical practice. However, serum CEA levels are elevated in only 17-47% of patients with CRC [14 - 16]. CEA can be elevated in many benign conditions, including benign liver and kidney disease, pancreatitis, inflammatory bowel disease, obstructive pulmonary disease and other malignancies including gastric, oesophageal, pancreatic, lung, breast and mesotheliomas. Levels may also be higher than the reference range in chronic smokers, and the cut-off point for the upper normal value is twice as for a non-smoker [17, 18]. Therefore, CEA is not used in isolation to diagnose CRC due to its lack of sensitivity and specificity. However, the presence of a high concentration of CEA can be useful in circumstances in which there is a high clinical probability of cancer, and the patient is not fit enough to undergo invasive investigations. Also, markedly raised serum CEA levels (>40μg/L) are usually indicative of metastatic disease [18].

Prediction of Prognosis

Although pathological staging of CRC is the most reliable prognostic predictor, serum CEA levels are routinely performed to reinforce decision-making. High CEA level during the preoperative period is correlated with poor prognosis [15, 18].

Follow up

Several studies have confirmed that intense post-treatment surveillance improves overall survival by detecting treatable metastasis [19, 20]. Along with imaging and endoscopic surveillance, serum CEA is a reliable tumour marker for the detection of recurrences in CRC patients. Up to 50% of patients who undergo curative resection for CRC can develop liver metastasis within 5 years. Resection of resectable liver metastasis is the only curative treatment apart from a liver transplant. Early detection of resectable liver metastasis improves the outcome significantly, and serial monitoring of CEA is extremely useful in that context. Similarly, the patients who develop metastasis are treatable with chemotherapy [21]. According to the National Comprehensive Cancer Network (NCCN) Guidelines, postoperative surveillance of CRC patients with pathological stages II, III and IV should include monitoring serum CEA levels every 3-6 months for 2 years, followed by 6 monthly tests for a total of 5 years. If serial CEA elevation is detected, the patient should be considered for subsequent investigations and treatment for metastasis [1]. Due to clonal changes in cancer cells, tumours secreting CEA at the beginning of the disease may develop metastatic disease, which does not secrete CEA. Therefore, a normal CEA level does not rule out the possibility of tumour recurrence or metastatic disease. Similarly, tumours that do not secrete CEA, in the beginning, may start producing it later due to clonal change, which is the rationale for monitoring those patient's CEA levels following curative intent treatment.

Markers for Breast Cancer

Breast cancer is the second most common cancer worldwide and the fifth cause for cancer-related death [22]. Early detection is of utmost importance, and it is mainly dependent on the clinical parameters. Although when positive, tumour markers provide a cost-effective and less invasive way of monitoring disease progression and treatment response, the utility of most tumour markers is questioned in the clinical setting due to the low sensitivity at the early stages of the disease [23]. A list of tumour markers related to breast cancer, which have clinical relevance, has been highlighted by the American Society of Clinical Oncology. They are CA 15-3, CA 27.29, CEA, Estrogen receptor (ER), Progesterone receptor (PR), Plasminogen activator inhibitor 1 (PAI-1), Human epidermal growth factor receptor 2 (HER2) and Urokinase plasminogen activator (uPA) [24].

However, the only tumour marker of clinical significance in breast cancer is CA15-3, which is mostly used to monitor disease in clinical settings. It is high molecular weight mucin, a carbohydrate-containing protein antigen. The gene responsible for CA15-3 is MUC1, and it is highly expressed in breast malignancies, making it a reliable marker for the assessment of prognosis [25]. However, the use of CA15-3 for screening is limited because it may be elevated in other malignancies such as ovarian, lung, pancreatic, and colon cancer and in benign conditions, including benign liver and breast diseases [26]. Therefore, tumour markers are not recommended for screening for breast cancer. CA15-3 is a reliable marker of prognosis and treatment efficacy as it has been observed that its serum concentration increases with the stage and size of cancer [27]. European

Group on Tumour Markers recommends serial monitoring of CEA and CA15-3 for early detection of recurrence, but it is not included in the standard post-treatment follow-up in guidelines NCCN guidelines. If measured, a 25% rise from the previous value is considered to be significant. To assess the chemotherapy response, CA 15-3 can be measured before every chemotherapy cycle. A reduction below 50% from the previous value is considered a satisfactory response [28].

In summary, none of the current clinical guidelines recommends the routine use of tumour markers in decision-making in breast cancer treatment.

Markers for Thyroid Cancer

Thyroid cancer is becoming increasingly common, especially among females. Differentiated thyroid cancers (DTC), which include Papillary, Follicular and Hurthle cell cancers, are by far the commonest, followed by Medullary and Anaplastic cancers. Thyroid tissue produces Thyroglobulin (Tg) as a precursor of active T3 and T4 hormones [29]. The serum Tg levels are proportional to the volume of active thyroid tissue. Therefore, it can be used to assess the cancer burden of DTC at presentation, adequacy of surgical clearance and monitor recurrences and treatment response [30].

Calcitonin is a hormone, which plays an important role in calcium homeostasis, is produced by parafollicular cells of the thyroid gland and is important as a tumour marker in medullary carcinoma.

Importance of Thyroglobulin in Differentiated Thyroid Cancer (DTC)

Surveillance after Thyroidectomy

Thyroglobulin is a useful marker for differentiated thyroid cancer. The definitive treatment modality for DTC is the surgical removal of the affected lobe (hemithyroidectomy) or the whole gland (total thyroidectomy), usually followed by radioactive iodine ablation of any residual thyroid tissue. It is not uncommon to leave some thyroid tissue behind, inadvertently or deliberately, during a total thyroidectomy due to various technical reasons. This residual thyroid tissue, if survived, may continue to produce Tg secondary to high TSH levels (lack of feedback inhibition). Therefore, measurement of serum Tg level is important in identifying residual thyroid tissue or recurrent disease [29]. Thus, serum Tg levels are routinely measured following total thyroidectomy (TT) as a component of the post-surgical evaluation to identify the residual, recurrent or metastatic disease [1, 29]. Serum Tg levels should be lower than the reference value of the index laboratory, following complete excision/ablation of thyroid tissue and should remain low if treatment is complete. The sensitivity of Tg measurement can be improved by either increasing the TSH value for >30 mIU/L by withholding thyroxin treatment or administering recombinant TSH. In the patient who had hemithyroidectomy or TT not followed by radioactive Iodine treatment, the interpretation of serum Tg values is less reliable due to the inability to differentiate between tumour and thyroid remnant, though the rising trend of Tg may be of clinical significance. Patients with persistently elevated Tg levels or upwardly trending Tg levels should be further evaluated for recurrence or metastatic disease, usually with Radio Iodine whole-body scan and cross-sectional imaging [31]. Nevertheless, 10-25% of patients develop antibodies against Tg (Anti-Tg antibodies), which can interfere with Tg measurement-based follow-up. Therefore, Thyroglobulin antibody (anti-Tg antibody) levels should also be evaluated along with Tg levels to exclude false-negative results secondary to the development of anti-Tg antibodies [29].

Determination of the Requirement of Radioactive Iodine Therapy

Thyroglobulin levels are useful in determining if radioactive iodine (RAI) treatment is required following thyroidectomy. In cases where there is no gross residual disease in the neck, typically RAI therapy is not required if all of the following conditions are met: the cancer is a classic papillary thyroid carcinoma, the largest primary tumour is less than 2cm in size, cancer is intrathyroidal, unifocal or multifocal with all foci are 1cm or less in size, negative post-operative ultrasound and a post-operative unstimulated thyroglobulin level of less than 1ng/ml confirmed 6-12 weeks following total thyroidectomy along with undetectable anti-Tg antibodies [1]. RAI should be selectively recommended if post-operative unstimulated Tg level is less than 5-10ng/ml measured 6-12 weeks following total thyroidectomy. If post-operative unstimulated Tg is more than 5-10ng/ml RAI treatment is recommended. However, care must be taken to exclude any normal thyroid remnant or gross residual disease by cross-sectional imaging such as computed tomography (CT) and magnetic resonance imaging (MRI) neck.

Importance of Calcitonin in Medullary Thyroid Carcinoma (MTC)

As mentioned earlier, MTC originates from parafollicular cells of the thyroid gland, hence it secretes excessive amounts of Calcitonin. Serum Calcitonin and CEA, to a lesser extent, are used as tumour markers in diagnosis, prognostication, assessment of treatment response and detection of recurrence/ residual disease in patients with MTC. Controversy exists on routine testing of Calcitonin levels in the evaluation of thyroid nodules and none of the guidelines recommends it. Using Calcitonin and CEA as a screening test in the setting of inherited MTC is abandoned due to lack of sensitivity. Calcitonin stimulation tests (with

Pentagastrin or Calcium) can be used to increase the positive predictive value [31].

Baseline Calcitonin and CEA levels should be checked in all diagnosed patients with MTC before surgical treatment. A level >400 ng/L predicts an increased risk of metastatic disease, especially in the presence of nodal disease, and cross-sectional imaging for staging is indicated. Lymph node (LN) metastasis is common in MTC, and LN clearance is an important component of curative-intent treatment. Calcitonin levels can be used to guide the extent of LN dissection as a biochemical cure can be achieved in >50% of patients with <1000 ng/L of calcitonin, if subjected to bilateral neck prophylactic LN dissection [31].

Serum Calcitonin and CEA levels should be checked in all patients following surgery, and it's not uncommon to have persistently elevated serum levels post-surgically. Doubling time for these markers can be used to get a more accurate picture of this group of patients. Further evaluation for recurrent or metastatic disease is required, especially if Calcitonin and CEA values are trending upward. Surgery is the only hope of achieving a cure for recurrent MTC, which emphasizes the importance of regular measurement of CEA and Calcitonin. However, there is a subgroup of people who have persistently elevated Calcitonin levels, yet are asymptomatic and imaging negative for recurrence or metastasis [31]. These patients do not require further treatment and can be followed up safely.

Marker for Hepatocellular Carcinoma

Hepatocellular carcinoma (HCC) is associated with chronic Hepatitis B and C infections, Aflatoxin B1 fungal toxin ingestion, alcoholic liver cirrhosis, autoimmune hepatitis *etc*. and HCC is the sixth most prevalent cancer in the world [32]. A number of tumour markers are being investigated for their potential applications in screening, diagnosis and predicting the prognosis of HCC. Out of them, only AFP (alpha-fetoprotein) is of current clinical relevance.

Screening

Patients with cirrhosis due to any reason and patients with hepatitis B infection (even without cirrhosis) are identified as being at high risk of developing HCC [1]. These patients should be screened for HCC by Ultrasound scanning (USS) and measurement of AFP levels. Even though AFP measurement cannot replace USS assessment, high or rising AFP levels are considered a prompt for CT or MRI scanning, regardless of USS results. Positive AFP levels or liver nodule/s of size 10mm or more in USS warrants further investigations to diagnose or exclude HCC [1]. If AFP and USS are negative, it is recommended to monitor with AFP and USS for another 6 months. If liver nodule/s less than 10mm in size are detected in USS, the patient should be followed up with a repeat USS and AFP levels in 3-6 months [1]. There is compelling evidence that screening with AFP and USS enables the detection of smaller HCCs at an earlier stage, thereby increasing the curability [33, 34].

Staging and Further Assessment

In patients with confirmed HCCs, comorbidity and liver reserve are assessed, and staging is determined by multidisciplinary evaluation. Alfa fetoprotein measurement is important for this staging process, along with evaluation of levels of bilirubin, liver transaminases, alkaline phosphatase, PT/INR, blood urea nitrogen (BUN), albumin, creatinine, platelets and chest X-ray *etc* [1].

Surveillance in HCC

Following definitive treatment for HCC, surveillance is done by monitoring AFP levels and imaging (multiphasic abdominopelvic MRI/ multiphasic CT) every 3-6 months during the first 2 years following surgery and 6 monthly thereafter [1]. Following adequate tumour resection, AFP levels should decline with a half-life of 3.5-4 days. Inadequate resection can be suspected when the half-life is longer or when AFP levels are not normalized following resection [34].

Markers for Gall Bladder and Cholangiocarcinoma

Gall bladder and biliary tract cancers are relatively rare, with worldwide age-standardized incidence rates of 2-3 per 100,000 population [35]. Gall bladder carcinomas are fatal, with only 10% of patients presenting at a surgically treatable stage of cancer [36]. Five-year survival of patients with cholangiocarcinoma range from 2-24%, with factors such as the location of tumour and the presence of distant metastasis playing an important role in determining the survival rate [1, 37]. CEA and CA 19-9 are the most used tumour markers in biliary tract carcinomas.

Screening

Both CEA and CA 19-9 are of importance in screening patients with biliary tract cancers. Even though the majority of patients with biliary cancers have elevated levels of CEA and CA 19-9, high levels of these tumour markers alone do not confirm the diagnosis [1]. Primary Sclerosing Cholangitis (PSC) is a known precursor for cholangiocarcinoma (CCA), with a lifetime risk of 15%. Therefore, diagnosed patients with PSC need screening for CCA, which includes regular measurement of CA 19.9 levels together with an abdominal ultrasound scan or

Magnetic Resonance Cholangiopancreatography (MRCP).

Diagnosis

Standard work-up for a suspected biliary duct/ gall bladder carcinoma includes, a thorough history and physical examination, liver function tests, multiphasic abdominopelvic CT/ MRI with intravenous contrast, MRCP (Magnetic resonance cholangiopancreatography) and tumour marker assessment with CEA and CA 19-9 [1].

Follow up

Both CEA and CA 19-9 are useful in post-surgical follow-up of patients with biliary tract cancers. The current NCCN guidelines suggest repeating CEA and CA 19-9 as clinically indicated in post-surgical patients, while conducting follow-up imaging every 3-6 months during the initial 2 years and every 6-12 months up to 5 years, to detect recurrences of the disease [1].

Markers for Pancreatic Carcinoma

Pancreatic cancer is a rare, fatal condition, of which the 5-year survival rate is just 9%, especially owing to the fact that the majority of patients are diagnosed after local or distant metastasis [38]. The majority of tumours (80-90%) are non-resectable at the time of clinical presentation, and even those tumours which are resected have a high recurrence rate [39]. CA 19-9 is the only tumour marker which is of clinical significance in pancreatic cancer. It has been found in colonic cancer tissue, normal pancreas, stomach, and biliary epithelium [40].

Screening

CA 19-9 is not useful for the screening of pancreatic cancer in asymptomatic patients due to; (a) benign conditions like chronic and acute pancreatitis, liver cirrhosis, cholangitis and obstructive jaundice are known to cause elevated CA19.9 levels, (b) being nonspecific to pancreatic adenocarcinoma and (c) not being expressed in Lewis a- b- genotype. Also, poorly differentiated and < 3cm size tumours may have normal CA19.9 levels, hence cannot be used as a substitute for histological diagnosis for pancreatic cancer. Nevertheless, it plays an important role in differentiating pancreatic cancer from chronic pancreatitis with high sensitivity (0.8-0.83) and specificity (0.79-0.82) [41].

Diagnosis and Workup

CA 19-9 is also important as a predictor of prognosis in patients with both resectable and non-resectable pancreatic cancer [42, 43]. The NCCN guidelines recommend measurement of CA 19-9 after adequate biliary drainage in patients with non-metastatic pancreatic carcinoma, along with assessment with chest and pelvic CT, endoscopic ultrasonography (EUS), MRI, endoscopic retrograde cholangiopancreatography (ERCP), liver function tests and germline testing [1]. As high preoperative values of CA 19-9 are associated with non-resectable disease, preoperative CA 19-9 levels are valuable for the surgeons to arrive at crucial therapeutic decisions.

Treatment algorithms have been developed using CA 19.9 values as a guide to the surgical approach. Resectability of the tumour is determined by preoperative imaging and "resectable" category is generally subjected to curative intent surgery in the form of Pancreaticoduodenectomy or total Pancreatectomy. Both procedures carry high morbidity and mortality. CA 19.9 of > 1000 kU/L is strongly suggestive of advanced disease even if the tumour may appear resectable. Therefore, diagnostic laparoscopy is indicated before embarking on major resections in this category of patients [44].

Follow up

High post-surgical CA 19-9 levels are indicative of residual disease [45]. Usually, in patients undergoing non-surgical treatment, the success of therapy is assessed by evaluation of tumour size by imaging, following chemotherapy and radiotherapy. However, this can be challenging in most patients due to the obscure margins of tumour and clinically non-apparent progression of cancer. In such instances, CA 19-9 measurement is of value to determine the treatment response [46]. Despite the advantages of CA 19-9 in pancreatic cancer, its use is limited in obstructive jaundice, as CA 19-9 bindings have been observed in about 28% of patients [40].

Markers for Ovarian Carcinoma

Ovarian masses are common in both pre-menopausal and post menopausal women and are typically found in asymptomatic women being investigated for another cause. It is only rarely that such a mass presents as malignant, but when it does it is usually a challenging disease to treat. Several tumour markers include CA-125, inhibin, beta-human chorionic gonadotrophin (βhCG), AFP, Lactate Dehydrogenase (LDH), CEA and CA 19-9, are useful in the clinical course of diagnosis, treatment and follow-up of ovarian cancer [1]. There are several histopathological types of ovarian neoplasms, epithelial ovarian cancer being the most common malignant ovarian cancer (90%). The rarer varieties include malignant germ cells and sex cord-stromal cell tumour [47, 48]. Epithelial type of ovarian neoplasm is the foremost cause of death due to gynaecological cancer and the fifth most commonest cause of cancer-related deaths in the USA. The five-year survival rate is 46.5%, mostly owing to delayed diagnosis due to less apparent symptoms [49].

Screening

Ovarian cancer is not routinely screened in the general population. However, high-risk patients, such as those with a positive family history or Breast Cancer Gene (BRCA) mutation, could be followed up using CA-125 levels and endovaginal ultrasound scan, though the validity of these screening tests is not certain up to date [1, 50, 51]. The use of CA-125 as a tool in early ovarian cancer detection is arguable due to its delayed increase in the course of the disease [52, 53]. Both Serum HE4 (Human Epididymis Protein 4) and CA-125 are found to be useful in differentiating a malignant pelvic mass from a benign tumour [54, 55]. Even though FDA has approved investigating HE4 and CA-125 levels for estimation of the risk of ovarian cancer in women with pelvic masses, the latest NCCN guidelines do not recommend these to conclude the status of an undiagnosed pelvic mass [1].

Diagnosis

A patient presenting with a suspicious pelvic mass with abdominal distension and ascites and/or with symptoms such as pelvic/ abdominal pain, bloating, anorexia, early satiety and urinary symptoms, without a clue of the source of malignancy, should be assessed with a thorough physical examination, Ultrasound / CT/ MRI scan, full blood count, liver function tests and CA-125 or any other tumour marker mentioned above [1].

Follow up

Upon determining the staging and delivering the appropriate treatment, the patient should be followed up to detect recurrences. CA-125 is an important component in the follow up of such patients. Recurrent disease is usually identified by clinical parameters such as abdominal/pelvic pain, raised CA-125 levels and with the use of imaging when indicated [1].

Patients with stage I, II, III and IV epithelial ovarian cancer are followed up initially every 2-4 months for two years, every 3-6 months in the next 3 years and annually afterwards. During the follow-up visit, CA-125 or any other tumour marker previously mentioned (depending on which tumour marker was initially elevated), should be evaluated along with a thorough physical examination, including a pelvic exam and imaging of chest/abdomen/pelvis [1]. The further management protocol is determined upon whether CA-125 is rising in a patient with a history of chemotherapy or naïve to chemotherapy [1].

The median period for clinical relapse is 2-6 months following the detection of an elevated CA-125 level (biochemical relapse). However, increasing CA-125 levels alone without signs and symptoms of recurrent disease, with negative pelvic examination and imaging of chest, abdomen and pelvis, brings about controversies in further management [56]. The latest data support the fact that immediate treatment for sole biochemical relapse does not provide an overall benefit to the patient, but decreases the quality of life [1]. Current recommendations following biochemical relapse (serially rising CA-125) with a previous history of chemotherapy, are enrolling the patient in a clinical trial, observation and delaying treatment until clinical relapse occurs, or immediate treatment according to category 2B recommendations in NCCN guidelines [1].

Markers for Testicular Carcinoma

Testicular cancer is relatively rare and represents less than 1% of all malignancies in men. The majority (95%) of malignant testicular cancers are testicular germ cell tumours (GCT) [1]. GCTs are categorized into two histological subtypes, seminoma and non-seminomas [57].

Tumour markers are of particular importance in predicting the treatment outcomes and prognosis patients with GCTs. The most widely used tumour markers are alpha-fetoprotein and (AFP), beta-human chorionic gonadotrophin (β-hCG) and lactate dehydrogenase (LDH). Serum levels of these markers should be determined prior to treatment and compared with the post-treatment values. Apart from that, AFP and β-hCG levels are specifically important in following up on all non-seminomas and stage II and III seminomas [1].

Beta-hCG (β-hCG)

Beta-hCG is a versatile tumour marker in testicular cancer as it is elevated in both seminomas and non-seminomas. Nevertheless, following circumstances of too high or too low β-hCG levels, may cause confusion: (a) initiating treatment in patients with mildly elevated β-hCG (less than 20IU/L), should be done with extra caution, since hyperthyroidism, hypogonadism and marijuana use could cause a mild elevation of β-hCG [58 - 60], (b) possibility of non-seminomatous GCT should be considered in a patient with seminoma and a β-hCG level of over 1000IU/L, (c) a post-orchidectomy β-hCG level of over 5000IU/L may indicate brain metastasis and a brain MRI scan should be performed. High β-hCG levels are also detected in adenocarcinomas, bladder cancer and lymphomas. Heterophile antibodies also cause an increase in β-hCG levels. Therefore in cases with absent radiographic evidence of disease with high β-hCG levels, indicating a false-positive result, the β-hCG test should be repeated using a different assay [1, 61, 62].

Lactate Dehydrogenase (LDH)

LDH is useful for assessment of prognosis and risk stratification of patients with disseminated non-seminomatous testicular cancers, who are about to start first-line chemotherapy [63]. There are several limitations to the use of LDH: it cannot be used for risk stratification of patients with pure seminomas; the specificity of LDH is much less than that of AFP and β-hCG, and therefore treatment decisions must not be based solely upon mildly elevated LDH levels (less than 3 x upper limit of normal LDH levels) [1].

Alpha-Fetoprotein (AFP)

Elevated serum AFP is usually detected with non-seminomas such as a yolk-sac tumour, embryonic carcinoma and teratoma. When a patient diagnosed with a pure seminoma presents with elevated AFP, the presence of an undetected non-seminoma component in the tumour is suspected, and management should be altered accordingly [63 - 66]. Thus, AFP is important in the diagnosis of pure seminomas, as the diagnosis is confirmed only with pure seminoma histology and normal serum AFP levels [1]. There are several limitations to the use of AFP in testicular cancer. A minority of patients have a chronic mild elevation of AFP levels, making it difficult to determine the presence of an actual recurrence. Further, other cancers such as gastric and hepatocellular carcinomas could cause an elevation in AFP levels, thereby making AFP nonspecific [1].

If a pure seminoma is diagnosed by histology and normal serum AFP levels as indicated previously, the serum β-hCG, AFP and LDH levels should be repeated, since the determination of precise TNM staging of tumour is based on post-orchidectomy levels [1]. If the tumour marker is declining, it should be followed up until normalization is achieved or plateaued.

Markers in Neuroendocrine Tumours

A number of tumor markers are under investigation for the management of neuroendocrine tumours. There is emerging evidence suggesting that mammalian target of rapamycin (mTOR) and CDKN1B (p27) expression may be of relevance to the prognostic assessment of neuroendocrine tumours [67, 68]. However, Chromogranin A is the only tumour marker which is being practically used in the clinical setup for neuroendocrine tumours. Neuroendocrine tumours show an elevated level of Chromogranin A, which is a protein secreted by the neuroendocrine cells.

Chromogranin A is of particular significance in the follow-up of patients following tumour resection. Elevated levels have been reported during the recurrence of disease, in several studies [69, 70]. However, an elevated Chromogranin A level alone is not sufficient for the diagnosis of a recurrence [1].

A high level of Chromogranin A is usually associated with poor prognosis in patients [1, 71]. Levels higher than twice the normal limit were found to be associated with shorter survival in patients with metastatic disease [72].

Thus, Chromogranin A is an important component in the follow-up and the determination of the prognosis of patients with neuroendocrine tumours.

Markers in Prostate Cancer

Prostate cancer accounted for 3.8% of all cancer-related deaths in 2020, around the globe [73]. Despite the increased incidence of PCa due to screening with (Prostate-specific antigen) PSA, the mortality due to PCa has declined due to advanced treatment options. Even though there are several other proteins which seem promising as prostate cancer markers, such as prostate stem cell antigen (PSCA), prostate-specific membrane antigen (PSMA), early prostate cancer antigen (EPCA), enhancer of zeste homolog gene 2 (EZH2), and urokinase plasminogen activator (uPA), none of them are used in the clinical setup [74, 75].

Among all the tumour markers related to any type of cancer, PSA is the oldest and most widely understood. Its use as a screening tool is questioned in recent years, yet it is invaluable in risk stratification and follow-up of PCa patients [76]. PSA is a glycoprotein serine protease enzyme produced by prostate epithelial cells, which is prostate-specific but not specific to prostate cancer. PSA could be significantly elevated in benign causes such as prostatitis, benign prostatic hyperplasia or recent instrumentation of the urinary tract and may be normal in patients with prostate cancer. Elevation of PSA after the digital rectal examination (DRE) is clinically insignificant.

Screening

Screening for PCa is one of the most controversial topics in current urological literature. This is mostly due to the heterogeneous nature of available evidence and partly due to the natural history of the disease. As a fact, most men with PCa who are co-morbid and elderly would die of causes other than PCa related, which raises the question of the value of screening. Screening for PCa with PSA is a much-debated area, but as of today, there is no clear evidence to support a PSA-based screening program. Few facts worth mentioning about screening for PCa are; a) screening is associated with an increased diagnosis of PCa, b) screening is associated with detection of more localised and less advanced PCa, c) no increase of PCa specific survival or overall survival was seen with PSA based screening.

Due to the heterogeneous nature of evidence, none of the major guidelines recommends PSA-based population screening for PCa, at the moment. However, a recent update from the European Urological Association states that "Offer early PSA testing to well-informed men who have a risk of having PCa" [77].

Diagnosis

PCa is usually suspected when DRE findings are combined with high PSA values and is confirmed by prostate biopsy. Normal PSA values may change according to age, but the risk of PCa is over 30% when PSA is above 3ng/ml. PSA over 100ng/ml is highly suggestive of metastatic PCa. Once diagnosed, risk stratification is done for treatment purposes, and PSA is an important parameter of this, together with the Gleason score and clinical staging [77].

Treatment

Decision-making in treatment for PCa not only depends on staging but also depends on the patient's life expectancy. Watchful waiting is an option for all stages of PCa in men who have a short life expectancy. These men will be followed up with infrequent PSA testing and will be subjected to palliative intent treatment upon the significant rise in PSA or development of symptoms. In men with early-stage PCa, deferring radical treatment until disease progression is called active surveillance [77]. Frequent PSA and prostate biopsies are done to pick up advancing diseases that will be subjected to radical treatment. Radical treatment is achieved with radiation therapy (RT) or prostatectomy, and PSA is used to follow-up these patients upon completion of treatment.

Follow up

Following RT, disease recurrence is defined as an elevation of PSA of >2 over the nadir PSA value and will be subjected to further curative-intent treatment. PSA levels should be undetectable following radical prostatectomy, and a rise over 0.2 ng/dl is considered a "biochemical recurrence" and should be evaluated further for recurrent or metastatic disease. Castrate Resistant Prostate Cancer (CRPC) is diagnosed when PSA continues to rise despite achieving castrate level testosterone, and this carries a poor prognosis [76, 77].

With the introduction of PSA indices, the accuracy of PSA testing in diagnostic and surveillance settings could be improved. PSA density refers to serum PSA value divided by prostate volume, and a higher value suggests a clinically significant PCa. PSA Kinetics such as PSA velocity and PSA doubling time could have a prognostic value but do not provide additional information compared to PSA alone [77].

New serum tests are available for PCa diagnosis, such as Prostate Health Index (PHI) test (combining free and total PSA and the [-2]pro-PSA isoform [p2PSA]) and the four kallikreins (4K) score test. Both tests are intended to reduce the number of unnecessary biopsies during screening [77]. Urine tests such as Prostate cancer gene 3 (PCA3), SelectMDX test, and TMPRSS2-ERG fusion test are still under evaluation and may be of clinical significance if proven to be superior to PSA testing or to be used in combination with PSA testing.

Table 1. Summary of the clinical utility of commonly used tumour markers.

Type of Cancer	Tumour Marker	Specific Use of the Marker
Colorectal	CEA	Diagnosis of cases with a high clinical probability of cancer, if the patient is not fit enough to undergo invasive investigations. Prediction of prognosis, Post-operative surveillance by being a reliable marker for the detection of recurrences.
Breast	CA15-3	Prognosis and treatment efficacy
Thyroid	Thyroglobulin	Assessment of cancer burden of differentiated thyroid cancers (DTCs) at presentation and adequacy of surgical clearance, monitor recurrences and treatment response.
	Calcitonin CEA	Diagnosis, prognostication, assessment of treatment response and detection of recurrence/ residual disease in patients with medullary thyroid carcinoma (MTC).
Hepatocellular	AFP	Screening, staging and further assessment, surveillance
Gall bladder and other biliary tracts	CEA CA 19-9	Screening, post-surgical follow up
Pancreatic	CA 19-9	Differentiating pancreatic cancer from chronic pancreatitis Prediction of prognosis in patients with both resectable and non-resectable tumours, Surgical decision making Determination of treatment response
Ovarian	CA-125	Differentiating a malignant pelvic mass from a benign one Post-surgical follow-up
	HE4	Differentiating a malignant pelvic mass from a benign one
Testicular	AFP	Diagnosis of pure seminomas Prediction of the treatment outcomes and prognosis Following up on all nonseminomas and stage II and III seminomas
	β-hCG	Prediction of treatment outcomes and prognosis Following up on all nonseminomas and stage II and III seminomas
	LDH	Assessment of prognosis, Risk stratification of patients with disseminated non-seminomatous testicular cancers, about to start first-line chemotherapy

(Table 1) cont.....

Type of Cancer	Tumour Marker	Specific Use of the Marker
Neuroendocrine tumours	Chromogranin A	Prediction of prognosis, Follow up
Prostate	PSA	Screening, Risk stratification, Follow-up

CONCLUSION

The biomarkers currently used in the clinical management of patients with cancer for screening, diagnosis, prognosis and therapy response provide critical information to the oncologist in guiding their care with some limitations. Thus, further development of specific and effective biomarkers would improve the quality and clinical outcome of patients with cancer.

CONSENT FOR PUBLICATION

Not applicable.

CONFLICT OF INTEREST

The authors declare no conflict of interest, financial or otherwise.

ACKNOWLEDGEMENTS

The authors acknowledge the Griffith University International Postgraduate Research Scholarship and Griffith University Postgraduate Research Scholarship, Australia and the Post Graduate Institute of Medicine, University of Colombo, Sri Lanka.

REFERENCES

[1] NCCN. 2020. https://www.nccn.org/professionals/physician_gls/default.aspx#site

[2] Abeloff MD, Armitage JO, Niederhuber JE, Kastan MB, McKenna WG. Abeloff's Clinical Oncology E-Book: Elsevier Health Sciences 2008.

[3] Sharma S. Tumor markers in clinical practice: General principles and guidelines. Indian J Med Paediatr Oncol 2009; 30(1): 1-8. [http://dx.doi.org/10.4103/0971-5851.56328] [PMID: 20668599]

[4] Rawla P, Sunkara T, Barsouk A. Epidemiology of colorectal cancer: incidence, mortality, survival, and risk factors. Prz Gastroenterol 2019; 14(2): 89-103. [http://dx.doi.org/10.5114/pg.2018.81072] [PMID: 31616522]

[5] Lech G, Słotwiński R, Słodkowski M, Krasnodębski IW. Colorectal cancer tumour markers and biomarkers: Recent therapeutic advances. World J Gastroenterol 2016; 22(5): 1745-55. [http://dx.doi.org/10.3748/wjg.v22.i5.1745] [PMID: 26855534]

[6] Jelski W, Mroczko B. Biochemical Markers of Colorectal Cancer – Present and Future. Cancer Manag Res 2020; 12: 4789-97. [http://dx.doi.org/10.2147/CMAR.S253369] [PMID: 32606968]

[7] Jelski W, Zalewski B, Chrostek L, Szmitkowski M. The activity of class I, II, III, and IV alcohol dehydrogenase isoenzymes and aldehyde dehydrogenase in colorectal cancer. Dig Dis Sci 2004; 49(6): 977-81.
[http://dx.doi.org/10.1023/B:DDAS.0000034557.23322.e0] [PMID: 15309886]

[8] Mroczko B, Szmitkowski M, Okulczyk B. Granulocyte-colony stimulating factor (G-CSF) and macrophagecolony stimulating factor (M-CSF) in colorectal cancer patients. Clin Chem Lab Med 2002; 40(4): 351-5.
[http://dx.doi.org/10.1515/CCLM.2002.056] [PMID: 12059074]

[9] Groblewska M, Mroczko B, Wereszczyńska-Siemiątkowska U, *et al.* Serum interleukin 6 (IL-6) and C-reactive protein (CRP) levels in colorectal adenoma and cancer patients. Clin Chem Lab Med 2008; 46(10): 1423-8.
[http://dx.doi.org/10.1515/CCLM.2008.278] [PMID: 18844497]

[10] Mroczko B, Szmitkowski M, WereszczyńSka-Siemiątkowska U, Okulczyk B. Stem cell factor (SCF) and interleukin 3 (IL-3) in the sera of patients with colorectal cancer. Dig Dis Sci 2005; 50(6): 1019-24.
[http://dx.doi.org/10.1007/s10620-005-2697-3] [PMID: 15986847]

[11] Galanzha E, Zharov V. Circulating Tumor Cell Detection and Capture by Photoacoustic Flow Cytometry *in Vivo* and *ex Vivo*. Cancers (Basel) 2013; 5(4): 1691-738.
[http://dx.doi.org/10.3390/cancers5041691] [PMID: 24335964]

[12] Li P, Stratton ZS, Dao M, Ritz J, Huang TJ. Probing circulating tumor cells in microfluidics. Lab Chip 2013; 13(4): 602-9.
[http://dx.doi.org/10.1039/c2lc90148j] [PMID: 23306378]

[13] Di Costanzo F, Pinzani P, Orlando C, *et al.* Circulating tumour cells in colorectal cancer. Eur J Cancer, Suppl 2008; 6(14): 52-9.
[http://dx.doi.org/10.1016/j.ejcsup.2008.06.097]

[14] Tarantino I, Warschkow R, Schmied BM, *et al.* Predictive Value of CEA for Survival in Stage I Rectal Cancer: a Population-Based Propensity Score-Matched Analysis. J Gastrointest Surg 2016; 20(6): 1213-22.
[http://dx.doi.org/10.1007/s11605-016-3137-8] [PMID: 27067235]

[15] Probst CP, Becerra AZ, Aquina CT, *et al.* Watch and Wait?—Elevated Pretreatment CEA Is Associated with Decreased Pathological Complete Response in Rectal Cancer. J Gastrointest Surg 2016; 20(1): 43-52.
[http://dx.doi.org/10.1007/s11605-015-2987-9] [PMID: 26546119]

[16] Cho WK, Choi DH, Park HC, *et al.* Elevated CEA is associated with worse survival in recurrent rectal cancer. Oncotarget 2017; 8(62): 105936-41.
[http://dx.doi.org/10.18632/oncotarget.22511] [PMID: 29285304]

[17] Koness RJ. CEA: is it of value in colorectal cancer? R I Med 1995; 78(6): 164-6.
[PMID: 7626815]

[18] Sturgeon CM. CHAPTER 42 - Tumour markers. In: Marshall WJ, Lapsley M, Day AP, Ayling RM, (Eds.). Clinical Biochemistry: Metabolic and Clinical Aspects (Third Edition): Churchill Livingstone 2014; 821-43.

[19] Velenik V. Post-treatment surveillance in colorectal cancer. Radiol Oncol 2010; 44(3): 135-41.
[http://dx.doi.org/10.2478/v10019-010-0018-8] [PMID: 22933905]

[20] van der Stok E, Spaander M, Grunhagen D, Verhoef C, Kuipers E. Surveillance after curative treatment for colorectal cancer. Nat Rev Clin Oncol 2016; 14.
[PMID: 27995949]

[21] Duffy MJ, van Dalen A, Haglund C, *et al.* Tumour markers in colorectal cancer: European Group on Tumour Markers (EGTM) guidelines for clinical use. Eur J Cancer 2007; 43(9): 1348-60.

[http://dx.doi.org/10.1016/j.ejca.2007.03.021] [PMID: 17512720]

[22] Latest global cancer data [press release]. 150 Cours Albert Thomas, 69372 Lyon CEDEX 08, France: WHO 2018.

[23] Marić P, Ozretić P, Levanat S, Oresković S, Antunac K, Beketić-Oresković L. Tumor markers in breast cancer--evaluation of their clinical usefulness. Coll Antropol 2011; 35(1): 241-7. [PMID: 21661378]

[24] Donepudi MS, Kondapalli K, Amos SJ, Venkanteshan P. Breast cancer statistics and markers. J Cancer Res Ther 2014; 10(3): 506-11. [PMID: 25313729]

[25] Kabel AM. Tumor markers of breast cancer: New prospectives. Journal of Oncological Sciences 2017; 3(1): 5-11. [http://dx.doi.org/10.1016/j.jons.2017.01.001]

[26] Bahrami-Ahmadi A, Makarian F, Mortazavizadeh MR, Yazdi MF, Chamani M. Symptomatic metastasis prediction with serial measurements of CA 15.3 in primary breast cancer patients. J Res Med Sci 2012; 17(9): 850.

[27] Shao Y, Sun X, He Y, Liu C, Liu H. Elevated levels of serum tumor markers CEA and CA15-3 are prognostic parameters for different molecular subtypes of breast cancer. PLoS One 2015; 10(7): e0133830. [http://dx.doi.org/10.1371/journal.pone.0133830] [PMID: 26207909]

[28] Molina R, Barak V, van Dalen A, *et al.* Tumor markers in breast cancer- European Group on Tumor Markers recommendations. Tumour Biol 2005; 26(6): 281-93. [http://dx.doi.org/10.1159/000089260] [PMID: 16254457]

[29] Xu J, Bergren R, Schneider D, Chen H, Sippel RS. Thyroglobulin antibody resolution after total thyroidectomy for cancer. J Surg Res 2015; 198(2): 366-70. [http://dx.doi.org/10.1016/j.jss.2015.03.094] [PMID: 25930167]

[30] Indrasena BSH. Use of thyroglobulin as a tumour marker. World J Biol Chem 2017; 8(1): 81-5. [http://dx.doi.org/10.4331/wjbc.v8.i1.81] [PMID: 28289520]

[31] Perros P, Boelaert K, Colley S, *et al.* Guidelines for the management of thyroid cancer. Clin Endocrinol (Oxf) 2014; 81(s1) (Suppl. 1): 1-122. [http://dx.doi.org/10.1111/cen.12515] [PMID: 24989897]

[32] Chu Y-J, Yang H-I, Wu H-C, *et al.* Aflatoxin B(1) exposure increases the risk of hepatocellular carcinoma associated with hepatitis C virus infection or alcohol consumption. European journal of cancer (Oxford, England : 1990) 2018; 94: 37-46.

[33] Toyoda H, Kumada T, Tada T, Sone Y, Kaneoka Y, Maeda A. Tumor Markers for Hepatocellular Carcinoma: Simple and Significant Predictors of Outcome in Patients with HCC. Liver Cancer 2015; 4(2): 126-36. [http://dx.doi.org/10.1159/000367735] [PMID: 26020034]

[34] Rich N, Singal AG. Hepatocellular carcinoma tumour markers: Current role and expectations. Best Pract Res Clin Gastroenterol 2014; 28(5): 843-53. [http://dx.doi.org/10.1016/j.bpg.2014.07.018] [PMID: 25260312]

[35] Bray F, Ferlay J, Soerjomataram I, Siegel RL, Torre LA, Jemal A. Global cancer statistics 2018: GLOBOCAN estimates of incidence and mortality worldwide for 36 cancers in 185 countries. CA Cancer J Clin 2018; 68(6): 394-424. [http://dx.doi.org/10.3322/caac.21492] [PMID: 30207593]

[36] Kanthan R, Senger JL, Ahmed S, Kanthan SC. Gallbladder Cancer in the 21st Century. J Oncol 2015; 2015: 1-26. [http://dx.doi.org/10.1155/2015/967472] [PMID: 26421012]

[37] Golan T, Raitses-Gurevich M, Kelley RK, *et al.* Overall survival and clinical characteristics of BRCA-associated cholangiocarcinoma: A multicenter retrospective study. Oncologist 2017; 22(7): 804-10. [http://dx.doi.org/10.1634/theoncologist.2016-0415] [PMID: 28487467]

[38] ASCO. Pancreatic cancer statistics 2020. https://www.cancer.net/cancer-types/pancreatic-cancer/statistics

[39] McGuigan A, Kelly P, Turkington RC, Jones C, Coleman HG, McCain RS. Pancreatic cancer: A review of clinical diagnosis, epidemiology, treatment and outcomes. World J Gastroenterol 2018; 24(43): 4846-61.
[http://dx.doi.org/10.3748/wjg.v24.i43.4846] [PMID: 30487695]

[40] Haglund MEU, Haglund U. Developments in serologic detection of human pancreatic adenocarcinoma. Scand J Gastroenterol 1999; 34(9): 833-44.
[http://dx.doi.org/10.1080/003655299750025273] [PMID: 10522599]

[41] Su SB, Qin SY, Chen W, Luo W, Jiang HX. Carbohydrate antigen 19-9 for differential diagnosis of pancreatic carcinoma and chronic pancreatitis. World J Gastroenterol 2015; 21(14): 4323-33.
[http://dx.doi.org/10.3748/wjg.v21.i14.4323] [PMID: 25892884]

[42] Steinberg W. The clinical utility of the CA 19-9 tumor-associated antigen. Am J Gastroenterol 1990; 85(4): 350-5.
[PMID: 2183589]

[43] Goonetilleke KS, Siriwardena AK. Systematic review of carbohydrate antigen (CA 19-9) as a biochemical marker in the diagnosis of pancreatic cancer. Eur J Surg Oncol 2007; 33(3): 266-70.
[http://dx.doi.org/10.1016/j.ejso.2006.10.004] [PMID: 17097848]

[44] Duffy MJ, Sturgeon C, Lamerz R, *et al.* Tumor markers in pancreatic cancer: a European Group on Tumor Markers (EGTM) status report. Ann Oncol 2010; 21(3): 441-7.
[http://dx.doi.org/10.1093/annonc/mdp332] [PMID: 19690057]

[45] Tian F, Appert H, Myles J, Howard JM. Prognostic value of serum CA 19-9 levels in pancreatic adenocarcinoma. Ann Surg 1992; 215(4): 350-5.
[http://dx.doi.org/10.1097/00000658-199204000-00008] [PMID: 1348409]

[46] Okusaka T, Yamada T, Maekawa M. Serum tumor markers for pancreatic cancer: the dawn of new era? JOP 2006; 7(4): 332-6.
[PMID: 16832130]

[47] Chan JK, Cheung MK, Husain A, *et al.* Patterns and progress in ovarian cancer over 14 years. Obstet Gynecol 2006; 108(3, Part 1): 521-8.
[http://dx.doi.org/10.1097/01.AOG.0000231680.58221.a7] [PMID: 16946210]

[48] Jelovac D, Armstrong DK. Recent progress in the diagnosis and treatment of ovarian cancer. CA Cancer J Clin 2011; 61(3): 183-203.
[http://dx.doi.org/10.3322/caac.20113] [PMID: 21521830]

[49] Siegel RL, Miller KD, Jemal A. Cancer statistics, 2018. CA Cancer J Clin 2018; 68(1): 7-30.
[http://dx.doi.org/10.3322/caac.21442] [PMID: 29313949]

[50] Hartge P. Designing early detection programs for ovarian cancer. J Natl Cancer Inst 2010; 102(1): 3-4.
[http://dx.doi.org/10.1093/jnci/djp450] [PMID: 20042718]

[51] Smith RA, Manassaram-Baptiste D, Brooks D, *et al.* Cancer screening in the United States, 2015: A review of current American Cancer Society guidelines and current issues in cancer screening. CA Cancer J Clin 2015; 65(1): 30-54.
[http://dx.doi.org/10.3322/caac.21261] [PMID: 25581023]

[52] Cramer DW, Bast RC Jr, Berg CD, *et al.* Ovarian cancer biomarker performance in prostate, lung, colorectal, and ovarian cancer screening trial specimens. Cancer Prev Res (Phila) 2011; 4(3): 365-74.
[http://dx.doi.org/10.1158/1940-6207.CAPR-10-0195] [PMID: 21372036]

[53] Anderson GL, McIntosh M, Wu L, *et al.* Assessing lead time of selected ovarian cancer biomarkers: a nested case-control study. J Natl Cancer Inst 2010; 102(1): 26-38. [http://dx.doi.org/10.1093/jnci/djp438] [PMID: 20042715]

[54] Romagnolo C, Leon AE, Fabricio ASC, *et al.* HE4, CA125 and risk of ovarian malignancy algorithm (ROMA) as diagnostic tools for ovarian cancer in patients with a pelvic mass: An Italian multicenter study. Gynecol Oncol 2016; 141(2): 303-11. [http://dx.doi.org/10.1016/j.ygyno.2016.01.016] [PMID: 26801941]

[55] Moore RG, Miller MC, Disilvestro P, *et al.* Evaluation of the diagnostic accuracy of the risk of ovarian malignancy algorithm in women with a pelvic mass. Obstet Gynecol 2011; 118(2): 280-8. [http://dx.doi.org/10.1097/AOG.0b013e318224fce2] [PMID: 21775843]

[56] Lindemann K, Kristensen G, Mirza MR, *et al.* Poor concordance between CA-125 and RECIST at the time of disease progression in patients with platinum-resistant ovarian cancer: analysis of the AURELIA trial. Ann Oncol 2016; 27(8): 1505-10. [http://dx.doi.org/10.1093/annonc/mdw238] [PMID: 27407100]

[57] Sarıcı H, Telli O, Arıcı M. Bilateral testicular germ cell tumors. Türk Üroloji Dergisi/Turkish Journal of Urology 2013; 39(4): 249-52. [http://dx.doi.org/10.5152/tud.2013.062] [PMID: 26328119]

[58] Ferraro S, Trevisiol C, Gion M, Panteghini M. Human Chorionic Gonadotropin Assays for Testicular Tumors: Closing the Gap between Clinical and Laboratory Practice. Clin Chem 2018; 64(2): 270-8. [http://dx.doi.org/10.1373/clinchem.2017.275263] [PMID: 29021329]

[59] Lempiäinen A, Hotakainen K, Blomqvist C, Alfthan H, Stenman UH. Increased human chorionic gonadotropin due to hypogonadism after treatment of a testicular seminoma. Clin Chem 2007; 53(8): 1560-1. [http://dx.doi.org/10.1373/clinchem.2007.088518] [PMID: 17644799]

[60] Morris MJ, Bosl GJ. Recognizing abnormal marker results that do not reflect disease in patients with germ cell tumors. J Urol 2000; 163(3): 796-801. [http://dx.doi.org/10.1016/S0022-5347(05)67807-X] [PMID: 10687980]

[61] Trojan A, Joller-Jemelka H, Stahel RA, Jacky E, Hersberger M. False-positive human serum chorionic gonadotropin in a patient with a history of germ cell cancer. Oncology 2004; 66(4): 336-8. [http://dx.doi.org/10.1159/000078336] [PMID: 15218303]

[62] Ballieux BEPB, Weijl NI, Gelderblom H, van Pelt J, Osanto S. False-positive serum human chorionic gonadotropin (HCG) in a male patient with a malignant germ cell tumor of the testis: a case report and review of the literature. Oncologist 2008; 13(11): 1149-54. [http://dx.doi.org/10.1634/theoncologist.2008-0159] [PMID: 18984875]

[63] Gilligan TD, Seidenfeld J, Basch EM, *et al.* American Society of Clinical Oncology Clinical Practice Guideline on uses of serum tumor markers in adult males with germ cell tumors. J Clin Oncol 2010; 28(20): 3388-404. [http://dx.doi.org/10.1200/JCO.2009.26.4481] [PMID: 20530278]

[64] Nazeer T, Ro JY, Amato RJ, Park YW, Ordonez NG, Ayala AG. Histologically pure seminoma with elevated alpha-fetoprotein: a clinicopathologic study of ten cases. Oncol Rep 1998; 5(6): 1425-9. [http://dx.doi.org/10.3892/or.5.6.1425] [PMID: 9769381]

[65] Salem M, Gilligan T. Serum tumor markers and their utilization in the management of germ-cell tumors in adult males. Expert Rev Anticancer Ther 2011; 11(1): 1-4. [http://dx.doi.org/10.1586/era.10.219] [PMID: 21166503]

[66] Kundu SD, Carver BS, Sheinfeld J. Retroperitoneal histologic findings of patients with elevated serum alpha-fetoprotein and pure seminoma at orchiectomy. Urology 2011; 78(4): 844-7. [http://dx.doi.org/10.1016/j.urology.2011.02.002] [PMID: 21782217]

[67] Qian ZR, Ter-Minassian M, Chan JA, *et al.* Prognostic significance of MTOR pathway component

expression in neuroendocrine tumors. J Clin Oncol 2013; 31(27): 3418-25.
[http://dx.doi.org/10.1200/JCO.2012.46.6946] [PMID: 23980085]

[68] Francis JM, Kiezun A, Ramos AH, *et al.* Somatic mutation of CDKN1B in small intestine neuroendocrine tumors. Nat Genet 2013; 45(12): 1483-6.
[http://dx.doi.org/10.1038/ng.2821] [PMID: 24185511]

[69] Massironi S, Rossi RE, Casazza G, *et al.* Chromogranin A in diagnosing and monitoring patients with gastroenteropancreatic neuroendocrine neoplasms: a large series from a single institution. Neuroendocrinology 2014; 100(2-3): 240-9.
[http://dx.doi.org/10.1159/000369818] [PMID: 25428270]

[70] Rossi RE, Ciafardini C, Sciola V, Conte D, Massironi S. Chromogranin A in the Follow-up of Gastroenteropancreatic Neuroendocrine Neoplasms. Pancreas 2018; 47(10): 1249-55.
[http://dx.doi.org/10.1097/MPA.0000000000001184] [PMID: 30325865]

[71] Oberg K, Janson ET, Eriksson B. Tumour markers in neuroendocrine tumours. Ital J Gastroenterol Hepatol 1999; 31 (Suppl. 2): S160-2.
[PMID: 10604122]

[72] Ter-Minassian M, Chan JA, Hooshmand SM, *et al.* Clinical presentation, recurrence, and survival in patients with neuroendocrine tumors: results from a prospective institutional database. Endocr Relat Cancer 2013; 20(2): 187-96.
[http://dx.doi.org/10.1530/ERC-12-0340] [PMID: 23319495]

[73] IARC. Global cancer observatory: WHO; 2020. https://gco.iarc.fr/

[74] Bradford TJ, Tomlins SA, Wang X, Chinnaiyan AM, Eds. Molecular markers of prostate cancer. Urologic Oncology: Seminars and Original Investigations. 2006.

[75] Shariat SF, Semjonow A, Lilja H, Savage C, Vickers AJ, Bjartell A. Tumor markers in prostate cancer I: blood-based markers. Acta oncologica 2011; 50(sup1): 61-75.

[76] Nelson K, Bennett P, Rance J. The experiences of giving and receiving social support for men with localised prostate cancer and their partners. Ecancermedicalscience 2019; 13(9): 989.
[http://dx.doi.org/10.3332/ecancer.2019.989] [PMID: 32010213]

[77] Gakis G, Bruins HM, Cathomas R, *et al.* European Association of Urology Guidelines on Primary Urethral Carcinoma—2020 Update. Eur Urol Oncol 2020; 3(4): 424-32.
[http://dx.doi.org/10.1016/j.euo.2020.06.003] [PMID: 32605889]

Part 2: DNA/RNA Biomarkers

CHAPTER 3

DNA Methylation Landscapes in Cancer and Non-Cancer Cells

Shaun Stangl[1,*] and **Vinod Gopalan**[1,*]

[1] *Cancer Molecular Pathology, School of Medicine and Dentistry, Griffith University, Gold Coast, Queensland 4222, Australia*

Abstract: Epigenetic modifications are heritable changes to gene expression without physical changes to the actual DNA sequence. The most widely studied epigenetic modification is DNA methylation, as it is influenced by aging, diet, diseases and the environment. DNA methylation involves direct chemical modification to the DNA and plays an important role in gene regulation by preventing proteins from binding to certain regions of the DNA, which causes these regions to be repressed. It is essential for normal development, cell differentiation and regulation of cellular biology. The DNA methylation landscape of each unique cell type helps to determine which genes are expressed and silenced. It is well known today that the accumulation of both genetic and epigenetic abnormalities contributes to the development of cancers. Aberrant DNA methylation is a hallmark of cancer. During cancer development and progression, the methylation landscape undergoes aberrant remodelling. Recently within cancer research, the advancements in DNA methylation mapping technologies have enabled methylation landscapes to be studied in greater detail, sparking new interest in how the methylation landscape undergoes a change in cancer and possible applications of DNA methylation. This chapter focuses on reviewing DNA methylation landscapes in normal cells and then how they are altered in cancer. It also discusses the applications of DNA methylation as cancer biomarkers.

Keywords: Biomarkers, Cancer, Demethylation, DNA, Epigenetics, Gene-bodies, Gene expression, Hypermethylation, Hypomethylation, Methylation, Promoter, Transcription.

INTRODUCTION

DNA methylation is a heritable epigenetic modification that plays an important role in regulating gene expression. It allows cells that are genetically identical to establish distinct cellular phenotypes without changing the actual DNA sequence.

* **Corresponding authors Vinod Gopalan:** Cancer Molecular Pathology, School of Medicine and Dentistry, Griffith University, Gold Coast, Queensland 4222, Australia; Email: v.gopalan@griffith.edu.au;
Shaun Stangel: Cancer Molecular Pathology, School of Medicine and Dentistry, Griffith University, Gold Coast, Queensland 4222, Australia; Email: shaun.stangl@alumni.griffithuni.edu.au

Farhadul Islam (Ed.)

Among all the different types of epigenetic mechanisms, DNA methylation is the most widely studied, as it is influenced by aging, diet, diseases and the environment. In mammalian genomes, DNA methylation is essential for normal development as well as several other biological processes, including cell differentiation, tissue-specific gene expression, maintaining genome stability, chromatin status, genomic imprinting, and silencing of potentially harmful genetic elements [1] and X-chromosome inactivation in females [2]. DNA methylation refers to the transfer of a methyl group (-CH3) from the S-adenosylmethionine (SAMe) molecule to the carbon-5 position of cytosine bases, to form 5-methylcytosine (5mC). The process is catalysed by three DNA methyltransferase enzymes (DNMTs) DNMT1, DNMT3A and DNMT3B. Maintenance DNA methyltransferase DNMT1, is responsible for maintaining DNA methylation patterns during cell division. DNMT1 copies the DNA methylation patterns of the parent strand onto the newly synthesised daughter strand of hemi-methylated DNA. The de novo DNA methyltransferases DNMT3A and DNMT3B, are mainly active during early development and help to establish new DNA methylation patterns on unmethylated DNA [3, 4].

DNA demethylation refers to the removal of methyl groups from 5mC. Recent studies have discovered that the ten-eleven translocation (TET) enzymes can oxidise 5mC, to produce 5-hydroxymethylcytosine (5hmC); 5hmC has been recognised as an important intermediate of DNA demethylation processes [5]. This recent discovery has generated new interest into the dynamics of how DNA methylation landscapes are remodelled with the contribution of DNA demethylation during early development, normal cell biology and cancer. Initially, oxidation of 5mC was hypothesised as a potential way of reactivating genes that had been silenced by DNA methylation [6, 7], however, this has since been ruled out [8 - 10]. DNA demethylation is achieved by both a passive and active process. Passive DNA demethylation occurs during DNA replication as a result of reduced DNMT1, causing each successful replication cycle to further dilute the content of 5mC in the genome as methylation patterns are not being copied onto newly replicated DNA [11]. Pathways of active DNA demethylation can occur independently of DNA replication. Active DNA demethylation uses three different enzyme families: (i) TET enzymes further oxidise 5hmC to form in order 5-formylcytosine (5fC) and 5-carboxylcytosine (5caC) [12]. (ii) The activation-induced cytidine deaminase/ apolipoprotein B editing complex (AID/APOBEC) family enzymes deaminate 5hmC to form 5-hydroxymethyluracil (5hmU) and 5mC to form thymine. (iii) Base excise repair (BER) glycosylase enzymes such as thymine DNA glycosylase (TDG) recognise and excise the damaged or incorrect base (*i.e.*, 5fC, 5caC, 5hmU and thymine), creating an abasic site (apurinic/apyrimidinic site; AP site). The AP site is then repaired with unmethylated cytosine by the BER pathway, concluding active DNA demethylation [13, 14].

Although there are still a lot of outstanding questions regarding cancer development, it is well known that age, diet, disease and the environment are capable of influencing changes to the epigenetic landscape, causing an increased risk of cancer development. It is well known that DNA methylation landscapes undergo aberrant changes during cancer development and progression. Patterns of DNA hypomethylation genome-wide accompanied by focal hypermethylation have been observed in all cancers ever studied [15]. With the recent advancements in DNA methylation mapping technologies combined with our growing knowledge of other epigenetic modifications, we are continuously improving our understanding of the role that DNA methylation plays in normal and disease states.

Normal DNA Methylation Location

The DNA methylation landscape of each cell type is different and plays an essential role in regulating patterns of gene expression. In mammals, DNA methylation predominantly occurs at cytosine-phosphate-guanine dinucleotides (CpG sites) [16]. In the human genome, CpG sites only make up approximately 1% of all dinucleotides, and this is because DNA methylation is mutagenic. CpG sites are under-represented in the human genome due to spontaneous deamination of 5mC to thymine [17]. CpG sites are not evenly distributed in the genome, and sequences that contain a high concentration of CpG sites are referred to as CpG islands (CGIs) [18]. CGIs are defined as short DNA sequences that are typically 500 to 1000 base pairs (bp) in length with a CpG content $\geq$ 50% and an observed to expected CpG ratio $\geq$ 60%. The majority of CGIs, approximately 50-70%, are located at gene promoters, especially the promoters of housekeeping genes. The methylation of promoter CGIs typically correlates with gene activity [19, 20].

In normal somatic cells, the majority of CpG sites are methylated, while CpG sites within promoter CGIs typically remain unmethylated and in a transcriptionally permissive chromatin state. The high frequency of unmethylated CpG sites in promoter CGIs increases the potential that transcription factors will bind, whereas DNA methylation of promoter CGIs along with chromatin folding leads to stable transcriptional silencing by physically blocking the binding of transcription factors to DNA. In addition, DNA methylation further indirectly inhibits transcription by the presence of methyl-CpG binding proteins (MBPs) that recruits chromatin-modifying proteins. Heterochromatin has a tightly packaged chromatin structure that is generally heavily methylated and transcriptionally silenced. In contrast, euchromatin has a lightly packaged chromatin structure that has less DNA methylation and is more easily accessed for transcription [21, 22]. Bordering CGIs are CGI shores, which are regions approximately two kilobases (kb) in length that have a lower density of CpG sites than CGIs. CGI shores typically have similar patterns of methylation to that of the neighbouring CGI. Recent studies have found that tissue-specific gene expression is strongly related to that of CGI shore methylation patterns rather than GCIs themselves. Similar to CGIs, methylation of CGI shores is associated with reduced transcriptional activity [23].

Gene-bodies, unlike most CGI promoters and shores, have an abundance of 5mC. However, research has observed a positive correlation between DNA methylation of gene-bodies and gene expression. A study that used mouse embryonic stem cells reported that DNA methylation of gene-bodies prevents the initiation of spurious intragenic transcription by RNA polymerase II. In addition, cell- and tissue-specific patterns of DNA methylation are observed more across gene-bodies than CGI promoters [24]. However, more investigation and evidence are required to further understand the relationship between patterns of DNA methylation in gene-bodies and gene expression [25].

In the human genome, intergenic regions that consist of harmful genetic elements are typically silenced by DNA methylated. DNA methylation of intergenic regions helps to maintain genomic stability. Cells that are DNMT1 null exhibit genomic instability because of aberrant patterns of hypomethylation at intergenic regions, which can lead to deletions, translocations and insertions [26].

Aberrant DNA Methylation in Cancer Genomes

Nowadays, cancer is recognised as a disease of both genetic and epigenetic alterations, with patterns of aberrant DNA methylation being recognised as a hallmark of cancer. Research has observed aberrant patterns of DNA methylation in all cancers ever studied; these alterations to the DNA methylation landscape contribute to carcinogenesis. In cancer, there are two frequently observed patterns of aberrant DNA methylation; they include global DNA hypomethylation and focal hypermethylation of promoter CGIs [15]. Global hypomethylation is associated with the aberrant activation and expression of previously silenced regions of the genome, resulting in increased transcriptional activity and genomic instability. Whereas focal hypermethylation that is observed at typically unmethylated promoter regions and is mainly associated with transcriptional silencing of tumour-suppressor genes (TSG), leading to uncontrolled cell division. Genomic instability and uncontrolled cell division are both key characteristics of cancer cells [27]. DNA methylation can also indirectly contribute to carcinogenesis by somatic mutation. 5mC has an increased tendency to undergo spontaneous deamination forming thymine. TpG mismatches in tumour-suppressor genes that are not successfully repaired by the BER pathway, can lead to transcriptional silencing and contribute to cancer development [22]. Somatic mutations in the TP53 gene are frequently reported in most human cancers [28]. Furthermore, in normal cells, the two opposing processes of DNA methylation and demethylation are tightly regulated. However, abnormal expression of DNMT enzymes is frequently observed in cancer, which can create a feedback loop that causes further alteration to the DNA methylation landscape [29].

In 1983, global hypomethylation was the earliest documented epigenetic abnormality observed in human cancers and refers to the loss of DNA methylation along the entire genome. Loss of DNA methylation is associated with aberrant expression of potentially harmful genetic elements and oncogenes. It is well known that DNA methylation plays an important role in regulating gene expression and maintaining genomic stability, whereas, in cancer, global DNA hypomethylation is suggested to contribute to increased transcriptional activity leading to widespread genomic instability. Recent genome-wide studies have established that patterns of global DNA hypomethylation occur to some extent in every type of human cancer. Hypomethylation has been observed both in early carcinogenesis and throughout cancer progression [30, 31]. Evidence that aberrant patterns of DNA hypomethylation are associated with genomic instability were observed in a study using mouse models. DNMT1 null embryos, embryos that have no DNMT1 expression, died around mid-gestation. In addition, adult mouse models with reduced or no DNMT1 expression in a particular tissue resulted in the animal developing cancer in that same tissue, this was because the cells were unable to maintain DNA methylation patterns and therefore, were unable to regulate normal patterns of gene expression [32]. Furthermore, genomic instability caused by DNA hypomethylation is a characteristic feature of immunodeficiency and cranio-facial defects (ICF) syndrome. ICF syndrome is the result of a mutation in the de novo DNMT3B gene, which leads to global hypomethylation to be observed at specific repetitive sequences found near the centromere [33]. In cancer cells, large regions of the genome that become hypomethylated are also strongly associated with changes to the chromatin status. Long interspersed nucleotide element-1 (LINE-1) is a class of repetitive sequences that make up approximately 17% of the human genome; because of the abundance of LINE-1, it is frequently used as a surrogate marker for global DNA methylation [34]. In normal somatic cells, LINE-1 sequences are heavily methylated and inactivated. Hypomethylation of LINE-1 sequences is frequently studied and has been associated with increased genomic instability of several human cancers, including colorectal, bladder, prostate and ovarian cancers. In addition, LINE-1 methylation status has been suggested as a potential diagnostic and prognostic biomarker for several different types of cancer [35, 36]. Short interspersed nuclear elements (SINEs) are another class of repetitive sequences that are generally methylated in normal cells, however, acute myeloid leukemia studies have reported a loss of DNA methylation of SINEs [37]. Although it is less frequent than promoter hypermethylation, promoter hypomethylation has also been observed in cancer cells. In cancer cells, the loss of methylation within promoter regions can result in the aberrant activation and expression of specific genes [30]. In melanoma, the MAGE-1 gene [38] in lung cancer, the engulfment and cell motility 3 (ELMO3) gene [39] and in breast and ovarian cancers, the SNCG gene are observed to have increased transcriptional activity accompanied by promoter hypomethylation [40]. Although, more testing is needed to further identify the link between promoter hypomethylation and aberrant gene expression, to ensure that it is not just a secondary feature of cancer cells.

Cancer cells have a unique ability to inactivate tumour-suppressor genes (TSGs), either genetically or epigenetically. Aberrant DNA hypermethylation frequently occurs within the unmethylated promoter regions of TSGs, resulting in transcriptional silencing in cancer cells. Recent studies have suggested that transcriptional silencing associated with CGI promoter hypermethylation is more frequent than silencing by mutation, in the majority of human cancers [41]. Silencing of a TSG by aberrant DNA hypermethylation can be regarded as one of the hits in terms of the Knudson hypothesis, also known as the two-hit hypothesis. Knudson proposed that majority of TSGs require both alleles to be silenced in order to cause a phenotypic change, just by silencing one allele of a TSG is generally insufficient to contribute to carcinogenesis as one functioning TSG can be sufficient to regulate cell proliferation [42]. DNA methylation is mitotically heritable, meaning that aberrant alterations to gene expression can be passed on to newly replicated cells. As time progresses, cells that continue to acquire aberrant DNA methylation associated with TSGs are more likely to divide rapidly and evade cell death, which is characteristic of cancer cells [29]. Recent genome-wide DNA methylation studies have reported that transcriptional silencing by aberrant hypermethylation of TSG promoter CGIs, varies depending on the type of cancer [43]. In prostate cancer, the Glutathione S-Transferase P (GSTP1) gene [22], retinoblastoma, the RB1 gene [44], in renal cell carcinoma, the VHL gene [45] and in breast and ovarian cancers, the BRCA1 gene [46] frequently display a loss of transcriptional activity due to aberrant promoter hypermethylation. These studies provide evidence that genes associated with carcinogenesis acquire aberrant methylation of promoter CGIs during cancer development, it has also highlighted that DNA hypermethylation of single genes has a similar silencing outcome as mutations. In addition, CGI shores are typically observed to become hypermethylated along with the bordering CGI. CGI shore hypermethylation was first observed in human colon cancer [23]. In some cancers, sets of TSGs are silenced by distinct patterns of extensive promoter hypermethylation; this phenomenon is referred to as the CpG island methylator phenotype (CIMP). In 1999 CIMP was first described in colorectal cancers (CRCs) by Toyota and colleagues, as another potential carcinogenic pathway driven by aberrant DNA hypermethylation. With the advancements in DNA methylation mapping technologies, the identification of CIMPs has enabled the stratification of cancer subtypes by specific DNA methylation patterns. CIMP-positive CRCs have several TSGs, including mismatch repair gene MLH1 transcriptionally silenced by promoter hypermethylation, which has been linked to BRAF mutations and microsatellite instability. Methylation of MLH1 promoter causes reduced expression and production of functional protein, preventing the cell from repairing mismatches along the genome, which increases the mutation rate [47]. CIMP has also been widely studied in gliomas. A recent study that analysed the DNA methylation data of human glioma samples from The Cancer Genome Atlas (TCGA) identified a glioma-CIMP (G-CIMP). Gliomas with observed G-CIMP were found to be tightly associated with IDH1 somatic mutations [48]. Other cancers where CIMP has been described include gastric cancer [49], neuroblastoma [50] and melanoma [51]. The methylation landscape of CIMP cancers is distinct from other cancer types and has been suggested as useful diagnostic, prognostic and therapeutic biomarkers in several human cancers.

Methylation-Based Biomarkers

Even with all the advancements in medicine and technology, cancer remains a major cause of morbidity and mortality worldwide. Early cancer detection and intervention is the most effective method that will improve patient outcomes. However, in the majority of cancers, tissue biopsies are what are typically used to determine a diagnosis. Non-invasive cancer detection is the challenge that researchers pursue [52]. In cancer, in addition to genetic changes, the epigenetic landscape is also altered and disrupted. DNA methylation changes are observed during both early stages of cancer development and throughout progression. With recent improvements to DNA methylation mapping technologies, there has been rapidly increasing interest into the applications of methylation-based biomarkers. Aberrant patterns of DNA methylation that are found in cancer genomes can be and have been used as sources of biomarkers for the early detection and diagnosis of cancer, prognosis, monitoring and can help predict response to therapy [15]. Methylation marks can be detected using several technologies in a variety of samples, not just fresh-frozen tissue and formalin-fixed paraffin-embedded (FFPE). Cancer cells can release cancer DNA into the blood and other body fluids, including saliva, urine and stool, all of which could be potentially utilised as non-invasive sources of cancer DNA. Peripheral blood and other blood fluids are referred to as liquid biopsies [53]. Currently, there is a lot of activity surrounding the detection of cancer-associated methylation changes in cell-free

DNA (cfDNA) released by tumours into the blood. cfDNA carries not just disease-associated genetic changes, but also patterns of DNA methylation. Studies have observed that DNA methylation patterns in cfDNA are consistent with the cells and or tissues from which they originated [54]. Therefore, implying that cfDNA can be used as a surrogate for cancer DNA as it reflects the primary tumour. In addition, applications of DNA methylation biomarkers have also been suggested to become useful for other diseases, including neurodegenerative and psychiatric disorders [55]. A study that compared DNA methylation of cfDNA in blood collected from patients with pancreatic cancer and chronic pancreatitis, showed that cancer and inflammatory disease produced different patterns of methylation [56].

Bladder Cancer

Bladder cancer is a common urogenital cancer, which is typically diagnosed after the patient presents with macroscopic haematuria. The current routine gold standard of bladder cancer diagnosis is by cystoscopy. However, cystoscopy involves using a telescope to look inside the bladder and biopsy the tumour, which is very expensive and invasive. As there is a high rate of recurrence, patients previously diagnosed with bladder cancer require frequent monitoring, hence the search for non-invasive methods of detecting bladder cancer. Recently, several studies have successfully examined aberrant DNA methylation in urine samples of bladder cancer patients, because urine samples are in direct contact with the tumour [57, 58]. Using quantitative methylation-specific PCR (QMSP), Wang *et al.* examined the methylation status of seven genes (EOMES, GDF15, NID2, PCDH17, POU4F2, TCF21, and ZNF154), and observed that the combination of *POU4F2* and *PCDH17* exhibited 90.00% sensitivity and 93.96% specificity in a cohort of 312 urine samples. This study collected urine samples from 130 urothelial cell carcinoma patients, 41 infected urinary calculi patients, 46 kidney cancer patients, 42 prostate cancer patients and 53 healthy controls [57].

Breast Cancer

Breast cancer is the most common type of cancer diagnosed in women worldwide and is one of the leading causes of cancer-related death among women. Detection of breast cancer in the early stages of the disease is the key to improving survival rates. However, small tumours are difficult to identify using mammography, which is pushing researchers to investigate new methods and technologies, including the analysis of DNA methylation using cfcDNA to screen for breast cancer [59]. Shan *et al.* used a high-throughput assay MethyLight to develop a panel test of six genes (SFN, P16, hMLH1, HOXD13, PCDHGB7 and RASSF1a) that exhibited aberrant patterns of methylation in cfcDNA of serum samples from breast cancer patients. Supporting the use of non-invasive DNA methylation biomarkers for the early diagnosis of breast cancer [60].

Colorectal Cancer

CRC is the third most common type of cancer and is a leading cause of cancer-related deaths world-wide [61]. To improve the patient prognosis of CRC, early detection by screening methods is important. Aberrant DNA hypermethylation of the Septin 9 (SEPT9) gene has been reported as an early event in several human cancers, including CRC. Methylated SEPT9 (mSEPT9) is used as a screening marker for CRC in tumour tissue and peripheral blood. However, early-stage CRC has low circulating tumour DNA (ctDNA) concentration. To increase the rate of detecting ctDNA panels of DNA methylation biomarkers could be screened at the same time, increasing the diagnostic and prognostic accuracy however, it also increases the cost and the testing complexity [62].

Lung Cancer

Lung cancer is the leading cause of cancer-related deaths worldwide, mainly due to the current limited diagnostic capabilities, with low rates of survival linked to late diagnosis. It is well known today that exposure to tobacco smoke is the main risk factor for lung cancer [63]. Studies have shown that generally, the earlier a diagnosis can be made, the higher the survival rate. However, only a very small proportion of lung cancer patients are fortunate to be diagnosed during the early stages of disease [64]. The currently recommended screening test for lung cancer is low-dose computed tomography (LDCT) however, benign lesions are commonly mistaken for lung cancer leading to risky and unnecessary follow-up tests and procedures [65]. Currently, there are several methylation marks under investigation for the early detection of lung cancers. The promoter region of the transmembrane protein with a single EGF-like and two follistatin domains (TMEFF2) gene is hypermethylated and inactivated in multiple cancer types. A study that analysed serum samples of 316 patients with non-small cell lung cancer (NSCLC) and 50 age-matched healthy controls, identified that hypermethylation of TMEFF2 was exclusively detected in 9.2% of patients with NSCLC. However, the biological function of TMEFF2 in carcinogenesis remains unknown, with conflicting studies reporting it functions as both an oncogene and TSG [66]. Sputum as a non-invasive surrogate of tumour DNA is gaining a lot of attention as it is a better representative of NSCLC than blood, because there is direct shedding of tumour DNA. A study published in 2007 compared the methylation status of 72 stage-III NSCLC patients using tissue, sputum and serum samples and identified four genes, p16, DAPK, PAX5 β, and GATA5, as potential methylation-based biomarkers [67 - 69].

Ovarian Cancer

Ovarian cancer (OC) is the most lethal gynaecological malignancy due to the majority of patients being diagnosed at a late stage. Current screening for OC includes the 'risk of malignancy index' that incorporates measuring serum levels of protein biomarker cancer antigen 125 (CA-125), however, its sensitivity and specificity are known to be poor, with only approximately 50% of stage-I OCs causing an increase of serum CA-125 [70]. Furthermore, aberrant elevated serum CA-125 has also been associated with several benign conditions and other malignancies [71, 72]. In the majority of OCs, along with other TSGs, the RAS association domain family protein 1A is hypermethylated and inactivated. Recently RASSF1A has been under investigation as a potential methylation biomarker to aid in the early diagnosis of OC. RASSF1A is a TSG that helps to regulate cell division. A study that assessed cell-free circulating DNA (cfcDNA) demonstrated 90.0% sensitivity and 86.7% specificity when comparing the methylation status of 3 gene promoters, including RASSF1A, between OC and health controls (HC). In addition, they reported that two gene promoters, including RASSF1A, were informative when differentiating between benign conditions and OC [73, 74]. Moving forward, more investigation into the applications of using non-invasive liquid biopsy testing to examine DNA methylation biomarkers for OC patients will ultimately improve upon current diagnosis, management and treatment methods [75].

Prostate Cancer

Prostate cancer is a leading cause of cancer-related deaths amongst men worldwide. Current diagnostic methods involve measuring levels of prostate-specific antigen (PSA) in serum, digital rectal examination and histological examination of needle biopsies [76]. Serum PSA is elevated in prostate cancer patients however, its sensitivity and specificity are poor as an individual biomarker, and the result is unnecessary biopsies are performed. Using QMSP, Brait *et al.* analysed the methylation status of ten genes (SSBP2, MCAM, ERα, ERβ, APC, CCND2, MGMT, GSTP1, p16 and RARβ2), previously associated with aberrant methylation in prostate cancer. This was to determine potential non-invasive methylation biomarkers for the early detection of prostate cancer. In this study, serum samples were collected from 84 prostate cancer patients, 30 health controls and 7 high-grade Prostatic Intraepithelial Neoplasia (HGPIN). Brait *et al.* developed a panel test of three methylated genes, MCAM, ERα and Erβ, that observed 75% sensitivity and 70% specificity, compared to PSA which had 77% sensitivity and 30% specificity [77].

CONCLUDING REMARKS

Over the past decade, there has been an increasing volume of reports about aberrant patterns of DNA methylation and its association with cancer. More recently, these include investigations into both cancer-associated DNA hypermethylation of TSG and genome-wide DNA hypomethylation. For a long time, cancer research has overlooked genome-wide hypomethylation for TSG promoter hypermethylation, as increased methylation is accompanied by transcriptional silencing and especially in terms of TSGs becoming inactivated. Even with the advancements made over the past decade, there is still a lot that is poorly understood. A lot of the underlying molecular mechanisms of aberrant DNA methylation landscape remodelling in cancer remain to be characterised. In cancer, why are some regions of the genome more susceptible to DNMT activity? How dynamic is the DNA methylation landscape during the initiation and progression of cancer, and how will those changes influence the progression of the disease? We know that aberrant DNA methylation is recognised as a hallmark of cancer, and with the advancements so far made towards DNA mapping technologies, there are methylation patterns being used nowadays as biomarkers for the detection and prognosis of cancer, as well as being used to predict responses to cancer therapies. With the increasing interest in developing DNA methylation-based *in vitro* diagnostic products (IVD), it is creating a competitive and innovative environment that will in turn, improve the cost and effectiveness, which ultimately will benefit cancer patients.

CONSENT OF PUBLICATION:

Not applicable.

CONFLICT OF INTEREST

The authors declare no conflict of interest, financial or otherwise.

ACKNOWLEDGMENTS

The authors would like to acknowledge and thank Dr. Farhadul Islam, Department of Biochemistry and Molecular Biology, University of Rajshahi, Rajshahi-6205, Bangladesh, for his continuous support of this chapter.

REFERENCES

[1] Hollister JD, Gaut BS. Epigenetic silencing of transposable elements: A trade-off between reduced transposition and deleterious effects on neighboring gene expression. Genome Res 2009; 19(8): 1419-

28.
[http://dx.doi.org/10.1101/gr.091678.109] [PMID: 19478138]

[2] Sharp AJ, Stathaki E, Migliavacca E, *et al.* DNA methylation profiles of human active and inactive X chromosomes. Genome Res 2011; 21(10): 1592-600.
[http://dx.doi.org/10.1101/gr.112680.110] [PMID: 21862626]

[3] Moore LD, Le T, Fan G. DNA methylation and its basic function. Neuropsychopharmacology 2013; 38(1): 23-38.
[http://dx.doi.org/10.1038/npp.2012.112] [PMID: 22781841]

[4] Zhang J, Yang C, Wu C, Cui W, Wang L. DNA Methyltransferases in Cancer: Biology, Paradox, Aberrations, and Targeted Therapy. Cancers (Basel) 2020; 12(8): 2123.
[http://dx.doi.org/10.3390/cancers12082123] [PMID: 32751889]

[5] Lu F, Liu Y, Jiang L, Yamaguchi S, Zhang Y. Role of Tet proteins in enhancer activity and telomere elongation. Genes Dev 2014; 28(19): 2103-19.
[http://dx.doi.org/10.1101/gad.248005.114] [PMID: 25223896]

[6] Ito S, D'Alessio AC, Taranova OV, Hong K, Sowers LC, Zhang Y. Role of Tet proteins in 5mC to 5hmC conversion, ES-cell self-renewal and inner cell mass specification. Nature 2010; 466(7310): 1129-33.
[http://dx.doi.org/10.1038/nature09303] [PMID: 20639862]

[7] Tahiliani M, Koh KP, Shen Y, *et al.* Conversion of 5-methylcytosine to 5-hydroxymethylcytosine in mammalian DNA by MLL partner TET1. Science 2009; 324(5929): 930-5.
[http://dx.doi.org/10.1126/science.1170116] [PMID: 19372391]

[8] Pastor WA, Pape UJ, Huang Y, *et al.* Genome-wide mapping of 5-hydroxymethylcytosine in embryonic stem cells. Nature 2011; 473(7347): 394-7.
[http://dx.doi.org/10.1038/nature10102] [PMID: 21552279]

[9] Williams K, Christensen J, Pedersen MT, *et al.* TET1 and hydroxymethylcytosine in transcription and DNA methylation fidelity. Nature 2011; 473(7347): 343-8.
[http://dx.doi.org/10.1038/nature10066] [PMID: 21490601]

[10] Wu H, D'Alessio AC, Ito S, *et al.* Dual functions of Tet1 in transcriptional regulation in mouse embryonic stem cells. Nature 2011; 473(7347): 389-93.
[http://dx.doi.org/10.1038/nature09934] [PMID: 21451524]

[11] Hahn MA, Szabó PE, Pfeifer GP. 5-Hydroxymethylcytosine: A stable or transient DNA modification? Genomics 2014; 104(5): 314-23.
[http://dx.doi.org/10.1016/j.ygeno.2014.08.015] [PMID: 25181633]

[12] Ito S, Shen L, Dai Q, *et al.* Tet proteins can convert 5-methylcytosine to 5-formylcytosine and 5-carboxylcytosine. Science 2011; 333(6047): 1300-3.
[http://dx.doi.org/10.1126/science.1210597] [PMID: 21778364]

[13] Talhaoui I, Couve S, Gros L, Ishchenko AA, Matkarimov B, Saparbaev MK. Aberrant repair initiated by mismatch-specific thymine-DNA glycosylases provides a mechanism for the mutational bias observed in CpG islands. Nucleic Acids Res 2014; 42(10): 6300-13.
[http://dx.doi.org/10.1093/nar/gku246] [PMID: 24692658]

[14] Bhutani N, Burns DM, Blau HM. DNA demethylation dynamics. Cell 2011; 146(6): 866-72.
[http://dx.doi.org/10.1016/j.cell.2011.08.042] [PMID: 21925312]

[15] Zhang W, Xu J. DNA methyltransferases and their roles in tumorigenesis. Biomark Res 2017; 5(1): 1.
[http://dx.doi.org/10.1186/s40364-017-0081-z] [PMID: 28127428]

[16] Ehrlich M, Gama-Sosa MA, Huang LH, *et al.* Amount and distribution of 5-methylcytosine in human DNA from different types of tissues or cells. Nucleic Acids Res 1982; 10(8): 2709-21.
[http://dx.doi.org/10.1093/nar/10.8.2709] [PMID: 7079182]

[17] Cooper DN, Mort M, Stenson PD, Ball EV, Chuzhanova NA. Methylation-mediated deamination of 5-methylcytosine appears to give rise to mutations causing human inherited disease in CpNpG trinucleotides, as well as in CpG dinucleotides. Hum Genomics 2010; 4(6): 406-10. [http://dx.doi.org/10.1186/1479-7364-4-6-406] [PMID: 20846930]

[18] Elango N, Yi SV. Functional relevance of CpG island length for regulation of gene expression. Genetics 2011; 187(4): 1077-83. [http://dx.doi.org/10.1534/genetics.110.126094] [PMID: 21288871]

[19] Sarda S, Hannenhalli S. Orphan CpG islands as alternative promoters. Transcription 2018; 9(3): 171-6. [http://dx.doi.org/10.1080/21541264.2017.1373209] [PMID: 29099304]

[20] Karlin S, Doerfler W, Cardon LR. Why is CpG suppressed in the genomes of virtually all small eukaryotic viruses but not in those of large eukaryotic viruses? J Virol 1994; 68(5): 2889-97. [http://dx.doi.org/10.1128/jvi.68.5.2889-2897.1994] [PMID: 8151759]

[21] Takai D, Jones PA. Comprehensive analysis of CpG islands in human chromosomes 21 and 22. Proc Natl Acad Sci USA 2002; 99(6): 3740-5. [http://dx.doi.org/10.1073/pnas.052410099] [PMID: 11891299]

[22] Skvortsova K, Stirzaker C, Taberlay P. The DNA methylation landscape in cancer. Essays Biochem 2019; 63(6): 797-811. [http://dx.doi.org/10.1042/EBC20190037] [PMID: 31845735]

[23] Irizarry RA, Ladd-Acosta C, Wen B, *et al.* The human colon cancer methylome shows similar hypo- and hypermethylation at conserved tissue-specific CpG island shores. Nat Genet 2009; 41(2): 178-86. [http://dx.doi.org/10.1038/ng.298] [PMID: 19151715]

[24] Maunakea AK, Nagarajan RP, Bilenky M, *et al.* Conserved role of intragenic DNA methylation in regulating alternative promoters. Nature 2010; 466(7303): 253-7. [http://dx.doi.org/10.1038/nature09165] [PMID: 20613842]

[25] Jjingo D, Conley AB, Yi SV, Lunyak VV, Jordan IK. On the presence and role of human gene-body DNA methylation. Oncotarget 2012; 3(4): 462-74. [http://dx.doi.org/10.18632/oncotarget.497] [PMID: 22577155]

[26] Rauscher GH, Kresovich JK, Poulin M, *et al.* Exploring DNA methylation changes in promoter, intragenic, and intergenic regions as early and late events in breast cancer formation. BMC Cancer 2015; 15(1): 816. [http://dx.doi.org/10.1186/s12885-015-1777-9] [PMID: 26510686]

[27] McMahon KW, Karunasena E, Ahuja N. The Roles of DNA Methylation in the Stages of Cancer. Cancer J 2017; 23(5): 257-61. [http://dx.doi.org/10.1097/PPO.0000000000000279] [PMID: 28926425]

[28] Olivier M, Hollstein M, Hainaut P. TP53 mutations in human cancers: origins, consequences, and clinical use. Cold Spring Harb Perspect Biol 2010; 2(1): a001008-8. [http://dx.doi.org/10.1101/cshperspect.a001008] [PMID: 20182602]

[29] Wajed SA, Laird PW, DeMeester TR. DNA methylation: an alternative pathway to cancer. Ann Surg 2001; 234(1): 10-20. [http://dx.doi.org/10.1097/00000658-200107000-00003] [PMID: 11420478]

[30] Ehrlich M. DNA hypomethylation in cancer cells. Epigenomics 2009; 1(2): 239-59. [http://dx.doi.org/10.2217/epi.09.33] [PMID: 20495664]

[31] Tsuda H, Takarabe T, Kanai Y, Fukutomi T, Hirohashi S. Correlation of DNA hypomethylation at pericentromeric heterochromatin regions of chromosomes 16 and 1 with histological features and chromosomal abnormalities of human breast carcinomas. Am J Pathol 2002; 161(3): 859-66. [http://dx.doi.org/10.1016/S0002-9440(10)64246-0] [PMID: 12213714]

[32] Hirasawa R, Chiba H, Kaneda M, *et al.* Maternal and zygotic Dnmt1 are necessary and sufficient for

the maintenance of DNA methylation imprints during preimplantation development. Genes Dev 2008; 22(12): 1607-16.
[http://dx.doi.org/10.1101/gad.1667008] [PMID: 18559477]

[33] Ehrlich M, Jackson K, Weemaes C. Immunodeficiency, centromeric region instability, facial anomalies syndrome (ICF). Orphanet J Rare Dis 2006; 1(1): 2.
[http://dx.doi.org/10.1186/1750-1172-1-2] [PMID: 16722602]

[34] Yang AS, Estécio MR, Doshi K, Kondo Y, Tajara EH, Issa JP. A simple method for estimating global DNA methylation using bisulfite PCR of repetitive DNA elements. Nucleic Acids Res 2004; 32(3): 38.
[http://dx.doi.org/10.1093/nar/gnh032] [PMID: 14973332]

[35] Ogino S, Nosho K, Kirkner GJ, *et al.* A cohort study of tumoral LINE-1 hypomethylation and prognosis in colon cancer. J Natl Cancer Inst 2008; 100(23): 1734-8.
[http://dx.doi.org/10.1093/jnci/djn359] [PMID: 19033568]

[36] Wolff EM, Byun HM, Han HF, *et al.* Hypomethylation of a LINE-1 promoter activates an alternate transcript of the MET oncogene in bladders with cancer. PLoS Genet 2010; 6(4): e1000917.
[http://dx.doi.org/10.1371/journal.pgen.1000917] [PMID: 20421991]

[37] Saied MH, Marzec J, Khalid S, *et al.* Genome wide analysis of acute myeloid leukemia reveal leukemia specific methylome and subtype specific hypomethylation of repeats. PLoS One 2012; 7(3): e33213.
[http://dx.doi.org/10.1371/journal.pone.0033213] [PMID: 22479372]

[38] Loriot A, De Plaen E, Boon T, De Smet C. Transient down-regulation of DNMT1 methyltransferase leads to activation and stable hypomethylation of MAGE-A1 in melanoma cells. J Biol Chem 2006; 281(15): 10118-26.
[http://dx.doi.org/10.1074/jbc.M510469200] [PMID: 16497664]

[39] Søes S, Daugaard IL, Sørensen BS, *et al.* Hypomethylation and increased expression of the putative oncogene ELMO3 are associated with lung cancer development and metastases formation. Oncoscience 2014; 1(5): 367-74.
[http://dx.doi.org/10.18632/oncoscience.42] [PMID: 25594031]

[40] Gupta A, Godwin AK, Vanderveer L, Lu A, Liu J. Hypomethylation of the synuclein gamma gene CpG island promotes its aberrant expression in breast carcinoma and ovarian carcinoma. Cancer Res 2003; 63(3): 664-73.
[PMID: 12566312]

[41] Ehrlich M. DNA hypermethylation in disease: mechanisms and clinical relevance. Epigenetics 2019; 14(12): 1141-63.
[http://dx.doi.org/10.1080/15592294.2019.1638701] [PMID: 31284823]

[42] Di Ruscio A, Welner RS, Tenen DG, Amabile G. The second hit of DNA methylation. Mol Cell Oncol 2016; 3(3): e1093690.
[http://dx.doi.org/10.1080/23723556.2015.1093690] [PMID: 27314082]

[43] Ongenaert M, Van Neste L, *et al.* PubMeth: a cancer methylation database combining text-mining and expert annotation. Nucleic Acids Research. 2007; 36(Database): D842-D846.
[http://dx.doi.org/10.1093/nar/gkm788]

[44] Choy KW, Lee TC, Cheung KF, *et al.* Clinical implications of promoter hypermethylation in RASSF1A and MGMT in retinoblastoma. Neoplasia 2005; 7(3): 200-6.
[http://dx.doi.org/10.1593/neo.04565] [PMID: 15799820]

[45] Kim BJ, Kim JH, Kim HS, Zang DY. Prognostic and predictive value of VHL gene alteration in renal cell carcinoma: a meta-analysis and review. Oncotarget 2017; 8(8): 13979-85.
[http://dx.doi.org/10.18632/oncotarget.14704] [PMID: 28103578]

[46] Azzollini J, Pesenti C, Pizzamiglio S, *et al.* Constitutive *BRCA1* Promoter Hypermethylation Can Be a Predisposing Event in Isolated Early-Onset Breast Cancer. Cancers (Basel) 2019; 11(1): 58.

[http://dx.doi.org/10.3390/cancers11010058] [PMID: 30634417]

[47] Yi JH. CpG island methylator phenotype in colorectal cancer. World Chin J Digestology 2016; 24(4): 558.
[http://dx.doi.org/10.11569/wcjd.v24.i4.558]

[48] Noushmehr H, Weisenberger DJ, Diefes K, *et al.* Identification of a CpG island methylator phenotype that defines a distinct subgroup of glioma. Cancer Cell 2010; 17(5): 510-22.
[http://dx.doi.org/10.1016/j.ccr.2010.03.017] [PMID: 20399149]

[49] Teodoridis JM, Hardie C, Brown R. CpG island methylator phenotype (CIMP) in cancer: Causes and implications. Cancer Lett 2008; 268(2): 177-86.
[http://dx.doi.org/10.1016/j.canlet.2008.03.022] [PMID: 18471961]

[50] Asada K, Abe M, Ushijima T. Clinical application of the CpG island methylator phenotype to prognostic diagnosis in neuroblastomas. J Hum Genet 2013; 58(7): 428-33.
[http://dx.doi.org/10.1038/jhg.2013.64] [PMID: 23739128]

[51] Tanemura A, Terando AM, Sim MS, *et al.* CpG island methylator phenotype predicts progression of malignant melanoma. Clin Cancer Res 2009; 15(5): 1801-7.
[http://dx.doi.org/10.1158/1078-0432.CCR-08-1361] [PMID: 19223509]

[52] Bray F, Ferlay J, Soerjomataram I, Siegel RL, Torre LA, Jemal A. Global cancer statistics 2018: GLOBOCAN estimates of incidence and mortality worldwide for 36 cancers in 185 countries. CA Cancer J Clin 2018; 68(6): 394-424.
[http://dx.doi.org/10.3322/caac.21492] [PMID: 30207593]

[53] Moss J, Magenheim J, Neiman D, *et al.* Comprehensive human cell-type methylation atlas reveals origins of circulating cell-free DNA in health and disease. Nat Commun 2018; 9(1): 5068.
[http://dx.doi.org/10.1038/s41467-018-07466-6] [PMID: 30498206]

[54] Huang J, Wang L. Cell-Free DNA Methylation Profiling Analysis—Technologies and Bioinformatics. Cancers (Basel) 2019; 11(11): 1741.
[http://dx.doi.org/10.3390/cancers11111741] [PMID: 31698791]

[55] Martínez-Iglesias O, Carrera I, Carril JC, Fernández-Novoa L, Cacabelos N, Cacabelos R. DNA Methylation in Neurodegenerative and Cerebrovascular Disorders. Int J Mol Sci 2020; 21(6): 2220.
[http://dx.doi.org/10.3390/ijms21062220] [PMID: 32210102]

[56] Liggett T, Melnikov A, Yi Q, *et al.* Differential methylation of cell-free circulating DNA among patients with pancreatic cancer *versus* chronic pancreatitis. Cancer 2010; 116(7): 1674-80.
[http://dx.doi.org/10.1002/cncr.24893] [PMID: 20143430]

[57] Wang Y, Yu Y, Ye R, *et al.* An epigenetic biomarker combination of PCDH17 and POU4F2 detects bladder cancer accurately by methylation analyses of urine sediment DNA in Han Chinese. Oncotarget 2016; 7(3): 2754-64.
[http://dx.doi.org/10.18632/oncotarget.6666] [PMID: 26700620]

[58] Friedrich MG, Weisenberger DJ, Cheng JC, *et al.* Detection of methylated apoptosis-associated genes in urine sediments of bladder cancer patients. Clin Cancer Res 2004; 10(22): 7457-65.
[http://dx.doi.org/10.1158/1078-0432.CCR-04-0930] [PMID: 15569975]

[59] Yang Y, Wu L, Shu XO, *et al.* Genetically Predicted Levels of DNA Methylation Biomarkers and Breast Cancer Risk: Data From 228 951 Women of European Descent. J Natl Cancer Inst 2020; 112(3): 295-304.
[http://dx.doi.org/10.1093/jnci/djz109] [PMID: 31143935]

[60] Shan M, Yin H, Li J, *et al.* Detection of aberrant methylation of a six-gene panel in serum DNA for diagnosis of breast cancer. Oncotarget 2016; 7(14): 18485-94.
[http://dx.doi.org/10.18632/oncotarget.7608] [PMID: 26918343]

[61] Jemal A, Bray F, Center MM, Ferlay J, Ward E, Forman D. Global cancer statistics. CA Cancer J Clin 2011; 61(2): 69-90.

[http://dx.doi.org/10.3322/caac.20107] [PMID: 21296855]

[62] Shen N, Wang T, Li D, Zhu Y, Xie H, Lu Y. Hypermethylation of the SEPT9 Gene Suggests Significantly Poor Prognosis in Cancer Patients: A Systematic Review and Meta-Analysis. Front Genet 2019; 10: 887.
[http://dx.doi.org/10.3389/fgene.2019.00887] [PMID: 31608117]

[63] Hecht SS, Szabo E. Fifty years of tobacco carcinogenesis research: from mechanisms to early detection and prevention of lung cancer. Cancer Prev Res (Phila) 2014; 7(1): 1-8.
[http://dx.doi.org/10.1158/1940-6207.CAPR-13-0371] [PMID: 24403288]

[64] Youlden DR, Cramb SM, Baade PD. The International Epidemiology of Lung Cancer: geographical distribution and secular trends. J Thorac Oncol 2008; 3(8): 819-31.
[http://dx.doi.org/10.1097/JTO.0b013e31818020eb] [PMID: 18670299]

[65] de Groot PM, Wu CC, Carter BW, Munden RF. The epidemiology of lung cancer. Transl Lung Cancer Res 2018; 7(3): 220-33.
[http://dx.doi.org/10.21037/tlcr.2018.05.06] [PMID: 30050761]

[66] Lee SM, Park JY, Kim DS. Methylation of TMEFF2 gene in tissue and serum DNA from patients with non-small cell lung cancer. Mol Cells 2012; 34(2): 171-6.
[http://dx.doi.org/10.1007/s10059-012-0083-5] [PMID: 22814847]

[67] Belinsky SA, Grimes MJ, Casas E, *et al.* Predicting gene promoter methylation in non-small-cell lung cancer by evaluating sputum and serum. Br J Cancer 2007; 96(8): 1278-83.
[http://dx.doi.org/10.1038/sj.bjc.6603721] [PMID: 17406356]

[68] Shen N, Du J, Zhou H, *et al.* A Diagnostic Panel of DNA Methylation Biomarkers for Lung Adenocarcinoma. Front Oncol 2019; 9: 1281.
[http://dx.doi.org/10.3389/fonc.2019.01281] [PMID: 31850197]

[69] Leygo C, Williams M, Jin HC, *et al.* DNA Methylation as a Noninvasive Epigenetic Biomarker for the Detection of Cancer. Dis Markers 2017; 2017: 1-13.
[http://dx.doi.org/10.1155/2017/3726595] [PMID: 29038612]

[70] Moss EL, Hollingworth J, Reynolds TM. The role of CA125 in clinical practice. J Clin Pathol 2005; 58(3): 308-12.
[http://dx.doi.org/10.1136/jcp.2004.018077] [PMID: 15735166]

[71] Singh A, Gupta S, Sachan M. Epigenetic Biomarkers in the Management of Ovarian Cancer: Current Prospectives. Front Cell Dev Biol 2019; 7: 182.
[http://dx.doi.org/10.3389/fcell.2019.00182] [PMID: 31608277]

[72] Petaja J, Pitkanen S, Vettenranta K, Fasth A, Heikinheimo M. Serum Tumor Marker CA 125 Is an Early and Sensitive Marker for Veno-Occlusive Disease in Children Undergoing Bone Marrow Transplantation. Pediatric Research. 1999; 45(4, Part 2 of 2): 151A-A.

[73] Liggett TE, Melnikov A, Yi Q, *et al.* Distinctive DNA methylation patterns of cell-free plasma DNA in women with malignant ovarian tumors. Gynecol Oncol 2011; 120(1): 113-20.
[http://dx.doi.org/10.1016/j.ygyno.2010.09.019] [PMID: 21056906]

[74] de Caceres II, Battagli C, Esteller M, *et al.* Tumor cell-specific BRCA1 and RASSF1A hypermethylation in serum, plasma, and peritoneal fluid from ovarian cancer patients. Cancer Res 2004; 64(18): 6476-81.
[http://dx.doi.org/10.1158/0008-5472.CAN-04-1529] [PMID: 15374957]

[75] S SK, Swamy SN, Premalatha CS, Pallavi VR, Gawari R. Aberrant Promoter Hypermethylation of RASSF1a and BRCA1 in Circulating Cell-Free Tumor DNA Serves as a Biomarker of Ovarian Carcinoma. Asian Pac J Cancer Prev 2019; 20(10): 3001-5.
[http://dx.doi.org/10.31557/APJCP.2019.20.10.3001] [PMID: 31653147]

[76] Graham J, Baker M, Macbeth F, Titshall V. Diagnosis and treatment of prostate cancer: summary of NICE guidance. BMJ 2008; 336(7644): 610-2.

[http://dx.doi.org/10.1136/bmj.39498.525706.AD] [PMID: 18340076]

[77] Brait M, Banerjee M, Maldonado L, *et al.* Promoter methylation of MCAM, ERα and ERβ in serum of early stage prostate cancer patients. Oncotarget 2017; 8(9): 15431-40. [http://dx.doi.org/10.18632/oncotarget.14873] [PMID: 28147335]

CHAPTER 4

Karyotyping and Chromosomal Aberrations in Cancer: Molecular and Diagnostic Biomarkers

Tracie T. Cheng[1,*], **Sujani M. K. Gamage**[1,2], **Sharmin Aktar**[1], **Vinod Gopalan**[1] and **Farhadul Islam**[3,4]

[1] *School of Medicine, Menzies Health Institute Queensland, Griffith University, Gold Coast, Australia*

[2] *Department of Anatomy, Faculty of Medicine, University of Peradeniya, Galaha Rd, 20400, Sri Lanka*

[3] *Griffith University, Institute for Glycomics, Gold Coast, Australia*

[4] *Department of Biochemistry and Molecular Biology, University of Rajshahi, Bangladesh*

Abstract: Chromosomal abnormalities induce genomic instability and are associated with cancer hallmarks. Chromosomal abnormalities can be categorised into structural and numerical aberrations and are seen under a light microscope. Given the ease of detecting and observing such changes using karyotyping, chromosomal aberrations may be a useful diagnostic tool. For example, the discovery of the Philadelphia chromosome was a cytogenetic hallmark of chronic myeloid leukaemia and acute lymphoblastic leukaemia. Thus, this chapter explores potential aberrations which have the potential to be used as cancer markers in a clinical setting. Recurrent structural aberrations with known genetic mutations are observed in cancers of the bones, lungs, salivary glands, soft tissue, stomach, thyroid, and uterus. The association of these genetic alterations with various cancers suggests a causative role of structural aberrations in carcinogenesis and is characteristic of some cancers. Additionally, mono- and tri-somies, known as aneuploidy, are common to all cancer types, however, their roles as a cause or consequence are difficult to establish due to the sheer loss or gain of genetic material, respectively. Cancers with the most frequent trisomies, include Ewing's sarcoma of the bone, astrocytoma of the brain, and renal adenocarcinoma. Common cancer monosomies include meningioma of the brain and ovarian adenocarcinoma. These chromosomal aberrations forge the path to a better understanding of cancer genetics. Though there are potential chromosome markers in cancer, the heterogeneity of cancer genetics makes this a challenging tool to incorporate into current oncological diagnostic guidelines.

Keywords: Aneuploidy, Biomarker, Cancer, Chromosomal aberrations, Clinical oncology, Cytogenetics, Diagnostic, Karyotype, Structural aberration.

[*] **Corresponding author Tracie T. Cheng:** School of Medicine, Menzies Health Institute Queensland, Griffith University, Gold Coast, Australia; Email: tracie.cheng@griffith.edu.au

Farhadul Islam (Ed.)

INTRODUCTION

Cancer is a common and deadly disease that continues to be diagnosed and treated at late stages. Early detection and accurate diagnoses are paramount to bettering prognoses and decreasing cancer-related morbidity. Although cancer cells are heterogeneous in nature and continually evolve and mutate, they are still a distinct population which exhibit targetable traits. These hallmarks of cancer (sustained proliferative signalling, evasion of growth suppressors, resistant to apoptosis, replicative immortality, promotion of angiogenesis, and metastasis) are underpinned by genomic instability, giving rise to aggressive and abnormal cellular behaviour [1]. Genomic instability refers to the rate of errors generated in a genome, and encompasses everything from a single point mutation to major chromosomal aberrations [2]. Genomic instability can arise from two distinct pathways; microsatellite instability (recessive trait) and chromosomal instability (dominant trait) [3]. This chapter focuses on chromosomal aberrations and biomarkers in clinical diagnostics.

Chromosomal aberrations describe any defect that compromises an organism's normal karyotype, and, therefore, can be detected using cytogenetic methods [4]. Karyotyping describes methods of organising and examining the chromosomal makeup of a cell to provide a holistic view of an organism's genetic material. Chromosomal instability (CIN) is a product of chromosomal aberrations, which can largely be grouped into structural or numerical abnormalities, describing the alteration of part of a chromosome and whole chromosomes, respectively [5]. Currently, cytogenetics plays an increasingly important role in cancer diagnostics, with physicians routinely using cytogenetic studies for cancer patients [6]. Whilst both benign and malignant tumours can express abnormal karyotypes, malignant tumours tend to show more numerous aberrations. Additionally, karyotypic complexity and numerous chromosome aberrations have been associated with aggressive clinical and poor histological features [7].

The Mitelman Database of Chromosome Aberrations and Gene Fusions in Cancer comprehensively collates literature regarding cancer cases and their associated cytogenetic changes [8]. Currently, over 70,000 cases involving more than 14,000 genes have been recorded, however, many aberrations are limited in the number of reported cases [8]. Due to the inherent heterogeneity of a tumour population, an almost infinite combination of chromosomal aberrations could exist. However, recurrent chromosomal aberrations are often found in certain cancers, and may be useful as a diagnostic marker, which can be easily identified using karyotyping and light microscopy [9].

CHROMOSOMAL ABERRATIONS AND CANCER

The Cell Cycle Condensed

Cancer cells and tumours are the consequence of inappropriate proliferation due to improper regulation of the cell cycle and the development of survival mechanisms. At any given time, many cells in the body remain in a quiescent state and only re-enter the cell cycle in response to appropriate stimuli [10]. Thus, inappropriate signalling to reactivate cell cycle progression is a major driver of tumorigenesis. In contrast, if a cell fails to re-enter quiescence and continuously progresses through the cell cycle, the result is a mass of uncontrolled proliferative cells [11]. Within the cell cycle itself, the cell must accurately replicate its DNA, and segregate and divide its genetic material accordingly amongst the two daughter cells with high fidelity. Progression through the cell cycle is dependent on levels of key molecules, which are altered through processes such as de/phosphorylation, SUMOylation, ubiquitin-dependent degradation, or acetylation [12]. Due to the sheer amount of information the cell must replicate and organise, a multitude of mechanisms exist to protect the cell from improper cell cycle progression. Cell cycle checkpoints are regulatory proteins, which exist at specific stages of the process and ensure the appropriate completion of previous stages before allowing the cell to continue through its replicative process [13].

Exiting the quiescent state (G0), a cell enters the first gap (G1) phase by passing through the restriction point, thus committing to the cell division process. Shortly after this, during the synthesis (S) phase of the cell cycle, chromosomes and some cellular components from the mother cell are replicated once to create two identical sets of genetic material. The cell then enters a longer gap phase (G2) before beginning the division process known as mitosis (M phase) [11, 14]. Dysfunctional replication of genetic material, particularly in S phase, may result in chromosomal translocations, inversions, and deletions (structural aberrations) [15].

Structural Aberrations and Associated Cancer Markers

Structural aberrations are the consequence of chromosome breakage and improper reunion or fusion [9]. Structural aberrations arise from errors in DNA replication in the synthesis phase of the cell cycle or failure to repair DNA/halt cell cycle progression at cell cycle checkpoints [16]. These aberrations depicted in Fig. (**1**) can be categorised into balanced and unbalanced translocations, which involve equal and unequal chromatin rearrangement across chromosomes, respectively; deletions which are a loss of a chromosome segment; inversions which result when two broken ends of the same chromosome are incorrectly re-joined; and isochromosomes which is the formation of a mirror image of a chromosome arm

(Fig. **1**) [17, 18]. Recurrent structural chromosomal aberrations are listed in Table **1** as extracted from the Mitelman database, with only the most common aberrations listed per tumour location, and may be useful as a potential chromosomal biomarker of cancers [8].

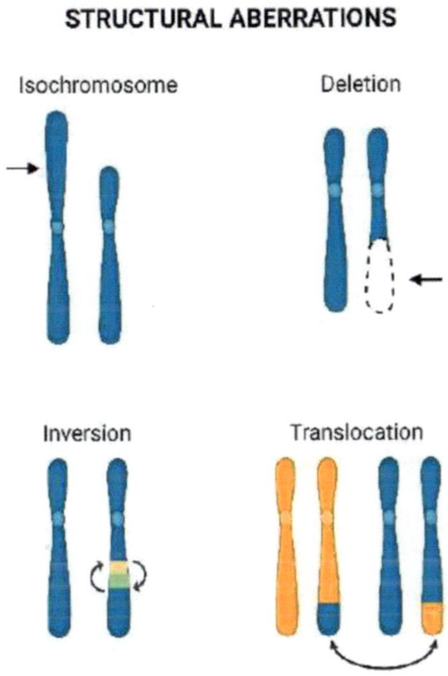

Fig. (1). Types of major structural chromosome aberrations.

Structural aberrations evidently play a role in tumorigenesis and cancer progression, however, only a limited number of genes have been directly linked to cancer-associated aberrations. Perhaps the most famous of which is the Philadelphia chromosome, whereby the translocation between chromosomes 9 and 22 creates a fusion *Bcr-Abl* oncogene in chronic myelogenous leukaemia [19]. In addition to a gain of function, carcinogenic aberrations can also be a consequence of a loss of function of a tumour suppressor gene, such as *PTEN* (*phosphatase and tensin homolog*) and *CDKN2A* (*cyclin-dependent kinase inhibitor 2A*) [20, 21]. The difficulty of deciphering chromosomal aberrations lies in the fact that such alterations are of such an immense scale, and many genes are affected, thus making it challenging to identify its molecular pathogenesis.

Table 1. Most frequently occurring structural chromosomal aberrations categorised by tumour sites.

Tumour site	Morphology	Type	Band	Aberration	Number of cases
Bladder	Transitional cell carcinoma	Unbalanced	5p10	i(5)(p10)	11
Bone	Ewing sarcoma	Balanced	11q24	t(11;22)(q24;q12)*	229
Brain	Astrocytoma, grade III-IV/Glioblastoma	Unbalanced	9p21	del(9)(p21)	15
		Unbalanced	9p13	del(9)(p13)	14
		Unbalanced	9p22	del(9)(p22)	14
		Unbalanced	19q13	add(19)(q13)	10
	Primitive neuroectodermal tumour/Medulloblastoma	Unbalanced	17q10	i(17)(q10)	15
	Meningioma	Unbalanced	1p13	del(1)(p13)	13
		Unbalanced	22q11	del(22)(q11)	11
Breast	Adenocarcinoma	Unbalanced	1q10	i(1)(q10)	58
		Unbalanced	1q10	der(1;16)(q10;p10)	54
		Unbalanced	16p10	der(1;16)(q10;p10)	54
Cerebellum	Primitive neuroectodermal tumour/Medulloblastoma	Unbalanced	17q10	i(17)(q10)	39
Eye	Retinoblastoma	Unbalanced	6p10	i(6)(p10)	46
	Malignant melanoma	Unbalanced	8q10	i(8)(q10)	46
Kidney	Adenocarcinoma	Unbalanced	3p13	der(3)t(3;5)(p13;q22)	44
		Unbalanced	5q22	der(3)t(3;5)(p13;q22)	44
		Balanced	1q21	t(X;1)(p11;q21)	30
	Wilms tumour	Unbalanced	1q10	i(1)(q10)	30
Large intestine	Adenocarcinoma	Unbalanced	8q10	i(8)(q10)	42
		Unbalanced	17q10	i(17)(q10)	36
		Unbalanced	13q10	i(13)(q10)	21
Lung	Adenocarcinoma	Unbalanced	5p10	i(5)(p10)	14
		Unbalanced	1q10	i(1)(q10)	12
	Squamous cell carcinoma	Unbalanced	3p13	del(3)(p13)	12
	Chondroid hamartoma	Balanced	6p21	t(6;14)(p21;q24)*	11
Oral cavity	Squamous cell carcinoma	Unbalanced	8q10	i(8)(q10)	18
		Unbalanced	5p10	i(5)(p10)	15
		Unbalanced	3q10	i(3)(q10)	12

(Table 1) cont.....

Tumour site	Morphology	Type	Band	Aberration	Number of cases
Ovary	Adenocarcinoma	Unbalanced	11p15	add(11)(p15)	33
		Unbalanced	19p13	add(19)(p13)	29
		Unbalanced	1p36	add(1)(p36)	28
		Unbalanced	19q13	add(19)(q13)	24
		Unbalanced	6q21	del(6)(q21)	23
Pancreas	Adenocarcinoma	Unbalanced	19q13	add(19)(q13)	15
		Unbalanced	1q10	i(1)(q10)	12
Pituitary gland	Adenoma	Unbalanced	1q10	i(1)(q10)	4
Pleura	Mesothelioma	Unbalanced	6q15	del(6)(q15)	8
		Unbalanced	9p21	del(9)(p21)	7
Prostate	Adenocarcinoma	Unbalanced	10q24	del(10)(q24)	8
		Unbalanced	7q22	del(7)(q22)	6
Salivary gland	Adenoma	Balanced	3p21	t(3;8)(p21;q12)*	77
Skin	Malignant melanoma	Unbalanced	1q10	i(1)(q10)	9
Soft tissue	Synovial sarcoma	Balanced	18q11	t(X;18)(p11;q11)*	139
	Liposarcoma, myxoid/round cell	Balanced	12q13	t(12;16)(q13;p11)*	91
	Alveolar rhabdomyosarcoma	Balanced	2q35	t(2;13)(q35;q14)	18
Stomach	Adenocarcinoma	Unbalanced	8q10	i(8)(q10)	11
	Extranodal marginal zone B-cell lymphoma	Balanced	11q21	t(11;18)*	10
Testis	Teratoma (mature and immature)	Unbalanced	12p10	i(12)(p10)	116
		Unbalanced	1p36	add(1)(p36)	18
		Unbalanced	12p13	add(12)(p13)	13
	Seminoma/ Dysgerminoma	Unbalanced	12p10	i(12)(p10)	48
	Combined germ cell tumours	Unbalanced	12p10	i(12)(p10)	43
Thyroid	Adenocarcinoma	Balanced	10q11	inv(10)(q11q21)*	6
	Adenoma	Balanced	2q13	t(2;3)(q13;p25)*	4
Tongue	Squamous cell carcinoma	Unbalanced	8q10	i(8)(q10)	19
		Unbalanced	3q10	i(3)(q10)	10

(Table 1) cont.....

Tumour site	Morphology	Type	Band	Aberration	Number of cases
Uterus (corpus)	Leiomyoma	Unbalanced	7q22	del(7)(q22q32)	42
		Unbalanced	7q32	del(7)(q22q32)	42
		Unbalanced	7q21	del(7)(q21q31)	35
		Unbalanced	7q31	del(7)(q21q31)	35
		Balanced	12q15	t(12;14)(q15;q24)*	31
	Endometrial stromal sarcoma	Balanced	10q22	t(10;17)(q22;p13)*	16
Vagina	Squamous cell carcinoma	Unbalanced	8q10	i(8)(q10)	17

The data are extracted from the Mitelman Database of Chromosome Aberrations and Gene Fusions [8]. Aberrations with a known gene association are indicated by an asterisk. Abbreviations: p, short arm; q, long arm; i, isochromosome; t, translocation; del, deletion; add, addition; der, derivative; inv, inversion.

Of the many listed recurrent structural chromosome aberrations listed in Table **1**, only selected few are associated with a known gene, as described below and indicated by an asterisk in Table **1**. These genes and their associated aberrations are listed in Table **2**.

Ewing sarcoma: *Ewing's sarcoma breakpoint region 1/Ewing sarcoma RNA binding protein 1* (*EWSR1*) and (*Friend leukaemia integration 1*) is a translocated gene fusion product of *EWSR1* and *FLI1*. EWS/FLI1 is an aberrant transcription factor, which drives this rare form of bone cancer [22]. Main targets of EWS/FLI1 include transcriptional regulators and secreted proteins, though its pathogenic role is not well understood [23].

Lung chondroid hamartoma: *high mobility group AT-hook-1* (*HMGA1*) encodes for a non-histone chromatin remodelling protein whilst *RAD51 paralog B* (*RAD51B*) encodes for a DNA repair protein [24, 25]. Though there is limited information on these genes in pulmonary chondroid hamartoma, translocations of these genes have been associated with increased proliferative activity and cell cycle dysregulation [26].

Salivary gland adenoma: *pleomorphic adenoma gene 1* (*PLAG1*) oncogene is a member of the PLAG family of zinc-finger transcription factors. Located on chromosome 8q12, this gene is associated with salivary gland adenomas. Also, it has been involved in lipoblastoma, hepatoblastoma, and acute myeloid leukaemia. This balanced translocation swaps the PLAG1 promoter gene with genes such as *CTNNB1* and *LIFR* [27, 28].

Synovial sarcoma: *synovial sarcoma translocation, chromosome 18* (*SS18*) is a gene encoding SSXT protein. *SSX family member 1/2/3* (*SSX1/2/3*) encodes for synovial sarcoma X breakpoint proteins. This translocation, as seen in virtually all cases of synovial sarcoma, involves the fusion of chromosomes 18/X to form an SS18-SSX gene product. There is evidence SS18-SSX regulates *AXIN2*, a key target of the *Wnt* signalling pathway. SS18-SSX may be able to activate Wnt signalling in the absence of Wnt ligand stimulation and/or β-catenin [29 - 31].

Liposarcoma, myxoid round cell: *DNA damage-inducible transcript 3* (*DDIT3*) is located on chromosome 12q13 [32]. *FUS RNA binding protein* (*FUS*) is found on chromosome 16p11 [33]. This *DDIT3-FUS* gene fusion product likely plays a role in liposarcoma by interacting with *NFKBIZ* and deregulates genes within the NF-κB pathway [34].

Extranodal marginal zone B-cell lymphoma: *Mucosa-associated lymphoid tissue 1* is the causative gene for MALT lymphoma [35]. MALT1 mutations have been associated with impaired lymphocyte activation and proliferation [36]. Furthermore, MALT1 complexes with CARD11 and BCL10 to form the CBM complex, which ultimately allows for NF-κB release and translocation to the nucleus [37]. MALT lymphoma presents with a *BIRC3-MALT1* fusion in ~30% cases, whilst trisomy 3 is observed in 60% of cases [38].

Thyroid adenocarcinoma: *Coiled-coil domain-containing 6 gene* (*CCDC6*) encodes for a DNA damage checkpoint protein. Its fusion with *rearranged during transfection* (*RET*) gene is a common oncogenic product in many cancer types [39]. This fusion is likely due to *CCDC6*'s locus at a fragile site [40]. *CCDC6-RET* is thought to confer tyrosine kinase activity to drive tumorigenesis [41].

Thyroid adenoma: *Paired-box gene 8* (*PAX8*) is a member of the PAX family of transcription factors [42]. *Peroxisome proliferator-activated receptor gamma* (*PPARG*) is a nuclear transcription factor playing a role as a master regulator of adipogenesis [43]. *PAX8-PPARG* fusion gene induces Wnt/TCF pathway activation to cause cellular transformation [44]. Leiomyoma: *RAD51B* mutation leads to impaired DNA repair pathways, and thus an increased likelihood of genomic instability [45].

Uterine adenocarcinoma: *tyrosine 3-monooxygenase/tryptophan 5-monooxyge nase activation protein epsilon* (*YWHAE*) encodes for 14-3-3 protein epsilon, which acts as a signal transduction mediator in processes such as cell division and insulin sensitivity [46]. This gene fusion product with *NUT family member 2B* (*NUTM2B*) is observed in soft tissue sarcoma, and kidney and uterine cancer in addition to uterine adenocarcinoma [47]. Aberrant 14-3-3 expression is likely the driver of proliferation, metabolism and differentiation of cancer cells [48].

Structural aberrations and their affected gene products are a driving force for carcinogenesis and cancer progression. Furthermore, such aberrations are characteristic of these cancers and can be microscopically detected, and thus are useful as potential markers with diagnostic significance.

Table 2. Genetic associations of structural aberrations in cancers.

Tumour site	Morphology	Type	Aberration	Gene
Bone	Ewing sarcoma	Balanced	t(11;22)(q24;q12)	*EWSR1* *FLI1*
Lung	Chondroid hamartoma	Balanced	t(6;14)(p21;q24)	*HMGA1* *RAD51B*
Salivary gland	Adenoma	Balanced	t(3;8)(p21;q12)	*PLAG1*
Soft tissue	Synovial sarcoma	Balanced	t(X;18)(p11;q11)	*SS18* *SSX1/2/3*
	Liposarcoma, myxoid/round cell	Balanced	t(12;16)(q13;p11)	*DDIT3* *FUS*
Stomach	Extranodal marginal zone B-cell lymphoma	Balanced	t(11;18)	*MALT1*
Thyroid	Adenocarcinoma	Balanced	inv(10)(q11q21)	*CCDC6* *RET*
	Adenoma	Balanced	t(2;3)(q13;p25)	*PAX8* *PPARG*
Uterus (corpus)	Leiomyoma	Balanced	t(12;14)(q15;q24)	*RAD51B*
	Adenocarcinoma	Balanced	t(10;17)(q22;p13)	*YWHAE* *NUTM2B*

The data are extracted from the Mitelman Database of Chromosome Aberrations and Gene Fusions [8].

Genetic Biomarkers for Structural Chromosome Aberrations

As aforementioned, structural aberrations arise from erroneous replication and/or incorrect checkpoint regulation, hence mutations in these types of machinery may act as genetic biomarkers of cancer cells. DNA replication is a tightly regulated process whose blueprint is prepared during late mitosis and G1 and executed during the S phase of the cell cycle [49]. Replication stress describes any factor which can alter replication machinery or dynamics [50]. In addition to intrinsic stressors such as telomeres, centromeres and common fragile sites, replicative stress can be brought on by exogenous stressors such as chemical compounds, radiation, metabolic by-products, and insufficient replicative factors [51]. Not only does replicative stress promote genomic instability and drive tumorigenesis, it can also lead to chromosomal instability as it compromises the integrity of the chromosomal material, consequently leading to breakage during mitosis and resulting in structural aberrations [50]. Common chromosomal fragile sites are genomic areas that are especially challenging to replicate due to their DNA sequence (usually A-T rich) and are more susceptible to breakage during mitosis [52]. These specific loci appear as breaks or gaps on metaphase chromosomes and are hotspots for rearrangement in cancer cells [53]. Several mechanisms exist to mitigate and minimise downstream consequences of replication stress, primarily the DNA damage checkpoint, restarting of the replication fork, and DNA repair [54]. Replication stress is a common feature in early carcinogenesis [55, 56]. Healthy cells generally do not exhibit replication stress, therefore, defective components of these cellular responses may be useful as cancer biomarkers.

DNA Damage Checkpoint

DNA damage checkpoints are functionally conserved points of surveillance during the cell cycle, whereby undetected DNA damage will trigger the checkpoint and ultimately lead to cell cycle arrest to allow for reparations [57]. DNA damage checkpoints coincide closely with cell cycle checkpoints and utilise the same machinery, thus mutations in key proteins can lead to defective DNA repair and also uncontrolled progression through the cell cycle [57]. Mutations in DNA damage proteins have been identified in many hereditary cancer syndromes, including ataxia telangiectasia (*ATM*), hereditary breast cancer (*BRCA1* and *BRCA2*), and Li-Fraumeni syndrome (*TP53*) [57]. The DNA damage response can halt the cell cycle at G1, intra-S or G2 phases by activating ATM (ataxia-telangiectasia mutated protein) and ATR (ataxia telantiectasia and Rad3-related protein) kinases, causing a cascade of events to occur [58]. Although, ATM and ATR are generally associated with double- and single-stranded breakages, respectively, their downstream effectors respond to both proteins, thus, the resultant pathways overlap and are not fully distinct from each other [59].

ATM and ATR are large serine/threonine kinases which only phosphorylate protein substrates [60]. Upon detecting DNA damage, ATM autophosphorylates from a multimer to an active monomeric form and is recruited to the site of damage along with the MRN complex (MRE11-RAD50-NBS1-complex) [61]. ATM then phosphorylates multiple substrates, the most studied being Chk2 (checkpoint kinase 2), resulting in a signal transduction cascade and checkpoint activation [60]. Unique substrates of Chk2 include BRCA1, PLK3, E2F1 and PML, subsequently promoting damage-induced transcription, DNA repair, cell cycle arrest and/or apoptosis [62 - 65]. ATR activation is a more complex process as the ATR-ATRIP (ATR-ATR interacting protein) is unable to directly associate with damaged DNA. RPA must directly interact with damaged DNA, and bring about localisation of the ATR-ATRIP complex to the site of damage [66]. ATR then activates Chk1 (checkpoint kinase 1) to lead to substrate-specific phosphorylation of TLK1/2, which acts to activate a chromatin remodelling pathway [66 - 68]. Chk1 and Chk2 also phosphorylate common downstream effectors, including MDM2, p53, CDC25A, and CDC25C, ultimately switching on checkpoint control of the cell cycle [69]. This DNA damage response is schematically depicted in Fig. (**2**).

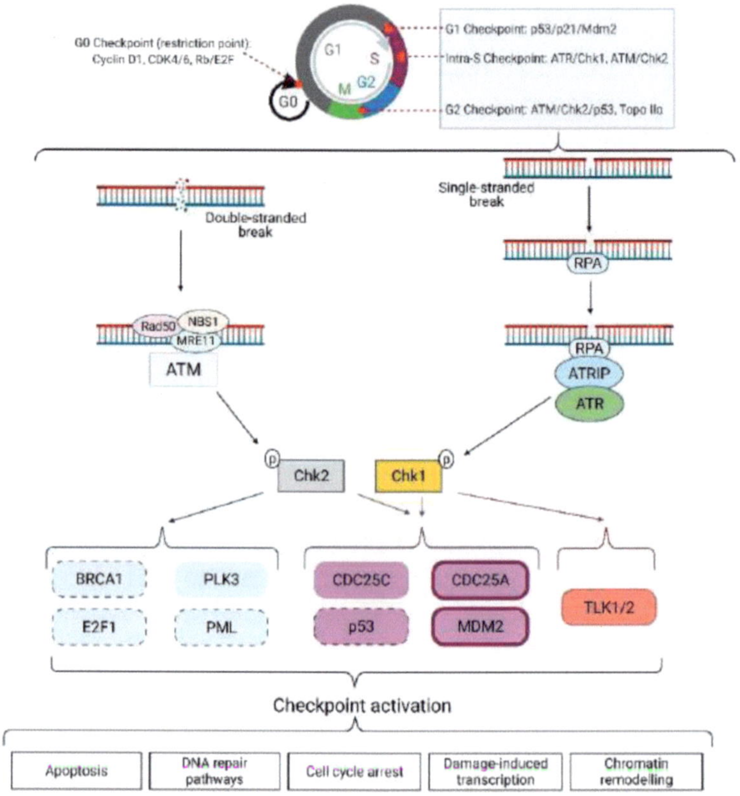

Fig. (2). DNA damage response following double- or single-stranded breaks. ATM and ATR are primary responders to activate a signalling cascade leading to checkpoint activation *via* Chk1 and Chk2. Effector proteins of Chk1 (red) and Chk2 (blue) and common effectors (purple) are shown here. Effectors with dashed borders and bolded borders are known as tumour suppressors and oncogenes, respectively.

Replication Fork

The synthesis phase of the cell cycle can be further broken down into three distinct processes; initiation, elongation and termination. Instances of DNA damage or intrinsically difficult regions to replicate (fragile sites) can alter the progression of DNA elongation at the region of the replication fork. Replication fork restart is the mechanism by which DNA synthesis is properly resumed after fork stalling or collapse [70]. Stalling of the replication fork is an unstable process and increases the likelihood of fork collapse, leading to uncoupling of helicase and polymerase enzymes, RPA (replication protein A) recruitment, and activation of ATR-ATRIP pathways [71]. Failures within the replication fork rescue machinery may promote genomic and chromosomal instability.

Regulation of the replication fork involves meticulous control of its speed, progression and accuracy. Upon sensing defective replication forks, the fork machinery must be stalled to allow time for repair prior to restart and progression. Through a process called PARPylation, PARP (poly (ADP-ribose) polymerase) proteins mediate pathways that are integral to the stalling of dysfunctional replication forks and fork reversal repair [45, 72]. PARP1 likely functions as a DNA nick sensor during synthesis and brings about stalling and p53-p2--mediated repair [73].

p53, perhaps the most studied tumour suppressor protein involved in DNA replication, also plays many regulatory roles in processes such as cellular metabolism, gene transcription, cell cycle checkpoints, and apoptosis [74]. Stalling of the replication fork promotes mutagenic RAD52 and POLθ pathway activation [75]. Suppression of these pathways is mediated by p53 and its recruitment of MRE11, a DNA replication restart nuclease, thus highlighting the importance of a functional p53 protein to facilitate proper replication fork restart [75, 76].

DNA Repair

DNA can undergo damage from either endogenous or exogenous sources, which trigger the cell's DNA damage response. At least six major DNA repair pathways, *i.e.,* base excision repair, mismatch repair, nucleotide excision repair, homologous recombination and non-homologous end joining, and translesional synthesis, have been identified [77, 78]. These repair pathways function to restore; damaged bases and single-stranded breaks, mismatched nucleotides, helix-distorting DNA lesions, double-stranded breaks, and DNA replication after adduct formation, respectively [78]. Defective DNA repair mechanisms promote tumorigenesis [79]. DNA repair genes which have been identified as mutated or affected in cancers are summarised in Table **3** [78].

Table 3. DNA repair genes and pathways in various cancers.

Cancer Type	Mutation in DNA Repair Gene	Altered Gene Expression	Defective Pathway
Turcot syndrome (brain and colon cancer)	*MSH2, MSH6, MLH1*	-	MMR
Hereditary non-polyposis colon cancer	*HNPCC*	-	MMR
Sporadic colorectal cancer	-	*-MSH2, -MLH1, -Ku70, -Ku86*	NER NHEJ
Xeroderma pigmentosum	*XPA, XPB, XPC, XPE, XPF, or XPG DNA pol E*	-	NER NHEJ
Testicular germ cell cancer	-	*-XPD*	NER
Lung cancer	*ERCC1, XPD*	*-BRCA1/2*	HR
Ovarian cancer	*BRCA1/2*	*-BRCA1/2* *+Pol β*	HR TLS
Prostate cancer	*BRCA1/2*	*-NBS1* *+Pol β*	HR TLS
Breast cancer	*BRCA1/2*	-	HR
Pancreatic cancer	*BRCA1/2*	-	HR
Gastric cancer	*BRCA1/2*	*+Pol β*	HR TLS
Fanconi anaemia	*FANC*	-	HR
Lig4 syndrome (leukaemia)	*DNA ligase IV*	-	NHEJ
Omenn syndrome (lymphoma)	*Artemis*	-	NHEJ
Cervical cancer	-	*-Ku70*	NHEJ
Uterine cancer	-	*+Pol β*	TLS

Characteristic Aneuploidy as a Cancer Marker and Its Associated Genes

Numerical aberrations, or aneuploidy, arise from errors during mitosis [16]. Like the rest of the cell cycle, mitosis is an exquisitely precise process regulated by a myriad of processes. Mitosis can be divided into five main stages; prophase, prometaphase, metaphase, anaphase, and telophase. Each phase is regulated by different proteins, resulting in nuclear and cytoplasmic division [80]. During this process, replicated genetic material from interphase (G1, S, G2) is condensed into recognisable chromosomes and segregated into respective daughter cells [81].

Whether aneuploidy is a cause or consequence of cancer is an unclear distinction and is likely to be mutually inclusive. Numerical aberrations are a distinguishing feature of cancer cells [82]. Recurrent aneusomies are listed in Table **4** as obtained from the Mitelman database [8]. Most commonly, aneuploidy results from non-disjunction, as seen in Fig. (**3**), including incorrect centrosome numbers, improper kinetochore-microtubule attachments, and defective spindle assembly checkpoint [81, 83].

Table 4. Most frequently occurring numerical chromosomal aberrations categorised by tumour site.

Tumour Site	Morphology	Type	Aberration	Number of Cases
Adrenal	Neuroblastoma	Monosomy	-X	42
		Monosomy	-17	28
		Monosomy	-19	28
		Trisomy	+7	28
		Monosomy	-10	27
		Monosomy	-11	27
		Trisomy	+17	26
Anus	Squamous cell carcinoma	Monosomy	-17	4
Bladder	Transitional cell carcinoma	Monosomy	-9	56
		Monosomy	-Y	33
		Trisomy	+7	21
Bone	Ewing sarcoma	Trisomy	+8	121
		Trisomy	+12	66
		Trisomy	+2	41
	Osteosarcoma, NOS	Monosomy	-13	51
		Monosomy	-10	45
		Monosomy	-9	42
		Monosomy	-17	42
		Monosomy	-15	38

(Table 4) cont.....

Tumour Site	Morphology	Type	Aberration	Number of Cases
Brain	Meningioma	Monosomy	-22	532
		Monosomy	-14	139
		Monosomy	-Y	120
		Monosomy	-X	75
		Monosomy	-18	69
	Astrocytoma, grade III-IV/ Glioblastoma	Trisomy	+7	210
		Monosomy	-10	196
		Monosomy	-Y	173
		Monosomy	-22	99
		Monosomy	-13	98
		Monosomy	-14	82
		Monosomy	-X	75
Breast	Adenocarcinoma	Monosomy	-X	113
		Monosomy	-22	106
		Monosomy	-13	105
Cerebellum	Meningioma	Monosomy	-22	22
	Primitive neuroectodermal tumour/Medulloblastoma	Monosomy	-22	19
Eye	Malignant melanoma	Monosomy	-3	67
		Monosomy	-Y	47
		Trisomy	+8	39
	Retinoblastoma	Monosomy	-16	30
Kidney	Adenocarcinoma	Trisomy	+7	445
		Monosomy	-Y	381
		Monosomy	-14	278
		Monosomy	-3	210
		Trisomy	+16	203
		Trisomy	+17	198
		Trisomy	+12	195
	Wilms tumour	Trisomy	+12	185
Large intestine	Adenocarcinoma	Monosomy	-18	105
		Trisomy	+7	103
		Monosomy	-Y	66
	Adenoma	Trisomy	+7	69

(Table 4) cont.....

Tumour Site	Morphology	Type	Aberration	Number of Cases
Larynx	Squamous cell carcinoma	Monosomy	-Y	52
		Monosomy	-21	23
Liver	Hepatoblastoma	Trisomy	+20	58
		Trisomy	+2	43
		Trisomy	+8	37
Lung	Squamous cell carcinoma	Monosomy	-Y	71
	Adenocarcinoma	Monosomy	-22	54
		Monosomy	-Y	54
		Monosomy	-13	51
Oral cavity	Squamous cell carcinoma	Monosomy	-Y	57
		Monosomy	-18	34
		Monosomy	-21	33
		Monosomy	-13	32
Oro- and hypopharynx	Squamous cell carcinoma	Monosomy	-Y	21
		Monosomy	-21	20
		Monosomy	-18	16
Ovary	Adenocarcinoma	Monosomy	-X	123
		Monosomy	-15	109
		Monosomy	-22	101
		Monosomy	-14	99
		Monosomy	-17	95
Pancreas	Adenocarcinoma	Monosomy	-18	75
		Monosomy	-17	48
		Monosomy	-21	47
		Monosomy	-6	41
Pituitary gland	Adenoma	Trisomy	+87	11
Pleura	Mesothelioma	Monosomy	-22	44
		Monosomy	-13	30
		Monosomy	-14	29
		Monosomy	-4	26
Prostate	Adenocarcinoma	Monosomy	-Y	67
		Trisomy	+7	23
Salivary gland	Adenoma	Trisomy	+8	14

(Table 4) cont.....

Tumour Site	Morphology	Type	Aberration	Number of Cases
Skin	Malignant melanoma	Monosomy	-10	37
		Monosomy	-21	25
		Trisomy	+20	24
	Basal cell carcinoma	Monosomy	-Y	23
Soft tissue	Non-neoplastic mesenchymal disorder/lesion	Trisomy	+7	50
	Malignant peripheral nerve sheath tumour/Triton	Monosomy	-17	38
		Monosomy	-9	36
		Monosomy	-10	36
		Monosomy	-X	36
		Monosomy	-13	34
		Monosomy	-16	31
	Synovial sarcoma	Trisomy	+12	33
	Undifferentiated pleomorphic sarcoma	Monosomy	-X	30
Spinal cord	Meningioma	Monosomy	-22	40
	Schwannoma	Monosomy	-22	10
	Ependymoma	Monosomy	-22	8
Stomach	Adenocarcinoma	Monosomy	-18	42
		Monosomy	-Y	32
		Monosomy	-22	31
Testis	Teratoma (mature and immature)	Monosomy	-18	85
		Monosomy	-13	75
		Monosomy	-4	74
		Monosomy	-10	74
		Monosomy	-11	73
Thyroid	Adenoma	Trisomy	+7	34
		Trisomy	+12	29
	Adenocarcinoma	Trisomy	+7	23
Tongue	Squamous cell carcinoma	Monosomy	-Y	30
		Monosomy	-21	29
		Monosomy	-14	22
		Monosomy	-18	21
		Monosomy	-22	21
Uterus (cervix)	Squamous cell carcinoma	Monosomy	-4	13

(Table 4) cont.....

Tumour Site	Morphology	Type	Aberration	Number of Cases
Uterus	Adenocarcinoma	Trisomy	+10	31
		Trisomy	+7	17
	Leiomyoma	Monosomy	-22	29
		Trisomy	+12	27
		Monosomy	-X	21
Vagina	Squamous cell carcinoma	Monosomy	-X	12
		Trisomy	+7	12

The data are extracted from the Mitelman Database of Chromosome Aberrations and Gene Fusions. (8) Minus and plus symbols denoting chromosome loss and gain respectively.

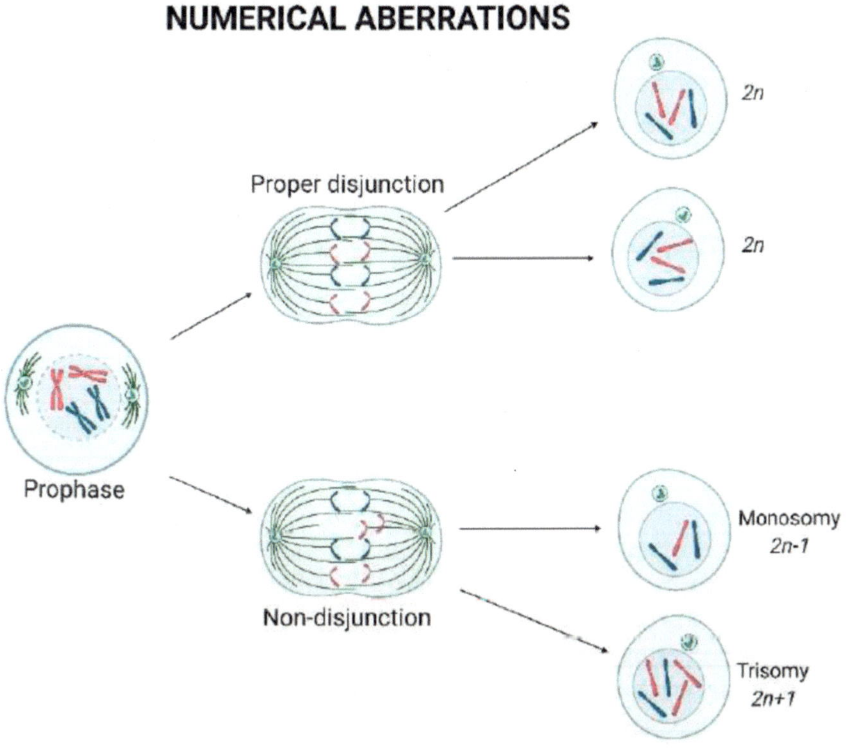

Fig. (3). Segregation of chromosomes during prophase, which can result in disomy (2n) or mono- and trisomy (2n-1, 2n+1) depending on the accuracy of disjunction processes.

In addition to a balanced translocation between chromosomes 11 and 22, Ewing's sarcoma also presents with trisomy 8 in half of the cases [84]. Taking both structural and numerical aberrations together can be a useful cytogenetic diagnostic characteristic of Ewing's sarcoma. Benign meningiomas often present with a full loss of chromosome 22 (Table **4**) or a partial deletion on chromosome 22 (Table **1**). Though it is not fully understood the extent of genetic loss in relation to cancer, monosomy 22 has been correlated to mutation of the *neurofibromin 2* (*NF2*) gene [85]. *NF2* encodes the merlin protein, which acts as a tumour suppressor [86], thus, loss of function of *NF2* may be a key step in meningioma tumorigenesis.

Trisomy 7 is a common occurrence in high-grade astrocytomas (glioblastomas), which are poorly differentiated and have poor prognoses. Interestingly, tumour recurrence was measured to be almost five times more likely in astrocytomas with trisomy 7 [87]. However, whilst this numerical aberration may provide clues to prognoses, trisomy 7 does not appear to be a glioblastoma-specific aberration [88]. Moreover, trisomy 7 was also a frequent numerical aberration in renal cell carcinoma, normal renal cells likely tend to gain an extra chromosome 7, which is retained by carcinoma cells and unlikely to be a tumour-specific genetic alteration [89].

Turner's syndrome is a genetic condition defined by the loss of chromosome X [90]. Whilst many cases of ovarian cancer are associated with monosomy X, individuals with Turner's syndrome are highly predisposed to ovarian failure, and as such, monosomy X is not likely a diagnostic marker for ovarian adenocarcinoma. Rather, the relationship is more likely that many cases of ovarian cancer are due to Turner's syndrome.

The Centrosome and the Centromere

In respect to chromosomes, the centrosome is an organelle which acts as a microtubule-organising centre and a regulator of the cell cycle. Duplication of the mother centrosome occurs during S phase in parallel to DNA replication, forming a structurally different, but functionally similar, daughter centrosome (Fig **4**) [91]. The replication of the centrosome must be tightly regulated such that the dividing cell will have two centrosomes to form bipolar mitotic spindles to dictate equal separation of genetic material [92]. The centrosome is composed of two centrioles surrounded by an electron-rich pericentriolar matrix (PCM) [93]. Its main roles include nucleating microtubules and serving as bipolar bodies to orient the dividing cell [93, 94]. Also, supplementary PCM recruitment occurs during the G2 phase [95]. These centrosome-nucleated microtubules attach to the centromere of the chromosome to form the kinetochore, which is required for segregation in anaphase [96]. The centrosome itself further matures to be a spindle pole to ensure correct chromosome segregation and govern the architecture of daughter cells [91]. Centrosome dysfunction has been shown to lead to incorrect spindle assembly and thus the abnormal formation of kinetochore-microtubule complexes [97].

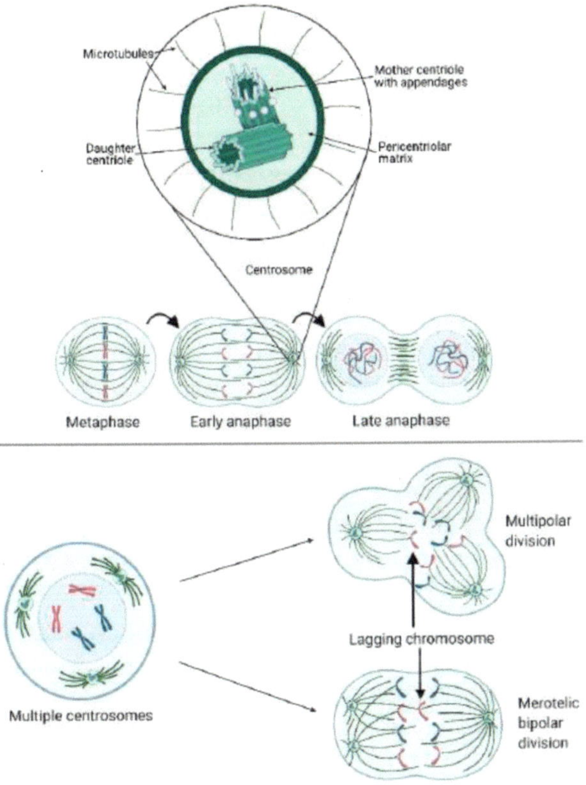

Fig. (4). The role of centrosomes in mitosis. The centrosome is an organelle which is replicated once during the cell cycle and plays a vital role in faithful cell division. Each centrosome contains a mother and daughter centriole. The two centrosomes migrate to opposite poles of the cell to ensure correct cellular segregation. Centrosome amplification can result in multipolar and merotelic division, both exhibiting lagging chromosomes, and leading to chromosomal aberrations.

Common to cancer cells, though its causal relationship remains unestablished, centrosome amplification is an umbrella term describing at least one of the following; larger than normal appearance of centrosomes, four or more centrioles present within a centrosome, and the presence of more than two centrosomes in the dividing cell [91, 98]. As seen in Fig. (**4**), centrosome amplification can lead to the multi-spindle formation and/or chromosome mis-segregation, ultimately leading to aneuploidy in daughter cells, thereby producing this hallmark of cancer [91, 96, 99]. A common visible feature of centrosome amplification is the existence of a lagging chromosome. This can be observed as a chromosome which trails behind the two masses of segregating chromosomes [100]. Lagging chromosomes are often a result of merotelic attachments, where a single kinetochore is bound by opposing mitotic spindles, thus experiencing pulling from both poles [101]. This promotes aberrant chromosome segregation.

The Kinetochore-Microtubule Complex

In the process of chromosome segregation, the centrosome attaches to the chromosome at the centromere *via* the formation of kinetochore-microtubule (k-MT) attachments. Throughout this incredibly dynamic process, many errors in attachment occur, therefore requiring a rigorous regulatory mechanism prior to advancement into the construction of the metaphase plate. The successful formation of such attachments is a result of a haphazard and random technique, whereby microtubules attach and reattach until each sister chromatid is securely captured from opposing spindles. Though the intricacies of the k-MT control network are not fully understood, several mechanisms which play a part include PLK1, Aurora kinases, and cyclin-CDK complexes, which serve to signal the un/satisfaction of the spindle assembly checkpoint [102]. During mitosis, myosin phosphatase targeting subunit1 (MYPT1) is phosphorylated by proline-directed kinases (*e.g.,* CDC2), which creates a binding motif for PLK1. Loss of PLK1 activity has been linked to mitotic arrest *via* decreased γ-tubulin recruitment to the centrosome and inhibiting centrosome maturation. However, depletion of both MYPT1 and PLK1 restores γ-tubulin at the centrosome and brings the cell out of mitotic arrest [103]. PLK1 functions to stabilise k-MT attachments during prometaphase. MYPT1 localisation to kinetochores is dependent on Cyclin A/Cdk1 activity.

Proper attachment of microtubules to kinetochores is partly ensured by Aurora B kinase and its regulation of Kinesin-13 mitotic centromere-associated kinesin (MCAK) [104]. As suggested by the name, kinesins are motor proteins, which primarily transport cargo along the length of a microtubule, whilst a subfamily of these, the MCAKs are able to destabilise microtubules directly [105]. Regulation of MCAK by Aurora B depends on the site of phosphorylation, whereby phosphorylation of T95 on MCAK promotes its localisation and association with chromosomal arms, but phosphorylation of S196 encourages dissociation from the chromosome arms. Importantly, dephosphorylation of T95 on MCAK correlates with the increased association with centrosomes [104]. Thus, Aurora B can control the degree of association of MCAK to appropriate parts of the chromosome and thereby regulate the stability of the microtubule.

The Spindle Assembly Checkpoint

Many checkpoints exist to regulate and control progression through the cell cycle. During the mitotic phase, the primary checkpoint is the spindle assembly checkpoint (SAC) as depicted in Fig (**5**). The SAC ensures the faithful segregation of sister chromatids by suspending the cell from entering anaphase until both conditions of this checkpoint, *i.e.,* the presence of microtubules bound to all kinetochores, and the presence of tension at the centromere-kinetochore complex are satisfied [106, 107].

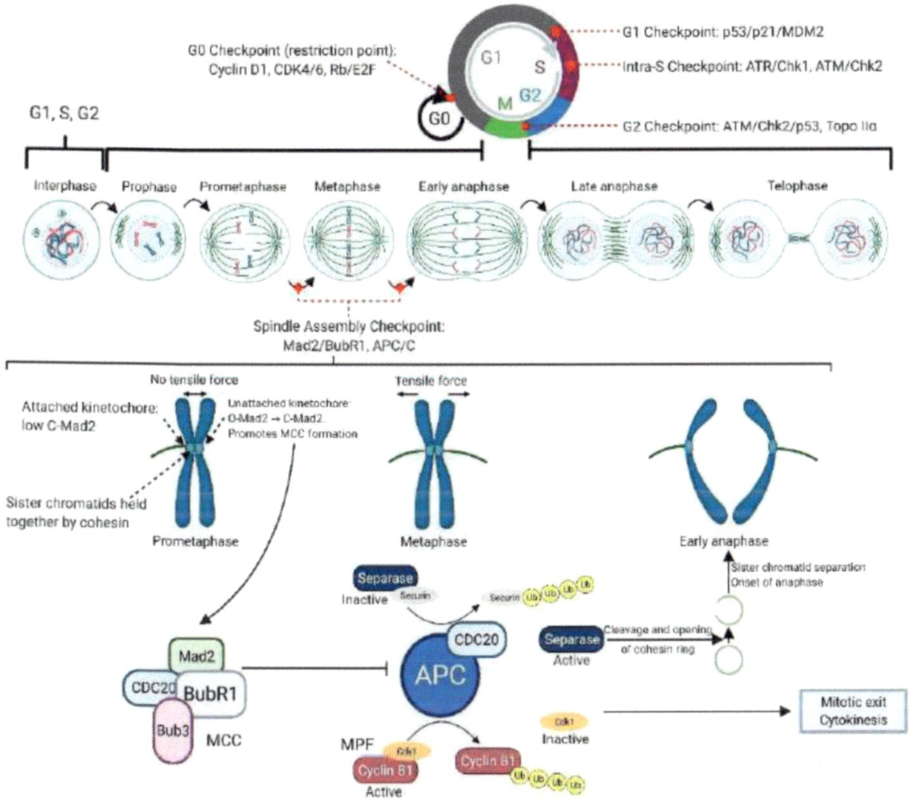

Fig. (5). Kinetochore-microtubule attachment dynamics regulating the spindle assembly checkpoint. The SAC acts to stop onset of anaphase upon sensing inappropriate k-MT attachments and lack of tension.

The SAC is in an active state during prometaphase due to the presence of unattached kinetochores and/or lack of tension catalysing the formation of the mitotic checkpoint complex (MCC) [108]. The rate-limiting step in the inactivation of the SAC is Mad2 (mitotic arrest deficient 2 protein) [109]. Specifically, in the region of the unattached kinetochore, cytosolic open-Mad2 (O-Mad2) is conformationally changed to closed-Mad2 (C-Mad2) by the

Mad1:C-Mad2 complex [110]. C-Mad2 then binds CDC20, to then further recruit the BubR1:Bub3 complex to form the MCC. The MCC acts to inhibit the actions of the E3 ubiquitin ligase, an anaphase-promoting complex or cyclosome (APC/C) [111].

Appropriate attachment of microtubules to kinetochores and application of tension at the centromere-kinetochore complex deters formation of C-Mad2 and the MCC, leading to the activation of APC. (112) Active APC is able to ubiquitinate cyclin B1 [112] and securin [113] and target these substrates for proteasomal degradation, thus inactivating and activating Cdk1 and separase, respectively. Active separase facilitates the cleavage of cohesin, and triggers separation of sister chromatids, and entry into anaphase [113]. Concurrently, degradation of cyclin B1 destroys the maturation promoting factor (MPF or the cyclin B1:Cdk1 complex), and pushes the cell out of mitosis towards cytokinesis [114].

A defect in this process may lead to an inappropriate progression into anaphase, and result in chromosome mis-segregation and aneuploidy, hence playing a potential role in tumorigenesis [115].

CONCLUDING REMARKS

The discovery and establishment of characteristic chromosomal aberrations is an important part of future cancer diagnostics. Although genetic abnormalities are common to all cancer cells, some cancer types are associated with observable aberrations using karyotyping. Often these chromosomal abnormalities play a role in cancer formation and progression and are, therefore, an identifiable and useful diagnostic characteristic. Whether chromosomal aberrations are a cause or a consequence of cancer is still unknown, though it has been shown to play both roles. In addition to using aberrations as a diagnostic tool, recurrent chromosomal errors also pave the way for understanding the molecular and genetic basis of cancer. The heterogeneous nature of cancer cells and their ability to replicate without maintaining chromosomal integrity makes it troublesome to pinpoint chromosomal aberrations as a diagnostic marker without better comprehension of cancer itself.

CONSENT FOR PUBLICATION

Not applicable.

CONFLICT OF INTEREST

The authors declare no conflict of interest, financial or otherwise.

ACKNOWLEDGEMENT

Figures in this chapter were created using BioRender.com.

REFERENCES

[1] Hanahan D, Weinberg RA. The hallmarks of cancer. Cell 2000; 100(1): 57-70. [http://dx.doi.org/10.1016/S0092-8674(00)81683-9] [PMID: 10647931]

[2] Sanjuán R, Pereira-Gómez M, Risso J. Genome Instability in DNA Viruses. In: Kovalchuk I, Kovalchuk O, Eds. Genome Stability. Boston: Academic Press 2016; pp. 37-47. [Internet] [http://dx.doi.org/10.1016/B978-0-12-803309-8.00003-3]

[3] Lengauer C, Kinzler KW, Vogelstein B. Genetic instability in colorectal cancers. Nature 1997; 386(6625): 623-7. [http://dx.doi.org/10.1038/386623a0] [PMID: 9121588]

[4] Preston RJ. Chromosome Aberrations. In: Wexler P, Ed. Encyclopedia of Toxicology 3rd ed. 2014; 955-8. [http://dx.doi.org/10.1016/B978-0-12-386454-3.00010-5]

[5] Alliance G, Screening Services TNY-M-AC for G and N. CHROMOSOMAL ABNORMALITIES [Internet]. Understanding Genetics: A New York, Mid-Atlantic Guide for Patients and Health Professionals. Genetic Alliance; 2009 [cited 2021 Jan 20]. Available from: https://www.ncbi.nlm.nih.gov/books/NBK115545/

[6] Knuutila S. Cytogenetics and molecular pathology in cancer diagnostics. Ann Med 2004; 36(3): 162-71. [http://dx.doi.org/10.1080/07853890310021733] [PMID: 15181972]

[7] Mitelman F, Johansson B, Mandahl N, Mertens F. Clinical significance of cytogenetic findings in solid tumors. Cancer Genet Cytogenet 1997; 95(1): 1-8. [http://dx.doi.org/10.1016/S0165-4608(96)00252-X] [PMID: 9140447]

[8] https://mitelmandatabase.isb-cgc.org/about

[9] Ferguson-Smith MA. Human Chromosome Aberrations. In: Maloy S, Hughes K, Eds. Brenner's Encyclopedia of Genetics. 2nd ed. San Diego: Academic Press 2013; pp. 546-9. http://www.sciencedirect.com/science/article/pii/B9780123749840002370 [Internet] [http://dx.doi.org/10.1016/B978-0-12-374984-0.00237-0]

[10] Cho IJ, Lui PP, Obajdin J, *et al.* Mechanisms, hallmarks, and implications of stem cell quiescence. Stem Cell Reports 2019; 12(6): 1190-200. [http://dx.doi.org/10.1016/j.stemcr.2019.05.012] [PMID: 31189093]

[11] Mercadante AA, Kasi A. Genetics, Cancer Cell Cycle Phases. StatPearls 2020. http://www.ncbi.nlm.nih.gov/books/NBK563158/ Internet

[12] Wenzel ES, Singh ATK. Cell-cycle Checkpoints and Aneuploidy on the Path to Cancer. Vivo Athens Greece 2018; 32(1): 1-5. [PMID: 29275292]

[13] Barnum KJ, O'Connell MJ. Cell cycle regulation by checkpoints. Methods Mol Biol 2014; 1170: 29-40. [http://dx.doi.org/10.1007/978-1-4939-0888-2_2] [PMID: 24906307]

[14] Malumbres M. 4 - Control of the Cell Cycle. In: Niederhuber JE, Armitage JO, Doroshow JH, Kastan MB, Tepper JE, editors. Abeloff's Clinical Oncology (Fifth Edition) [Internet]. Philadelphia: Churchill Livingstone; 2014 [cited 2021 Jan 22]. p. 52-68.e6. Available from: http://www.sciencedirect.com/science/article/pii/B9781455728657000047

[15] Vargas-Rondón N, Villegas V, Rondón-Lagos M. The role of chromosomal instability in cancer and

therapeutic responses. Cancers (Basel) 2017; 10(1): 4. [http://dx.doi.org/10.3390/cancers10010004] [PMID: 29283387]

[16] Mrózek K, Bloomfield CD. Chromosome Aberrations. In: Bertino JR, Ed. Encyclopedia of Cancer 2nd ed. 2002; 485-96. http://www.sciencedirect.com/science/article/pii/B0122275551005050 [Internet] [http://dx.doi.org/10.1016/B0-12-227555-1/00505-0]

[17] Harel T, Pehlivan D, Caskey CT, Lupski JR. Mendelian, Non-Mendelian, Multigenic Inheritance, and Epigenetics. In: Rosenberg RN, Pascual JM, Eds. Rosenberg's Molecular and Genetic Basis of Neurological and Psychiatric Disease 5th ed. 2015; 3-27. http://www.sciencedirect.com/science/article/pii/B9780124105294000012 [Internet] [http://dx.doi.org/10.1016/B978-0-12-410529-4.00001-2]

[18] Moore C, Best R. Chromosomal Genetic Disease: Structural aberrations;. Charleen M. Moore and Robert G. Best; Encyclopedia of life sciences, 2001, John Wiley & Sons, Ltd.

[19] Nowell C. The minute chromosome (Ph1) in chronic granulocytic leukemia. Blut 1962; 8(2): 65-6. [http://dx.doi.org/10.1007/BF01630378] [PMID: 14480647]

[20] Li J, Yen C, Liaw D, *et al.* PTEN, a putative protein tyrosine phosphatase gene mutated in human brain, breast, and prostate cancer. Science 1997; 275(5308): 1943-7. [http://dx.doi.org/10.1126/science.275.5308.1943] [PMID: 9072974]

[21] Orlow I, Lacombe L, Hannon GJ, *et al.* Deletion of the p16 and p15 genes in human bladder tumors. J Natl Cancer Inst 1995; 87(20): 1524-9. [http://dx.doi.org/10.1093/jnci/87.20.1524] [PMID: 7563186]

[22] Lee J, Nguyen PT, Shim HS, *et al.* EWSR1, a multifunctional protein, regulates cellular function and aging via genetic and epigenetic pathways. Biochim Biophys Acta BBA - Mol Basis Dis. 2019; 1865(7): 1938-45.

[23] Cidre-Aranaz F, Alonso J. EWS/FLI1 Target Genes and Therapeutic Opportunities in Ewing Sarcoma. Front Oncol 2015; 5: 162. https://www.frontiersin.org/articles/10.3389/fonc.2015.00162/full [http://dx.doi.org/10.3389/fonc.2015.00162] [PMID: 26258070]

[24] HMGA1 high mobility group AT-hook 1 [Homo sapiens (human)] - Gene - NCBI [Internet]. [cited 2021 Feb 4]. Available from: https://www.ncbi.nlm.nih.gov/gene/3159

[25] RAD51B RAD51 paralog B [Homo sapiens (human)] - Gene - NCBI [Internet]. [cited 2021 Feb 4]. Available from: https://www.ncbi.nlm.nih.gov/gene/5890

[26] Unachukwu U, Chada K, D'Armiento J. High Mobility Group AT-Hook 2 (HMGA2) Oncogenicity in Mesenchymal and Epithelial Neoplasia. Int J Mol Sci 2020; 21(9): 3151. [http://dx.doi.org/10.3390/ijms21093151] [PMID: 32365712]

[27] Juma AR, Damdimopoulou PE, Grommen SVH, Van de Ven WJM, De Groef B. Emerging role of PLAG1 as a regulator of growth and reproduction. J Endocrinol 2016; 228(2): R45-56. [http://dx.doi.org/10.1530/JOE-15-0449] [PMID: 26577933]

[28] Van Dyck F, Declercq J, Braem C, Van de Ven W. PLAG1, the prototype of the PLAG gene family: Versatility in tumour development (Review). Int J Oncol 2007; 30(4): 765-74. [http://dx.doi.org/10.3892/ijo.30.4.765] [PMID: 17332914]

[29] Cironi L, Petricevic T, Fernandes Vieira V, *et al.* The fusion protein SS18-SSX1 employs core Wnt pathway transcription factors to induce a partial Wnt signature in synovial sarcoma. Sci Rep 2016; 6(1): 22113. [http://dx.doi.org/10.1038/srep22113] [PMID: 26905812]

[30] Ladanyi M. Fusions of the SYT and SSX genes in synovial sarcoma. Oncogene 2001; 20(40): 5755-62. [http://dx.doi.org/10.1038/sj.onc.1204601] [PMID: 11607825]

[31] Yang K, Lui WO, Xie Y, *et al.* Co-existence of SYT-SSX1 and SYT-SSX2 fusions in synovial

sarcomas. Oncogene 2002; 21(26): 4181-90.
[http://dx.doi.org/10.1038/sj.onc.1205569] [PMID: 12037676]

[32] DDIT3 DNA damage inducible transcript 3 [Homo sapiens (human)] - Gene - NCBI [Internet]. [cited 2021 Feb 7]. Available from: https://www.ncbi.nlm.nih.gov/gene/1649

[33] FUS FUS RNA binding protein [Homo sapiens (human)] - Gene - NCBI [Internet]. [cited 2021 Feb 7]. Available from: https://www.ncbi.nlm.nih.gov/gene/2521

[34] Göransson M, Andersson MK, Forni C, *et al.* The myxoid liposarcoma FUS-DDIT3 fusion oncoprotein deregulates NF-κB target genes by interaction with NFKBIZ. Oncogene 2009; 28(2): 270-8.
[http://dx.doi.org/10.1038/onc.2008.378] [PMID: 18850010]

[35] Schreuder MI, van den Brand M, Hebeda KM, Groenen PJTA, van Krieken JH, Scheijen B. Novel developments in the pathogenesis and diagnosis of extranodal marginal zone lymphoma. J Hematop 2017; 10(3-4): 91-107.
[http://dx.doi.org/10.1007/s12308-017-0302-2] [PMID: 29225710]

[36] Su HC, Lenardo MJ. Chapter - 5: Combined Immune Deficiencies. In: Sullivan KE, Stiehm ER, (Eds.), Stiehm's Immune Deficiencies [Internet]. Amsterdam: Academic Press; 2014 [cited 2021 Feb 7]. p. 143–69. Available from: https://www.sciencedirect.com/science/article/pii/B9780124055469000054

[37] Roifman CM. 35 - Primary T-Cell Immunodeficiencies. In: Rich RR, Fleisher TA, Shearer WT, Schroeder HW, Frew AJ, Weyand CM, Eds. Clinical Immunology 5th ed. 2019; 489-508.e1. https://www.sciencedirect.com/science/article/pii/B9780702068966000351 [Internet]
[http://dx.doi.org/10.1016/B978-0-7020-6896-6.00035-1]

[38] Extranodal Marginal Zone Lymphoma of Mucosa-Associated Lymphoid Tissue (MALT Lymphoma) - ScienceDirect [Internet]. [cited 2021 Feb 7]. Available from: https://www.sciencedirect.com/science/article/pii/B9780123851833000334

[39] Cerrato A, Merolla F, Morra F, Celetti A. CCDC6: the identity of a protein known to be partner in fusion. Int J Cancer 2018; 142(7): 1300-8.
[http://dx.doi.org/10.1002/ijc.31106] [PMID: 29044514]

[40] Gandhi M, Dillon LW, Pramanik S, Nikiforov YE, Wang Y-H. DNA breaks at fragile sites generate oncogenic RET/PTC rearrangements in human thyroid cells. Oncogene 2010; 29(15): 2272-80.
[http://dx.doi.org/10.1038/onc.2009.502] [PMID: 20101222]

[41] Mejia Saldarriaga M, Steinberg A, Severson EA, Binder A. A Case of *CCDC6-RET* Fusion Mutation in Adult Acute Lymphoblastic Leukemia (ALL), a Known Activating Mutation Reported in ALL. Front Oncol 2019; 9: 1303. https://www.ncbi.nlm.nih.gov/pmc/articles/PMC6901674/
[http://dx.doi.org/10.3389/fonc.2019.01303] [PMID: 31850206]

[42] Xiang LI, Kong B. PAX8 is a novel marker for differentiating between various types of tumor, particularly ovarian epithelial carcinomas. Oncol Lett 2013; 5(3): 735-8.
[http://dx.doi.org/10.3892/ol.2013.1121] [PMID: 23425942]

[43] Wafer R, Tandon P, Minchin JEN. The Role of Peroxisome Proliferator-Activated Receptor Gamma (*PPARG*) in Adipogenesis: Applying Knowledge from the Fish Aquaculture Industry to Biomedical Research. Front Endocrinol (Lausanne) 2017; 8: 102. https://www.frontiersin.org/articles/10.3389/fendo.2017.00102/full
[http://dx.doi.org/10.3389/fendo.2017.00102] [PMID: 28588550]

[44] Vu-Phan D, Grachtchouk V, Yu J, Colby LA, Wicha MS, Koenig RJ. The thyroid cancer PAX8–PPARG fusion protein activates Wnt/TCF-responsive cells that have a transformed phenotype. Endocr Relat Cancer 2013; 20(5): 725-39.
[http://dx.doi.org/10.1530/ERC-13-0058] [PMID: 24025583]

[45] Zellweger R, Dalcher D, Mutreja K, *et al.* Rad51-mediated replication fork reversal is a global

response to genotoxic treatments in human cells. J Cell Biol 2015; 208(5): 563-79.
[http://dx.doi.org/10.1083/jcb.201406099] [PMID: 25733714]

[46] PubChem. https://pubchem.ncbi.nlm.nih.gov/gene/YWHAE/human

[47] https://www.cancer-genetics.org/NUTM2B.htm

[48] Lee CH, Ou WB, Mariño-Enriquez A, *et al.* 14-3-3 fusion oncogenes in high-grade endometrial stromal sarcoma. Proc Natl Acad Sci USA 2012; 109(3): 929-34.
[http://dx.doi.org/10.1073/pnas.1115528109] [PMID: 22223660]

[49] Fragkos M, Ganier O, Coulombe P, Méchali M. DNA replication origin activation in space and time. Nat Rev Mol Cell Biol 2015; 16(6): 360-74.
[http://dx.doi.org/10.1038/nrm4002] [PMID: 25999062]

[50] Wilhelm T, Said M, Naim V. DNA Replication Stress and Chromosomal Instability: Dangerous Liaisons. Genes (Basel) 2020; 11(6): 642. https://www.ncbi.nlm.nih.gov/pmc/articles/PMC7348713/
[http://dx.doi.org/10.3390/genes11060642] [PMID: 32532049]

[51] Mazouzi A, Velimezi G, Loizou JI. DNA replication stress: Causes, resolution and disease. Exp Cell Res 2014; 329(1): 85-93.
[http://dx.doi.org/10.1016/j.yexcr.2014.09.030] [PMID: 25281304]

[52] Voutsinos V, Munk SHN, Oestergaard VH. Common Chromosomal Fragile Sites—Conserved Failure Stories. Genes (Basel) 2018; 9(12): 580. https://www.ncbi.nlm.nih.gov/pmc/articles/PMC6315858/
[http://dx.doi.org/10.3390/genes9120580] [PMID: 30486458]

[53] Durkin SG, Glover TW. Chromosome fragile sites. Annu Rev Genet 2007; 41(1): 169-92.
[http://dx.doi.org/10.1146/annurev.genet.41.042007.165900] [PMID: 17608616]

[54] Gaillard H, García-Muse T, Aguilera A. Replication stress and cancer. Nat Rev Cancer 2015; 15(5): 276-89.
[http://dx.doi.org/10.1038/nrc3916] [PMID: 25907220]

[55] Bartkova J, Rezaei N, Liontos M, *et al.* Oncogene-induced senescence is part of the tumorigenesis barrier imposed by DNA damage checkpoints. Nature 2006; 444(7119): 633-7.
[http://dx.doi.org/10.1038/nature05268] [PMID: 17136093]

[56] Bartkova J, Hořejší Z, Koed K, *et al.* DNA damage response as a candidate anti-cancer barrier in early human tumorigenesis. Nature 2005; 434(7035): 864-70.
[http://dx.doi.org/10.1038/nature03482] [PMID: 15829956]

[57] Laiho M, Latonen L. Cell cycle control, DNA damage checkpoints and cancer. Ann Med 2003; 35(6): 391-7.
[http://dx.doi.org/10.1080/07853890310014605] [PMID: 14572162]

[58] Medema RH, Macůrek L. Checkpoint control and cancer. Oncogene 2012; 31(21): 2601-13.
[http://dx.doi.org/10.1038/onc.2011.451] [PMID: 21963855]

[59] Patil M, Pabla N, Dong Z. Checkpoint kinase 1 in DNA damage response and cell cycle regulation. Cell Mol Life Sci 2013; 70(21): 4009-21.
[http://dx.doi.org/10.1007/s00018-013-1307-3] [PMID: 23508805]

[60] Smith J, Mun Tho L, Xu N. Chapter 3 - The ATM–Chk2 and ATR–Chk1 Pathways in DNA Damage Signaling and Cancer. In: Vande Woude GF, Klein G, editors. Advances in Cancer Research [Internet]. Academic Press; 2010 [cited 2021 Feb 3]. p. 73–112. http://www.sciencedirect.com/science/article/pii/B9780123808882000030

[61] Bakkenist CJ, Kastan MB. DNA damage activates ATM through intermolecular autophosphorylation and dimer dissociation. Nature 2003; 421(6922): 499-506.
[http://dx.doi.org/10.1038/nature01368] [PMID: 12556884]

[62] Yang S, Kuo C, Bisi JE, Kim MK. PML-dependent apoptosis after DNA damage is regulated by the checkpoint kinase hCds1/Chk2. Nat Cell Biol 2002; 4(11): 865-70.

[http://dx.doi.org/10.1038/ncb869] [PMID: 12402044]

[63] Yarden RI, Pardo-Reoyo S, Sgagias M, Cowan KH, Brody LC. BRCA1 regulates the G2/M checkpoint by activating Chk1 kinase upon DNA damage. Nat Genet 2002; 30(3): 285-9. [http://dx.doi.org/10.1038/ng837] [PMID: 11836499]

[64] Xie S, Wu H, Wang Q, *et al.* Genotoxic stress-induced activation of Plk3 is partly mediated by Chk2. Cell Cycle 2002; 1(6): 424-9. [http://dx.doi.org/10.4161/cc.1.6.271] [PMID: 12548019]

[65] Stevens C, Smith L, La Thangue NB. Chk2 activates E2F-1 in response to DNA damage. Nat Cell Biol 2003; 5(5): 401-9. [http://dx.doi.org/10.1038/ncb974] [PMID: 12717439]

[66] Awasthi P, Foiani M, Kumar A. ATM and ATR signaling at a glance. J Cell Sci 2015; 128(23): jcs.169730. [http://dx.doi.org/10.1242/jcs.169730] [PMID: 26567218]

[67] Bartek J, Lukas J. Chk1 and Chk2 kinases in checkpoint control and cancer. Cancer Cell 2003; 3(5): 421-9. [http://dx.doi.org/10.1016/S1535-6108(03)00110-7] [PMID: 12781359]

[68] Groth A, Lukas J, Nigg EA, *et al.* Human Tousled like kinases are targeted by an ATM- and Chk1-dependent DNA damage checkpoint. EMBO J 2003; 22(7): 1676-87. [http://dx.doi.org/10.1093/emboj/cdg151] [PMID: 12660173]

[69] Lukas C, Falck J, Bártková J, Bartek J, Lukas J. Distinct spatiotemporal dynamics of mammalian checkpoint regulators induced by DNA damage. Nat Cell Biol 2003; 5(3): 255-60. [http://dx.doi.org/10.1038/ncb945] [PMID: 12598907]

[70] Alexander JL, Orr-Weaver TL. Replication fork instability and the consequences of fork collisions from rereplication. Genes Dev 2016; 30(20): 2241-52. [http://dx.doi.org/10.1101/gad.288142.116] [PMID: 27898391]

[71] Byun TS, Pacek M, Yee M, Walter JC, Cimprich KA. Functional uncoupling of MCM helicase and DNA polymerase activities activates the ATR-dependent checkpoint. Genes Dev 2005; 19(9): 1040-52. [http://dx.doi.org/10.1101/gad.1301205] [PMID: 15833913]

[72] Berti M, Ray Chaudhuri A, Thangavel S, *et al.* Human RECQ1 promotes restart of replication forks reversed by DNA topoisomerase I inhibition. Nat Struct Mol Biol 2013; 20(3): 347-54. [http://dx.doi.org/10.1038/nsmb.2501] [PMID: 23396353]

[73] Merchut-Maya JM, Bartek J, Maya-Mendoza A. Regulation of replication fork speed: Mechanisms and impact on genomic stability. DNA Repair (Amst) 2019; 81: 102654. [http://dx.doi.org/10.1016/j.dnarep.2019.102654] [PMID: 31320249]

[74] Toufektchan E, Toledo F. The Guardian of the Genome Revisited: p53 Downregulates Genes Required for Telomere Maintenance, DNA Repair, and Centromere Structure. Cancers. 2018; 10(5): 135.

[75] Roy S, Tomaszowski K-H, Luzwick JW, Park S, Li J, Murphy M, *et al.* p53 orchestrates DNA replication restart homeostasis by suppressing mutagenic RAD52 and POLθ pathways. Powell S, editor. eLife 2018; 7: e31723.

[76] Yeo CQX, Alexander I, Lin Z, *et al.* p53 Maintains Genomic Stability by Preventing Interference between Transcription and Replication. Cell Rep 2016; 15(1): 132-46. [http://dx.doi.org/10.1016/j.celrep.2016.03.011] [PMID: 27052176]

[77] Chatterjee N, Walker GC. Mechanisms of DNA damage, repair, and mutagenesis. Environ Mol Mutagen 2017; 58(5): 235-63. [http://dx.doi.org/10.1002/em.22087] [PMID: 28485537]

[78] D'Andrea AD. 4 - DNA Repair Pathways and Human Cancer. In: Mendelsohn J, Gray JW, Howley PM, Israel MA, Thompson CB, editors. The Molecular Basis of Cancer (Fourth Edition) [Internet]. Philadelphia: W.B. Saunders; 2015 [cited 2021 Feb 7]. p. 47-66.e2. Available from: https://www.sciencedirect.com/science/article/pii/B9781455740666000044

[79] Torgovnick A, Schumacher B. DNA repair mechanisms in cancer development and therapy. Front Genet 2015; 6: 157. https://www.frontiersin.org/articles/10.3389/fgene.2015.00157/full#B23 [http://dx.doi.org/10.3389/fgene.2015.00157] [PMID: 25954303]

[80] Bavle RM. Mitosis at a glance. J Oral Maxillofac Pathol 2014; 18 (Suppl. 1): S2-5. [PMID: 25364173]

[81] Sansregret L, Swanton C. The Role of Aneuploidy in Cancer Evolution. Cold Spring Harb Perspect Med 2017; 7(1): a028373. https://www.ncbi.nlm.nih.gov/pmc/articles/PMC5204330/ [http://dx.doi.org/10.1101/cshperspect.a028373] [PMID: 28049655]

[82] Sen S. Aneuploidy and cancer. Curr Opin Oncol 2000; 12(1): 82-8. [http://dx.doi.org/10.1097/00001622-200001000-00014] [PMID: 10687734]

[83] Compton DA. Mechanisms of aneuploidy. Curr Opin Cell Biol 2011; 23(1): 109-13. [http://dx.doi.org/10.1016/j.ceb.2010.08.007] [PMID: 20810265]

[84] Mugneret F, Lizard S, Aurias A, Turc-Carel C. Chromosomes in Ewing's sarcoma. II. Nonrandom additional changes, trisomy 8 and der(16)t(1;16). Cancer Genet Cytogenet 1988; 32(2): 239-45. [http://dx.doi.org/10.1016/0165-4608(88)90286-5] [PMID: 3163262]

[85] Domingues P, González-Tablas M, Otero Á, *et al.* Genetic/molecular alterations of meningiomas and the signaling pathways targeted. Oncotarget 2015; 6(13): 10671-88. [http://dx.doi.org/10.18632/oncotarget.3870] [PMID: 25965831]

[86] Stamenkovic I, Yu Q. CHAPTER 5 - CD44 Meets Merlin and Ezrin: Their Interplay Mediates the Pro-Tumor Activity of CD44 and Tumor-Suppressing Effect of Merlin. In: Stern R, Ed. Hyaluronan in Cancer Biology. San Diego: Academic Press 2009; pp. 71-87. https://www.sciencedirect.com/science/article/pii/B9780123741783100055 [Internet] [http://dx.doi.org/10.1016/B978-012374178-3.10005-5]

[87] Roth JJ, Fierst TM, Waanders AJ, Yimei L, Biegel JA, Santi M. Whole chromosome 7 gain predicts higher risk of recurrence in pediatric pilocytic astrocytomas independently from KIAA1549-BRAF fusion status. J Neuropathol Exp Neurol 2016; 75(4): 306-15. [http://dx.doi.org/10.1093/jnen/nlw001] [PMID: 26945035]

[88] Lindström E, Salford LG, Heim S, *et al.* Trisomy 7 and sex chromosome loss need not be representative of tumor parenchyma cells in malignant glioma. Genes Chromosomes Cancer 1991; 3(6): 474-9. [http://dx.doi.org/10.1002/gcc.2870030610] [PMID: 1663782]

[89] Limon J, Mrózek K, Heim S, *et al.* On the significance of trisomy 7 and sex chromosome loss in renal cell carcinoma. Cancer Genet Cytogenet 1990; 49(2): 259-63. [http://dx.doi.org/10.1016/0165-4608(90)90150-9] [PMID: 2208062]

[90] Simpson JL, Qin Y, Chen Z-J. Germ Cell Failure and Ovarian Resistance: Human Genes and Disorders. In: Leung PCK, Adashi EY, Eds. The Ovary. 3rd ed. Academic Press 2019; pp. 461-84. https://www.sciencedirect.com/science/article/pii/B9780128132098000285 [Internet] [http://dx.doi.org/10.1016/B978-0-12-813209-8.00028-5]

[91] Chan JY. A clinical overview of centrosome amplification in human cancers. Int J Biol Sci 2011; 7(8): 1122-44. [http://dx.doi.org/10.7150/ijbs.7.1122] [PMID: 22043171]

[92] Kellogg DR. Organizing cytoplasmic events. Nature 1989; 340(6229): 99-100. [http://dx.doi.org/10.1038/340099a0] [PMID: 2500602]

[93] Vertii A, Hehnly H, Doxsey S. The Centrosome, a Multitalented Renaissance Organelle. Cold Spring Harb Perspect Biol 2016; 8(12): a025049. https://www.ncbi.nlm.nih.gov/pmc/articles/PMC5131770/ [http://dx.doi.org/10.1101/cshperspect.a025049] [PMID: 27908937]

[94] Wu Q, Li B, Liu L, Sun S, Sun S. Centrosome dysfunction: a link between senescence and tumor immunity. Signal Transduct Target Ther 2020; 5(1): 107. [http://dx.doi.org/10.1038/s41392-020-00214-7] [PMID: 32606370]

[95] Banterle N, Gönczy P. Centriole biogenesis: from identifying the characters to understanding the plot. Annu Rev Cell Dev Biol 2017; 33(1): 23-49. [http://dx.doi.org/10.1146/annurev-cellbio-100616-060454] [PMID: 28813178]

[96] Gemble S, Simon A, Pennetier C, *et al.* Centromere dysfunction compromises mitotic spindle pole integrity. Curr Biol 2019; 29(18): 3072-3080.e5. [http://dx.doi.org/10.1016/j.cub.2019.07.052] [PMID: 31495582]

[97] Castellanos E, Dominguez P, Gonzalez C. Centrosome dysfunction in Drosophila neural stem cells causes tumors that are not due to genome instability. Curr Biol 2008; 18(16): 1209-14. [http://dx.doi.org/10.1016/j.cub.2008.07.029] [PMID: 18656356]

[98] D'Assoro AB, Lingle WL, Salisbury JL. Centrosome amplification and the development of cancer. Oncogene 2002; 21(40): 6146-53. [http://dx.doi.org/10.1038/sj.onc.1205772] [PMID: 12214243]

[99] Santaguida S, Amon A. Short- and long-term effects of chromosome mis-segregation and aneuploidy. Nat Rev Mol Cell Biol 2015; 16(8): 473-85. [http://dx.doi.org/10.1038/nrm4025] [PMID: 26204159]

[100] Ganem NJ, Pellman D. Linking abnormal mitosis to the acquisition of DNA damage. J Cell Biol 2012; 199(6): 871-81. [http://dx.doi.org/10.1083/jcb.201210040] [PMID: 23229895]

[101] Thompson SL, Compton DA. Chromosome missegregation in human cells arises through specific types of kinetochore–microtubule attachment errors. Proc Natl Acad Sci USA 2011; 108(44): 17974-8. [http://dx.doi.org/10.1073/pnas.1109720108] [PMID: 21997207]

[102] Godek KM, Kabeche L, Compton DA. Regulation of kinetochore–microtubule attachments through homeostatic control during mitosis. Nat Rev Mol Cell Biol 2015; 16(1): 57-64. [http://dx.doi.org/10.1038/nrm3916] [PMID: 25466864]

[103] Yamashiro S, Yamakita Y, Totsukawa G, *et al.* Myosin phosphatase-targeting subunit 1 regulates mitosis by antagonizing polo-like kinase 1. Dev Cell 2008; 14(5): 787-97. [http://dx.doi.org/10.1016/j.devcel.2008.02.013] [PMID: 18477460]

[104] Zhang X, Lan W, Ems-McClung SC, Stukenberg PT, Walczak CE. Aurora B phosphorylates multiple sites on mitotic centromere-associated kinesin to spatially and temporally regulate its function. Mol Biol Cell 2007; 18(9): 3264-76. [http://dx.doi.org/10.1091/mbc.e07-01-0086] [PMID: 17567953]

[105] Moore A, Wordeman L. The mechanism, function and regulation of depolymerizing kinesins during mitosis. Trends Cell Biol 2004; 14(10): 537-46. [http://dx.doi.org/10.1016/j.tcb.2004.09.001] [PMID: 15450976]

[106] Pinsky BA, Biggins S. The spindle checkpoint: tension *versus* attachment. Trends Cell Biol 2005; 15(9): 486-93. [http://dx.doi.org/10.1016/j.tcb.2005.07.005] [PMID: 16084093]

[107] Musacchio A, Salmon ED. The spindle-assembly checkpoint in space and time. Nat Rev Mol Cell Biol 2007; 8(5): 379-93. [http://dx.doi.org/10.1038/nrm2163] [PMID: 17426725]

[108] Lara-Gonzalez P, Westhorpe FG, Taylor SS. The spindle assembly checkpoint. Curr Biol 2012;

22(22): R966-80.
[http://dx.doi.org/10.1016/j.cub.2012.10.006] [PMID: 23174302]

[109] Sironi L, Mapelli M, Knapp S, De Antoni A, Jeang K-T, Musacchio A. Crystal structure of the tetrameric Mad1-Mad2 core complex: implications of a 'safety belt' binding mechanism for the spindle checkpoint. EMBO J 2002; 21(10): 2496-506.
[http://dx.doi.org/10.1093/emboj/21.10.2496] [PMID: 12006501]

[110] Mapelli M, Musacchio A. MAD contortions: conformational dimerization boosts spindle checkpoint signaling. Curr Opin Struct Biol 2007; 17(6): 716-25.
[http://dx.doi.org/10.1016/j.sbi.2007.08.011] [PMID: 17920260]

[111] Alfieri C, Zhang S, Barford D. Visualizing the complex functions and mechanisms of the anaphase promoting complex/cyclosome (APC/C). Open Biol 2017; 7(11): 170204.
[http://dx.doi.org/10.1098/rsob.170204] [PMID: 29167309]

[112] Pines J. Cubism and the cell cycle: the many faces of the APC/C. Nat Rev Mol Cell Biol 2011; 12(7): 427-38.
[http://dx.doi.org/10.1038/nrm3132] [PMID: 21633387]

[113] Nasmyth K, Haering CH. Cohesin: its roles and mechanisms. Annu Rev Genet 2009; 43(1): 525-58.
[http://dx.doi.org/10.1146/annurev-genet-102108-134233] [PMID: 19886810]

[114] Chesnel F, Bazile F, Pascal A, Kubiak JZ. Cyclin B dissociation from CDK1 precedes its degradation upon MPF inactivation in mitotic extracts of Xenopus laevis embryos. Cell Cycle 2006; 5(15): 1687-98.
[http://dx.doi.org/10.4161/cc.5.15.3123] [PMID: 16921258]

[115] Kops GJPL. The kinetochore and spindle checkpoint in mammals. Front Biosci 2008; Volume(13): 3606-20.
[http://dx.doi.org/10.2741/2953] [PMID: 18508459]

CHAPTER 5

Tumour DNA Sequencing

Farhadul Islam[1,*]

[1] *Department of Biochemistry and Molecular Biology, University of Rajshahi, Rajshahi-6205, Bangladesh*

Abstract: Cancer pathogenesis is a multistep process involving the accumulation of complex genetic and epigenetic alterations. The disease can be sporadic or familial in nature. The genes associated with much familial cancer or inherited cancer susceptible syndrome have already been identified. Thus, genetic testing for pathogenic variants of these genes could predict whether an individual has a high risk of developing cancer in their lifetime. Also, tumour DNA sequencing in patients with cancer can be used for therapy selection and to predict treatment outcomes. The recent development of high throughput sequencing enables the exploration of whole genome profiling, including mutations, structural variations, transcriptomes, splicing events, *etc*., in patients with cancer, thereby providing guidelines for personalized precision medicine in clinical practice. However, the translation of cancer genome sequencing information into the clinical treatment plan is highly complicated, needs multidisciplinary expert panels and is not cost-effective for mass application. Further development in sequencing analysis and data interpretation are imperative for point-of-care settings applications. This chapter outlines the clinical significance of tumour DNA testing and genomic sequencing in various cancers.

Keywords: Tumour DNA, Genetic testing, Genomic sequencing, Cancer genome sequencing, High-throughput sequencing, Sporadic cancer, Familial cancer, Cancer predisposition, Structural variation, Somatic mutation, Hereditary cancer, Cancer syndrome, Breast cancer, Ovarian cancer, Colorectal cancer, Skin cancer, Prostate cancer, Lung cancer, Thyroid cancer, Pancreatic cancer, Next-generation sequencing.

INTRODUCTION

Cancer is a genetic and cellular disease caused by the abnormal growth and proliferation of cells. The process of carcinogenesis is multi-facet and involves a series of complex genetic and epigenetic alterations that lead to the transformation of a normal cell into a cancerous cell [1 - 4]. The changes can be identified by tu-

* **Corresponding author Farhadul Islam:** Department of Biochemistry and Molecular Biology, University of Rajshahi, Rajshahi-6205, Bangladesh; E-mail: farhad_bio83@ru.ac.bd

mour profiling- a laboratory test used to detect specific genes or gene mutations and /or alterations, proteins or other biomarkers in a patient with cancer [5]. This molecular profiling of tumour could help in guiding personalised treatment decisions and can predict the metastasis and recurrence of cancer.

The presence of extensive genetic heterogeneity (both intertumoural and intratumoural) in cancer has significant implications for the selection of cancer biomarkers to guide decision-making in cancer treatment [6]. Therefore, cancer genome sequencing or tumour DNA sequencing permits oncologists and clinicians to identify the specific and unique alterations a patient has undergone during the development of their cancer [7]. This information could guide the personalized therapeutic options for the patients.

Numerous mutations underlie the development of each cancer, and it is reported that mutations in more than 1% of human genes (*i.e.,* cancer genes) contribute to cancer pathogenesis [8]. Also, 90% of the cancer genes showed somatic mutations, 20% showed germline, while 10% cancer genes showed both somatic and germline mutations [8]. The germline alterations (*i. e.,* mutations) associated with various cancer, especially familial cancer, have already been identified (Table **1**). For example, mutations in *BRCA1* and *BRCA2* genes cause HBOC syndrome, a known risk factor for the development of breast and ovarian cancer [9]. Patients with HBOC syndrome have a chance (50 to 85%) to develop breast cancer in their lifetime [9]. Thus, direct sequencing of *BRCA1* and *BRCA2* has been done to screen women suspicious for hereditary cancers. In addition, mutations in many other genes, such as *ATM, BRCA1, BRCA2, CDH1, CHEK2, NBN, NF1, PALB2, PTEN, STK11*, and *TP53,* are associated with the pathogenesis of breast cancer. Most importantly, somatic mutations in genes involved in cell proliferation, survival and death, such as *p53*, *RAS* family *etc*., are associated with the development of various cancer [8]. For instance, more than 50% cancers had shown *p53* somatic or acquired mutations [10]. Also, mutations in RAS have been identified in different types of cancers, including pancreas (90%), colorectal (50%), thyroid (50%), lung (30%), ovarian (15%), bladder (6%), breast, liver, skin, kidney and leukaemia [11]. Hence, tumour DNA sequencing could provide insightful, personalized information for molecular characterization of cancer along with susceptibility screening.

Additionally, in the context of personalised-precision medicine, discovery, development and validation of clinically useful biomarkers are prerequisites for better management of patients with cancer. Cancer biomarkers for susceptibility assessment, screening (early detection), stratification of cancer, the prognosis of the disease, the decision of appropriate therapeutics and duration of treatment, monitoring of therapy response and cancer recurrence are needed. Tumour DNA sequencing, especially cancer genome sequencing, could be useful in therapy selection, response monitoring and cancer risk prediction. Therefore, the clinical implication (such as early detection, therapy selection, and response monitoring and cancer risk assessment) of tumour DNA sequencing is described in this chapter.

Table 1. Mutations associated with hereditary cancers.

Cancer	Genes
Breast cancer in women	ATM, BARD1, BRCA1, BRCA2, BRIP1, CHEK2, CDH1, NF1, NBN, PALB2, PTEN, RAD51C, RAD51D, STK11, TP53
Breast cancer in men	BRCA1, BRCA2, CHEK2, PALB2
Colorectal cancer	APC, EPCAM, MLH1, MSH2, MSH6, PMS2, CHEK2, PTEN, STK11, TP53, MUTYH
Endometrial cancer	EPCAM, MLH1, MSH2, MSH6, PMS2, PTEN, STK11
Fallopian tube, ovarian, primary peritoneal cancer	ATM, BRCA1, BRCA2, BRIP1, EPCAM, MLH1, MSH2, MSH6, NB, PALB2, RAD51C, RAD51D, STK11
Gastric cancer	CDH1, STK11, EPCAM, MLH1, MSH2, MSH6, PMS2
Melanoma	BAP1, BRCA2 CDK4, CDKN2A, PTEN, TP53
Pancreatic cancer	ATM, BRCA1, BRCA2, CDKN2A, EPCAM, MLH1, MSH2, MSH6, PALB2, STK11, TP53
Prostate cancer	ATM, BRCA1, BRCA2, CHEK2,HOXB13, PALB2, EPCAM, MLH1, MSH2, MSH6, PMS2

Genetic Alterations in Cancer

Cancer genomes encompass a number of genetic changes, including chromosomal structural alterations, nucleotide changes, transcriptome changes, *etc.* Gross chromosomal structural changes in cancer can be accomplished by amplification, deletion, translocation and/or inversion of chromosomal segments or entire chromosomes. These structural changes, of course, duly alter genes in a number of ways, which in turn could be critical to the onset or progression of the disease [12]. Therefore, the identification and characterization of chromosomal structural variations associated with cancer could provide valuable information with increased clinical significance.

Alterations in certain nucleotides in tumour DNA have also been reported in various cancer pathogenesis [13, 14]. Targeted sequencing followed by amplification of tumour DNA is a powerful approach to successfully identify the key somatic mutations in cancer genomes. The targeted tumour DNA sequencing can characterize hundreds of genes, even the entire exome (all the protein-coding exons), to detect the variants that significantly contributed to carcinogenesis in a given cancer type. For example, in the sequencing of a large number of lung adenocarcinoma and glioblastoma multiforme (GBM) (similar pathological stage and histological grade) tumour, novel genes mutations or mutations panel have been identified in each type of cancer [13, 15]. Also, targeted tumour DNA sequencing provides information on cellular pathways putatively affected by the mutation types. For instance, signalling network-associated MAPK, p53 and mTOR pathways are impacted by the combination of point mutations, copy number changes, and loss of heterozygosity in lung adenocarcinomas [15]. On the other hand, sequencing of GBM samples revealed some commonly mutated genes that affected novel pathways, such as *IDH1* mutations (>80% GBM patients) affecting the Krebs cycle and cellular homeostasis [16]. Clinically, *IDH1* mutations are more prevalent in secondary GBM (73%) than primary (3.7%) patients with GBM. Also, *IDH1* mutations are associated with younger age (33 *versus* 53 years) and a favourable prognosis for patients with GBM [17, 18]. Furthermore, targeted tumour DNA sequencing could identify candidate cancer genes (CAN-genes), thereby providing information to detect driving mutations associated with carcinogenesis, *i.e.,* drivers and passenger (no impact) mutations, by integrating gene expression, somatic mutations and copy number changes information.

In addition, sequencing of RNA (RNA-seq) extracted from cancer cells can give a better insight of tumour profiling that has developed during the disease progression [19]. Cancer genome characterization by RNA-seq generates comprehensive, complete transcriptomic information of a given tumour along with a correlation to the known genetic alterations such as structural changes, copy number variation, insertion and /or deletion, translocation, and point mutations. Also, it produces data that can enhance the understanding of the transcriptome in cancer. RNA-seq data can identify allele-specific expression in the context of known mutations, verify the impact of a nonsense mutation or lead to finding novel mutations in cancers [20]. Furthermore, RNA-seq data can identify alternate splicing isoforms, novel genes that previously have not been annotated due to lack of ESTs or missed by *in silico* prediction, fusion transcripts and micro-RNAs (miRNAs) in a cancer genome [21 - 24]. These RNA-seq data can predicts the prognosis of patients with various cancers.

Genetic Tests for Cancer

Cancer genetic testing helps to estimate the chance of developing cancer in an individual in a lifetime by examining the specific types of alterations in genes, chromosomes or proteins [25]. Currently, genetic tests are available for several types of cancers, including breast, ovarian, colorectal, thyroid, prostate, pancreatic, kidney, stomach cancers, melanoma and sarcomas [25]. Genetic testing may predict the risk of developing specific cancer, and inheritance of mutant genes and provide information to guide personalized health care. However, no genetic test can predict that an individual can develop cancer for sure, though it can predict that the individual has a higher chance than most people [25]. In addition, genetic testing will be increasingly important in cancer diagnosis and personalised treatment for better clinical outcomes. Most commonly used genetic tests for various cancer types are summarized in the following sections.

Breast Cancer

Currently, tumour profiling for genetic and genomic variation has become a critical part of the management of patients with breast cancer, especially advanced breast cancer. In cancer patients with a family history of breast cancer or other cancer, genetic testing is imperative to determine whether a hereditary cancer syndrome is associated with cancer development. In advanced breast cancer, detection of targetable mutations, such as *PIK3CA, HER2* or other tyrosine kinase inhibitors, could provide information for therapy selection [26]. Also, analysis of transcriptome-based expression can be used in the management of early-stage estrogen receptor-positive breast cancer. Thus, tumour DNA profiling provides prognostic significance in the clinical setting for adjuvant endocrine therapy and could be useful in predicting the benefit of adjuvant chemotherapy in patients with breast cancer.

Additionally, a number of genes, such as *BRCA1/2, PTEN, TP53, STK11, CDH1* and *PALB2* have been associated with the increased risk of developing breast cancer [27, 28]. Among these genes, mutations in *BRCA1/2* are high penetrance for breast cancer, accounting for the majority of hereditary breast cancer, 5-10% of all patients with breast cancers [28, 29]. The presence of cancer-predisposing mutations in patient's sample (blood, tissues or saliva) can be identified by a number of commercially available genetic testing, thereby predicting the risk of developing breast cancer in an individual in a lifetime. Therefore, genetic testing is an integral part of the clinical management of the majority of patients with breast cancer.

Ovarian Cancer

Germline mutations in *BRCA1/2* have been associated with 15% of ovarian cancer, while somatic *BRCA1/2* mutations and epigenetic inactivation of *BRCA1/2* have been associated with 6% and 10.8% of ovarian cancer, respectively [30]. In addition, mutations in other genes, such as mismatch repair (10-15%), and homologous recombination pathways genes, have been implicated in ovarian carcinogenesis [30]. Furthermore, 23% of high-grade serous ovarian carcinoma had shown *BRCA1/2* germline mutations [31]. Hence, genetic testing of the susceptible gene or genes panel could effectively use to screed patients with ovarian cancer.

The genetic testing of ovarian cancer also has prognostic and predictive significance. For example, patients with *BRCA1/2* mutations or homologous recombination deficiency treated with poly(ADP-ribose) polymerase (PARP) inhibitors provide improved progression-free survival [30, 32]. Also, in the case of cancer relapse, patients carrying *BRCA1/2* mutations respond to both platin/non-platin-based regimens more frequently when compared to the mutations negative patients [32]. Patients carry somatic *BRCA1/2* mutations in response to the multiple cycles of platin-based chemotherapies [32]. Thus, mutation status may be useful in decision-making for systemic therapy selection in the clinical setting. However, it was reported that annual genetic screening with a high sensitivity could not reduce ovarian cancer-related mortality by more than 50%, and frequent screening has a low positive predictive value in practical applications. Therefore, the research outcome remains promising; adaptation of genetic and genomic testing into clinical applications needs further development and validation.

Colorectal Cancer

Pathogenesis of colorectal cancer (CRC) is a multistep process involving a series of histological, morphological, epigenetics and genetic alterations that accumulated over time [32]. In CRC, about 30% of cases had shown familial clustering- patients having potentially identifiable genetic components [33]. In addition, 3-5% of CRC patients are associated with high-risk, inherited colon cancer syndrome such as Lunch syndrome, inflammatory bowel disease and familial adenomatous polyposis (FAP). Detection of genetic changes of the genes associated with CRC syndrome coupled with other genetic insights into the clinical course has led to the development of specific management guidelines and genetic tests that can identify these familial disorders in patients susceptible to develop CRC [34]. Also, genetic profiling of CRC provides insight into the changes underlying the development of CRC, which in turn could identify predisposed, asymptomatic patients at early-stage precancerous polyps before becoming malignant, thereby may lead to a substantial reduction of CRC burden [34]. Genetic testing and counselling could be life-saving not for the affected people but also for the family members of the patients with CRC.

A non-invasive multi-target stool (mt-sDNA) test has been developed and approved to detect abnormal DNA and occult blood in stool samples to screen patients with CRC [35, 36]. In this test, alterations in genes (ten genes) associated with CRC, haemoglobin biomarkers were examined and combined with a diagnostic algorithm to provide a single composite positive or negative outcome. A composite of abnormal DNA and /or blood indicates the potential of a cancerous or precancerous lesion. The individuals are referred for a diagnostic colonoscopy for further examination and treatments. The mt-sDNA test has high analytical sensitivity (92.3%) and specificity (86.6%), whereas it has extremely high negative predictive values (99.94%) in the case of individuals' exhibiting the negative result of the mt-sDNA test. The likelihood of having a missed CRC was only 0.06%, and only 5.2% of patients have a risk of developing advanced adenomas [37].

In CRC, tumour DNA sequencing for identification of mutations in key genes, *Ras* family and *TP53,* for example, could provide prognostic implications [38]. Mutations of *KRAS* in patients with advanced CRC were associated with a poorer prognosis, and mutated patients had significantly shorter progression-free and overall survival rates. Also, advanced colorectal cancer samples with *TP53* mutations had shown the worst survival and poorer prognosis, along with reduced chemotherapy response in multivariate analysis [38]. Thus, these mutations were associated with the biological aggressiveness of cancer.

Additionally, multigene panel testing by parallel sequencing could identify Lynch syndrome, FAM, hereditary inflammatory bowel disease and cancer at an early stage, generating information for precision cancer treatment by providing new strategies for surveillance and chemoprevention opportunities [39]. Targeted immunotherapy for the treatment of mismatch repair deficient and hyper-mutated CRC individuals with genetic predisposition can be identified by genetic testing.

Thyroid Cancer

The genetic mutations and molecular changes in different types of thyroid cancers, *i.e.,* papillary thyroid cancer (PTC), follicular thyroid cancer (FTC), anaplastic thyroid cancer (ATC), medullary thyroid cancer (MTC) and rare Hurthle cell cancer can be identified in fine-needle aspiration (FNA) from thyroid nodules by genetic testing [40, 41]. Tumour profiling could successfully ameliorate cancer diagnosis and management of patients with thyroid malignancy by providing personalised information in clinical settings. For example, PTC (accounting for 85-90% thyroid cancer) patients can be diagnosed by analysing FNA samples for a panel mutation in *TERT, BRAF, PAX8/ PPARγ*, *RAS* and *RET* using genetic testing. Detection of these mutations in PTC samples provides a strong indication of the presence of malignancy and guides the clinical management for a significant proportion of patients with indeterminate cytology [41].

Mutations in *TERT, BRAF, PAX8/ PPARγ*, *RAS* and *RET* affect the MAPK signalling pathway, thereby providing opportunities to develop targeted therapies against thyroid cancer. In PTC, about 50% of patients had shown BRAF(V600E) mutations associated with biological aggressive and cancer recurrence [42]. Thus, preoperative analysis of *BRAF(V600E)* in low-risk patients may provide significant prognostic implications and intensive management of these patients could be beneficial. Also, *BRAF*-targeted therapies and other kinase inhibitors and/or combinations with other regimens could be helpful in treating advanced thyroid cancer patients.

Medullary thyroid cancer (MTC) accounts for 10% of all thyroid cancers and can be both sporadic and familial [43]. In familial MTC, the malignancy can occur alone or as a component of multiple endocrine neoplasia type 2A (MEN 2A), consisting of MTC, pheochromocytoma and hyperparathyroidism. It can also occur as a component of MEN 2B, comprising MTC, pheochromocytoma and mucosal neuromas [43]. Genetic testing for MTC was first established and was used for predicting thyroid cancer risk and making preventive surgery at an early stage [40]. It was noted that mutations in *RET*, a proto-oncogene, affect subjects from MEN 2 and lead to MTC pathogenesis. Therefore, identification of *RET* mutations in the risk group provided preventive surgery for the subjects, resulting in no cancer development. Thus, genetic testing currently used to screen thyroid cancer provides key information on the diagnosis, risk stratification and personalized care of patients with thyroid cancer.

Prostate Cancer

Development of a significant proportion of prostate cancer (10-20%) has been attributed strongly to hereditary/ family components, thus, germline genetic testing and somatic genomic profiling could identify personalised precision therapeutics and/or clinical care, especially in advanced prostate cancer patients [44 - 46]. Individuals with multiple single-gene polymorphisms and a family history of prostate cancer have a significantly higher risk of prostate carcinogenesis. Recent advancements in sequencing technologies identify a number of high-risk alterations in several genes, including *BRCA1/2, MLH1, MSH2/6, PMS2, HOXB13, CHEK2, NBN, BRIP1* and *ATM* [47]. Also, the development and approval of targeted therapeutics, such as olaparib for *BRCA1/2, ATM*-mutated, metastatic and castrate-resistant prostate cancer, indicate that genetic testing has critical implications in therapeutic management. Thus, referral of genetic testing based on clinical features, family history and ethnicity could provide cost-effective genetic profiling of patients and their family members with an increased risk of developing prostate cancer. This can help inform prostate cancer screening and choose therapeutic options in clinical settings.

Pancreatic Cancer

Pancreatic cancer, either familial or sporadic, is the most deadly cancer, with a 5-year survival rate of approximately 5% both in men and women [48]. Due to its fast progression and prognosis, identification of high-risk groups and early lesions detection could improve the clinical outcome. Understanding the risk factors and genetic predisposition has important implications not only for cancer prevention but also for screening and personalized therapeutic management. In pancreatic cancer, about 10% of cases have familial inheritance and several hereditary syndromes such as pancreatitis, breast and ovarian cancer syndrome, familial atypical mole and multiple melanoma, Lynch syndrome *etc*., and family history of pancreatic cancer attributed to the development of pancreatic cancer [49, 50]. Individuals with increased risk for pancreatic cancer screening should be tested for the candidate genes, including *PRSS1, BRCA1/2, CDKN2, ATM* and *PALB2* for germline mutations.

Genetic testing for familial pancreatic cancer in women who underwent breast imaging can identify the high-risk group in the retrospective analysis [51]. A 10.4% of subjects were classified at high risk for familial pancreatic cancer development. Another study noted that genetic testing for the hereditary syndrome, endoscopic ultrasound, and fine needle aspiration in high risk patients can identify pancreatic cancer at early stages [52], potentially improving the clinical outcome in patients with pancreatic cancer. However, significant emphasis should be given to screening patients for hereditary cancer syndromes to get optimum benefits from genetic risk prediction testing.

Lung Cancer

Recent advancements in molecular profiling of lung cancer enrich our understanding of cancer initiation, maintenance and progression, thus, providing critical insights for targeted therapies. Genetic testing for the identification of diver mutation or resistance mutations of heterogeneous lung tumours radically changed the clinical management and outcome of the disease by opening new horizons to the discovery and development of a variety of novel targeted therapies [52, 53]. The benefit of genetic testing in patients with lung cancer, especially advanced stage non-small cell lung cancer (NSCL), is evidenced by shifting the standard care from empirically based on patient's clinicopathological factors to use biomarker-driven treatment algorithms based on the molecular profiling of patient's tumour in therapy selection [54]. For example, genetic testing is being used to treat patients with advanced NSCL harbouring gain-of-function mutations in *EGFR* or *ALK* gene rearrangements by first-line tyrosine kinase inhibitors and provide genotype-based personalised targeted therapies [53].

Traditional sequencing approaches have identified the presence of drive and/or resistance mutations, amplification in *EGFR*, *KRAS*, *BRAF*, *MET*, *EML4-ALK1*, *DDR2*, *FGFR1* and *HER2* along with *ALK* and *ROS1* fusions in lung cancer [53 - 55]. Multiplex genotyping and high-throughput profiling by next-generation sequencing provide a rapid and comprehensive analysis of the cancer genome of individual patients with lung cancer, thereby categorizing the patients into molecular subsets for targeted therapy in clinical settings. In addition, the detection of specific mutations could provide predictive implications on the outcome of targeted therapies and have prognostic significance in the clinical management of patients with lung cancer [53, 54].

Additionally, in lung cancer, genetic testing for driver mutations is useful to identify patients who are likely to respond to the targeted therapy [56, 57]. For example, the presence of mutations in *EGFR* gene, especially in exon 18-21 in patients with lung cancer, responded to the targeted therapy gefitinib and erlotinib in a prospective study [57]. However, prognostic and predictive values of *EGFR* mutations need to be validated using randomised trials. Thus, the genetic testing appeared to be useful in the diagnosis and stratification of cancer patients, at least for lung cancer patients.

Skin Cancer

Genetic predisposition plays important roles in both melanoma and non-melanoma skin cancer development [58]. For example, specific alleles of the gene encoding melanocortin 1 receptor can predict skin cancer risk and act as an independent risk factor regardless of hair colour or skin types [58]. Also, since impaired UVA and UVB defence mechanisms are associated with the skin cancer risk, thus, examining the genetic predisposition may be helpful in the care of patients undergoing psoralen plus UVA (PUVA) or UVB treatments for cutaneous disorders such as psoriasis, vitiligo and eczema [58]. Therefore, genetic testing in high-risk populations, along with family and medical history, could play an important role in the diagnosis of skin cancer.

Tumour DNA profiling of melanoma, the deadliest and most common skin cancer with a rapid rate of incidence, revealed that a number of specific genetic and genomic abnormalities are associated with carcinogenesis. Most of the genetic and genomic driving changes are noted in a number of genes, including *NRAS*, *BRAF*, *KIT*, *PTEN*, *GNAQ/GNA11* and *MAP2K1/2* (*MEK1/2*) [59]. Identification of genetic signature of melanomas permits the development of targeted therapies directed against KIT, MEK1/2 and mutated BRAF, such as the development and clinical approval of vemurafenib in the treatment of patients with BRAF-mutated melanomas [60]. As one-half of the advanced, *i.e.,* unresectable or metastatic melanomas carrying *BRAF* (V600E) mutations, the targeted therapy against BRAF and MEK by molecular inhibitors provides significant long-term benefits in the majority of skin cancer patients [61]. Also, genetic testing shows that mutational load is associated with tumour progression and provides evolutionary trajectories of different subtypes of melanomas. Furthermore, it gives insights regarding of development of acquired resistance to BRAF and MEK inhibitors in patients with advanced melanomas. Therefore, genetic testing for *BRAF* is critical in the management of patients with melanomas.

In familial melanoma (10% cases), a number of inherited mutations were identified in genes such as *MITF, CDKN2A, BRCA1, BAP1, CXC, TERT, POT1, TERTF2IP, ACD* and *CDK4* as the susceptible for cancer development [62]. In addition, mutations in *MC1R* and *MITF* predict a moderately increased risk for melanoma development [62]. Thus, genetic counselling and testing for melanoma predisposition mutations could be useful in clinical applications, especially for treatment selections in patients with advanced disease stages.

Additionally, hereditary cancer predisposition syndrome, especially cutaneous tumours are associated with a number of cancer development (Table **2**). For instance, alterations in *PTEN* associated with Cowden syndrome, predisposition to the trichilemmoma, acral keratosis, lipomas, and milia skin disorders, which in turn can act as a risk factor for the development of breast, thyroid and endometrial cancers [63, 64]. Also, mutations in *APC* (Gardner's syndrome) predisposed to pilomatrixoma, epidermoid cysts with features of pilomatrixoma that can act as a risk factor for colon cancer, desmoid tumours, osteomas and endocrine tumours development [63, 64]. Therefore, genetic testing for these hereditary skin tumours could predict the risk associated with a number of fatal cancers.

Table 2. Hereditary cutaneous tumours syndromes and associated cancers.

Name of syndrome	Gene	Skin tumour	Associated cancer
Birt-Hogg-Dubé syndrome	*FLCN*	Fibrofolliculoma Trichodiscoma	Renal cancer, Lung cysts Pneumothoraces
Cowden syndrome	*PTEN*	Trichilemmoma Acral keratoses Lipomas, Milia	Breast cancer, Thyroid cancer Endometrial cancer
Familial leiomyomas	*FH*	Piloleiomyoma Angioleiomyoma	Renal cancer (Type 2 papillary RCC)

(Table 2) cont.....

Name of syndrome	Gene	Skin tumour	Associated cancer
Muir-Torre syndrome	*MSH2* *MLH1*	Sebaceous adenoma Sebaceous epithelioma Sebaceous carcinoma Keratoacanthoma	Colorectal cancer Genitourinary cancer
Tuberous sclerosis	*TSC1* *TSC2*	Hypopigmented macules Facial angiofibroma Shagreen patch Periungual fibroma	Neurological abnormalities: epilepsy, autism, intellectual disability, Renal abnormalities Multi-organ hamartomatous overgrowth
CYLD cutaneous syndrome	*CYLD*	Cylindroma, Spiradenoma, Trichoepithelioma, milia	Salivary gland tumour – membranous basal cell adenoma
Gardner's syndrome	*APC*	Pilomatrixoma Epidermoid cysts with features of pilomatrixoma	Colon cancer, Desmoid tumours, Osteomas, Endocrine tumours
Naevoid basal cell carcinoma syndrome	*PTCH* *SUFU*	Basal cell carcinoma	Medulloblastoma
Melanoma pancreatic cancer syndrome	*CDKN2A*	Melanoma	Pancreatic cancer

Cancer Genome Sequencing: The Future of Precision Medicine

In the past decade, genome sequencing has been developed exponentially from a rare research tool to an approach with broad applications in clinical settings. In sequencing technologies, the transition from targeted gene sequencing to whole exome sequencing (WES) to whole genome sequencing (WGS) has been possible due to the massive advancements in technologies and bioinformatics analysis. Genomic profiling has revealed the etiopathology of previously un-diagnosable diseases and conditions, identifying drive variants and the pathophysiology of various diseases, including cancer [65].

Cancer genome sequencing is the whole genome sequencing for the identification and characterization of DNA or RNA sequence of a single, homogenous or heterogeneous group of cancer cell(s). In cancer genome sequencing, primary tumour tissue, adjacent or distant normal tissues, the microenvironment component, such as fibroblasts/stromal cells or metastatic tumour tissue are directly sequenced to generate information of any changes of nucleotide bases (DNA or RNA), copy number, mutations status and structural variations in cancer samples. Also, it profiles gene expression patterns and miRNA expressions, and can identify alternative splicing events [66]. Thus, cancer genome sequencing has fundamentally improved our understanding of the underlying mechanism of the disease, thereby has provided strategies and approaches for characterizing, monitoring, guiding and evaluating the treatment in clinical settings.

The application and scope of tumour DNA sequencing have already been brought into the clinics, and targeted genomic panels for susceptible genes (germline mutations) and actionable somatic mutations for specific cancer types are becoming routine analyses in many cancer centres [67]. The high-throughput sequencing of larger-gene panels is also seen in routine analysis in many clinical managements, which could drive the discovery of novel variants associated with cancer pathogenesis along with well-characterized mutations in cancer genes [68]. For example, whole genome analysis of tongue adenocarcinoma identified genomic amplification and concurrent abundant expression of a novel oncogene (*RET*), the potential driver of the disease and kinase inhibitor targeting RET protein provided a new horizon of personalized treatment of patients with cancer [69]. In addition, post-treatment sample analysis provides insights into the disease progression and evolution of cancer to circumvent the treatment regimen, which led to a pilot Personalized OncoGenomics clinical trial with the aim of intern-t--treat based on the genomic information of individuals [70]. Developing sequencing pipelines for larger sample analysis and comprehensive interpretation tools could provide framework for cancer-specific unbiased approaches for whole genome sequencing.

Recent developments in next-generation sequencing enable long-read sequencing along with short-read and linked-read sequencing, which allows haplotype phasing and improved structural variants detection and de novo assembly analysis [71]. Thus, substantially improving the resolution of complex genomic events, providing precise and comprehensive digital karyotypes of cancer. Clinical cancer genome sequencing also includes cancer clonal sequencing, which in turn generates mutational clonality load of a cancer type, unveiling the tumour heterogeneity. Since tumour heterogeneity and cancer metastasis are associated with therapy response and the survival of cancer patients, thus, analysis of heterogeneity and driving events in cancer metastasis by genome profiling can predict drug resistance in an individual patient.

Additionally, the complete genomic information, in combination with extensive clinical information, will provide unprecedented research and clinical management platform to understand the underlying mechanisms of therapeutic response, acquired drug resistance, therapy failure and cancer recurrence. Also, whole genome and transcriptome analysis at various points of the disease course can provide a real-time view of the cancer progression and therapy response. These analyses will provide a feedback loop, which could be critical for examining the patients as the data are related to the improved cancer stratification and personalised therapeutic intervention in clinics. In addition, annotation of clinical management (therapy selection, course of therapy, response to the given therapy *etc.*) would feed into large-scale analysis in the preclinical research for further understanding of carcinogenesis and identification of rational cancer biomarkers for diagnosis and prognosis along with the development of new drugs for better management of patients with cancers.

CONCLUSION

Cancer genetic and genomic sequencing has become more common and sophisticated in cancer research and clinical utilities with the advancement of sequencing technologies and data analysis platforms. Cancer genomic profiling provides abundant information to understand the explicit biology of carcinogenesis in individual cancer, thereby providing the guidelines for personalized management of patients in care centres. In addition, genetic testing and counselling in susceptible populations could predict the genetic predisposition of the cancer risk, resulting in improved diagnosis and therapy selection in clinical settings.

CONSENT FOR PUBLICATION

Not applicable.

CONFLICT OF INTEREST

The author declares no conflict of interest, financial or otherwise.

ACKNOWLEDGEMENT

The author thanks the University of Rajshahi, Bangladesh, for providing the technical support.

REFERENCES

[1] Kinzler KW, Vogelstein B. Lessons from hereditary colorectal cancer. Cell 1996; 87(2): 159-70. [http://dx.doi.org/10.1016/S0092-8674(00)81333-1] [PMID: 8861899]

[2] Baylin SB. The cancer epigenome: its origins, contributions to tumorigenesis, and translational implications. Proc Am Thorac Soc 2012; 9(2): 64-5. [http://dx.doi.org/10.1513/pats.201201-001MS] [PMID: 22550245]

[3] Ting AH, McGarvey KM, Baylin SB. The cancer epigenome—components and functional correlates. Genes Dev 2006; 20(23): 3215-31. [http://dx.doi.org/10.1101/gad.1464906] [PMID: 17158741]

[4] Jones PA, Baylin SB. The epigenomics of cancer. Cell 2007; 128(4): 683-92. [http://dx.doi.org/10.1016/j.cell.2007.01.029] [PMID: 17320506]

[5] Harnan S, Tappenden P, Cooper K, *et al.* Tumour profiling tests to guide adjuvant chemotherapy decisions in early breast cancer: a systematic review and economic analysis. Health Technol Assess 2019; 23(30): 1-328. [http://dx.doi.org/10.3310/hta23300] [PMID: 31264581]

[6] Burrell RA, McGranahan N, Bartek J, Swanton C. The causes and consequences of genetic

heterogeneity in cancer evolution. Nature 2013; 501(7467): 338-45.
[http://dx.doi.org/10.1038/nature12625] [PMID: 24048066]

[7] Roychowdhury S, Iyer MK, Robinson DR, *et al.* Personalized oncology through integrative high-throughput sequencing: a pilot study. Sci Transl Med 2011; 3(111): 111ra121.
[http://dx.doi.org/10.1126/scitranslmed.3003161] [PMID: 22133722]

[8] Futreal PA, Coin L, Marshall M, *et al.* A census of human cancer genes. Nat Rev Cancer 2004; 4(3): 177-83.
[http://dx.doi.org/10.1038/nrc1299] [PMID: 14993899]

[9] Nielsen FC, van Overeem Hansen T, Sørensen CS. Hereditary breast and ovarian cancer: new genes in confined pathways. Nat Rev Cancer 2016; 16(9): 599-612.
[http://dx.doi.org/10.1038/nrc.2016.72] [PMID: 27515922]

[10] Olivier M, Hollstein M, Hainaut P. TP53 mutations in human cancers: origins, consequences, and clinical use. Cold Spring Harb Perspect Biol 2010; 2(1): a001008.
[http://dx.doi.org/10.1101/cshperspect.a001008] [PMID: 20182602]

[11] Prior IA, Hood FE, Hartley JL. The frequency of ras mutations in cancer. Cancer Res 2020; 80(14): 2969-74.
[http://dx.doi.org/10.1158/0008-5472.CAN-19-3682] [PMID: 32209560]

[12] Wang WJ, Li LY, Cui JW. Chromosome structural variation in tumorigenesis: mechanisms of formation and carcinogenesis. Epigenetics Chromatin 2020; 13(1): 49.
[http://dx.doi.org/10.1186/s13072-020-00371-7] [PMID: 33168103]

[13] Comprehensive genomic characterization defines human glioblastoma genes and core pathways. Nature 2008; 455(7216): 1061-8.
[http://dx.doi.org/10.1038/nature07385] [PMID: 18772890]

[14] Ross JA, Rosen GD. The molecular biology of lung cancer. Curr Opin Pulm Med 2002; 8(4): 265-9.
[http://dx.doi.org/10.1097/00063198-200207000-00004] [PMID: 12055387]

[15] Ding L, Getz G, Wheeler DA, *et al.* Somatic mutations affect key pathways in lung adenocarcinoma. Nature 2008; 455(7216): 1069-75.
[http://dx.doi.org/10.1038/nature07423] [PMID: 18948947]

[16] Han S, Liu Y, Cai SJ, *et al.* IDH mutation in glioma: molecular mechanisms and potential therapeutic targets. Br J Cancer 2020; 122(11): 1580-9.
[http://dx.doi.org/10.1038/s41416-020-0814-x] [PMID: 32291392]

[17] Nobusawa S, Watanabe T, Kleihues P, Ohgaki H. IDH1 mutations as molecular signature and predictive factor of secondary glioblastomas. Clin Cancer Res 2009; 15(19): 6002-7.
[http://dx.doi.org/10.1158/1078-0432.CCR-09-0715] [PMID: 19755387]

[18] Yan H, Parsons DW, Jin G, *et al.* IDH1 and IDH2 mutations in gliomas. N Engl J Med 2009; 360(8): 765-73.
[http://dx.doi.org/10.1056/NEJMoa0808710] [PMID: 19228619]

[19] Mardis ER, Wilson RK. Cancer genome sequencing: a review. Hum Mol Genet 2009; 18(R2): R163-8.
[http://dx.doi.org/10.1093/hmg/ddp396] [PMID: 19808792]

[20] Shah SP, Köbel M, Senz J, *et al.* Mutation of FOXL2 in granulosa-cell tumors of the ovary. N Engl J Med 2009; 360(26): 2719-29.
[http://dx.doi.org/10.1056/NEJMoa0902542] [PMID: 19516027]

[21] Wang J, Dean DC, Hornicek FJ, Shi H, Duan Z. RNA sequencing (RNA-Seq) and its application in ovarian cancer. Gynecol Oncol 2019; 152(1): 194-201.
[http://dx.doi.org/10.1016/j.ygyno.2018.10.002] [PMID: 30297273]

[22] Maher CA, Kumar-Sinha C, Cao X, *et al.* Transcriptome sequencing to detect gene fusions in cancer. Nature 2009; 458(7234): 97-101.

[http://dx.doi.org/10.1038/nature07638] [PMID: 19136943]

[23] Wyman SK, Parkin RK, Mitchell PS, *et al.* Repertoire of microRNAs in epithelial ovarian cancer as determined by next generation sequencing of small RNA cDNA libraries. PLoS One 2009; 4(4): e5311.
[http://dx.doi.org/10.1371/journal.pone.0005311] [PMID: 19390579]

[24] Cancer.Net/Genetic testing for cancer risk (https://www.cancer.net/navigating-cancer-care/canc-r-basics/genetics/genetic-testing-cancer-risk)

[25] Litton JK, Burstein HJ, Turner NC. Molecular testing in breast cancer. Am Soc Clin Oncol Educ Book 2019; 39(39): e1-7.
[http://dx.doi.org/10.1200/EDBK_237715] [PMID: 31099622]

[26] Lynch JA, Venne V, Berse B. Genetic tests to identify risk for breast cancer. Semin Oncol Nurs 2015; 31(2): 100-7.
[http://dx.doi.org/10.1016/j.soncn.2015.02.007] [PMID: 25951739]

[27] Campeau PM, Foulkes WD, Tischkowitz MD. Hereditary breast cancer: new genetic developments, new therapeutic avenues. Hum Genet 2008; 124(1): 31-42.
[http://dx.doi.org/10.1007/s00439-008-0529-1] [PMID: 18575892]

[28] Gage M, Wattendorf D, Henry LR. Translational advances regarding hereditary breast cancer syndromes. J Surg Oncol 2012; 105(5): 444-51.
[http://dx.doi.org/10.1002/jso.21856] [PMID: 22441895]

[29] Fostira F, Papadimitriou M, Papadimitriou C. Current practices on genetic testing in ovarian cancer. Ann Transl Med 2020; 8(24): 1703.
[http://dx.doi.org/10.21037/atm-20-1422] [PMID: 33490215]

[30] Alsop K, Fereday S, Meldrum C, *et al.* BRCA mutation frequency and patterns of treatment response in BRCA mutation-positive women with ovarian cancer: a report from the Australian Ovarian Cancer Study Group. J Clin Oncol 2012; 30(21): 2654-63.
[http://dx.doi.org/10.1200/JCO.2011.39.8545] [PMID: 22711857]

[31] Balchen V, Simon K. Colorectal cancer development and advances in screening. Clin Interv Aging 2016; 11: 967-76.
[http://dx.doi.org/10.2147/CIA.S109285] [PMID: 27486317]

[32] Kaz AM, Brentnall TA. Genetic testing for colon cancer. Nat Clin Pract Gastroenterol Hepatol 2006; 3(12): 670-9.
[http://dx.doi.org/10.1038/ncpgasthep0663] [PMID: 17130877]

[33] Calland JF, Adams RB, DePrince K, Foley EF, Powell SM. Genetic syndromes and genetic tests in colorectal cancer. Semin Gastrointest Dis 2000; 11(4): 207-18.
[PMID: 11057948]

[34] Levin B, Lieberman DA, McFarland B, *et al.* Screening and surveillance for the early detection of colorectal cancer and adenomatous polyps, 2008: a joint guideline from the American Cancer Society, the US Multi-Society Task Force on Colorectal Cancer, and the American College of Radiology. Gastroenterology 2008; 134(5): 1570-95.
[http://dx.doi.org/10.1053/j.gastro.2008.02.002] [PMID: 18384785]

[35] Binefa G, Rodríguez-Moranta F, Teule A, Medina-Hayas M. Colorectal cancer: From prevention to personalized medicine. World J Gastroenterol 2014; 20(22): 6786-808.
[http://dx.doi.org/10.3748/wjg.v20.i22.6786] [PMID: 24944469]

[36] Imperiale TF, Ransohoff DF, Itzkowitz SH, *et al.* Multitarget stool DNA testing for colorectal-cancer screening. N Engl J Med 2014; 370(14): 1287-97.
[http://dx.doi.org/10.1056/NEJMoa1311194] [PMID: 24645800]

[37] Russo A, Bazan V, Agnese V, Rodolico V, Gebbia N. Prognostic and predictive factors in colorectal cancer: Kirsten Ras in CRC (RASCAL) and TP53CRC collaborative studies. Ann Oncol 2005; 16

(Suppl. 4): iv44-9.
[http://dx.doi.org/10.1093/annonc/mdi907] [PMID: 15923428]

[38] Valle L, Vilar E, Tavtigian SV, Stoffel EM. Genetic predisposition to colorectal cancer: syndromes, genes, classification of genetic variants and implications for precision medicine. J Pathol 2019; 247(5): 574-88.
[http://dx.doi.org/10.1002/path.5229] [PMID: 30584801]

[39] Milne D. Genetic tests predict thyroid cancer risk, making preventive surgery possible. J Natl Cancer Inst 1994; 86(17): 1268-70.
[http://dx.doi.org/10.1093/jnci/86.17.1268] [PMID: 7914936]

[40] Ferrari SM, Fallahi P, Ruffilli I, *et al.* Molecular testing in the diagnosis of differentiated thyroid carcinomas. Gland Surg 2018; 7(S1) (Suppl. 1): S19-29.
[http://dx.doi.org/10.21037/gs.2017.11.07] [PMID: 30175060]

[41] Tang KT, Lee CH. BRAF mutation in papillary thyroid carcinoma: pathogenic role and clinical implications. J Chin Med Assoc 2010; 73(3): 113-28.
[http://dx.doi.org/10.1016/S1726-4901(10)70025-3] [PMID: 20230995]

[42] Utiger RD. Medullary thyroid carcinoma, genes, and the prevention of cancer. N Engl J Med 1994; 331(13): 870-1.
[http://dx.doi.org/10.1056/NEJM199409293311309] [PMID: 7915823]

[43] Mulligan LM, Eng C, Healey CS, *et al.* Specific mutations of the RET proto-oncogene are related to disease phenotype in MEN 2A and FMTC. Nat Genet 1994; 6(1): 70-4.
[http://dx.doi.org/10.1038/ng0194-70] [PMID: 7907913]

[44] Cheng H, Powers J, Schaffer K, Sartor O. Practical Methods for Integrating Genetic Testing Into Clinical Practice for Advanced Prostate Cancer. Am Soc Clin Oncol Educ Book 2018; 38(38): 372-81.
[http://dx.doi.org/10.1200/EDBK_205441] [PMID: 30231311]

[45] Brandão A, Paulo P, Teixeira MR. Hereditary Predisposition to Prostate Cancer: From Genetics to Clinical Implications. Int J Mol Sci 2020; 21(14): 5036.
[http://dx.doi.org/10.3390/ijms21145036] [PMID: 32708810]

[46] Zhen JT, Syed J, Nguyen KA, *et al.* Genetic testing for hereditary prostate cancer: Current status and limitations. Cancer 2018; 124(15): 3105-17.
[http://dx.doi.org/10.1002/cncr.31316] [PMID: 29669169]

[47] Reznik R, Hendifar AE, Tuli R. Genetic determinants and potential therapeutic targets for pancreatic adenocarcinoma. Front Physiol 2014; 5: 87.
[http://dx.doi.org/10.3389/fphys.2014.00087] [PMID: 24624093]

[48] Ghiorzo P. Genetic predisposition to pancreatic cancer. World J Gastroenterol 2014; 20(31): 10778 89.
[http://dx.doi.org/10.3748/wjg.v20.i31.10778] [PMID: 25152581]

[49] Rustgi AK. Familial pancreatic cancer: genetic advances. Genes Dev 2014; 28(1): 1-7.
[http://dx.doi.org/10.1101/gad.228452.113] [PMID: 24395243]

[50] Kartal K, Guan Z, Tang R, *et al.* Familial pancreatic cancer: who should be considered for genetic testing? Ir J Med Sci 2022; 191: 641-50.
[http://dx.doi.org/10.1007/s11845-021-02572-9] [PMID: 33733397]

[51] Parikh AR. Lung Cancer Genomics. Acta Med Acad 2019; 48(1): 78-83.
[http://dx.doi.org/10.5644/ama2006-124.244] [PMID: 31264435]

[52] Fois SS, Paliogiannis P, Zinellu A, Fois AG, Cossu A, Palmieri G. Molecular epidemiology of the main druggable genetic alterations in non-small cell lung cancer. Int J Mol Sci 2021; 22(2): 612.
[http://dx.doi.org/10.3390/ijms22020612] [PMID: 33435440]

[53] Li T, Kung HJ, Mack PC, Gandara DR. Genotyping and genomic profiling of non-small-cell lung

cancer: implications for current and future therapies. J Clin Oncol 2013; 31(8): 1039-49. [http://dx.doi.org/10.1200/JCO.2012.45.3753] [PMID: 23401433]

[54] Popper HH, Ryska A, Tímár J, Olszewski W. Molecular testing in lung cancer in the era of precision medicine. Transl Lung Cancer Res 2014; 3(5): 291-300. [PMID: 25806314]

[55] Lazarus DR, Ost DE. How and when to use genetic markers for nonsmall cell lung cancer. Curr Opin Pulm Med 2013; 19(4): 1. [http://dx.doi.org/10.1097/MCP.0b013e328362075c] [PMID: 23715289]

[56] Cadranel J, Zalcman G, Sequist L. Genetic profiling and epidermal growth factor receptor-directed therapy in nonsmall cell lung cancer. Eur Respir J 2011; 37(1): 183-93. [http://dx.doi.org/10.1183/09031936.00179409] [PMID: 21030453]

[57] Lynde CW, Sapra S. Predictive testing of the melanocortin 1 receptor for skin cancer and photoaging. Skin Therapy Lett 2010; 15(1): 5-7. [PMID: 20066389]

[58] Wilson MA, Nathanson KL. Molecular testing in melanoma. Cancer J 2012; 18(2): 117-23. [http://dx.doi.org/10.1097/PPO.0b013e31824f11bf] [PMID: 22453011]

[59] Chapman PB, Hauschild A, Robert C, *et al.* Improved survival with vemurafenib in melanoma with BRAF V600E mutation. N Engl J Med 2011; 364(26): 2507-16. [http://dx.doi.org/10.1056/NEJMoa1103782] [PMID: 21639808]

[60] Cheng L, Lopez-Beltran A, Massari F, MacLennan GT, Montironi R. Molecular testing for BRAF mutations to inform melanoma treatment decisions: a move toward precision medicine. Mod Pathol 2018; 31(1): 24-38. [http://dx.doi.org/10.1038/modpathol.2017.104] [PMID: 29148538]

[61] Potrony M, Badenas C, Aguilera P, *et al.* Update in genetic susceptibility in melanoma. Ann Transl Med 2015; 3(15): 210. [PMID: 26488006]

[62] Gabree M, Seidel M. Genetic testing by cancer site: skin. Cancer J 2012; 18(4): 372-80. [http://dx.doi.org/10.1097/PPO.0b013e3182624664] [PMID: 22846740]

[63] Brown S, Brennan P, Rajan N. Inherited skin tumour syndromes. Clin Med (Lond) 2017; 17(6): 562-7. [http://dx.doi.org/10.7861/clinmedicine.17-6-562] [PMID: 29196359]

[64] Prokop JW, May T, Strong K, *et al.* Genome sequencing in the clinic: the past, present, and future of genomic medicine. Physiol Genomics 2018; 50(8): 563-79. [http://dx.doi.org/10.1152/physiolgenomics.00046.2018] [PMID: 29727589]

[65] Meyerson M, Gabriel S, Getz G. Advances in understanding cancer genomes through second-generation sequencing. Nat Rev Genet 2010; 11(10): 685-96. [http://dx.doi.org/10.1038/nrg2841] [PMID: 20847746]

[66] Bosdet IE, Docking TR, Butterfield YS, *et al.* A clinically validated diagnostic second-generation sequencing assay for detection of hereditary BRCA1 and BRCA2 mutations. J Mol Diagn 2013; 15(6): 796-809. [http://dx.doi.org/10.1016/j.jmoldx.2013.07.004] [PMID: 24094589]

[67] Zehir A, Benayed R, Shah RH, *et al.* Erratum: Mutational landscape of metastatic cancer revealed from prospective clinical sequencing of 10,000 patients. Nat Med 2017; 23(8): 1004. [http://dx.doi.org/10.1038/nm0817-1004c] [PMID: 28777785]

[68] Jones SJM, Laskin J, Li YY, *et al.* Evolution of an adenocarcinoma in response to selection by targeted kinase inhibitors. Genome Biol 2010; 11(8): R82. [http://dx.doi.org/10.1186/gb-2010-11-8-r82] [PMID: 20696054]

[69] Jackman SD, Vandervalk BP, Mohamadi H, *et al.* ABySS 2.0: resource-efficient assembly of large

genomes using a Bloom filter. Genome Res 2017; 27(5): 768-77.
[http://dx.doi.org/10.1101/gr.214346.116] [PMID: 28232478]

[70] Laskin J, Jones S, Aparicio S, *et al.* Lessons learned from the application of whole-genome analysis to the treatment of patients with advanced cancers. Molecular Case Studies 2015; 1(1): a000570.
[http://dx.doi.org/10.1101/mcs.a000570] [PMID: 27148575]

[71] Zhao EY, Jones M, Jones SJM. Whole-Genome Sequencing in Cancer. Cold Spring Harb Perspect Med 2019; 9(3): a034579.
[http://dx.doi.org/10.1101/cshperspect.a034579] [PMID: 29844223]

CHAPTER 6

Circulating Tumour DNA: A Promising Cancer Biomarker

Sharmin Aktar[1,2], **Plabon Kumar Das**[3], **Vinod Gopalan**[1], **Alfred King-yin Lam**[1,4] and **Farhadul Islam**[5,*]

[1] *School of Medicine, Menzies Health Institute Queensland, Griffith University, Gold Coast, Australia*

[2] *Department of Biochemistry and Molecular Biology, Mawlana Bhashani Science and Technology University, Tangail-1902, Bangladesh*

[3] *Institute for Glycomics, Griffith University, Gold Coast, Australia*

[4] *Pathology Queensland, Gold Coast University Hospital, Gold Coast, Australia*

[5] *Department of Biochemistry and Molecular Biology, University of Rajshahi, Rajshahi-6205, Bangladesh*

Abstract: Liquid biopsies, such as tumor-relevant proteins, miRNAs, circulating tumour cells (CTC) and cell-free DNA (cfDNA), have all been shown to have promising potential to be used as cancer biomarkers. However, the sensitivity and specificity of these biomarkers are currently insufficient, prohibiting their widespread application in clinical practice. Circulating tumour DNA (ctDNA) has received a lot of attention in recent years as a potential diagnostic and prognostic tool. Since tumours release genetic material, (*i. e.* ctDNA) into the bloodstream before they are apparent on imaging or cause symptoms, thus, ctDNA is one of the most promising liquid biopsy biomarkers for early diagnosis, prognosis, and treatment monitoring of patients with cancer. Accordingly, extensive preclinical and clinical research support that ctDNA has the potential to be considered a novel tool in early cancer diagnosis and prognosis. Also, ctDNA analysis can reliably predict tumour growth and treatment efficacy, as well as can aid in targeted therapy. Herein, this chapter will discuss the clinical significance of ctDNA in the management of patients with cancer as a potential liquid biopsy biomarker.

Keywords: Cancer biomarkers, Circulating tumour DNA (ctDNA), Early cancer detection, Liquid biopsy, Prognosis, Risk of relapse, Treatment efficacy.

[*] **Corresponding author Farhadul Islam:** Department of Biochemistry and Molecular Biology, University of Rajshahi, Rajshahi-6205, Bangladesh; Email: farhad_bio83@ru.ac.bd

INTRODUCTION

A number of traditional pathological examinations, such as tissue biopsy and imaging technologies, are used to diagnose cancers in clinical settings presently. Though tissue biopsy and imaging-based tumour diagnosis are considered the gold standard, they have numerous limitations, such as being ineffective for early-stage tumours or residual lesions detection. Also, limited application in assessing the treatment efficacy and prognosis of the disease [1]. As a result, a new branch of oncology research has emerged in recent years that focuses on cancer-derived components that circulate in the bloodstream [2].

Hence, over the last few years, a novel diagnostic approach known as "liquid biopsy"— the analysis of tumours using biomarkers circulating in peripheral blood such as circulating tumour cells (CTCs) and circulating cell-free tumour DNA (ctDNA) as well as exosomes, Tumour-relevant protein molecules and miRNAs- has gotten a lot of attention [2 - 9]. Liquid biopsy currently has a high specificity, allowing for the collection of consistent and reliable data from a blood sample in a simple and non-invasive manner [10]. Liquid biopsies are more convenient than traditional biopsies, and they pose no risk to the patient [4, 11]. Therefore, it is becoming increasingly popular as emerging tumour-specific markers for diagnosis and prognosis. Tumour-relevant protein molecules and miRNAs as well as circulating tumour cells (CTC), have all been demonstrated to be acceptable tumour biomarkers as a liquid biopsy in different cancers [5 - 9]. For example, large-scale clinical investigations have focused on the use of CTC counts as prognosis and monitoring therapy response in various cancer patients in recent years [3, 4]. However, the sensitivity and specificity of these biomarkers are currently inadequate, preventing their broader use in clinical practise. As a result, the development of new, highly sensitive, and specific tumour biomarkers is needed for better management of patients with cancer.

At the early stage of cancer, the tumours are small, less complex, and non-metastatic; milder therapy is more likely to be effective and could improve the survival of patients along with their quality of life [12]. Thus, there is a great need to develop accurate tests for the early detection of cancer. During tumour apoptosis or necrosis, tumour cells and CTCs may release their genetic materials into the bloodstream which is called ctDNA [13]. Since ctDNA is released into the circulation before tumours are visible on imaging or produce symptoms, *i. e.,* at early stages, hence ctDNA is considered one of the most promising biomarkers among liquid biopsy for early cancer diagnosis [14]. As the mutations of the original tumour are preserved, researchers have discovered that screening genetic lesions using ctDNA is very sensitive and specific, implying that employing ctDNA as a liquid biopsy could greatly improve current tumour diagnosis and prognosis outcome [1]. For example, ctDNA levels are higher in patients at advanced stages of breast, colorectal, pancreatic and gastro-esophageal cancer than in early-stage patients [1, 15]. ctDNA analysis can also reliably predict tumour growth and prognosis, as well as aid in targeted therapy [16 - 18]. Furthermore, as a result of recent breakthroughs in ctDNA analysis, a number of studies have recently described the potential efficacy of their application in cancer management [4, 19]. Herein, the focus of this chapter is on the clinical implications of ctDNA as a critical component of liquid biopsies in cancer patients.

CIRCULATING TUMOR DNA (CTDNA)

Biology of ctDNA

Tumor DNA can be discharged into the bloodstream of cancer patients by primary tumours, CTCs, micrometastasis, or overt metastases during disease progression [1, 4, 13]. The majority of this ctDNA comes from tumour cells that have died or necrotized and released their fragmented DNA into the bloodstream [13]. ctDNA makes up only a small percentage of the total cell-free DNA (cfDNA), generally inferred by the detection of somatic variants [10]. In 1948, Mandel and Métais discovered non-cellular nucleic acids in the bloodstream of cancer patients [20], and this was the first time cfDNA was reported [3]. cfDNA may present outside of cells in body fluids such as plasma, urine, and cerebrospinal fluid (CSF) [21]. The majority of cfDNA in plasma originates from leukocytes, while only a minor percentage is tumour□derived (ctDNA) [21].

ctDNA fragments are slightly shorter nucleosome-associated fragments (80-200bp) [22]. However, the size of ctDNA fragments is still unknown, some researchers believe it is longer than its corresponding non-tumor cell-free DNA (cfDNA), while others believe it is shorter [1]. Recently Jiang *et al.* noted that the plasma of liver cancer patients had both long and short DNA molecules (<150 bp, 150-180 bp, and >180 bp), with the short fragments containing the tumor-relevant copy number aberrations [23]. The proportion of DNA fragments shorter than 150 bp and the tumour DNA fraction in plasma had a positive correlation, whereas the proportion of DNA fragments with sizes between 150 and 180 bp and tumor DNA fraction in plasma had no correlation. The proportion of DNA longer than 180 bp and the tumour DNA fraction in plasma were found to have a negative correlation. A similar phenomenon was also described by Madhavan *et al.* in patients with breast cancer [24].

In plasma or serum, ctDNA can be found as single-stranded or double-stranded DNA [1]. In principle, ctDNA contains genetic abnormalities that are identical to those found in tumour cells [25]. Plasma samples are preferred over serum samples for ctDNA analysis as plasma samples may become contaminated with the DNA released into the bloodstream from lysed background cells (leukocytes) during the clotting process [3]. Though the half-life of ctDNA is yet unknown, some cfDNA studies have highlighted its short lifespan (16 min to 2.5 h) [22, 26, 27]. The short half-life of ctDNA, ctDNA levels can provide a 'real-time' assessment of entire solid tumor mass presence in patients [1, 22, 28]. However, the plasma clearance of cfDNA *via* the liver, spleen, and kidney, lead researchers to examine ctDNA in urine to better understand the potential utility of urine sample for the detection of the tumor [29]. Furthermore, blood enzymes, such as DNases, may digest circulating DNA, allowing it to be partially cleared from the bloodstream at the time of examination [29].

The Mechanism of ctDNA Entry into the Bloodstream

A growing body of information indicated the potential of ctDNA as a cancer biomarker, however, the processes by which tumour DNA reaches the bloodstream remain largely unknown. Apoptosis, necrosis, CTC lysis, and active secretion from tumour cells have all been proposed as routes for ctDNA release into the circulation [13]. Apoptosis, also known as programmed cell death, causes the death of cells to release ctDNA in the form of nucleosome-associated fragments (-166 bp), as evidenced by electrophoresis [1]. The macrophages consume and digest the majority of freed nucleosomes; however, this clearance system can become overburdened or compromised as a result of tumour growth and increased cell death, resulting in excessive amounts of nucleosomes entering the bloodstream [1]. ctDNA may also be released *via* necrosis, especially the partially digested circulating DNA [1]. Cancer patients in advanced stages with a substantial number of necrotic tumour cells have more plasma ctDNA than those in early stages [30].

However, apoptotic or necrotic tumour cells are not the only sources of ctDNA. Evidences showed *that* living tumour cells can also release ctDNA into circulation [31]. This could explain patients with early-stage cancer can also have detectable ctDNA [1]. Furthermore, levels of ctDNA presence in the blood rise with tumour growth [13], implying that ctDNA is released from active tumour cells [32]. Evidence also supports that CTC might be another source of ctDNA [30], as ctDNA and CTC contain identical mutational copies of genes. CTCs are able to evade the phagocytic activity of macrophages and consequently can be shed into the bloodstream [1]. These cells undergo lysis and release circulating DNA into the bloodstream. However, CTC is only found in a small percentage of peripheral blood, thus, ctDNA from CTC may not be the primary source (Fig. **1**) [1].

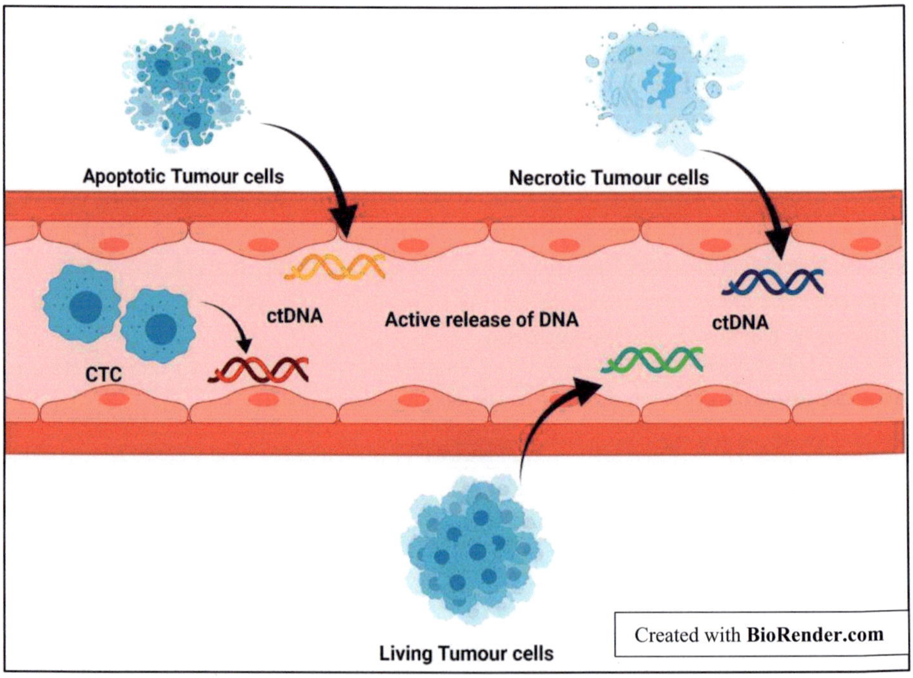

Fig. (1). Entry of ctDNA into the Bloodstream. Apoptosis, necrosis, living tumour cells and CTC lysis release ctDNA into circulation. Cells, which have died due to apoptosis or necrosis, released their fragmented DNA into the bloodstream. Also, in living tumour cells, CTCs can release ctDNA directly into circulation. CTCs may undergo lysis due to the phagocytic activity of macrophages and release circulating DNA into the bloodstream.

Detection of ctDNA

ctDNA contains the same mutations as the corresponding genomic DNA in the primary tumour, thus, researchers have tried to take advantage of this fact to develop assays that could be used in cancer management in clinical settings. As ctDNA makes up a very small percentage of total cfDNA, often less than 0.01% [26, 33], hence more sensitive and specific technologies need to be established for ctDNA detection and analysis. Over the past few years, extensive research has been performed on the development of effective technologies for ctDNA detection and analysis. Both tumour-dependent and independent methods have been developed and used for ctDNA analysis. For tumour dependent approach, tumor-guided analysis of plasma DNA is performed, which needs prior knowledge of mutations specific to the corresponding primary tumor [34]. Generally, this is accomplished by analysing a biopsy or tumour specimen, selecting markers to probe (*i.e.*, to detect mutations), and evaluating those markers in plasma [34]. This assay is mainly performed using PCR (*e.g.*, digital PCR, droplet digital PCR,

BEAMing (beads, emulsion, amplification, and magnetics), digital PCR, and amplification-refractory mutation system (ARMS)-PCR) [35, 36]. In the case of tumor-independent analysis, which requires no prior knowledge of mutations in the original tumour [34]. Sanger sequencing, next-generation sequencing (NGS) are the most commonly used methods for untargeted ctDNA analysis [35]. In some circumstances, pre-existing knowledge of frequent mutations seen in cancer subtypes, such as mutations in the KRAS2, CDKN2A, and TP53 genes for pancreatic cancer, guides such investigation [34]. The latter approach can be useful for early cancer detection if a large panel of the most frequently mutated genes for the relevant malignancy could be utilised for cancer screening [34].

Despite being exceedingly sensitive, fast, and relatively inexpensive, PCR-based assays are constrained by low multiplexing capacity, allowing only a limited number of loci to be analysed concurrently [36]. Hence, the second approach, especially Sanger sequencing, is used to identify plasma ctDNA. However, several drawbacks to Sanger-based ctDNA detection, including low throughput, time-consuming methods, expensive, and the possibility of PCR bias, which limit their potential application in point-of-care facilities [1, 32]. Thus, numerous viable and convenient alternatives to Sanger sequencing, such as BEAMing, CAPP-seq, and NGS technologies, have been developed in the recent decade [1].

The BEAMing is a tumour-dependent technique, in which the DNA fragment is amplified with primers that contain known tag sequences and then covalently bonded to magnetic beads [26]. Flow cytometry is then used to sort the beads that carry the mutation. CAPP-seq (cancer personalised profiling by deep sequencing) is another new technology developed by Newman *et al.* for quantifying ctDNA, where a probe panel with biotinylated DNA oligonucleotides has been used to target recurrently mutated areas in the tumour [31]. Using this technique, ctDNA was found in 100% of stage II-IV and 50% of stage I NSCLC patients, with 96% specificity for mutant allele fractions down to ~0.02% [32]. These new techniques have much higher sensitivity for detecting ctDNA than prior methods. They are also low-cost and high throughput. Thus, these "second generation" sequencing techniques have improved the evaluation of the clinical potential of ctDNA analysis. Additionally, Third-generation sequencing approaches, such as NGS-based technologies, have been intended to be highly sensitive, inexpensive and have the potential to speed up the widespread use of ctDNA detection in routine analysis of patients with cancer. These unique techniques, however, have some limitations. For example, NGS-based approaches yield an informative diagnosis in around 50% of early-stage patients, implying that sensitivity needs to be improved [32, 33]. Furthermore, the expenses are still very high, which limits their use in clinical practice.

ctDNA as a Promising Biomarker in Cancer Diagnosis and Prognosis

The extremely heterogeneous and constantly evolving nature of tumors causes more often tissue biopsy-based tests to fail to predict tumor progression accurately [1]. In addition, small and residual lesions followed by therapeutic intervention are not detected by tissue biopsy-based techniques. Thus, in recent years, plasma-based biomarkers with minimal invasion and satisfactory conformity, have held the promise to predict tumor occurrence, progression, and monitoring therapy response and recurrence [6]. However, these plasma-based biomarkers approaches have limited sensitivity and specificity and, thus, often fail to meet the clinical requirements [30, 33]. Considering the limitations of all existing plasma-based methods, analysing ctDNA is a clinically accepted replacement of tissue biopsies with the ability to provide information about the molecular make-up of the entire tumor burden more accurately [34, 35]. Also, ctDNA has the potential to be used where the primary location of tumour is unknown, particularly in late-stage disease diagnostic settings [34]. Preclinical studies and clinical trials are pointing out towards extremely promising capacity of ctDNA as a very dynamic tool for detecting metastases, monitoring treatment efficacy, and even in the determination of suitable therapeutic strategies. The role of ctDNA as a promising biomarker in cancer diagnosis, prognosis, treatment decision and disease monitoring is described below.

ctDNA as Diagnostic Biomarker

ctDNA may offer a non-invasive, low-risk and easy to be performed test for the early detection of cancer, thus, it could provide a better opportunity to treat patients as the disease is more treatable if diagnosed early [28, 37]. Also, the levels of ctDNA correlated with the advancement of cancer, thus, it could be used to stratify patients with cancer. For example, patients with advanced gastro-esophageal, pancreatic, breast and colorectal cancers had higher levels of ctDNA when compared to patients with early stages of those diseases [30]. Furthermore, ctDNAs hold more promise than protein biomarkers as ctDNAs may be more informative, accurate, and specific [38]. For instance, a clinical test performance for the blood-based diagnostic gene signature suggested that ctDNA analysis is a specific, non-invasive test when compared with conventional clinical histopathology reporting of the resected tissues in patients with lung cancer [37]. The sensitivity of ctDNA analysis was 75% (95% CI, 67%-81%) and specificity was 89% (95% CI, 70%-98%), while the positive predictive value was 98% (95% CI, 93%-100%), and the negative predictive value was 35% (95% CI, 24%-48%). Another study by Bettegowda *et al.* investigated the roles of ctDNA in tumour identification in patients with diverse cancer types [30]. It was noted that ctDNA was detected in more than 75% of individuals with localised disease, when their chances of a good outcome are the best. Even in individuals with stage I, where surgery is usually invariably curative, 47% of patients had measurable quantities of ctDNA in their blood samples. More than two-thirds of patients with stage III disease, which are curable in certain forms of cancer, had detectable ctDNA. They also found ctDNA in patients without detectable circulating tumor cells [30]. In a separate cohort of 206 patients with metastatic colorectal cancers, they showed that the sensitivity of ctDNA for detection of clinically relevant *KRAS* mutations was 87.2%, and its specificity was 99.2% [30]. Another study conducted by Dawson *et al.*, comparing the efficacy of ctDNA, CTC, and CA15-3, in 30 metastatic breast cancer patients, suggested that the detection rate of ctDNA was 97%, higher than CTC (78%) and CA15-3 (87%) [39].

Detection of ctDNA along with other markers such as protein markers in cancer patients might be more efficient than using those markers alone. A recent study noted a better diagnosis of patients with various types of cancer when they combined potential protein biomarkers with ctDNA in the detection of cancer [40]. They described a multi-analytes blood test, called CancerSEEK, that uses combined assays for determining the levels of circulating proteins and mutations in ctDNA and may not only detect the presence of early malignancies but also pinpoint the organ of these tumour origin . About 78% for stage III cancers, 73% of sensitivity for stage II, cancers and 43% for stage I cancers with almost 100% specificity were found when they used this CancerSEEK blood test [40]. Considering the lower sensitivity of ctDNA marker in early-stage cancer than in advanced stages, the clinical utility of ctDNA in the diagnosis of early-stage cancer is less promising [41]. Furthermore, methylated epigenetic ctDNA markers may play a role as the most promising candidates for screening of patients with various cancers [42].

ctDNA as Prognostic Biomarker

Along with its potential diagnostic benefits, ctDNA analysis could be used as a promising prognostic tool in cancer management [28]. It was noted that poorer survival rates were associated with patients with a detectable amount of ctDNA in their plasma when compared to patients without ctDNA [43, 44]. For example, in pancreatic cancer, 50% of patients (N = 52) had shown detectable ctDNA levels and had significantly worse overall and progression-free survival than ctDNA negative patients (8.4 *vs.* 16 months for overall; 3.2 *vs.* 7.9 months for progression-free survival) [45]. In another study, ctDNA showed prognostic significance in early stage (I-III) CRC patients (n=25). The study found that 68% patients had two-year recurrence-free survival when ctDNA was detected. On the other hand, recurrence-free survival rate was 100% for the patients with no detectable ctDNA [46]. Also, a higher disease control rate (42%) was noted in patients with lower ctDNA levels (<25% quartile) when compared to almost 0% disease control rate with higher ctDNA levels (>75% quartile) [47]. Moreover, higher levels of ctDNA were reported with higher tumour load [46, 48, 49].

Additionally, as quantitative ctDNA analysis reflects disease progression, thus, ctDNA analysis is suitable for monitoring treatment response [28]. Short half-life (16 min to 2.5 h) of ctDNA lead rapidly drop, followed by surgical removal of tumor tissue [26, 50], and this biological property allows ctDNA to be used as a marker for disease monitoring and treatment response [1, 22, 28]. A study reported the potential of ctDNA to detect minimal residual disease in 1046 plasma samples from a prospective cohort of 230 patients with resected stage II colon cancer [51]. In patients who did not receive adjuvant chemotherapy, ctDNA was found in 14 of 178 patients (7.9%), and recurrence was found in 11 of these 14 patients during follow-up (78.6%). The presence of ctDNA following chemotherapy was likewise linked to a shorter recurrence-free survival in patients who had had chemotherapy [51]. Also, in another study, ctDNA was detected in patients with stage I-III colorectal carcinomas and higher levels of ctDNA were associated with shorter relapse-free survival within 3 months after surgery [52, 53].. Therefore, the detection of ctDNA levels, in both pre and post-operative stages of cancer, could be utilized as a potential prognostic marker. In addition, in a randomized phase III clinical trial (NCT01103323), as a pre-treatment and alternative modality, the utility of circulating DNA as a prognostic parameter was demonstrated in metastatic CRC (mCRC) [54]. It was noted that high baseline circulating DNA concentrations were associated with shorter median overall survival and progression-free survival in placebo-treated patients, whereas treatment with regorafenib provides a consistent overall and progression-free survival benefit in a variety of subgroups of patients with metastatic colorectal cancer. These findings illustrate the value of circulating tumour DNA in determining tumour genotype in clinical decision-making. Furthermore, higher ctDNA levels contribute to treatment resistance in numerous cancer types [30, 39, 55 - 57]. Thus, ctDNA analysis can be useful in predicting the risk of disease relapse. In colorectal cancer, detection of ctDNA could potentially predict post-surgery relapse of disease with nearly 100% sensitivity and specificity [58]. Therefore, ctDNA could be used as a potential diagnostic and prognostic tool in cancer, along with its implications in measuring therapy response.

Challenges

Despite the promising diagnostic and prognostic significance of ctDNA, there are a number of challenges that limit their application in clinical practices. The limitations include a lack of standardized procedures for collecting and extracting ctDNA from serum or plasma, the need for prior knowledge of specific mutations of the particular tumour types, *etc*. Pre-analytical variables, such as incorrect specimen collection or blood processing methods, have varying effects on cfDNA level, quality, and downstream molecular applications, which could reduce the levels of ctDNA in the samples [21]. Lysis of cfDNA during the clotting process of blood cells in collection tubes, some studies have identified substantially higher cfDNA levels in serum than in plasma [3, 59, 60], posing additional problems for detecting low-level somatic mutations [21].

Beyond the above issues, ctDNA-based assays also face a number of difficulties, including a lower fraction of ctDNA in total cfDNA in the peripheral blood (sometimes 1% or even less < 0.01%) [26, 33] and need prior knowledge of specific mutations, which can be difficult to obtain in point-of-care settings [1]. Furthermore, despite the potential of ctDNA in early cancer diagnosis, one of the key obstacles to using ctDNA testing as a screening tool is the risk of overdiagnosis due to false positive tests [29]. Cancer-associated mutations can appear even in people as they get older who never get cancer during their lives [4]. For example, mutations in both TP53 and KRAS have been found in skin biopsies of healthy people who have never had cancer [61]. As a result, developing methods for detecting ctDNA that improve specificity and sensitivity is critical for clinical usage of ctDNA. Hence, appropriate standards and guidelines must be addressed before broad clinical applications.

Another challenge is that ctDNA is found to be higher in the majority of stage II–IV diseases [32, 40]. For instance, Newman *et al.* detected ctDNA in 100% of patients with stage II-IV NSCLC and only in 50% of patients with stage I. The abundance of ctDNA in patients with stage I tumors was 10 times lower than the patients in an advanced stage of the disease [32]. Thus, technological improvements are warranted to reach an acceptable sensitivity for early cancer detection using ctDNA.

CONCLUSION

In the realm of precision oncology, ctDNA analysis is a rapidly growing and promising technique as a non-invasive blood-based biomarker with the potential for considerable clinical effect. Despite some discrepancies, due to its non-invasive nature, ctDNA analysis may offer potential applications in disease diagnosis, monitoring therapy efficacy and patient response to treatment over time. In late-stage disease diagnostic settings, ctDNA has the potential to be routinely utilised to make a clinical decision, especially when biopsies are difficult to obtain or when the main location of the cancer is uncertain. In the future, it can also be used in early-stage disease diagnosis. Hence, extensive studies still need to improve the ctDNA detection techniques, which will minimize the limitations as well as for broad clinical implementation.

CONSENT FOR PUBLICATION

Not applicable.

CONFLICT OF INTEREST

The authors declare no conflict of interest, financial or otherwise.

ACKNOWLEDGEMENT

The authors would like to thank Griffith University for providing technical and logistic assistance. The authors also wish to thank other members of the cancer molecular pathology group, Griffith University, Australia, for their valuable suggestions.

REFERENCES

[1] Cheng F, Su L, Qian C. Circulating tumor DNA: a promising biomarker in the liquid biopsy of cancer. Oncotarget 2016; 7(30): 48832-41. [http://dx.doi.org/10.18632/oncotarget.9453] [PMID: 27223063]

[2] Siravegna G, Marsoni S, Siena S, Bardelli A. Integrating liquid biopsies into the management of cancer. Nat Rev Clin Oncol 2017; 14(9): 531-48. [http://dx.doi.org/10.1038/nrclinonc.2017.14] [PMID: 28252003]

[3] Osumi H, Shinozaki E, Yamaguchi K, Zembutsu H. Clinical utility of circulating tumor DNA for colorectal cancer. Cancer Sci 2019; 110(4): 1148-55. [http://dx.doi.org/10.1111/cas.13972] [PMID: 30742729]

[4] Alix-Panabières C, Pantel K. Clinical applications of circulating tumor cells and circulating tumor DNA as liquid biopsy. Cancer Discov 2016; 6(5): 479-91. [http://dx.doi.org/10.1158/2159-8290.CD-15-1483] [PMID: 26969689]

[5] Ballehaninna UK, Chamberlain RS. Serum CA 19-9 as a biomarker for pancreatic cancer—a comprehensive review. Indian J Surg Oncol 2011; 2(2): 88-100. [http://dx.doi.org/10.1007/s13193-011-0042-1] [PMID: 22693400]

[6] Mäbert K, Cojoc M, Peitzsch C, Kurth I, Souchelnytskyi S, Dubrovska A. Cancer biomarker discovery: Current status and future perspectives. Int J Radiat Biol 2014; 90(8): 659-77. [http://dx.doi.org/10.3109/09553002.2014.892229] [PMID: 24524284]

[7] Kosaka N, Iguchi H, Ochiya T. Circulating microRNA in body fluid: a new potential biomarker for cancer diagnosis and prognosis. Cancer Sci 2010; 101(10): 2087-92. [http://dx.doi.org/10.1111/j.1349-7006.2010.01650.x] [PMID: 20624164]

[8] Yap TA, Lorente D, Omlin A, Olmos D, de Bono JS. Circulating tumor cells: a multifunctional biomarker. Clin Cancer Res 2014; 20(10): 2553-68. [http://dx.doi.org/10.1158/1078-0432.CCR-13-2664] [PMID: 24831278]

[9] Shen J, Hu Q, Schrauder M, *et al.* Circulating miR-148b and miR-133a as biomarkers for breast cancer detection. Oncotarget 2014; 5(14): 5284-94. [http://dx.doi.org/10.18632/oncotarget.2014] [PMID: 25051376]

[10] Crowley E, Di Nicolantonio F, Loupakis F, Bardelli A. Liquid biopsy: monitoring cancer-genetics in the blood. Nat Rev Clin Oncol 2013; 10(8): 472-84. [http://dx.doi.org/10.1038/nrclinonc.2013.110] [PMID: 23836314]

[11] Merker JD, Oxnard GR, Compton C, *et al.* Circulating tumor DNA analysis in patients with cancer: American Society of Clinical Oncology and College of American Pathologists joint review. Arch Pathol Lab Med 2018; 142(10): 1242-53. [http://dx.doi.org/10.5858/arpa.2018-0901-SA] [PMID: 29504834]

[12] Aravanis AM, Lee M, Klausner RD. Next-generation sequencing of circulating tumor DNA for early cancer detection. Cell 2017; 168(4): 571-4. [http://dx.doi.org/10.1016/j.cell.2017.01.030] [PMID: 28187279]

[13] Stroun M, Maurice P, Vasioukhin V, *et al.* The origin and mechanism of circulating DNA. Ann N Y Acad Sci 2000; 906(1): 161-8. [http://dx.doi.org/10.1111/j.1749-6632.2000.tb06608.x] [PMID: 10818614]

[14] Fiala C, Kulasingam V, Diamandis EP. Circulating tumor dna for early cancer detection. J Appl Lab Med 2018; 3(2): 300-13. [http://dx.doi.org/10.1373/jalm.2018.026393] [PMID: 33636948]

[15] Bettegowda C, Sausen M, Leary RJ, *et al.* Detection of circulating tumor DNA in early-and late-stage human malignancies . Science translational medicine. 2014;6(224):224ra24-ra24.

[16] Martignetti JA, Camacho-Vanegas O, Priedigkeit N, *et al.* Personalized ovarian cancer disease surveillance and detection of candidate therapeutic drug target in circulating tumor DNA. Neoplasia 2014; 16(1): 97-W29. [http://dx.doi.org/10.1593/neo.131900] [PMID: 24563622]

[17] Bidard FC, Madic J, Mariani P, *et al.* Detection rate and prognostic value of circulating tumor cells and circulating tumor DNA in metastatic uveal melanoma. Int J Cancer 2014; 134(5): 1207-13. [http://dx.doi.org/10.1002/ijc.28436] [PMID: 23934701]

[18] Romero D. Tracking ctDNA to evaluate relapse risk. Nat Rev Clin Oncol 2015; 12(11): 624. [http://dx.doi.org/10.1038/nrclinonc.2015.159] [PMID: 26370605]

[19] Lebofsky R, Decraene C, Bernard V, *et al.* Circulating tumor DNA as a non-invasive substitute to metastasis biopsy for tumor genotyping and personalized medicine in a prospective trial across all tumor types. Mol Oncol 2015; 9(4): 783-90. [http://dx.doi.org/10.1016/j.molonc.2014.12.003] [PMID: 25579085]

[20] Mandel P, Metais P. Nuclear Acids In Human Blood Plasma. C R Seances Soc Biol Fil 1948; 142(3-4): 241-3. [PMID: 18875018]

[21] Stewart CM, Kothari PD, Mouliere F, *et al.* The value of cell-free DNA for molecular pathology. J Pathol 2018; 244(5): 616-27. [http://dx.doi.org/10.1002/path.5048] [PMID: 29380875]

[22] Wan JCM, Massie C, Garcia-Corbacho J, *et al.* Liquid biopsies come of age: towards implementation of circulating tumour DNA. Nat Rev Cancer 2017; 17(4): 223-38. [http://dx.doi.org/10.1038/nrc.2017.7] [PMID: 28233803]

[23] Jiang P, Chan CWM, Chan KCA, *et al.* Lengthening and shortening of plasma DNA in hepatocellular carcinoma patients. Proc Natl Acad Sci USA 2015; 112(11): E1317-25. [http://dx.doi.org/10.1073/pnas.1500076112] [PMID: 25646427]

[24] Madhavan D, Wallwiener M, Bents K, *et al.* Plasma DNA integrity as a biomarker for primary and metastatic breast cancer and potential marker for early diagnosis. Breast Cancer Res Treat 2014; 146(1): 163-74. [http://dx.doi.org/10.1007/s10549-014-2946-2] [PMID: 24838941]

[25] Bardelli A, Pantel K. Liquid biopsies, what we do not know (yet). Cancer Cell 2017; 31(2): 172-9. [http://dx.doi.org/10.1016/j.ccell.2017.01.002] [PMID: 28196593]

[26] Diehl F, Schmidt K, Choti MA, *et al.* Circulating mutant DNA to assess tumor dynamics. Nat Med 2008; 14(9): 985-90. [http://dx.doi.org/10.1038/nm.1789] [PMID: 18670422]

[27] Lo YMD, Zhang J, Leung TN, Lau TK, Chang AMZ, Hjelm NM. Rapid clearance of fetal DNA from maternal plasma. Am J Hum Genet 1999; 64(1): 218-24. [http://dx.doi.org/10.1086/302205] [PMID: 9915961]

[28] Marcuello M, Vymetalkova V, Neves RPL, *et al.* Circulating biomarkers for early detection and clinical management of colorectal cancer. Mol Aspects Med 2019; 69: 107-22. [http://dx.doi.org/10.1016/j.mam.2019.06.002] [PMID: 31189073]

[29] Kunnath AP, Priyashini T. Potential applications of circulating tumor dna technology as a cancer diagnostic tool. Cureus 2019; 11(6): e4907. [http://dx.doi.org/10.7759/cureus.4907] [PMID: 31423385]

[30] Bettegowda C, Sausen M, Leary RJ, *et al.* Detection of circulating tumor DNA in early- and late-stage human malignancies. Sci Transl Med 2014; 6(224): 224ra24. [http://dx.doi.org/10.1126/scitranslmed.3007094] [PMID: 24553385]

[31] van der Vaart M, Pretorius PJ. The origin of circulating free DNA. Clin Chem 2007; 53(12): 2215. [http://dx.doi.org/10.1373/clinchem.2007.092734] [PMID: 18267930]

[32] Newman AM, Bratman SV, To J, *et al.* An ultrasensitive method for quantitating circulating tumor DNA with broad patient coverage. Nat Med 2014; 20(5): 548-54. [http://dx.doi.org/10.1038/nm.3519] [PMID: 24705333]

[33] Yong E. Cancer biomarkers: Written in blood. Nature 2014; 511(7511): 524-6. [http://dx.doi.org/10.1038/511524a] [PMID: 25079538]

[34] Campos-Carrillo A, Weitzel JN, Sahoo P, *et al.* Circulating tumor DNA as an early cancer detection tool. Pharmacol Ther 2020; 207: 107458. [http://dx.doi.org/10.1016/j.pharmthera.2019.107458] [PMID: 31863816]

[35] Li J, Han X, Yu X, *et al.* Clinical applications of liquid biopsy as prognostic and predictive biomarkers in hepatocellular carcinoma: circulating tumor cells and circulating tumor DNA. J Exp Clin Cancer Res 2018; 37(1): 213. [http://dx.doi.org/10.1186/s13046-018-0893-1] [PMID: 30176913]

[36] De Rubis G, Rajeev Krishnan S, Bebawy M. Liquid biopsies in cancer diagnosis, monitoring, and prognosis. Trends Pharmacol Sci 2019; 40(3): 172-86. [http://dx.doi.org/10.1016/j.tips.2019.01.006] [PMID: 30736982]

[37] Leung M, Freidin MB, Freydina DV, *et al.* Blood-based circulating tumor DNA mutations as a diagnostic and prognostic biomarker for lung cancer. Cancer 2020; 126(8): 1804-9. [http://dx.doi.org/10.1002/cncr.32699] [PMID: 31999831]

[38] Han X, Wang J, Sun Y. Circulating tumor dna as biomarkers for cancer detection. Genomics Proteomics Bioinformatics 2017; 15(2): 59-72. [http://dx.doi.org/10.1016/j.gpb.2016.12.004] [PMID: 28392479]

[39] Dawson SJ, Tsui DWY, Murtaza M, *et al.* Analysis of circulating tumor DNA to monitor metastatic breast cancer. N Engl J Med 2013; 368(13): 1199-209. [http://dx.doi.org/10.1056/NEJMoa1213261] [PMID: 23484797]

[40] Cohen JD, Li L, Wang Y, *et al.* Detection and localization of surgically resectable cancers with a multi-analyte blood test. Science 2018; 359(6378): 926-30. [http://dx.doi.org/10.1126/science.aar3247] [PMID: 29348365]

[41] Phallen J, Sausen M, Adleff V, *et al.* Direct detection of early-stage cancers using circulating tumor

DNA. Sci Transl Med 2017; 9(403): eaan2415.
[http://dx.doi.org/10.1126/scitranslmed.aan2415] [PMID: 28814544]

[42] Petit J, Carroll G, Gould T, Pockney P, Dun M, Scott RJ. Cell-free DNA as a diagnostic blood-based biomarker for colorectal cancer: a systematic review. J Surg Res 2019; 236: 184-97.
[http://dx.doi.org/10.1016/j.jss.2018.11.029] [PMID: 30694754]

[43] El Messaoudi S, Mouliere F, Du Manoir S, *et al.* Circulating DNA as a strong multimarker prognostic tool for metastatic colorectal cancer patient management care. Clin Cancer Res 2016; 22(12): 3067-77.
[http://dx.doi.org/10.1158/1078-0432.CCR-15-0297] [PMID: 26847055]

[44] Spindler KG, Appelt AL, Pallisgaard N, Andersen RF, Jakobsen A. KRAS-mutated plasma DNA as predictor of outcome from irinotecan monotherapy in metastatic colorectal cancer. Br J Cancer 2013; 109(12): 3067-72.
[http://dx.doi.org/10.1038/bjc.2013.633] [PMID: 24263065]

[45] Uesato Y, Sasahira N, Ozaka M, Sasaki T, Takatsuki M, Zembutsu H. Evaluation of circulating tumor DNA as a biomarker in pancreatic cancer with liver metastasis. PLoS One. 2020; 15(7): e0235623-e.

[46] Lecomte T, Berger A, Zinzindohoué F, *et al.* Detection of free-circulating tumor-associated DNA in plasma of colorectal cancer patients and its association with prognosis. Int J Cancer 2002; 100(5): 542-8.
[http://dx.doi.org/10.1002/ijc.10526] [PMID: 12124803]

[47] Spindler KLG, Pallisgaard N, Vogelius I, Jakobsen A. Quantitative cell-free DNA, KRAS, and BRAF mutations in plasma from patients with metastatic colorectal cancer during treatment with cetuximab and irinotecan. Clin Cancer Res 2012; 18(4): 1177-85.
[http://dx.doi.org/10.1158/1078-0432.CCR-11-0564] [PMID: 22228631]

[48] Gautschi O, Huegli B, Ziegler A, *et al.* Origin and prognostic value of circulating KRAS mutations in lung cancer patients. Cancer Lett 2007; 254(2): 265-73.
[http://dx.doi.org/10.1016/j.canlet.2007.03.008] [PMID: 17449174]

[49] Gray ES, Rizos H, Reid AL, *et al.* Circulating tumor DNA to monitor treatment response and detect acquired resistance in patients with metastatic melanoma. Oncotarget 2015; 6(39): 42008-18.
[http://dx.doi.org/10.18632/oncotarget.5788] [PMID: 26524482]

[50] Muhanna N, Di Grappa MA, Chan HHL, *et al.* Cell-free dna kinetics in a pre-clinical model of head and neck cancer. Sci Rep 2017; 7(1): 16723.
[http://dx.doi.org/10.1038/s41598-017-17079-6] [PMID: 29196748]

[51] Tie J, Wang Y, Tomasetti C, *et al.* Circulating tumor DNA analysis detects minimal residual disease and predicts recurrence in patients with stage II colon cancer. Sci Transl Med 2016; 8(346): 346ra92.
[http://dx.doi.org/10.1126/scitranslmed.aaf6219] [PMID: 27384348]

[52] Spindler KLG. Methodological, biological and clinical aspects of circulating free DNA in metastatic colorectal cancer. Acta Oncol 2017; 56(1): 7-16.
[http://dx.doi.org/10.1080/0284186X.2016.1253861] [PMID: 28010185]

[53] Schøler LV, Reinert T, Ørntoft MBW, *et al.* Clinical implications of monitoring circulating tumor dna in patients with colorectal cancer. Clin Cancer Res 2017; 23(18): 5437-45.
[http://dx.doi.org/10.1158/1078-0432.CCR-17-0510] [PMID: 28600478]

[54] Tabernero J, Lenz HJ, Siena S, *et al.* Analysis of circulating DNA and protein biomarkers to predict the clinical activity of regorafenib and assess prognosis in patients with metastatic colorectal cancer: a retrospective, exploratory analysis of the CORRECT trial. Lancet Oncol 2015; 16(8): 937-48.
[http://dx.doi.org/10.1016/S1470-2045(15)00138-2] [PMID: 26184520]

[55] Parkinson CA, Gale D, Piskorz AM, *et al.* Exploratory analysis of tp53 mutations in circulating tumour dna as biomarkers of treatment response for patients with relapsed high-grade serous ovarian carcinoma: a retrospective study. PLoS Med 2016; 13(12): e1002198.
[http://dx.doi.org/10.1371/journal.pmed.1002198] [PMID: 27997533]

[56] Lipson EJ, Velculescu VE, Pritchard TS, *et al.* Circulating tumor DNA analysis as a real-time method for monitoring tumor burden in melanoma patients undergoing treatment with immune checkpoint blockade. J Immunother Cancer 2014; 2(1): 42.
[http://dx.doi.org/10.1186/s40425-014-0042-0] [PMID: 25516806]

[57] Oshiro C, Kagara N, Naoi Y, *et al.* PIK3CA mutations in serum DNA are predictive of recurrence in primary breast cancer patients. Breast Cancer Res Treat 2015; 150(2): 299-307.
[http://dx.doi.org/10.1007/s10549-015-3322-6] [PMID: 25736040]

[58] Reinert T, Schøler LV, Thomsen R, *et al.* Analysis of circulating tumour DNA to monitor disease burden following colorectal cancer surgery. Gut 2016; 65(4): 625-34.
[http://dx.doi.org/10.1136/gutjnl-2014-308859] [PMID: 25654990]

[59] Lee TH, Montalvo L, Chrebtow V, Busch MP. Quantitation of genomic DNA in plasma and serum samples: higher concentrations of genomic DNA found in serum than in plasma. Transfusion 2001; 41(2): 276-82.
[http://dx.doi.org/10.1046/j.1537-2995.2001.41020276.x] [PMID: 11239235]

[60] Jung M, Klotzek S, Lewandowski M, Fleischhacker M, Jung K. Changes in concentration of DNA in serum and plasma during storage of blood samples. Clin Chem 2003; 49(6): 1028-9.
[http://dx.doi.org/10.1373/49.6.1028] [PMID: 12766024]

[61] Gormally E, Vineis P, Matullo G, *et al.* TP53 and KRAS2 mutations in plasma DNA of healthy subjects and subsequent cancer occurrence: a prospective study. Cancer Res 2006; 66(13): 6871-6.
[http://dx.doi.org/10.1158/0008-5472.CAN-05-4556] [PMID: 16818665]

CHAPTER 7

Circulating Tumour Cells in Solid Cancer

Sharmin Aktar[1,2], **Tracie T. Cheng**[1], **Sujani M. K. Gamage**[1,3], **Vinod Gopalan**[1] and **Farhadul Islam**[3,4,*]

[1] *School of Medicine, Menzies Health Institute Queensland, Griffith University, Gold Coast, Australia*

[2] *Department of Biochemistry and Molecular Biology, Mawlana Bhashani Science and Technology University, Tangail-1902, Bangladesh*

[3] *Department of Anatomy, Faculty of Medicine, University of Peradeniya, Galaha Rd, 20400, Sri Lanka*

[4] *Griffith University, Institute for Glycomics, Gold Coast, Australia*

[5] *Department of Biochemistry and Molecular Biology, University of Rajshahi, Rajshahi-6205, Bangladesh*

Abstract: Circulating tumour cells (CTCs), as 'liquid biopsy", has a major benefit over traditional tissue biopsy and has the potential to become a less invasive and more cost effective cancer biomarker. The presence of CTCs in the circulation indicates the presence of a tumour and the possibility of metastatic spread. Hence, the characterisation of CTCs is expected to provide crucial insights into the mechanisms of metastasis. It can also provide useful information about the future use of CTCs as a surrogate endpoint biomarker in diagnosis, prognosis, and treatment response prediction by minimizing the limitations of tissue biopsies. Also, it provides a new horizon for the development of novel targeted therapies. However, the lack of specific and effective methods is the key limitation in CTC detection and isolation in patients with cancer. Therefore, more responsive methods and approaches may be needed to improve the accuracy of CTC measurements. Herein, this book chapter will provide a current picture of CTCs as surrogate biomarkers for disease diagnosis, prognosis and predicting therapy response, along with the risk of relapse in cancers.

Keywords: Circulating tumour cells (CTCs), Diagnosis, Liquid biopsy, Overall Survival, Prognosis, Progression Free Survival, Risk of Relapse, Therapeutic Targets.

INTRODUCTION

Cancer was the second leading cause of death globally in 2020 [1]. The high mor-

* **Corresponding author Farhadul Islam:** Department of Biochemistry and Molecular Biology, University of Rajshahi, Rajshahi-6205, Bangladesh; E-mail: farhad_bio83@ru.ac.bd

tality rate of this disease is mostly attributed to its late diagnosis and the emergence of anti-therapy resistance [2]. Circulating tumor cells (CTCs) are cells that escape from a primary tumour into the vasculature or lymphatics and seed at distant sites to metastasize [3]. CTCs had recently been gaining widespread attention as an alternative and a promising non-invasive biomarker with minimal cost and risk over the current traditional disease assessment methods [4]. The discovery of CTCs in peripheral blood was first reported by Thomas Ashworth in 1869 [5]. However, their clinical implications for better management of cancer patients have come into focus in recent years. For example, a number of studies have demonstrated that CTCs had the potential to be used as a "liquid biopsy" and could be used in clinical settings for better diagnosis and predictor of clinical prognosis and treatment efficacy of the disease [6, 7].

CTCs are very rare cells (1 CTC per 10^5–10^7 peripheral blood mononuclear cells) [8], however, they can be isolated from blood by non-invasive approaches, such as using their distinctive physical (size, density, *etc.*) characteristics or biological (immunoaffinity-based, *e.g.*, cell surface antigens-EpCAM, HER2, and MUC1]) properties or combinations of these features [9, 10]. As CTCs are believed to be a key player in the process of metastasis, they can be used to monitor the progression of cancer over time in patients with advanced stages. This can provide insightful information to better understand tumour cells' dissemination during metastasis [7, 11]. In addition, studies showed that CTCs have uniquely attributed to therapy resistance, thereby, studying CTCs could provide a better understanding of therapy resistance, leading to establishing better therapeutic strategies. Furthermore, analysis of CTCs has a promising potential for patients with early stages [7, 12]. As CTCs can be detected in patients with early-stage of cancer and have been reported to become a potential diagnostic biomarker and an independent prognostic factor for reduced progression-free survival (PFS) and overall survival (OS) [13 - 16]. Tumour-derived CTCs in the peripheral fluids of patients with cancers have the potential to be used as independent prognostic biomarkers for predicting metastatic relapse, monitoring treatment efficacy, as well as understanding metastasis development in various cancers, including breast, prostate, lung, colorectal, ovarian, pancreatic, head and neck, bladder cancer and melanoma as well as haematological malignancies [7, 10, 17]. For instance, patients with metastatic breast cancer had shown basal CTC count equal to five or more than five in 7.5 ml of blood [18]. These patients had shown shorter progression-free and overall survival when compared with patients having less than five CTC counts in 7.5 ml of blood [18]. For routine clinical implementation, however, adequate clinical and technological validation for specificity and sensitivity have not yet been achieved. Thus, a promising and reliable outcome is still scarce for the potential use of CTCs as surrogate endpoint biomarkers in cancer patients. Extensive research is going on to overcome technological limitations. This chapter will focus on the potential role of CTCs as a novel biomarker and their effectiveness as an important diagnostic and prognostic tool in different types of cancer.

Circulating Tumour Cells (CTCs): Cytomorphology, Biology and Isolation Techniques

Circulating tumour cells (CTCs) leave the primary or metastatic tumour site, invade and circulate into the circulation, and if they survive, they migrate to secondary organs, where they can seed metastasis [3]. CTCs are a highly dynamic and heterogeneous subpopulation. The heterogeneity of CTCs is due to the accumulation of various genetic and epigenetic changes in its different subpopulations [19]. Also, the phenotypic and genotypic characteristics of CTCs can change during the course of the disease by microenvironmental factors and /or therapeutic selective pressures [20]. These cells are very rare cells, approximately 1 CTC per 10^5–10^7 peripheral blood mononuclear cells or even lower in solid tumours during local growth (8). They can be found as a single cells or clusters of cells containing an aggregation of a heterogeneous population of 3 or more cancer cells [21]. These clusters of CTCs are known as circulating tumor microemboli (CTM). It is thought that CTMs appear from the aggregation of adjacent cells within the primary tumour mass, rather than from single CTCs aggregating together after shedding [22].

Currently, there is no uniform information regarding the morphological characteristics of CTCs, and recent studies have showed the morphological heterogeneity of CTCs [23 - 25]. For example, a recent study reported that CTCs have a relatively larger dense basophilic and irregular nucleus (generally 13 to 15 µm in diameter) compared to leukocytes, a high nucleus-to-cell ratio, and a pale-bluish ring of cytoplasm encircling the nucleus [23]. Another study noted that CTCs have a relatively big nucleus (more than 8 µm) and prominent nucleoli [25]. It is very difficult to propagate *in vitro* culture of CTCs due to high transcriptional activities, and they usually survive up to 14 days [26].

CTCs are involved in the metastatic cascade, starting from the dissemination of tumour cells into the bloodstream and then e-seed for metastasis [11]. During this process, disseminating tumour cells (CTCs) must fight against several mechanical or environmental factors, such as shear forces, oxidative stress in the bloodstream, and the immune surveillance to extravasate into the distant site and colonize locally to form metastasis or remain dormant [20, 27]. The complete process of metastasis is unclear, however, it is believed that CTCs undergo the epithelial-mesenchymal transition (EMT) [28]. EMT is a normal physiological phenomenon that occurs during embryogenesis. During EMT, the epithelial cells lose the cell-

cell adhesion (Loss of epithelial and cell adhesion markers) and apical-basal polarity and obtain mesenchymal markers, which allows the cells to migrate and intravasate through the extracellular matrix (ECM) membrane into the circulation. After intravasation, the CTCs circulate into the vessel and regain their epithelial phenotype, a reverse process of EMT known as mesenchymal-epithelial transition (MET), to successfully seed and form metastasis in a secondary site. Thus, CTCs disseminate from their epithelial origin to colonize the distant organs by EMT and MET process (Fig. **1**).

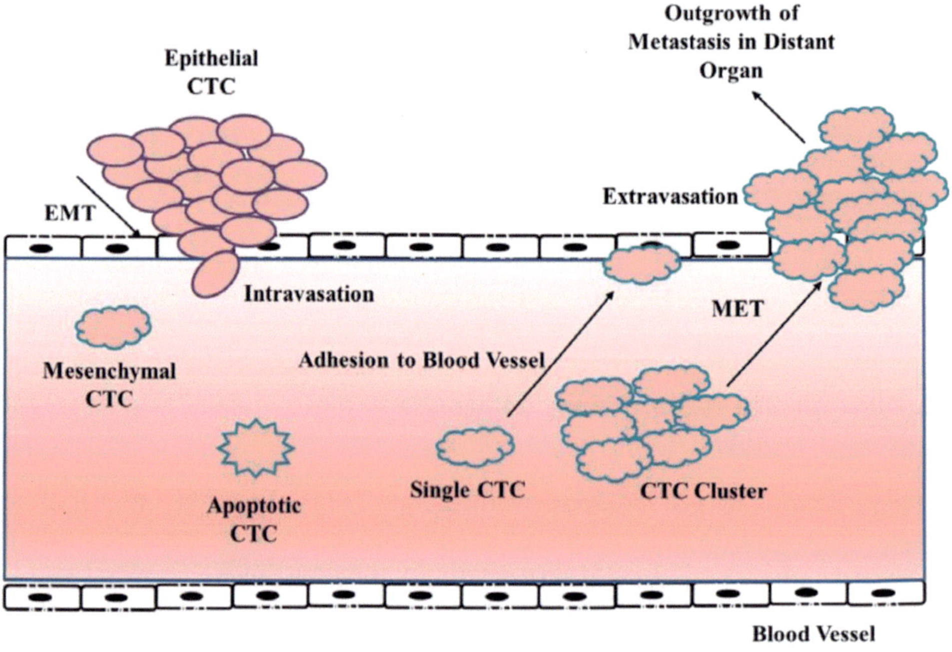

Fig. (1). Biology of circulating tumour cells. Circulating tumour cells (CTCs) undergo epithelial-mesenchymal transition (EMT), intravasate into the bloodstream and then undergo a mesenchymal-epithelial transition (MET) to disseminate and form metastasis in the secondary site. Disseminating tumour cells must fight against the shear stress in the bloodstream, and the immune surveillance to extravasate into the distant site, undergo MET, and colonize locally to form metastasis or remain dormant. CTCs can exist as individual cells or cell clusters; the latter show increased metastatic potential compared to individual CTCs.

Over the past few years, a number of CTC isolation technologies have been developed. In essence, these methods can be categorized into two main groups: label□dependent technologies, which utilize antigenic expression of the CTCs (cell surface antigens e. g., EpCAM, HER2, and MUC1 *etc.*) and label□independent techniques, which exploit distinct physical properties (size, density, electrical properties, *etc.*) (Fig. **2**). CellSearch, AdnaTest, magnetic□activated cell sorting (MACS), microfluidic chip methods, and enzyme□linked immune absorbent spot (ELISpot) assay are most extensively used as label□dependent methods, whereas CellCollector, size of epithelial tumour cell technique (ISET), CellSieve and Parsortix, are label□independent methods used to isolate CTCs (Fig. **2**). Among these technologies and methods, CellSearch is the only CTC isolation method that has been approved by the US Food and Drug Administration (FDA) in 2004 [29], although other antigen-based CTC isolation technologies are continuously emerging [30]. There are limitations to using both categories of isolation technologies. For example, CTCs may completely lose epithelial markers, including EpCAM expression, which have undergone the EMT transition process, hence making isolation impossible using label□dependent methods [10]. In contrast, label□independent techniques can be used to isolate CTCs even after EMT [10]. However, the size-based technology may also lose the smaller CTCs as this technology use a particular pore size filter to isolate CTCs. Therefore, further technological developments are imperative to develop effective methods for the efficient isolation of CTCs.

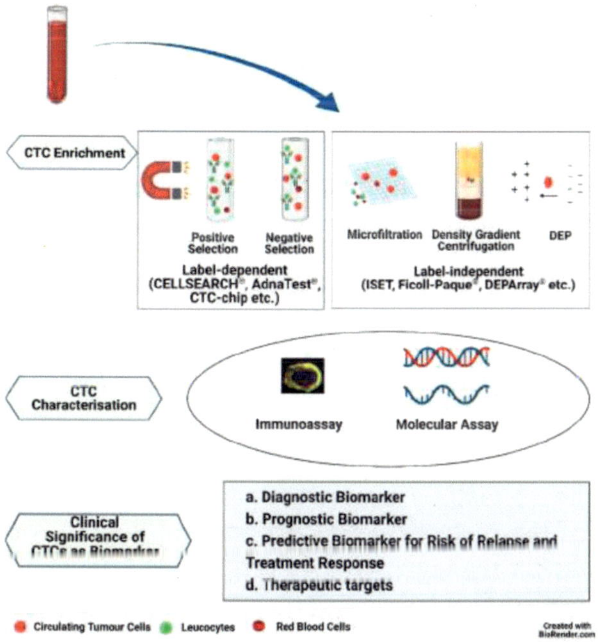

Fig. (2). Overview of CTCs Enrichment, Characterisation, and Their Clinical Applications. Enrichment technologies of CTCs can be categorized into two main groups: label□dependent that utilizes antigenic expression of the CTCs (cell surface antigens [eg, EpCAM, Vimentin, HER2, and MUC1 *etc.*) and label□independent techniques that exploit distinct physical properties (size, density, electrical properties *etc.*). CTCs are found to be a potentially useful marker for diagnosis, prognosis, and predicting therapy response and risk of relapse, as well as designing therapeutic targets.

CTCs in Solid Cancers

CTCs are associated with the key steps in metastasis, thus, CTCs can provide important information regarding individual cancer by a simple blood test [10]. CTC analysis can act as a real-time non-invasive liquid biopsy, which has a significant advantage over conventional biopsy and might become a less invasive and more cost-effective alternative to tissue biopsy [3, 7]. Also, as the CTCs counts correlate with the tumour burden of the disease, they could have the potential to be a more accurate method for the real-time monitoring of cancers than many other commonly used soluble biomarkers [31, 32]. Although CTC counts have been useful for clinical prognosis, however, the true extent of their use will be limited until the cells can be characterized in terms of their individual biological properties [10]. Thus, the progression of the disease and its response to treatment can be very well-monitored by characterizing CTCs, which are disseminated from the primary tumour [33]. Accordingly, recent studies have focused on evaluating the biological characterization of CTCs for a better understanding of this disease progression, cure and the effects of these phenotypic differences on clinical parameters [3, 33 - 35]. A study reported the clinical relevance of epithelial, mesenchymal and epithelial-mesenchymal CTCs in colorectal cancer and found that only mesenchymal and epithelial-mesenchymal CTCs, not epithelial CTCs, correlated with clinical stage and metastasis of patients with colorectal cancers [34]. Similarly, mesenchymal CTCs associated with the clinical stage and treatment efficacy in esophageal squamous cell carcinoma [35].

Molecular characterization, particularly genetic and proteomic characterization, has been on the rise as the clinical utility of CTCs for personalized-therapy has become more apparent in the expression profiling of CTCs. Genetic characterization explores the presence of a specific mutation or activation of an oncogene [36]. These characterizations of CTCs can identify specific genetic events during the metastatic process, thus helping in better understanding of crucial aspects of the metastatic process and holding a promise for cancer drug development or better management of the diseases [19, 37, 38]. In recent years, a growing number of studies have performed expression profiling of CTCs in order to identify clinically relevant gene signatures that may help to predict disease progression and guide therapeutic decisions [39, 40].

In solid cancers, both CTCs and CTMs in the blood have been proportionally correlated with patients' prognoses [28]. Between them, CTMs are more strongly correlated with patient outcomes [22, 41]. It was demonstrated that CTMs have prognostic significance and higher numbers are related to shorter PFS and OS in breast [42], lung [41] melanoma [43], ovarian cancer [44], gastric [45], colorectal

[46], liver [47], and pancreatic ductal adenocarcinomas [48]. Also, CTCs have significant prognostic implications in various cancers, such as breast cancer, lung cancer, colorectal cancer and gastric cancers.

Breast Cancer

Breast cancer has now surpassed lung cancer as the most frequently diagnosed cancer worldwide in 2020 [1]. In breast cancer, CTC clearance could possibly be used as a "surrogate" marker for potentially improved survival of patients [7].

Several methods have been developed for isolating CTCs from both early and metastatic breast cancer patients. Regardless of cancer subtypes, CTCs could be detected in 76% of breast cancer patients with all stages, and their counts are correlated to the tumour burden [18, 49]. CTCs detection may be affected due to the loss of epithelial markers on CTCs as a result of EMT [50]. Hence CTCs characterisation with additional markers during EMT may provide potential predictive information for prognosis and therapeutic intervention. The CTCs simultaneously expressed epithelial and mesenchymal markers along with tumour stem cell markers in both metastatic and early breast cancer [51, 52]. The expression of mesenchymal and epithelial markers such as EMT regulators, including transforming growth factor (TGF)-β pathway components and FOXC1 (a transcription factor) in CTCs of patients with breast cancer was associated with the disease progression [53]. Moreover, CTCs expressing EMT□inducing transcription factors that characterize CTCs during partial or complete EMT may facilitate the monitoring of therapeutic agents capable of targeting CTCs [50]. In addition, a study reported the apoptotic and proliferative status of CTCs in breast cancer patients and noted that CTCs originated from patients with metastatic disease had substantially less apoptotic CTCs than patients with early breast cancer patients. Also, adjuvant chemotherapy decreased the counts of CTCs inpatient as well as the number of proliferating CTCs in breast cancers [54]. Clinical trials with various drugs based on different designs are currently being performed to determine the potential of CTC targeting therapeutics for routine applications in breast cancer patients [7].

Lung Cancer

Lung cancer is the world's second most common cancer and the leading cause of cancer death [1]. In lung cancer, CTCs could be detected even before angiogenesis, and they can be found in the bloodstream for a long time before the disease is diagnosed Thus, they have the potential to become a biomarker for early disease diagnosis in symptomatic patients [55]. However, lung cancer diagnosis using CTC as a biomarker is still in progress. Also, CTC counts can be used to predict the survival of patients with both small cell lung cancer and non–small cell lung cancer [56, 57].

Gastrointestinal Tract Cancers

Among gastrointestinal (GI) tract cancers, colorectal cancer (CRC) is one of the most commonly diagnosed malignancies and one of the leading causes of cancer-related morbidity and mortality throughout the world [1]. CRC patients had very low levels of CTCs in peripheral circulation when compared to breast cancer or prostate cancer patients [58]. In CRC, the CTCs counts can be used for assessing cancer staging [16, 25]. However, the majority of studies did not find a correlation between CTC counts and cancer staging in CRC [59, 60]. Thus, there should be more evidence to support the identification of CTCs as a marker for early CRC diagnosis. Also, CTCs levels are often found to be related to a poor prognosis in patients with CRC [58]. For example, patients who have three or more CTCs/7.5 mL of blood have a lower survival rate [60]. On the other hand, Bessa *et al.* did not find any association between CTC counts and prognosis in postoperative CRC patients [61].

In gastric cancer (GC), higher CTC levels have been related to a lower overall survival rate, and CTC counts can predict the presence of metastasis in GC patients [62, 63]. The stem-like properties of CTCs in patients with GC play a key role in metastasis. For instance, CD44+ CTCs can predict both metastasis and disease recurrence in patients with GC [64]. Similarly EpCAM, being considered a predictive tool for peritoneal metastasis in patients with gastric cancer [65]. CTMs, along with CTCs, have recently been shown promising for gastric cancer prognosis [66].

Patients with pancreatic cancer have a poor prognosis due to the frequent and early spread of the disease, as well as late diagnosis due to unspecific and late symptoms of the disease [7]. Detection of CTCs in peripheral blood may be a promising biomarker for the detection and prognosis of pancreatic cancer [67, 68]. The clinical relevance of CTC detection in pancreatic cancer has been reviewed by Tjensvoll *et al.*, which reveals the presence of CTCs correlates with an unfavourable outcome in patients with pancreatic cancer [69].

Hepatocellular carcinoma (HCC), is another GI tract cancer and a common form of primary liver cancer with complicated aetiology and treatment options [7]. CTCs in HCC have prognostic significance and have potential implications for future treatment stratification [70 - 73]. A study reported emerging CTC detection methodologies and the clinical implications of CTC in HCC patients [74]. They found that patients with increased postoperative CTC counts (from preoperative

CTC < 2 to postoperative CTC ≥ 2) had significantly reduced disease-free survival (DFS) and OS [75].

Another common and deadly GI tract cancer is esophageal squamous cell carcinoma. The disease has shown early metastasis and recurrence, thus, the prognostic information is particularly essential for better management of patients with esophageal squamous cell carcinoma [10]. The presence of CTCs has the potential to be a strong, independent prognostic biomarker for tumour recurrence in esophageal squamous cell carcinoma. However, pathological characteristics such as tumour position, tumour size, TNM stage, differentiation grade, tumour depth, lymph node metastasis, and lymphatic or venous invasion are unrelated to the CTC counts [76, 77].

Bladder cancer, which can be non–muscle-invasive or muscle-invasive, is another common GI tract cancer CTCs counts, exhibited prognostic and predictive significance for cancer recurrence and oncological outcomes in patients with both forms of bladder cancer [78, 79]. However, a study noted that in patients with cT2 bladder cancer, CTC status is unlikely to be clinically useful for guiding therapeutic decisions [80].

Head and Neck Cancer

Head and neck cancer is the seventh most prevalent cancer worldwide [81]. These cancers usually originate from the squamous cells lining the moist, mucosal surfaces inside the head and neck (for example, surfaces of the mouth, the nose, and the throat). Most of the head and neck cancers are squamous cell carcinomas (HNSCC) [82]. Several clinical studies indicate that CTCs can be used as a real-time liquid biopsy to monitor disease progression and the early response to chemotherapy in patients with HNSCC [83, 84]. Also, CTCs can be used in patients with thyroid cancer for disease monitoring and prognosis, in particular for characterisation of clinicopathological features, predicting metastases and treatment response [85, 86].

Prostate Cancer

Prostate cancer represents the most common cancer type in men [87]. Several studies have suggested non-invasive blood tests for CTCs in patients with prostate cancer, and have reported a correlation between the presence of CTCs and early carcinogenesis, cancer progression and effectiveness of treatment [87]. Currently, a number of methods are being explored, focusing on the identification, isolation, capture, and characterisation of CTCs in the blood of PC patients [88, 89].

Renal Carcinoma

CTCs have been studied far less in patients with renal carcinoma compared to those with bladder and prostate cancer, as CTCs in renal cancer patients lack the expression of the EpCAM surface protein, which is used as "gold-standard" marker for the enrichment and detection of CTCs [10]. Despite these shortcomings in detection, there have been some evidences of CTCs having a prognostic value in renal carcinoma [90, 91]. For example, a robust multicenter prospective cohort of first-line metastatic patients with renal carcinoma study reported that the presence of 3 or more CTCs predicts a significantly shorter PFS and OS [92]. Another study detected CTC with distinct profiles such as epithelial, mesenchymal, stem cell-like or mixed-cell characteristics at different time points during anti-angiogenic therapy. They noted that the presence and number of N-cadherin-positive or CD133-positive CTC were associated with inferior PFS [93].

Other Cancers

CTCs have both diagnostic and prognostic significance in ovarian cancer and cervical cancer, the deadliest of the gynecologic cancers [94 - 98]. Obermayr *et al.* reported a panel of six genes that can be used to identify CTCs in patients using PCR and were able to identify 44% of cervical cancer, 64% of endometrial cancer, and 19% of ovarian cancer patients [99]. Also, novel CTC markers in patients with epithelial ovarian cancer were identified and assessed their implications for clinical outcomes [100]. In this study, CTCs were significantly found more often six months after completion of adjuvant chemotherapy in platinum-resistant patients, predicting an adverse outcome independent from classical prognostic parameters.

Patients with melanoma could be assayed for improvement and therapy response using CTC counts [101 - 103]. However, the difficulty in isolating CTCs and the heterogeneity of CTCs in melanoma have hindered the usefulness of CTCs as a prognostic tool [104]. New methods are currently being developed to improve the isolation and monitoring of CTCs in melanoma [105]. Molecular characterisation of CTCs may also provide insight into the clinical implications as well as new approaches to therapeutic options that would benefit personalised melanoma management [106, 107]. CTCs have also been demonstrated to be substantially associated with tumour load, the extent of disease, the initiation of new metastases, and OS and PFS in other solid tumours such as neuroendocrine cancers and CNS cancers [108, 109]. Studies on clinical applications of CTCs as liquid biopsy in CNS metastases are still limited. Most of them are retrospective and comprise small, heterogeneous patient cohorts. Hence, the optimal use of CTCs as a surrogate for tissue biopsy in diagnosis, prognosis, monitoring, and guidance of treatment decisions has yet to be defined.

In hematologic cancer such as leukemia, multiple myeloma and several lymphoma, including aggressive B□cell lymphoma, non□Hodgkin lymphomas, and Hodgkin lymphoma, there is little pre-clinical/clinical research exists regarding the clinical use of CTCs [110, 111]. According to the preliminary studies, CTCs tend to be promising as both prognostic and predictive biomarkers for disease recurrence and therapy response in hematologic cancers [10]. The natural state of leukemic cells is circulating in the blood, which makes it unique among cancers. However, the presence of CTCs from other cancers, such as breast cancer, may be confused with those from leukaemia, presenting a problem for other cancers.

CTCs as Surrogate Biomarker in Clinical Application

Liquid biopsy is a quick, non-invasive, and cost-effective method of monitoring disease status or treatment response. CTCs, as a "liquid biopsy", can thus stir up the prediction of disease aggressiveness and the monitoring of therapeutic response in patients with a minimally invasive biopsy. As a result, changes in disease detection and patient-specific management will be significantly improved. In the last decade, studies have shown the predictive value of CTCs for prognosis in patients with cancers. A summary of the studies in different solid cancers that suggested the potential application of CTCs as a useful marker for diagnosis, prognosis, and predicting therapy response and risk of relapse is discussed in the following sections.

CTCs as Diagnostic Biomarkers

Accumulating information suggests that CTCs have the potential to be used as a biomarker for the early diagnosis of various cancers (Table **1**). For example, a recent meta-analysis reported that CTCs showed a high diagnostic implication for lung cancer [112]. Also, CTCs can be useful for determining tumour staging at the time of diagnosis. The percentage of CTCs from 4 mL blood was found to be elevated in patients with advanced-stage breast cancer. Average CTC count at the cancer stage from 0 to III were 1, 2.17, 2.59, and 3.25, respectively [113]. CTCs can diagnose and predicts the staging of patients with pancreatic ductal adenocarcinoma (PDAC) as well as prostate cancer [114, 115], while in another study, CTCs were not found to be effective for the staging of patients with gastric cancer [116].

Furthermore, the presence of more than 3 CTCs counts in 4 mL of blood indicated the presence of local/regional metastasis in patients with PDAC [114]. Fan *et al.* reported a cancer stem cell (CSC) multi-markers panel, including EpCAM, CD90,

CD133, and CK19, for CTC detection to diagnose hepatitis B virus-related hepatocellular carcinoma. The panel can detect hepatitis B virus-related hepatocellular carcinoma at an early stage and enable to distinguish between liver cirrhosis, chronic hepatitis B infection, and benign hepatic lesion [117]. A recent study demonstrated that folate receptor positive CTCs (FR^+-CTCs) with maximum tumour diameter is a reliable method to differentiate the malignancy of small-sized, indeterminate solitary pulmonary nodules in non-invasive lung adenocarcinoma [118]. A study noted that the combination of CTCs and serum CEA biomarkers may be a valuable diagnostic marker in patients with colorectal cancer [16]. Since CTCs can be identified before they spread, their detection, isolation and analysis in various cancer can allow more accurate early diagnosis and staging of patients, thus serving as a better diagnostic tool for therapy decision-making—one that can be obtained quickly, reproducibly, and repeatedly through a fluid biopsy from cancer patients [119].

Table 1. CTCs as Diagnostic Biomarker for patients with various cancer.

Type of Cancers	Findings	References
Breast Cancer	CTCs could be used as a biomarker for early cancer screening, and staging	[113, 120]
Lung cancer	Presence of CTCs can diagnose early lung cancer. Also, CTC counts correlated with stage, size of primary tumour.	[121]
Prostate cancer	CTCs showed great potential for early diagnosis of prostate cancer.	[122, 123]
CRC	CTCs have the potential for diagnosis of different cancer stages. Also, in combination with CEA, CTCs could act as more potential early diagnostic biomarker.	[16, 25]
Gastric cancer	CTCs have potential as an early diagnostic biomarker, however, ineffective for staging of cancer	[116]
Pancreatic cancer	Vimentin+ CTCs could be useful in diagnosis, monitoring the tumour burden	[124]
Ovarian Cancer	Detection of CTCs allows early diagnosis	[97]
Cervical cancer	Detection of CTC is helpful for the early diagnosis of cervical cancer micro-metastasis and for the assessment of disease status.	[98]
ESCC	CTCs count were correlated with the T stage but not with the N or M stage. CTCs may improve accuracy of preoperative staging in EC	[76, 125]

CRC: Colorectal cancer; ESCC: Esophageal squamous cell carcinoma.

CTCs as Prognostic Biomarkers for Survival Analysis

CTC-liquid biopsy has made considerable progress in recent years and has become an insightful method for providing detailed information on patient's prognosis *via* a non-invasive process (Table **2**). Therefore, the researchers are increasingly aware of the significance of CTCs in cancer care, including understanding the abilities of CTCs in cancer prediction, diagnosis, and prognosis [126]. This progress could have the potential to change the technologies of cancer detection and patient's management. The information also will help to guide the selection of suitable therapeutic targets and provide new insights into the mechanism of these therapies. Studies on CTCs demonstrated that CTC counts are correlated with the prognosis of patients in a number of cancer such as breast, colorectal, prostate, melanoma, gastric, ovarian, lung cancer *etc*. (Table **2**). The prognostic significance of CTCs has been most extensively studied in breast cancer (Table **2**). CTCs can be used as a surrogate biomarker by defining a minimum threshold value to determine the prognostic outcome. It was noted that patients with 5 CTCs/7.5 mL of blood have an "unfavourable" prognosis, whereas those with 4 CTCs/7.5 mL of blood have a more "favourable" survival. Using the CellSearch Method (Veridex, South Raritan, NJ), for example, a cut-off value of 5 or more than 5 CTCs in 7.5 mL of blood was calculated retrospectively to suggest poor prognosis based on the survival of patients with metastatic breast cancer [18]. These results paved the way for the FDA to approve the CellSearch assay for CTC detection and isolation, which is standardised, semi-automated, and free of pre-analytical errors, revolutionising the clinical use of CTCs in a variety of cancers [7]. Similarly, retrospective studies noted that the determination of CTC cut-off values in clinical trials for metastatic prostate cancer had shown prognostic significance (Table **2**) [127, 128]. Patients with ≥5 CTCs in their 7.5 mL of blood have a worse prognosis in comparison with patients having <5 CTCs [127, 128]. While other studies found that the higher the CTC number, the worse the patient's overall survival, regardless of cut-off values [129, 130]. A meta-analysis of patients with prostate cancer also suggested a significant association between CTC counts and overall survival and relapse-free survival/disease-free survival [131].

In lung cancer, the CTC count has been found useful in assessing the prognosis (Table **2**) [132, 133]. Patients with higher CTCs counts at the time of diagnosis or after one cycle of chemotherapy have a poor prognosis [134]. A persistently elevated CTC count after one cycle of chemotherapy has stronger predictive significance. Patients with more CTCs (>300) had a worse prognosis than patients with fewer 2 CTCs (<2) [135]. Interestingly, the expression of unique markers in CTCs could also be useful as a prognostic marker in lung cancer. For example, the expression of programmed cell death protein 1 (PD1) receptor and its ligand (programmed death–ligand 1; PDL1) in CTCs can act as a prognostic marker for non-small-cell lung carcinoma (NSCLC) [136, 137]. Assessing the expression of these proteins over time *via* tissue biopsy can be difficult, however using the minimally invasive "liquid biopsy" method of CTC detection *via* blood draw can become feasible [10].

The prognostic significance of CTCs has also been reported in colorectal cancer (CRC) (Table **2**) [138 - 141]. A recent study noted that the presence of CTCs was correlated to poor survival in patients with advanced CRC stage [140]. In the cases where CEA or other markers are not substantially increased in advanced-stage CRC, the presence of CTCs may be used to track disease progression more effectively, followed by chemotherapy [142].

A number of studies have demonstrated the prognostic implication of CTCs in patients with squamous cell carcinoma of the head and neck (SCCHN), esophageal squamous cell carcinoma (ESCC), thyroid cancer (Table **2**).

For example, a multivariate analysis of CTC status in patients with HNSCC during concurrent chemoradiotherapy reported that in chemoradiotherapy responders, CTCs are significantly reduced [143]. CTC decline within the first month indicates a longer PFS and OS. The prognostic significance of CTCs in other cancers such as ovarian, cervical, melanoma, and renal cancer, including CNS metastasis, is yet to be established, however, many studies have identified associations between CTCs and poor prognosis [92, 94, 95, 144]. Thus, CTCs have the potential to be used as a prognostic biomarker in patients with cancer.

Table 2. CTCs as Prognostic Biomarker for patients with various cancer.

Type of Cancers	Findings	References
Metastatic breast cancer	CTCs were found to be correlated with poor progression□free and overall survival	[145 - 148]
NSCLC	CTC count has a strong predictive value for PFS and OS.	[56]
SCLC	Higher CTCs counts are associated with worse PFS and OS independent of all other factors	[57]
CRC	CTCs may serve as an effective and potential prognostic indicator for overall and progression-free survival.	[16, 149]
mCRPC	CTCs were elevated and correlated with poor survival rates	[150 - 153]
HNSCC	CTCs counts were strongly correlated with patients' survival	[154 - 156]
Skin cancer: Merkel cell carcinoma	The presence of CTCs was associated with poor survival	[157]
HCC	Number of CTCs after surgery correlates with prognosis	[158]
Pancreatic cancer	The presence of CTCs was correlated with overall survival and progression□free survival rates	[159]
ESCC	CTC numbers were found to correlate with disease prognosis	[76, 125, 160]
Cervical cancer	Serum CTC and squamous cell carcinoma antigen (SCC-Ag) levels are potentially useful biomarkers for the prediction of prognosis and their combination significantly improves the predictive ability for survival.	[95]

(Table 2) cont.....

Type of Cancers	Findings	References
Ovarian Cancer	Expression of EpCAM in CTC-positive patients predicts prognosis	[97]
Thyroid Cancer	CTCs can help predict the prognosis of patients with thyroid cancer	[85, 86]

CRC, Colorectal cancer; mCRPC, Metastatic castration-resistant prostate cancer; NSCLC, Non-small cell lung cancer; SCLC, Small cell lung cancer; HNSCC, Head and neck squamous cell carcinoma; HCC, Hepatocellular carcinoma; ESCC, Esophageal squamous cell carcinoma.

CTCS AS A PREDICTIVE BIOMARKER

In Treatment Monitoring

CTC enumeration has the potential to be used as an exploratory predictor of effectiveness and a measurement of treatment response (Table **3**) [161 - 163]. The traditional imaging methods are often paired with blood tumour marker levels to track chemotherapy treatment, but these indicators can take several months to indicate different drug responses [164, 165]. CTC levels in the blood, on the other hand, have been shown to predict changes in just a few weeks, well before the onset of symptoms, and tend to have a higher degree of accuracy [164]. The clinical usefulness of CTC enumeration is enhancing clinicians' ability to reliably determine treatment benefit and expediting the identification of appropriate treatment regimens for particular patients [166]. Given the evidence for CTC numbers and their relation to outcomes, there's been a drive to look at CTC sub-populations that can help direct therapies and boost cancer survival predictions [167].

CTCs have been shown to predict patient response during treatment in a number of breast cancer clinical trials [168 - 170]. Wallwiener *et al.*, for example, noted that consistent high CTC counts after one cycle of chemotherapy predict shorter survival in metastatic breast cancer, CTCs can thus be useful in modifying systemic therapies [171]. Furthermore, CTC HER2 status may assist in deciding the best treatment options based on the HER2 profile in HER2-positive patients [172]. At least 50% of hormone receptor-positive breast cancer recurrences have a latency period of ≥5 years [173]. The clinical utility of CTC count as an objective decision method has been demonstrated in a recent study when considering 1st line therapy in ER^+ $HER2^-$ metastatic breast cancer [168]. CTC count confirmed a priori clinical decision in the majority of patients; however, trial findings indicate that in some cases, CTC count can be trusted for either escalating (considering Chemotherapy (CT) in patients with a high CTC count) or de-escalating (considering hormone therapy (HT) in patients with a low CTC count) 1st line therapy [168]. Trapp *et al.* assessed the CTC counts before and 2 years after chemotherapy in patients with high-risk, early-stage breast cancer [174]. At 2 years after chemotherapy, 198 (18.2%) of 1,087 patients had detectable CTCs, and a positive CTC status at this time point was predictive of shorter disease-free survival (DFS) and overall survival (OS). Another multivariate analysis showed that the detection of CTCs is associated with a 13.1-fold higher risk of recurrence [175].

In prostate cancer patients, CTC counts showed promise as an early efficacy endpoint in systemic or local therapy treatment response (Table **3**). For example, if chemotherapy (taxane) is used, patients with metastatic prostate cancer who test positive for nuclear-localized androgen receptor splice variant 7 (AR-V7) protein in CTCs are more likely to live longer [176]. Furthermore, telomere in CTC among high-risk cases of localised prostate cancer after 6 months of androgen deprivation therapy (ADT), 6 months after completion of radiotherapy (RT), and 36 months after initial care revealed differences in treatment efficacy, suggesting the potential utility of CTCs in monitoring the efficacy of treatment among patients [177].

In lung cancer, CTCs counts may predict to approve their current treatment and recommend any necessary improvements [55]. For example, Pailler *et al.* showed that CTCs might predict crizotinib efficacy, and after treatment with crizotinib, patients with NSCLC, showed increased survival and decreased CTC sub-populations [178]. If the variations of CTCs counts are shown to have an effect on therapy responses, results such as the above studies may have significant consequences for treatment. Also, the rise in CTCs counts may happen due to the patient's medication being unsuccessful, necessitating a shift in treatment choices or therapeutic medications based on the CTC count during chemotherapy [164]. As a result, CTCs derived from cancer patients may be used as a complex biomarker to demonstrate how cancer drugs affect their therapeutic targets.

Table 3. CTCs as a predictive biomarker for monitoring the effectiveness of therapy.

Type of Cancers	Findings	References
Breast cancer	CTC status may predict response to therapy	[13, 175]
CRC	CTCs could be used as predictive markers for therapy response or for a risk of a therapy failure.	[179, 180]
NSCLC	The changes in CTC counts could predict chemotherapy response	[181]
SCLC	CTCs could be useful for monitoring treatment efficacy	[182]
Prostate Cancer	The expression of specific genes in CTCs could have the potential to predict the therapy response	[176, 183 - 186]
HNSCC	CTCs could be used to monitor patient's responses to the treatment	[84, 187]
ESCC	CTCs might serve as a reference indicator for the treatment effects	[188]

(Table 3) cont.....

Type of Cancers	Findings	References
Rectal cancer	CTCs may be useful in identifying a response to neoadjuvant chemo-radiation therapy	[189]

CRC, Colorectal cancer; NSCLC, Non-small cell lung cancer; SCLC, Small cell lung cancer; HNSCC, Head and neck squamous cell carcinoma; ESCC, Esophageal squamous cell carcinoma; HCC, Hepatocellular carcinoma.

In Risk of Disease Relapse

CTCs may serve as an indicator of disease relapse (Table **4**). A multicentre study conducted on early breast cancer patients found that patients with ≥5 CTCs/30 mL of blood had the worst prognosis, and CTC detection before and after chemotherapy was linked to a higher risk of relapse [190]. In addition, a randomised secondary clinical trial reported that a single positive CTC assay can produce independent prognostic details for late clinical recurrence (after 5 years of diagnosis) of hormone receptor-positive breast cancer, providing proof of concept that CTCs can be used to stratify for late recurrence and direct therapy [175]. A predictive correlation of CTC counts with metastatic relapse has also been found in prostate, colorectal, lung and bladder cancer as well as in other cancer (Table **4**) [191 - 194]. Thus, monitoring for CTCs in patients with early-stage cancer before and after surgery is thought to be helpful to identify patients who are at risk of disease recurrence and would benefit from adjuvant therapy [195].

Table 4. CTCs as predictive biomarker for metastasis and risk of relapse.

Type of Cancers	Findings	References
Breast cancer	A positive CTC assay result was associated with a 13.1-fold higher risk of recurrence	[175]
NSCLC	The presence of CTCs after surgery was significantly associated with early recurrence.	[196]
Prostate Cancer	CTC may contribute to predicting metastases and exploring the mechanisms of therapy resistance	[197 - 199]
Ovarian cancer	CTCs were found to correlate with metastases to the ovary rather than ovarian cancer itself	[200]
Malignant melanoma	Patients with higher numbers of CTCs had a significantly higher risk of relapse	[103]
Pancreatic cancer	Vimentin^{+} CTCs could be useful to predict tumour recurrence.	[124]
ESCC	A CTC count >2 was a strong independent prognostic indicator of tumour recurrence	[76]

NSCLC, Non-small cell lung cancer; ESCC, Esophageal squamous cell carcinoma.

Current Challenges in CTC Clinical Research

Although CTC research has progressed significantly in recent years, the effective methods for the detection and isolation of CTCs are yet to be standardized in many malignancies. The most used method, the CellSearch device, comes with several drawbacks. Its detection rate and prognostic importance are both adequate, but its failure to detect CTCs that have lost epithelial markers or its incompatibility with tumours of non-epithelial origin is still debated. The technical issues encountered during the isolation of CTCs using current EpCAM-dependent approaches may lead to lower CTC detection rates, which did not appear to be significant for survival, whereas EpCAM-independent approaches had higher detection rates [201]. Also, there are a plethora of technological variables that add further contradictions to the current stand. Thus, the lack of a common reference standard, as well as the limitation of fixed cells stained for limited biomarkers, sample size and volume, and sample preparation time, have resulted in inconsistent findings. These barriers have an effect on the identification rate, patient positivity, and prognostic implications [28]. Thus, further development of effective and sensitive methods could improve the potential of CTCs as an effective cancer biomarker.

CONCLUSION

In the context of the above discussion, we can infer that research into the characterisation of CTCs is still ongoing, with the potential to provide crucial insights into the mechanisms of metastasis and help in the production of novel targeted therapies. It can also provide useful information about the future use of CTCs as a surrogate endpoint biomarker in diagnosis, prognosis, and treatment response prediction, and it may help address the limitations of tissue biopsies. Therefore, more responsive methods and alternative approaches may be needed to improve the accuracy of CTC measurements.

CONSENT FOR PUBLICATION

Not applicable.

CONFLICT OF INTEREST

The authors declare no conflict of interest, financial or otherwise.

ACKNOWLEDGEMENT

The authors are thankful to the Molecular and Cellular Pathology, School of Medicine and Dentistry, Griffith University, Gold Coast, Australia, for providing the technical support for the work.

REFERENCES

[1] IARC IAfRoC. All cancers 2020. https://gco.iarc.fr/today/data/factsheets/cancers/20-Breast-fa-t-sheet.pdf

[2] Shin DS, Zaretsky JM, Escuin-Ordinas H, *et al.* Primary Resistance to PD-1 Blockade Mediated by *JAK1/2* Mutations. Cancer Discov 2017; 7(2): 188-201. [http://dx.doi.org/10.1158/2159-8290.CD-16-1223] [PMID: 27903500]

[3] Alix-Panabières C, Pantel K. Circulating tumor cells: liquid biopsy of cancer. Clin Chem 2013; 59(1): 110-8. [http://dx.doi.org/10.1373/clinchem.2012.194258] [PMID: 23014601]

[4] Alves Martins BA, de Bulhões GF, Cavalcanti IN, Martins MM, de Oliveira PG, Martins AMA. Biomarkers in Colorectal Cancer: The Role of Translational Proteomics Research. Front Oncol 2019; 9(1284): 1284. [http://dx.doi.org/10.3389/fonc.2019.01284] [PMID: 31828035]

[5] Ashworth T. A case of cancer in which cells similar to those in the tumours were seen in the blood after death. Aust Med J 1869; 14: 146.

[6] Yang C, Xia BR, Jin WL, Lou G. Circulating tumor cells in precision oncology: clinical applications in liquid biopsy and 3D organoid model. Cancer Cell Int 2019; 19(1): 341. [http://dx.doi.org/10.1186/s12935-019-1067-8] [PMID: 31866766]

[7] Lianidou ES, Strati A, Markou A. Circulating tumor cells as promising novel biomarkers in solid cancers. Crit Rev Clin Lab Sci 2014; 51(3): 160-71. [http://dx.doi.org/10.3109/10408363.2014.896316] [PMID: 24641350]

[8] Alix-Panabières C, Pantel K. Challenges in circulating tumour cell research. Nat Rev Cancer 2014; 14(9): 623-31. [http://dx.doi.org/10.1038/nrc3820] [PMID: 25154812]

[9] Bankó P, Lee SY, Nagygyörgy V, *et al.* Technologies for circulating tumor cell separation from whole blood. J Hematol Oncol 2019; 12(1): 48. [http://dx.doi.org/10.1186/s13045-019-0735-4] [PMID: 31088479]

[10] Jin KT, Chen XY, Lan HR, *et al.* Current progress in the clinical use of circulating tumor cells as prognostic biomarkers. Cancer Cytopathol 2019; 127(12): 739-49. [http://dx.doi.org/10.1002/cncy.22189] [PMID: 31589381]

[11] Pantel K, Speicher MR. The biology of circulating tumor cells. Oncogene 2016; 35(10): 1216-24. [http://dx.doi.org/10.1038/onc.2015.192] [PMID: 26050619]

[12] Ding Y, Li W, Wang K, Xu C, Hao M, Ding L. Perspectives of the Application of Liquid Biopsy in Colorectal Cancer. BioMed Res Int 2020; 2020: 1-13. [http://dx.doi.org/10.1155/2020/6843180] [PMID: 32258135]

[13] Goodman CR, Seagle BLL, Friedl TWP, *et al.* Association of Circulating Tumor Cell Status With Benefit of Radiotherapy and Survival in Early-Stage Breast Cancer. JAMA Oncol 2018; 4(8)e180163 [http://dx.doi.org/10.1001/jamaoncol.2018.0163] [PMID: 29800954]

[14] Thorsteinsson M, Jess P. The clinical significance of circulating tumor cells in non-metastatic colorectal cancer--a review. Eur J Surg Oncol. 2011; 37(6): 459-65.

[15] Lowes LE, Lock M, Rodrigues G, *et al.* Circulating tumour cells in prostate cancer patients receiving salvage radiotherapy. Clin Transl Oncol 2012; 14(2): 150-6. [http://dx.doi.org/10.1007/s12094-012-0775-5] [PMID: 22301405]

[16] Yu H, Ma L, Zhu Y, Li W, Ding L, Gao H. Significant diagnostic value of circulating tumour cells in colorectal cancer. Oncol Lett 2020; 20(1): 317-25. [http://dx.doi.org/10.3892/ol.2020.11537] [PMID: 32565958]

[17] Pantel K, Alix-Panabières C, Riethdorf S. Cancer micrometastases. Nat Rev Clin Oncol 2009; 6(6): 339-51.
[http://dx.doi.org/10.1038/nrclinonc.2009.44] [PMID: 19399023]

[18] Cristofanilli M, Budd GT, Ellis MJ, *et al.* Circulating tumor cells, disease progression, and survival in metastatic breast cancer. N Engl J Med 2004; 351(8): 781-91.
[http://dx.doi.org/10.1056/NEJMoa040766] [PMID: 15317891]

[19] Micalizzi DS, Maheswaran S, Haber DA. A conduit to metastasis: circulating tumor cell biology. Genes Dev 2017; 31(18): 1827-40.
[http://dx.doi.org/10.1101/gad.305805.117] [PMID: 29051388]

[20] Manicone M, Poggiana C, Facchinetti A, Zamarchi R. Critical issues in the clinical application of liquid biopsy in non-small cell lung cancer. J Thorac Dis 2017; 9(S13) (Suppl. 13): S1346-58.
[http://dx.doi.org/10.21037/jtd.2017.07.28] [PMID: 29184673]

[21] Torino F, Bonmassar E, Bonmassar L, *et al.* Circulating tumor cells in colorectal cancer patients. Cancer Treat Rev 2013; 39(7): 759-72.
[http://dx.doi.org/10.1016/j.ctrv.2012.12.007] [PMID: 23375250]

[22] Aceto N, Bardia A, Miyamoto DT, *et al.* Circulating tumor cell clusters are oligoclonal precursors of breast cancer metastasis. Cell 2014; 158(5): 1110-22.
[http://dx.doi.org/10.1016/j.cell.2014.07.013] [PMID: 25171411]

[23] Cleris L, Daidone MG, Fina E, Cappelletti V. The Detection and Morphological Analysis of Circulating Tumor and Host Cells in Breast Cancer Xenograft Models. Cells 2019; 8(7): 683.
[http://dx.doi.org/10.3390/cells8070683] [PMID: 31284534]

[24] Bobek V, Matkowski R, Gürlich R, *et al.* Cultivation of circulating tumor cells in esophageal cancer. Folia Histochem Cytobiol 2014; 52(3): 171-7.
[http://dx.doi.org/10.5603/FHC.2014.0020] [PMID: 25308732]

[25] Baek DH, Kim GH, Song GA, *et al.* Clinical Potential of Circulating Tumor Cells in Colorectal Cancer: A Prospective Study. Clin Transl Gastroenterol 2019; 10(7)e00055.
[http://dx.doi.org/10.14309/ctg.0000000000000055] [PMID: 31246593]

[26] Lu X, Mu E, Wei Y, *et al.* VCAM-1 promotes osteolytic expansion of indolent bone micrometastasis of breast cancer by engaging α4β1-positive osteoclast progenitors. Cancer Cell 2011; 20(6): 701-14.
[http://dx.doi.org/10.1016/j.ccr.2011.11.002] [PMID: 22137794]

[27] Lozar T, Gersak K, Cemazar M, Kuhar CG, Jesenko T. The biology and clinical potential of circulating tumor cells. Radiol Oncol 2019; 53(2): 131-47.
[http://dx.doi.org/10.2478/raon-2019-0024] [PMID: 31104002]

[28] Bailey P, Martin S. Insights on CTC Biology and Clinical Impact Emerging from Advances in Capture Technology. Cells 2019; 8(6): 553.
[http://dx.doi.org/10.3390/cells8060553] [PMID: 31174404]

[29] Riethdorf S, Fritsche H, Müller V, *et al.* Detection of circulating tumor cells in peripheral blood of patients with metastatic breast cancer: a validation study of the CellSearch system. Clin Cancer Res 2007; 13(3): 920-8.
[http://dx.doi.org/10.1158/1078-0432.CCR-06-1695] [PMID: 17289886]

[30] Castro-Giner F, Aceto N. Tracking cancer progression: from circulating tumor cells to metastasis. Genome Med 2020; 12(1): 31.
[http://dx.doi.org/10.1186/s13073-020-00728-3] [PMID: 32192534]

[31] Sefrioui D, Blanchard F, Toure E, *et al.* Diagnostic value of CA19.9, circulating tumour DNA and circulating tumour cells in patients with solid pancreatic tumours. Br J Cancer 2017; 117(7): 1017-25.
[http://dx.doi.org/10.1038/bjc.2017.250] [PMID: 28772284]

[32] Krebs MG, Sloane R, Priest L, *et al.* Evaluation and prognostic significance of circulating tumor cells

in patients with non-small-cell lung cancer. J Clin Oncol 2011; 29(12): 1556-63. [http://dx.doi.org/10.1200/JCO.2010.28.7045] [PMID: 21422424]

[33] Bidard FC, Vincent-Salomon A, Sigal-Zafrani B, *et al.* Prognosis of women with stage IV breast cancer depends on detection of circulating tumor cells rather than disseminated tumor cells. Ann Oncol 2008; 19(3): 496-500. [http://dx.doi.org/10.1093/annonc/mdm507] [PMID: 18187488]

[34] Zhao R, Cai Z, Li S, *et al.* Expression and clinical relevance of epithelial and mesenchymal markers in circulating tumor cells from colorectal cancer. Oncotarget 2017; 8(6): 9293-302. [http://dx.doi.org/10.18632/oncotarget.14065] [PMID: 28030836]

[35] Chen W, Li Y, Yuan D, Peng Y, Qin J. Practical value of identifying circulating tumor cells to evaluate esophageal squamous cell carcinoma staging and treatment efficacy. Thorac Cancer 2018; 9(8): 956-66. [http://dx.doi.org/10.1111/1759-7714.12771] [PMID: 29893036]

[36] Mamdouhi T, Twomey JD, McSweeney KM, Zhang B. Fugitives on the run: circulating tumor cells (CTCs) in metastatic diseases. Cancer Metastasis Rev 2019; 38(1-2): 297-305. [http://dx.doi.org/10.1007/s10555-019-09795-4] [PMID: 31053984]

[37] Pantel K, Alix-Panabières C. Circulating tumour cells and cell-free DNA in gastrointestinal cancer. Nat Rev Gastroenterol Hepatol 2017; 14(2): 73-4. [http://dx.doi.org/10.1038/nrgastro.2016.198] [PMID: 28096542]

[38] Magbanua MJM, Park JW. Advances in genomic characterization of circulating tumor cells. Cancer Metastasis Rev 2014; 33(2-3): 757-69. [http://dx.doi.org/10.1007/s10555-014-9503-7] [PMID: 24867683]

[39] Sergeant G, van Eijsden R, Roskams T, Van Duppen V, Topal B. Pancreatic cancer circulating tumour cells express a cell motility gene signature that predicts survival after surgery. BMC Cancer 2012; 12(1): 527. [http://dx.doi.org/10.1186/1471-2407-12-527] [PMID: 23157946]

[40] Kwan TT, Bardia A, Spring LM, *et al.* A digital RNA signature of circulating tumor cells predicting early therapeutic response in localized and metastatic breast cancer. Cancer Discov 2018; 8(10): 1286-99. [http://dx.doi.org/10.1158/2159-8290.CD-18-0432] [PMID: 30104333]

[41] Hou JM, Krebs MG, Lancashire L, *et al.* Clinical significance and molecular characteristics of circulating tumor cells and circulating tumor microemboli in patients with small-cell lung cancer. J Clin Oncol 2012; 30(5): 525-32. [http://dx.doi.org/10.1200/JCO.2010.33.3716] [PMID: 22253462]

[42] Wang C, Mu Z, Chervoneva I, *et al.* Longitudinally collected CTCs and CTC-clusters and clinical outcomes of metastatic breast cancer. Breast Cancer Res Treat 2017; 161(1): 83-94. [http://dx.doi.org/10.1007/s10549-016-4026-2] [PMID: 27771841]

[43] Long E, Ilie M, Bence C, *et al.* High expression of TRF2, SOX10, and CD10 in circulating tumor microemboli detected in metastatic melanoma patients. A potential impact for the assessment of disease aggressiveness. Cancer Med 2016; 5(6): 1022-30. [http://dx.doi.org/10.1002/cam4.661] [PMID: 26945789]

[44] Lee M, Kim EJ, Cho Y, *et al.* Predictive value of circulating tumor cells (CTCs) captured by microfluidic device in patients with epithelial ovarian cancer. Gynecol Oncol 2017; 145(2): 361-5. [http://dx.doi.org/10.1016/j.ygyno.2017.02.042] [PMID: 28274569]

[45] Zheng X, Fan L, Zhou P, *et al.* Detection of circulating tumor cells and circulating tumor microemboli in gastric cancer. Transl Oncol 2017; 10(3): 431-41. [http://dx.doi.org/10.1016/j.tranon.2017.02.007] [PMID: 28448959]

[46] Zhang D, Zhao L, Zhou P, *et al.* Circulating tumor microemboli (CTM) and vimentin+ circulating

tumor cells (CTCs) detected by a size-based platform predict worse prognosis in advanced colorectal cancer patients during chemotherapy. Cancer Cell Int 2017; 17(1): 6.
[http://dx.doi.org/10.1186/s12935-016-0373-7] [PMID: 28070168]

[47] Vona G, Estepa L, Béroud C, *et al.* Impact of cytomorphological detection of circulating tumor cells in patients with liver cancer. Hepatology 2004; 39(3): 792-7.
[http://dx.doi.org/10.1002/hep.20091] [PMID: 14999698]

[48] Chang MC, Chang YT, Chen JY, *et al.* Clinical significance of circulating tumor microemboli as a prognostic marker in patients with pancreatic ductal adenocarcinoma. Clin Chem 2016; 62(3): 505-13.
[http://dx.doi.org/10.1373/clinchem.2015.248260] [PMID: 26861552]

[49] Lucci A, Hall CS, Lodhi AK, *et al.* Circulating tumour cells in non-metastatic breast cancer: a prospective study. Lancet Oncol 2012; 13(7): 688-95.
[http://dx.doi.org/10.1016/S1470-2045(12)70209-7] [PMID: 22677156]

[50] Mego M, Mani SA, Lee BN, *et al.* Expression of epithelial-mesenchymal transition-inducing transcription factors in primary breast cancer: The effect of neoadjuvant therapy. Int J Cancer 2012; 130(4): 808-16.
[http://dx.doi.org/10.1002/ijc.26037] [PMID: 21387303]

[51] Aktas B, Tewes M, Fehm T, Hauch S, Kimmig R, Kasimir-Bauer S. Stem cell and epithelial-mesenchymal transition markers are frequently overexpressed in circulating tumor cells of metastatic breast cancer patients. Breast Cancer Res 2009; 11(4): R46.
[http://dx.doi.org/10.1186/bcr2333] [PMID: 19589136]

[52] Kallergi G, Papadaki MA, Politaki E, Mavroudis D, Georgoulias V, Agelaki S. Epithelial to mesenchymal transition markers expressed in circulating tumour cells of early and metastatic breast cancer patients. Breast Cancer Res 2011; 13(3): R59.
[http://dx.doi.org/10.1186/bcr2896] [PMID: 21663619]

[53] Yu M, Bardia A, Wittner BS, *et al.* Circulating breast tumor cells exhibit dynamic changes in epithelial and mesenchymal composition. science. 2013; 339(6119): 580-4.

[54] Kallergi G, Konstantinidis G, Markomanolaki H, *et al.* Apoptotic circulating tumor cells in early and metastatic breast cancer patients. Mol Cancer Ther 2013; 12(9): 1886-95.
[http://dx.doi.org/10.1158/1535-7163.MCT-12-1167] [PMID: 23778153]

[55] Potdar P, Lotey N. Role of circulating tumor cells in future diagnosis and therapy of cancer. J Cancer Metastasis Treat 2015; 1(2): 44-56.
[http://dx.doi.org/10.4103/2394-4722.158803]

[56] Tong B, Xu Y, Zhao J, *et al.* Prognostic role of circulating tumor cells in patients with *EGFR* -mutated or *ALK* -rearranged non-small cell lung cancer. Thorac Cancer 2018; 9(5): 640-5.
[http://dx.doi.org/10.1111/1759-7714.12631] [PMID: 29582563]

[57] Tay RY, Fernández-Gutiérrez F, Foy V, *et al.* Prognostic value of circulating tumour cells in limited-stage small-cell lung cancer: analysis of the concurrent once-daily *versus* twice-daily radiotherapy (CONVERT) randomised controlled trial. Ann Oncol 2019; 30(7): 1114-20.
[http://dx.doi.org/10.1093/annonc/mdz122] [PMID: 31020334]

[58] Mathai R, Vidya R, Reddy B, *et al.* Potential Utility of Liquid Biopsy as a Diagnostic and Prognostic Tool for the Assessment of Solid Tumors: Implications in the Precision Oncology. J Clin Med 2019; 8(3): 373.
[http://dx.doi.org/10.3390/jcm8030373] [PMID: 30889786]

[59] Uen YH, Lu CY, Tsai HL, *et al.* Persistent presence of postoperative circulating tumor cells is a poor prognostic factor for patients with stage I-III colorectal cancer after curative resection. Ann Surg Oncol 2008; 15(8): 2120-8.
[http://dx.doi.org/10.1245/s10434-008-9961-7] [PMID: 18481151]

[60] Wang JY, Wu CH, Lu CY, *et al.* Molecular detection of circulating tumor cells in the peripheral blood

of patients with colorectal cancer using RT-PCR: significance of the prediction of postoperative metastasis. World J Surg 2006; 30(6): 1007-13.
[http://dx.doi.org/10.1007/s00268-005-0485-z] [PMID: 16736329]

[61] Bessa X, Piñol V, Castellví-Bel S, *et al.* Prognostic value of postoperative detection of blood circulating tumor cells in patients with colorectal cancer operated on for cure. Ann Surg 2003; 237(3): 368-75.
[http://dx.doi.org/10.1097/01.SLA.0000055223.27623.F3] [PMID: 12616121]

[62] Hiraiwa K, Takeuchi H, Hasegawa H, *et al.* Clinical significance of circulating tumor cells in blood from patients with gastrointestinal cancers. Ann Surg Oncol 2008; 15(11): 3092-100.
[http://dx.doi.org/10.1245/s10434-008-0122-9] [PMID: 18766405]

[63] Matsusaka S, Chìn K, Ogura M, *et al.* Circulating tumor cells as a surrogate marker for determining response to chemotherapy in patients with advanced gastric cancer. Cancer Sci 2010; 101(4): 1067-71.
[http://dx.doi.org/10.1111/j.1349-7006.2010.01492.x] [PMID: 20219073]

[64] Zhou J, Ma X, Bi F, Liu M. Clinical significance of circulating tumor cells in gastric cancer patients. Oncotarget 2017; 8(15): 25713-20.
[http://dx.doi.org/10.18632/oncotarget.14879] [PMID: 28147337]

[65] Imano M, Itoh T, Satou T, *et al.* High expression of epithelial cellular adhesion molecule in peritoneal metastasis of gastric cancer. Target Oncol 2013; 8(4): 231-5.
[http://dx.doi.org/10.1007/s11523-012-0239-4] [PMID: 23161021]

[66] Abdallah EA, Braun AC, Flores BCTCP, *et al.* The potential clinical implications of circulating tumor cells and circulating tumor microemboli in gastric cancer. Oncologist 2019; 24(9): e854-63.
[http://dx.doi.org/10.1634/theoncologist.2018-0741] [PMID: 30846515]

[67] Han L, Chen W, Zhao Q. Prognostic value of circulating tumor cells in patients with pancreatic cancer: a meta-analysis. Tumour Biol 2014; 35(3): 2473-80.
[http://dx.doi.org/10.1007/s13277-013-1327-5] [PMID: 24218336]

[68] Bidard FC, Huguet F, Louvet C, *et al.* Circulating tumor cells in locally advanced pancreatic adenocarcinoma: the ancillary CirCe 07 study to the LAP 07 trial. Ann Oncol 2013; 24(8): 2057-61.
[http://dx.doi.org/10.1093/annonc/mdt176] [PMID: 23676420]

[69] Tjensvoll K, Nordgård O, Smaaland R. Circulating tumor cells in pancreatic cancer patients: Methods of detection and clinical implications. Int J Cancer 2014; 134(1): 1-8.
[http://dx.doi.org/10.1002/ijc.28134] [PMID: 23447365]

[70] von Felden J, Schulze K, Krech T, *et al.* Circulating tumor cells as liquid biomarker for high HCC recurrence risk after curative liver resection. Oncotarget 2017; 8(52): 89978-87.
[http://dx.doi.org/10.18632/oncotarget.21208] [PMID: 29163804]

[71] Nel I, Baba HA, Ertle J, *et al.* Individual profiling of circulating tumor cell composition and therapeutic outcome in patients with hepatocellular carcinoma. Transl Oncol 2013; 6(4): 420-8.
[http://dx.doi.org/10.1593/tlo.13271] [PMID: 23908685]

[72] Schulze K, Gasch C, Staufer K, *et al.* Presence of EpCAM-positive circulating tumor cells as biomarker for systemic disease strongly correlates to survival in patients with hepatocellular carcinoma. Int J Cancer 2013; 133(9): 2165-71.
[http://dx.doi.org/10.1002/ijc.28230] [PMID: 23616258]

[73] Sun YF, Xu Y, Yang XR, *et al.* Circulating stem cell-like epithelial cell adhesion molecule-positive tumor cells indicate poor prognosis of hepatocellular carcinoma after curative resection. Hepatology 2013; 57(4): 1458-68.
[http://dx.doi.org/10.1002/hep.26151] [PMID: 23175471]

[74] Zhang Y, Li J, Cao L, Xu W, Yin Z, Eds. Circulating tumor cells in hepatocellular carcinoma: detection techniques, clinical implications, and future perspectives. Seminars in oncology. 2012. Elsevier.

[75] Yu J, Xiao W, Dong S, *et al.* Effect of surgical liver resection on circulating tumor cells in patients with hepatocellular carcinoma. BMC Cancer 2018; 18(1): 835. [http://dx.doi.org/10.1186/s12885-018-4744-4] [PMID: 30126375]

[76] Han L, Li YJ, Zhang WD, Song PP, Li H, Li S. Clinical significance of tumor cells in the peripheral blood of patients with esophageal squamous cell carcinoma. Medicine (Baltimore) 2019; 98(6)e13921. [http://dx.doi.org/10.1097/MD.0000000000013921] [PMID: 30732126]

[77] Wang S, Du H, Li G. Significant prognostic value of circulating tumor cells in esophageal cancer patients: A meta-analysis. Oncotarget 2017; 8(9): 15815-26. [http://dx.doi.org/10.18632/oncotarget.15012] [PMID: 28178659]

[78] Busetto GM, Ferro M, Del Giudice F, *et al.* The prognostic role of circulating tumor cells (CTC) in high-risk non–muscle-invasive bladder cancer. Clin Genitourin Cancer 2017; 15(4): e661-6. [http://dx.doi.org/10.1016/j.clgc.2017.01.011] [PMID: 28188046]

[79] Anantharaman A, Friedlander T, Lu D, *et al.* Programmed death-ligand 1 (PD-L1) characterization of circulating tumor cells (CTCs) in muscle invasive and metastatic bladder cancer patients. BMC Cancer 2016; 16(1): 744. [http://dx.doi.org/10.1186/s12885-016-2758-3] [PMID: 27658492]

[80] Guzzo TJ, McNeil BK, Bivalacqua TJ, Elliott DJ, Sokoll LJ, Schoenberg MP, Eds. The presence of circulating tumor cells does not predict extravesical disease in bladder cancer patients prior to radical cystectomy Urologic Oncology: Seminars and Original Investigations 2012.

[81] Kulasinghe A, Hughes BGM, Kenny L, Punyadeera C. An update: circulating tumor cells in head and neck cancer. Expert Rev Mol Diagn 2019; 19(12): 1109-15. [http://dx.doi.org/10.1080/14737159.2020.1688145] [PMID: 31680565]

[82] Perumal V, Corica T, Dharmarajan A, *et al.* Circulating Tumour Cells (CTC), Head and Neck Cancer and Radiotherapy; Future Perspectives. Cancers (Basel) 2019; 11(3): 367. [http://dx.doi.org/10.3390/cancers11030367] [PMID: 30875950]

[83] Liu K, Chen N, Wei J, Ma L, Yang S, Zhang X. Clinical significance of circulating tumor cells in patients with locally advanced head and neck squamous cell carcinoma. Oncol Rep 2020; 43(5): 1525-35. [http://dx.doi.org/10.3892/or.2020.7536] [PMID: 32323844]

[84] Garrel R, Mazel M, Perriard F, *et al.* Circulating Tumor Cells as a Prognostic Factor in Recurrent or Metastatic Head and Neck Squamous Cell Carcinoma: The CIRCUTEC Prospective Study. Clin Chem 2019; 65(10): 1267-75. [http://dx.doi.org/10.1373/clinchem.2019.305904] [PMID: 31387885]

[85] Ehlers M, Allelein S, Schwarz F, *et al.* Increased numbers of circulating tumor cells in thyroid cancer patients. Horm Metab Res 2018; 50(8): 602-8. [http://dx.doi.org/10.1055/a-0651-4913] [PMID: 30081408]

[86] Qiu ZL, Wei WJ, Sun ZK, *et al.* Circulating tumor cells correlate with clinicopathological features and outcomes in differentiated thyroid cancer. Cell Physiol Biochem 2018; 48(2): 718-30. [http://dx.doi.org/10.1159/000491898] [PMID: 30025398]

[87] Pantel K, Hille C, Scher HI. Circulating Tumor Cells in Prostate Cancer: From Discovery to Clinical Utility. Clin Chem 2019; 65(1): 87-99. [http://dx.doi.org/10.1373/clinchem.2018.287102] [PMID: 30602476]

[88] Ried K, Tamanna T, Matthews S, Eng P, Sali A. New Screening Test Improves Detection of Prostate Cancer Using Circulating Tumor Cells and Prostate-Specific Markers. Front Oncol 2020; 10(582): 582. [http://dx.doi.org/10.3389/fonc.2020.00582] [PMID: 32391268]

[89] Ried K, Eng P, Sali A. Screening for circulating tumour cells allows early detection of cancer and monitoring of treatment effectiveness: an observational study. Asian Pacific journal of cancer

prevention. APJCP 2017; 18(8): 2275-85.
[PMID: 28843267]

[90] Gorin MA, Verdone JE, van der Toom E, Bivalacqua TJ, Allaf ME, Pienta KJ. Circulating tumour cells as biomarkers of prostate, bladder, and kidney cancer. Nat Rev Urol 2017; 14(2): 90-7.
[http://dx.doi.org/10.1038/nrurol.2016.224] [PMID: 27872478]

[91] Nagaya N, Kanayama M, Nagata M, Horie S. The Surge in the Number of Circulating Tumor Cells Following Treatment with Sunitinib for Metastatic Renal Cell Carcinoma: A Case Report 2018.
[http://dx.doi.org/10.2169/internalmedicine.0663-17]

[92] Basso U, Facchinetti A, Rossi E, *et al.* Prognostic role of circulating tumor cells-CTCs in metastatic renal cell carcinoma. J Clin Oncol 2017; 35(15_suppl) (Suppl.): 4568.
[http://dx.doi.org/10.1200/JCO.2017.35.15_suppl.4568]

[93] Nel I, Gauler TC, Bublitz K, *et al.* Circulating Tumor Cell Composition in Renal Cell Carcinoma. PLoS One 2016; 11(4)e0153018
[http://dx.doi.org/10.1371/journal.pone.0153018] [PMID: 27101285]

[94] Chebouti I, Kasimir-Bauer S, Buderath P, *et al.* EMT-like circulating tumor cells in ovarian cancer patients are enriched by platinum-based chemotherapy. Oncotarget 2017; 8(30): 48820-31.
[http://dx.doi.org/10.18632/oncotarget.16179] [PMID: 28415744]

[95] Wen YF, Cheng TT, Chen XL, *et al.* Elevated circulating tumor cells and squamous cell carcinoma antigen levels predict poor survival for patients with locally advanced cervical cancer treated with radiotherapy. PLoS One 2018; 13(10)e0204334.
[http://dx.doi.org/10.1371/journal.pone.0204334] [PMID: 30303986]

[96] Takakura M, Matsumoto T, Nakamura M, *et al.* Detection of circulating tumor cells in cervical cancer using a conditionally replicative adenovirus targeting telomerase-positive cells. Cancer Sci 2018; 109(1): 231-40.
[http://dx.doi.org/10.1111/cas.13449] [PMID: 29151279]

[97] Zhang X, Li H, Yu X, *et al.* Analysis of Circulating Tumor Cells in Ovarian Cancer and Their Clinical Value as a Biomarker. Cell Physiol Biochem 2018; 48(5): 1983-94.
[http://dx.doi.org/10.1159/000492521] [PMID: 30092594]

[98] Pan L, Yan G, Chen W, Sun L, Wang J, Yang J. Distribution of circulating tumor cell phenotype in early cervical cancer. Cancer Manag Res 2019; 11: 5531-6.
[http://dx.doi.org/10.2147/CMAR.S198391] [PMID: 31354357]

[99] Obermayr E, Sanchez-Cabo F, Tea MKM, *et al.* Assessment of a six gene panel for the molecular detection of circulating tumor cells in the blood of female cancer patients. BMC Cancer 2010; 10(1): 666.
[http://dx.doi.org/10.1186/1471-2407-10-666] [PMID: 21129172]

[100] Obermayr E, Castillo-Tong DC, Pils D, *et al.* Molecular characterization of circulating tumor cells in patients with ovarian cancer improves their prognostic significance — A study of the OVCAD consortium. Gynecol Oncol 2013; 128(1): 15-21.
[http://dx.doi.org/10.1016/j.ygyno.2012.09.021] [PMID: 23017820]

[101] Tanaka R, Koyanagi K, Narita N, Kuo C, Hoon DSB. Prognostic molecular biomarkers for cutaneous malignant melanoma. J Surg Oncol 2011; 104(4): 438-46.
[http://dx.doi.org/10.1002/jso.21969] [PMID: 21557225]

[102] Xu MJ, Dorsey JF, Amaravadi R, *et al.* Circulating Tumor Cells, DNA, and mRNA: Potential for Clinical Utility in Patients With Melanoma. Oncologist 2016; 21(1): 84-94.
[http://dx.doi.org/10.1634/theoncologist.2015-0207] [PMID: 26614709]

[103] Pachmann K, Willecke-Hochmuth R, Schneider K, Kaatz M. Circulating epithelial tumor cells as a prognostic tool for malignant melanoma. Melanoma Res 2018; 28(1): 37-43.
[http://dx.doi.org/10.1097/CMR.0000000000000407] [PMID: 29076925]

[104] De Souza LM, Robertson BM, Robertson GP. Future of circulating tumor cells in the melanoma clinical and research laboratory settings. Cancer Lett 2017; 392: 60-70. [http://dx.doi.org/10.1016/j.canlet.2017.01.023] [PMID: 28163189]

[105] Po JW, Ma Y, Balakrishna B, *et al.* Immunomagnetic isolation of circulating melanoma cells and detection of PD-L1 status. PLoS One 2019; 14(2)e0211866 [http://dx.doi.org/10.1371/journal.pone.0211866] [PMID: 30735560]

[106] Klinac D, Gray ES, Millward M, Ziman M. Advances in personalized targeted treatment of metastatic melanoma and non-invasive tumor monitoring. Front Oncol 2013; 3: 54. [http://dx.doi.org/10.3389/fonc.2013.00054] [PMID: 23515890]

[107] Hoshimoto S, Faries MB, Morton DL, *et al.* Assessment of prognostic circulating tumor cells in a phase III trial of adjuvant immunotherapy after complete resection of stage IV melanoma. Ann Surg 2012; 255(2): 357-62. [http://dx.doi.org/10.1097/SLA.0b013e3182380f56] [PMID: 22202581]

[108] Behnan J, Finocchiaro G, Hanna G. The landscape of the mesenchymal signature in brain tumours. Brain 2019; 142(4): 847-66. [http://dx.doi.org/10.1093/brain/awz044] [PMID: 30946477]

[109] Boire A, Brandsma D, Brastianos PK, *et al.* Liquid biopsy in central nervous system metastases: a RANO review and proposals for clinical applications. Neuro-oncol 2019; 21(5): 571-84. [http://dx.doi.org/10.1093/neuonc/noz012] [PMID: 30668804]

[110] Mishima Y, Paiva B, Shi J, *et al.* The Mutational Landscape of Circulating Tumor Cells in Multiple Myeloma. Cell Rep 2017; 19(1): 218-24. [http://dx.doi.org/10.1016/j.celrep.2017.03.025] [PMID: 28380360]

[111] Huhn S, Weinhold N, Nickel J, *et al.* Circulating tumor cells as a biomarker for response to therapy in multiple myeloma patients treated within the GMMG-MM5 trial. Bone Marrow Transplant 2017; 52(8): 1194-8. [http://dx.doi.org/10.1038/bmt.2017.91] [PMID: 28504661]

[112] Ye Y, Li SL, Wang JJ, Liu B. The diagnostic value of circulating tumor cells for lung cancer. Medicine (Baltimore) 2019; 98(12)e14936. [http://dx.doi.org/10.1097/MD.0000000000014936] [PMID: 30896658]

[113] Jin L, Zhao W, Zhang J, *et al.* Evaluation of the diagnostic value of circulating tumor cells with CytoSorter ® CTC capture system in patients with breast cancer. Cancer Med 2020; 9(5): 1638-47. [http://dx.doi.org/10.1002/cam4.2825] [PMID: 31908156]

[114] Ankeny JS, Court CM, Hou S, *et al.* Circulating tumour cells as a biomarker for diagnosis and staging in pancreatic cancer. Br J Cancer 2016; 114(12): 1367-75. [http://dx.doi.org/10.1038/bjc.2016.121] [PMID: 27300108]

[115] Agerbæk MØ, Bang-Christensen SR, Yang MH, *et al.* The VAR2CSA malaria protein efficiently retrieves circulating tumor cells in an EpCAM-independent manner. Nat Commun 2018; 9(1): 3279. [http://dx.doi.org/10.1038/s41467-018-05793-2] [PMID: 30115931]

[116] Kang HM, Kim GH, Jeon HK, *et al.* Circulating tumor cells detected by lab-on-a-disc: Role in early diagnosis of gastric cancer. PLoS One 2017; 12(6)e0180251. [http://dx.doi.org/10.1371/journal.pone.0180251] [PMID: 28662130]

[117] Guo W, Sun YF, Shen MN, *et al.* Circulating Tumor Cells with Stem-Like Phenotypes for Diagnosis, Prognosis, and Therapeutic Response Evaluation in Hepatocellular Carcinoma. Clin Cancer Res 2018; 24(9): 2203-13. [http://dx.doi.org/10.1158/1078-0432.CCR-17-1753] [PMID: 29374055]

[118] Zhou Q, Geng Q, Wang L, *et al.* Value of folate receptor-positive circulating tumour cells in the clinical management of indeterminate lung nodules: A non-invasive biomarker for predicting malignancy and tumour invasiveness. EBioMedicine 2019; 41: 236-43.

[http://dx.doi.org/10.1016/j.ebiom.2019.02.028] [PMID: 30872130]

[119] Thiele JA, Bethel K, Králíčková M, Kuhn P. Circulating Tumor Cells: Fluid Surrogates of Solid Tumors. Annu Rev Pathol 2017; 12(1): 419-47.
[http://dx.doi.org/10.1146/annurev-pathol-052016-100256] [PMID: 28135562]

[120] Hu X, Zhu D, Chen M, *et al.* Precise and non-invasive circulating tumor cell isolation based on optical force using homologous erythrocyte binding. Lab Chip 2019; 19(15): 2549-56.
[http://dx.doi.org/10.1039/C9LC00361D] [PMID: 31263813]

[121] Fiorelli A, Accardo M, Carelli E, Angioletti D, Santini M, Di Domenico M. Circulating Tumor Cells in Diagnosing Lung Cancer: Clinical and Morphologic Analysis. Ann Thorac Surg 2015; 99(6): 1899-905.
[http://dx.doi.org/10.1016/j.athoracsur.2014.11.049] [PMID: 25678504]

[122] Wong KHK, Tessier SN, Miyamoto DT, *et al.* Whole blood stabilization for the microfluidic isolation and molecular characterization of circulating tumor cells. Nat Commun 2017; 8(1): 1733.
[http://dx.doi.org/10.1038/s41467-017-01705-y] [PMID: 29170510]

[123] Ren X, Foster BM, Ghassemi P, Strobl JS, Kerr BA, Agah M. Entrapment of Prostate Cancer Circulating Tumor Cells with a Sequential Size-Based Microfluidic Chip. Anal Chem 2018; 90(12): 7526-34.
[http://dx.doi.org/10.1021/acs.analchem.8b01134] [PMID: 29790741]

[124] Wei T, Zhang X, Zhang Q, *et al.* Vimentin-positive circulating tumor cells as a biomarker for diagnosis and treatment monitoring in patients with pancreatic cancer. Cancer Lett 2019; 452: 237-43.
[http://dx.doi.org/10.1016/j.canlet.2019.03.009] [PMID: 30905814]

[125] Reeh M, Effenberger KE, Koenig AM, *et al.* Circulating Tumor Cells as a Biomarker for Preoperative Prognostic Staging in Patients With Esophageal Cancer. Ann Surg 2015; 261(6): 1124-30.
[http://dx.doi.org/10.1097/SLA.0000000000001130] [PMID: 25607767]

[126] Li X-Y, Dong M, Zang X-Y, *et al.* The emerging role of circulating tumor cells in cancer management. Am J Transl Res 2020; 12(2): 332-42.
[PMID: 32194887]

[127] Moreno JG, Miller MC, Gross S, Allard WJ, Gomella LG, Terstappen LWMM. Circulating tumor cells predict survival in patients with metastatic prostate cancer. Urology 2005; 65(4): 713-8.
[http://dx.doi.org/10.1016/j.urology.2004.11.006] [PMID: 15833514]

[128] de Bono JS, Scher HI, Montgomery RB, *et al.* Circulating tumor cells predict survival benefit from treatment in metastatic castration-resistant prostate cancer. Clin Cancer Res 2008; 14(19): 6302-9.
[http://dx.doi.org/10.1158/1078-0432.CCR-08-0872] [PMID: 18829513]

[129] Olmos D, Arkenau HT, Ang JE, *et al.* Circulating tumour cell (CTC) counts as intermediate end points in castration-resistant prostate cancer (CRPC): a single-centre experience. Ann Oncol 2009; 20(1): 27-33.
[http://dx.doi.org/10.1093/annonc/mdn544] [PMID: 18695026]

[130] Danila DC, Heller G, Gignac GA, *et al.* Circulating tumor cell number and prognosis in progressive castration-resistant prostate cancer. Clin Cancer Res 2007; 13(23): 7053-8.
[http://dx.doi.org/10.1158/1078-0432.CCR-07-1506] [PMID: 18056182]

[131] Ma X, Xiao Z, Li X, *et al.* Prognostic role of circulating tumor cells and disseminated tumor cells in patients with prostate cancer: a systematic review and meta-analysis. Tumour Biol 2014; 35(6): 5551-60.
[http://dx.doi.org/10.1007/s13277-014-1731-5] [PMID: 24563278]

[132] Tognela A, Spring KJ, Becker T, *et al.* Predictive and prognostic value of circulating tumor cell detection in lung cancer: A clinician's perspective. Crit Rev Oncol Hematol 2015; 93(2): 90-102.
[http://dx.doi.org/10.1016/j.critrevonc.2014.10.001] [PMID: 25459665]

[133] Zhu WF, Li J, Yu LC, *et al.* Prognostic value of EpCAM/MUC1 mRNA-positive cells in non-small

cell lung cancer patients. Tumour Biol 2014; 35(2): 1211-9.
[http://dx.doi.org/10.1007/s13277-013-1162-8] [PMID: 24061641]

[134] Hiltermann TJN, Pore MM, van den Berg A, *et al.* Circulating tumor cells in small-cell lung cancer: a predictive and prognostic factor. Ann Oncol 2012; 23(11): 2937-42.
[http://dx.doi.org/10.1093/annonc/mds138] [PMID: 22689177]

[135] Hou JM, Greystoke A, Lancashire L, *et al.* Evaluation of circulating tumor cells and serological cell death biomarkers in small cell lung cancer patients undergoing chemotherapy. Am J Pathol 2009; 175(2): 808-16.
[http://dx.doi.org/10.2353/ajpath.2009.090078] [PMID: 19628770]

[136] Kloten V, Lampignano R, Krahn T, Schlange T. Circulating Tumor Cell PD-L1 Expression as Biomarker for Therapeutic Efficacy of Immune Checkpoint Inhibition in NSCLC. Cells 2019; 8(8): 809.
[http://dx.doi.org/10.3390/cells8080809] [PMID: 31374957]

[137] Wang Y, Kim TH, Fouladdel S, *et al.* PD-L1 Expression in Circulating Tumor Cells Increases during Radio(chemo)therapy and Indicates Poor Prognosis in Non-small Cell Lung Cancer. Sci Rep 2019; 9(1): 566.
[http://dx.doi.org/10.1038/s41598-018-36096-7] [PMID: 30679441]

[138] Tan Y, Wu H. The significant prognostic value of circulating tumor cells in colorectal cancer: A systematic review and meta-analysis. Curr Probl Cancer 2018; 42(1): 95-106.
[http://dx.doi.org/10.1016/j.currproblcancer.2017.11.002] [PMID: 29277243]

[139] Messaritakis I, Sfakianaki M, Papadaki C, *et al.* Prognostic significance of CEACAM5mRNA-positive circulating tumor cells in patients with metastatic colorectal cancer. Cancer Chemother Pharmacol 2018; 82(5): 767-75.
[http://dx.doi.org/10.1007/s00280-018-3666-9] [PMID: 30094617]

[140] Wang L, Zhou S, Zhang W, *et al.* Circulating tumor cells as an independent prognostic factor in advanced colorectal cancer: a retrospective study in 121 patients. Int J Colorectal Dis 2019; 34(4): 589-97.
[http://dx.doi.org/10.1007/s00384-018-03223-9] [PMID: 30627849]

[141] Rahbari NN, Aigner M, Thorlund K, Mollberg N, Motschall E, Jensen K, *et al.* Meta-analysis shows that detection of circulating tumor cells indicates poor prognosis in patients with colorectal cancer 2010.
[http://dx.doi.org/10.1053/j.gastro.2010.01.008]

[142] Huang MY, Tsai HL, Huang JJ, Wang JY. Clinical Implications and Future Perspectives of Circulating Tumor Cells and Biomarkers in Clinical Outcomes of Colorectal Cancer. Transl Oncol 2016; 9(4): 340-7.
[http://dx.doi.org/10.1016/j.tranon.2016.06.006] [PMID: 27567958]

[143] Mohamed A, Twardy B, Zordok MA, *et al.* Concurrent chemoradiotherapy with weekly *versus* triweekly cisplatin in locally advanced squamous cell carcinoma of the head and neck: Comparative analysis. Head Neck 2019; 41(5): 1490-8.
[http://dx.doi.org/10.1002/hed.25379] [PMID: 30835900]

[144] Patel AS, Allen JE, Dicker DT, *et al.* Identification and enumeration of circulating tumor cells in the cerebrospinal fluid of breast cancer patients with central nervous system metastases. Oncotarget 2011; 2(10): 752-60.
[http://dx.doi.org/10.18632/oncotarget.336] [PMID: 21987585]

[145] Ignatiadis M, Litière S, Rothe F, *et al.* Trastuzumab *versus* observation for HER2 nonamplified early breast cancer with circulating tumor cells (EORTC 90091-10093, BIG 1-12, Treat CTC): a randomized phase II trial. Ann Oncol 2018; 29(8): 1777-83.
[http://dx.doi.org/10.1093/annonc/mdy211] [PMID: 29893791]

[146] Guan X, Ma F, Li C, *et al.* The prognostic and therapeutic implications of circulating tumor cell

phenotype detection based on epithelial-mesenchymal transition markers in the first-line chemotherapy of HER2-negative metastatic breast cancer. Cancer Commun (Lond) 2019; 39(1): 1. [http://dx.doi.org/10.1186/s40880-018-0346-4] [PMID: 30606259]

[147] Horimoto Y, Tokuda E, Murakami F, *et al.* Analysis of circulating tumour cell and the epithelial mesenchymal transition (EMT) status during eribulin-based treatment in 22 patients with metastatic breast cancer: a pilot study. J Transl Med 2018; 16(1): 287. [http://dx.doi.org/10.1186/s12967-018-1663-8] [PMID: 30342534]

[148] Paoletti C, Schiavon G, Dolce EM, *et al.* Circulating Biomarkers and Resistance to Endocrine Therapy in Metastatic Breast Cancers: Correlative Results from AZD9496 Oral SERD Phase I Trial. Clin Cancer Res 2018; 24(23): 5860-72. [http://dx.doi.org/10.1158/1078-0432.CCR-18-1569] [PMID: 30082476]

[149] Nanduri LK, Hissa B, Weitz J, Schölch S, Bork U. The prognostic role of circulating tumor cells in colorectal cancer. Expert Rev Anticancer Ther 2019; 19(12): 1077-88. [http://dx.doi.org/10.1080/14737140.2019.1699065] [PMID: 31778322]

[150] Vogelzang NJ, Fizazi K, Burke JM, *et al.* Circulating Tumor Cells in a Phase 3 Study of Docetaxel and Prednisone with or without Lenalidomide in Metastatic Castration-resistant Prostate Cancer. Eur Urol 2017; 71(2): 168-71. [http://dx.doi.org/10.1016/j.eururo.2016.07.051] [PMID: 27522164]

[151] Heller G, Fizazi K, McCormack R, *et al.* The Added Value of Circulating Tumor Cell Enumeration to Standard Markers in Assessing Prognosis in a Metastatic Castration-Resistant Prostate Cancer Population. Clin Cancer Res 2017; 23(8): 1967-73. [http://dx.doi.org/10.1158/1078-0432.CCR-16-1224] [PMID: 27678453]

[152] Lorente D, Olmos D, Mateo J, *et al.* Circulating tumour cell increase as a biomarker of disease progression in metastatic castration-resistant prostate cancer patients with low baseline CTC counts. Ann Oncol 2018; 29(7): 1554-60. [http://dx.doi.org/10.1093/annonc/mdy172] [PMID: 29741566]

[153] Miyamoto DT, Lee RJ, Kalinich M, *et al.* An RNA-Based Digital Circulating Tumor Cell Signature Is Predictive of Drug Response and Early Dissemination in Prostate Cancer. Cancer Discov 2018; 8(3): 288-303. [http://dx.doi.org/10.1158/2159-8290.CD-16-1406] [PMID: 29301747]

[154] Strati A, Koutsodontis G, Papaxoinis G, *et al.* Prognostic significance of PD-L1 expression on circulating tumor cells in patients with head and neck squamous cell carcinoma. Ann Oncol 2017; 28(8): 1923-33. [http://dx.doi.org/10.1093/annonc/mdx206] [PMID: 28838214]

[155] Wang HM, Wu MH, Chang PH, *et al.* The change in circulating tumor cells before and during concurrent chemoradiotherapy is associated with survival in patients with locally advanced head and neck cancer. Head Neck 2019; 41(8): hed.25744. [http://dx.doi.org/10.1002/hed.25744.] [PMID: 30903634]

[156] Oliveira TB, Braun AC, Nicolau UR, *et al.* Prognostic impact of baseline circulating tumor cells (CTCs) detected by the isolation by size of epithelial tumor cells (ISET) in locally advanced head and neck squamous cell carcinoma (LAHNSCC): Results of a prospective study. J Clin Oncol 2019; 37(15_suppl) (Suppl.): 6061. [http://dx.doi.org/10.1200/JCO.2019.37.15_suppl.6061]

[157] Riethdorf S, Hildebrandt L, Heinzerling L, *et al.* Detection and Characterization of Circulating Tumor Cells in Patients with Merkel Cell Carcinoma. Clin Chem 2019; 65(3): 462-72. [http://dx.doi.org/10.1373/clinchem.2018.297028] [PMID: 30626636]

[158] Wang L, Li Y, Xu J, *et al.* Quantified postsurgical small cell size CTCs and $EpCAM^+$ circulating tumor stem cells with cytogenetic abnormalities in hepatocellular carcinoma patients determine cancer relapse. Cancer Lett 2018; 412: 99-107.

[http://dx.doi.org/10.1016/j.canlet.2017.10.004] [PMID: 29031565]

[159] Effenberger KE, Schroeder C, Hanssen A, *et al.* Improved Risk Stratification by Circulating Tumor Cell Counts in Pancreatic Cancer. Clin Cancer Res 2018; 24(12): 2844-50. [http://dx.doi.org/10.1158/1078-0432.CCR-18-0120] [PMID: 29559560]

[160] Zhang Y, Li J, Wang L, *et al.* Clinical significance of detecting circulating tumor cells in patients with esophageal squamous cell carcinoma by EpCAM-independent enrichment and immunostaining-fluorescence *in situ* hybridization. Mol Med Rep 2019; 20(2): 1551-60. [http://dx.doi.org/10.3892/mmr.2019.10420] [PMID: 31257510]

[161] Eigl BJ, Chi K, Tu D, *et al.* A randomized phase II study of pelareorep and docetaxel or docetaxel alone in men with metastatic castration resistant prostate cancer: CCTG study IND 209. Oncotarget 2018; 9(8): 8155-64. [http://dx.doi.org/10.18632/oncotarget.24263] [PMID: 29487723]

[162] Kulasinghe A, Kapeleris J, Kimberley R, *et al.* The prognostic significance of circulating tumor cells in head and neck and non-small-cell lung cancer. Cancer Med 2018; 7(12): 5910-9. [http://dx.doi.org/10.1002/cam4.1832] [PMID: 30565869]

[163] Pantel K, Alix-Panabières C. Liquid biopsy and minimal residual disease — latest advances and implications for cure. Nat Rev Clin Oncol 2019; 16(7): 409-24. [http://dx.doi.org/10.1038/s41571-019-0187-3] [PMID: 30796368]

[164] Sharma S, Zhuang R, Long M, *et al.* Circulating tumor cell isolation, culture, and downstream molecular analysis. Biotechnol Adv 2018; 36(4): 1063-78. [http://dx.doi.org/10.1016/j.biotechadv.2018.03.007] [PMID: 29559380]

[165] Budd GT, Cristofanilli M, Ellis MJ, *et al.* Circulating tumor cells *versus* imaging--predicting overall survival in metastatic breast cancer. Clin Cancer Res 2006; 12(21): 6403-9. [http://dx.doi.org/10.1158/1078-0432.CCR-05-1769] [PMID: 17085652]

[166] Matsusaka S, Suenaga M, Mishima Y, *et al.* Circulating tumor cells as a surrogate marker for determining response to chemotherapy in Japanese patients with metastatic colorectal cancer. Cancer Sci 2011; 102(6): 1188-92. [http://dx.doi.org/10.1111/j.1349-7006.2011.01926.x] [PMID: 21401804]

[167] Snow A, Chen D, Lang JE. The current status of the clinical utility of liquid biopsies in cancer. Expert Rev Mol Diagn 2019; 19(11): 1031-41. [http://dx.doi.org/10.1080/14737159.2019.1664290] [PMID: 31482746]

[168] Bidard F-C, Jacot W, Dureau S, *et al.* Abstract GS3-07: Clinical utility of circulating tumor cell count as a tool to chose between first line hormone therapy and chemotherapy for ER+ HER2- metastatic breast cancer: Results of the phase III STIC CTC trial. Cancer Res 2019; 79(4_Supplement) (Suppl.).GS3-07. [http://dx.doi.org/10.1158/1538-7445.SABCS18-GS3-07]

[169] Iwata H, Masuda N, Yamamoto D, *et al.* Circulating tumor cells as a prognostic marker for efficacy in the randomized phase III JO21095 trial in Japanese patients with HER2-negative metastatic breast cancer. Breast Cancer Res Treat 2017; 162(3): 501-10. [http://dx.doi.org/10.1007/s10549-017-4138-3] [PMID: 28181129]

[170] Riethdorf S, Müller V, Loibl S, *et al.* Prognostic Impact of Circulating Tumor Cells for Breast Cancer Patients Treated in the Neoadjuvant "Geparquattro" Trial. Clin Cancer Res 2017; 23(18): 5384-93. [http://dx.doi.org/10.1158/1078-0432.CCR-17-0255] [PMID: 28679772]

[171] Wallwiener M, Riethdorf S, Hartkopf AD, *et al.* Serial enumeration of circulating tumor cells predicts treatment response and prognosis in metastatic breast cancer: a prospective study in 393 patients. BMC Cancer 2014; 14(1): 512. [http://dx.doi.org/10.1186/1471-2407-14-512] [PMID: 25015676]

[172] Masuda T, Hayashi N, Iguchi T, Ito S, Eguchi H, Mimori K. Clinical and biological significance of

circulating tumor cells in cancer. Mol Oncol 2016; 10(3): 408-17. [http://dx.doi.org/10.1016/j.molonc.2016.01.010] [PMID: 26899533]

[173] Pan H, Gray R, Braybrooke J, *et al.* 20-year risks of breast-cancer recurrence after stopping endocrine therapy at 5 years. N Engl J Med 2017; 377(19): 1836-46. [http://dx.doi.org/10.1056/NEJMoa1701830] [PMID: 29117498]

[174] Trapp E, Janni W, Schindlbeck C, *et al.* Presence of circulating tumor cells in high-risk early breast cancer during follow-up and prognosis. J Natl Cancer Inst 2019; 111(4): 380-7. [http://dx.doi.org/10.1093/jnci/djy152] [PMID: 30312434]

[175] Sparano J, O'Neill A, Alpaugh K, *et al.* Association of Circulating Tumor Cells With Late Recurrence of Estrogen Receptor–Positive Breast Cancer. JAMA Oncol 2018; 4(12): 1700-6. [http://dx.doi.org/10.1001/jamaoncol.2018.2574] [PMID: 30054636]

[176] Graf RP, Hullings M, Barnett ES, Carbone E, Dittamore R, Scher HI. Clinical Utility of the Nuclear-localized AR-V7 Biomarker in Circulating Tumor Cells in Improving Physician Treatment Choice in Castration-resistant Prostate Cancer. Eur Urol 2020; 77(2): 170-7. [http://dx.doi.org/10.1016/j.eururo.2019.08.020] [PMID: 31648903]

[177] Wark L, Quon H, Ong A, Drachenberg D, Rangel-Pozzo A, Mai S. Long-Term Dynamics of Three Dimensional Telomere Profiles in Circulating Tumor Cells in High-Risk Prostate Cancer Patients Undergoing Androgen-Deprivation and Radiation Therapy. Cancers (Basel) 2019; 11(8): 1165. [http://dx.doi.org/10.3390/cancers11081165] [PMID: 31416141]

[178] Pailler E, Oulhen M, Borget I, *et al.* Circulating Tumor Cells with Aberrant *ALK* Copy Number Predict Progression-Free Survival during Crizotinib Treatment in *ALK* -Rearranged Non–Small Cell Lung Cancer Patients. Cancer Res 2017; 77(9): 2222-30. [http://dx.doi.org/10.1158/0008-5472.CAN-16-3072] [PMID: 28461563]

[179] Kaifi JT, Kunkel M, Dicker DT, *et al.* Circulating tumor cell levels are elevated in colorectal cancer patients with high tumor burden in the liver. Cancer Biol Ther 2015; 16(5): 690-8. [http://dx.doi.org/10.1080/15384047.2015.1026508] [PMID: 25785486]

[180] Lankiewicz S, Zimmermann S, Hollmann C, Hillemann T, Greten TF. Circulating tumour cells as a predictive factor for response to systemic chemotherapy in patients with advanced colorectal cancer. Mol Oncol 2008; 2(4): 349-55. [http://dx.doi.org/10.1016/j.molonc.2008.09.001] [PMID: 19383356]

[181] Shishido SN, Carlsson A, Nieva J, *et al.* Circulating tumor cells as a response monitor in stage IV non-small cell lung cancer. J Transl Med 2019; 17(1): 294. [http://dx.doi.org/10.1186/s12967-019-2035-8] [PMID: 31462312]

[182] Aggarwal C, Wang X, Ranganathan A, *et al.* Circulating tumor cells as a predictive biomarker in patients with small cell lung cancer undergoing chemotherapy. Lung Cancer 2017; 112: 118-25. [http://dx.doi.org/10.1016/j.lungcan.2017.08.008] [PMID: 29191584]

[183] Armstrong AJ, Halabi S, Luo J, *et al.* Prospective Multicenter Validation of Androgen Receptor Splice Variant 7 and Hormone Therapy Resistance in High-Risk Castration-Resistant Prostate Cancer: The PROPHECY Study. J Clin Oncol 2019; 37(13): 1120-9. [http://dx.doi.org/10.1200/JCO.18.01731] [PMID: 30865549]

[184] Wark L, Klonisch T, Awe J, *et al.* Dynamics of three-dimensional telomere profiles of circulating tumor cells in patients with high-risk prostate cancer who are undergoing androgen deprivation and radiation therapies. Urol Oncol 2017; 35(3): 112.e1-112.e11. [http://dx.doi.org/10.1016/j.urolonc.2016.10.018] [PMID: 27956006]

[185] Autio KA, Dreicer R, Anderson J, *et al.* Safety and Efficacy of BIND-014, a Docetaxel Nanoparticle Targeting Prostate-Specific Membrane Antigen for Patients With Metastatic Castration-Resistant Prostate Cancer. JAMA Oncol 2018; 4(10): 1344-51. [http://dx.doi.org/10.1001/jamaoncol.2018.2168] [PMID: 29978216]

[186] de Kruijff IE, Sieuwerts AM, Onstenk W, *et al.* Circulating Tumor Cell Enumeration and Characterization in Metastatic Castration-Resistant Prostate Cancer Patients Treated with Cabazitaxel. Cancers (Basel) 2019; 11(8): 1212.
[http://dx.doi.org/10.3390/cancers11081212] [PMID: 31434336]

[187] Zheng W, Zhang Y, Guo L, *et al.* Evaluation of therapeutic efficacy with CytoSorter®, circulating tumor cell–capture system in patients with locally advanced head and neck squamous cell carcinoma. Cancer Manag Res 2019; 11: 5857-69.
[http://dx.doi.org/10.2147/CMAR.S208409] [PMID: 31303792]

[188] Qiao Y, Li J, Shi C, *et al.* Prognostic value of circulating tumor cells in the peripheral blood of patients with esophageal squamous cell carcinoma. OncoTargets Ther 2017; 10: 1363-73.
[http://dx.doi.org/10.2147/OTT.S129004] [PMID: 28424552]

[189] Troncarelli Flores BC, Souza e Silva V, Ali Abdallah E, *et al.* Molecular and kinetic analyses of circulating tumor cells as predictive markers of treatment response in locally advanced rectal cancer patients. Cells 2019; 8(7): 641.
[http://dx.doi.org/10.3390/cells8070641] [PMID: 31247977]

[190] Rack B, Schindlbeck C, Jückstock J, *et al.* Circulating tumor cells predict survival in early average-to-high risk breast cancer patients. J Natl Cancer Inst 2014; 106(5): dju066.
[http://dx.doi.org/10.1093/jnci/dju066.] [PMID: 24832787]

[191] Thalgott M, Rack B, Horn T, *et al.* Detection of Circulating Tumor Cells in Locally Advanced High-risk Prostate Cancer During Neoadjuvant Chemotherapy and Radical Prostatectomy. Anticancer Res 2015; 35(10): 5679-85.
[PMID: 26408743]

[192] Gazzaniga P, de Berardinis E, Raimondi C, *et al.* Circulating tumor cells detection has independent prognostic impact in high-risk non-muscle invasive bladder cancer. Int J Cancer 2014; 135(8): 1978-82.
[http://dx.doi.org/10.1002/ijc.28830] [PMID: 24599551]

[193] Wang D, Yang Y, Jin L, *et al.* Prognostic models based on postoperative circulating tumor cells can predict poor tumor recurrence-free survival in patients with stage II-III colorectal cancer. J Cancer 2019; 10(19): 4552-63.
[http://dx.doi.org/10.7150/jca.30512] [PMID: 31528219]

[194] Wu CY, Lee CL, Wu CF, *et al.* Circulating Tumor Cells as a Tool of Minimal Residual Disease Can Predict Lung Cancer Recurrence: A longitudinal, Prospective Trial. Diagnostics (Basel) 2020; 10(3): 144.
[http://dx.doi.org/10.3390/diagnostics10030144] [PMID: 32155787]

[195] Hardingham JE, Grover P, Winter M, Hewett PJ, Price TJ, Thierry B. Detection and Clinical Significance of Circulating Tumor Cells in Colorectal Cancer--20 Years of Progress. Mol Med. 2015; 21(Suppl 1(uppl 1)S)S25-31.

[196] Bayarri-Lara C, Ortega FG, Cueto Ladrón de Guevara A, *et al.* Circulating Tumor Cells Identify Early Recurrence in Patients with Non-Small Cell Lung Cancer Undergoing Radical Resection. PLoS One 2016; 11(2)e0148659
[http://dx.doi.org/10.1371/journal.pone.0148659] [PMID: 26913536]

[197] Cieślikowski WA, Budna-Tukan J, Świerczewska M, *et al.* Circulating Tumor Cells as a Marker of Disseminated Disease in Patients with Newly Diagnosed High-Risk Prostate Cancer. Cancers (Basel) 2020; 12(1): 160.
[http://dx.doi.org/10.3390/cancers12010160] [PMID: 31936460]

[198] Josefsson A, Larsson K, Freyhult E, Damber JE, Welén K. Gene Expression Alterations during Development of Castration-Resistant Prostate Cancer Are Detected in Circulating Tumor Cells. Cancers (Basel) 2019; 12(1): 39.
[http://dx.doi.org/10.3390/cancers12010039] [PMID: 31877738]

[199] Huaman J, Naidoo M, Zang X, Ogunwobi OO. Fibronectin Regulation of Integrin B1 and SLUG in Circulating Tumor Cells. Cells 2019; 8(6): 618. [http://dx.doi.org/10.3390/cells8060618] [PMID: 31226820]

[200] Lou E, Vogel RI, Teoh D, *et al.* Assessment of Circulating Tumor Cells as a Predictive Biomarker of Histology in Women With Suspected Ovarian Cancer. Lab Med 2018; 49(2): 134-9. [http://dx.doi.org/10.1093/labmed/lmx084] [PMID: 29361118]

[201] Fabisiewicz A, Szostakowska-Rodzos M, Zaczek AJ, Grzybowska EA. Circulating Tumor Cells in Early and Advanced Breast Cancer; Biology and Prognostic Value. Int J Mol Sci 2020; 21(5): 1671. [http://dx.doi.org/10.3390/ijms21051671] [PMID: 32121386]

Part 3: Protein/Enzyme Biomarkers

CHAPTER 8

Protein Cancer Biomarkers

Sarath S. Joseph[1], Dan H. V. Tran[1], Farhadul Islam[2] and Vinod Gopalan[1,*]

[1] *Molecular and Cellular Pathology, School of Medicine and Dentistry, Griffith University, Gold Coast, Australia*

[2] *Department of Biochemistry and Molecular Biology, University of Rajshahi, Rajshahi-6205, Bangladesh*

Abstract: Cancer is one of the leading causes of death worldwide and it is becoming increasingly important to be able to efficiently identify and map the progression of cancers. The study of the diagnostic, predictive and prognostic value of protein biomarkers has become one of the main aspects at the forefront of cancer research. The diversity of various biomarkers for different cancers and their varying roles in each disease presents a continual challenge for researchers to understand, with new biomarkers still being discovered today. Understanding the role of protein biomarkers ensures patients are diagnosed with greater confidence and helps clinicians with treatment regimes. This chapter aims to discuss the clinical significance of various protein biomarkers in terms of their diagnostic, prognostic, and predictive value in the treatment of their respective cancers.

Keywords: Biomarker, BRCA, Cancer, Calretinin, CD117, Desmin, Diagnosis, ER/PR receptor, GFAP, HER2, Inhibin, Keratin, Protein, Prognosis, Predictive marker, S100 protein, TTF-1.

INTRODUCTION

Even with advancements in therapeutic interventions, the prognostic outcome of most cancers is poor. The low survivability of cancer can be mainly attributed to the difficulty in detecting it at an early stage and the insufficient tools available to map the progression of the disease. At the time of clinical presentation, more often than not, the tumour has metastasized, making it difficult to excise. Imaging, such as mammography with high sensitivity for breast cancer [1], is routinely utilised as screening tools to detect a select range of common tumours before they metastasize. However, the diagnostic and prognostic utility of imaging is questionable for other cancers, not to mention other limitations, including difficulty in tracing macro and micro metastasis. Current limitations result in poor

* **Corresponding author Vinod Gopalan:** Molecular and Cellular Pathology, School of Medicine and Dentistry, Griffith University, Gold Coast, Australia; Email: v.gopalan@griffith.edu.au

surveillance of identified tumours, often resulting in a lack of understanding of the progression of cancer and the regrettable late-stage detection of cancer spread.

The involvement of protein-encoding genes and proteins in tumour growth has been established as a promising front for understanding the development of cancer. Utilising proteins generated from mutated genes during cancer pathogenesis can reveal a great amount of information regarding the identity of the tumour, its origin and its progression. This potentially opens a role for these protein biomarkers to act as predictive markers in clinical use and could offer a real-time assessment of therapeutic efficacy, revolutionising the prognostic role of a simple serum sample. Thirty-seven well-established proteins in today's literature that act as biomarkers (Table **1**), with significant diagnostic, prognostic and clinical value, will be discussed in this chapter.

Table 1. Summary of the diagnostic and prognostic biomarkers with their associated cancers.

Protein Biomarkers	Associated Cancers	References
α-SMA	Oral tongue squamous cell carcinoma, Lung adenocarcinoma, Ovarian cancer	[1, 2, 3, 4, 6]
BRAF	Colon adenocarcinoma, Melanoma, Lung adenocarcinoma, Thyroid papilloma	[7, 9, 10, 11, 12, 13, 14]
BRCA1,BRCA2	Breast cancer, Ovarian cancer, Prostate cancer, Fallopian tube cancer, Endometrial cancer, Pancreatic cancer, Prostate cancer, Colorectal cancer, Melanoma	[17, 18, 19, 20, 21, 22, 23, 24, 25]
Calretinin	Epithelial pleural mesothelioma	[27, 28, 29, 30]
CD117	Gastrointestinal stromal tumour	[32, 33, 34, 35, 36]
CD20	B cell lymphoma, Leukemia	[40,41,42,44]
CD30	B Cell lymphoma	[46, 47, 48]
Chromogranin A	Neuroendocrine tumour	[52, 53, 54]
Cytokeratin (TPA, TPS & CYFRA 21.1)	Lung cancer, Squamous cell carcinoma of Oesophagus, Metastatic breast cancer, Colorectal cancer	[57, 58, 60]
Desmin	Colorectal cancer, Gastrointestinal stromal tumour, Embryonal sarcoma, Gall bladder cancer	[62,63, 64, 65, 66, 67]
EGFR	Lung adenocarcinoma, Glioblastoma, Breast cancer, Colon adenocarcinoma	[68, 69, 70, 71]
EML4/ALK	Lung adenocarcinoma	[72, 73 74]
ER/PR	Breast cancer, Endometrial cancer, Ovarian cancer	[75, 76, 77, 79, 80, 85]
FIP1L1-PDGFRα	Chronic eosinophilic leukemia	[86, 87]
FLI-1 protein	Ewing sarcoma, Vascular tumour, Lymphoblastic lymphoma	[88, 89]

(Table 1) cont.....

Protein Biomarkers	Associated Cancers	References
GFAP	Glioma, Glioblastoma	[91, 92, 93]
GCDFP-15	Breast cancer	[94, 95, 96]
HER2/neu	Breast cancer, Gastric cancer	[97, 98, 99, 100, 101, 102]
hPG80	Colorectal cancer, Renal cell carcinoma, Hepatocellular carcinoma	[103, 104, 107]
HMB-45	Melanoma	[108, 109]
Inhibin	Ovarian cancer	[110]
Keratin-17	Gastric cancer, Breast cancer, Ovarian cancer, Endometrial cancer, High-grade cervical cancer, Bladder cancer	[112, 113, 114, 115, 116, 117]
Keratin-19	Breast cancer, Hepatocellular carcinoma	[118, 119]
KRAS	Lung adenocarcinoma, Pancreatic adenocarcinoma, Colon adenocarcinoma	[122, 123, 124, 125, 126]
Mart-1	Melanoma	[127, 128, 129]
MyoD1	Rhabdomyosarcoma, Breast cancer, Colorectal cancer, Gastric cancer, Head and neck cancer, Lung cancer, Retinoblastoma, Medulloblastoma, Colorectal cancer	[130, 131, 133]
MSA	Paediatric rhabdomyosarcoma, Laryngeal leiomyosarcoma	[134, 135]
Neurofilament	Breast cancer, Gastric cancer, Prostate cancer, Brain metastases from lung cancer	[136, 137, 138, 139]
PDGFR	Ovarian cancer, Breast cancer, Gastrointestinal stromal tumour	[140, 141, 143, 144]
PML/RARα	Promyelocytic leukemia	[148, 149]
S100 protein	Melanoma, Ovarian cancer, Pancreatic cancer, Colorectal cancer, Glioblastoma	[150, 151, 152, 154]
Synaptophysin	Paraganglioma, Pheochromocytoma, Neuroendocrine epithelial tumours	[155, 156]
TTF 1	Thyroid cancer, Lung adenocarcinoma	[157, 158, 159, 161]
Vimentin	Thyroid cancer, Breast cancer, Melanoma, Renal Cell carcinoma, Central neuron system cancer, Gastrointestinal cancer, Cervical cancer, Endometrial cancer, Hepatocellular cancer, Non-small cell lung cancer	[162, 163, 164, 165, 166]

PROTEIN BIOMARKERS

α-Smooth Muscle Actin (α-SMA)

α-SMA is overexpressed in several cancers. Firstly, α-SMA is overexpressed in myofibroblasts in oral tongue squamous cell carcinoma (OTSCC) and acts as an important prognostic biomarker for OTSCC progression, metastasis and patient survival [2]. In a study by Smitha *et al.*, α-SMA was expressed in myofibroblasts in all tissues of OTSCC whilst no α-SMA was detected in the normal oral mucosa or pre-cancerous oral leukoplakia [3]. An increase in α-SMA expression was also detected in OTSCC with lymph node metastasis compared to those without [3].

In lung adenocarcinoma cells, α-SMA also regulates c-MET and FAK expression, which positively upregulates its metastatic potential [4]. α-SMA is subsequently used as an important prognostic biomarker and potential therapeutic target for better management of lung adenocarcinoma [4].

However, in ovarian cancer, the prognostic value of α-SMA as a biomarker is currently debated. For example, a study by Da Silva *et al.*, indicated that there was no significant difference in α-SMA expression between malignant and benign ovarian neoplasms [5]. However, a study by Anggorowati *et al.* described that tumour cells that exhibited α-SMA were predicted to be more invasive, more likely to metastasise and have a worse prognosis [6]. To further complicate this point, Anggorowati *et al.*'s study also detailed that regardless of the location, α-SMA was higher in the stroma of benign ovarian tumours compared to malignant ones [6]. Further research is required to fully understand the nature of α-SMA in ovarian cancer.

BRAF

The BRAF gene encodes for the BRAF protein, which is involved in cell growth and differentiation through the epidermal growth factor receptor (EGFR)-medicated mitogen-activated protein kinase (MAPK) pathway [7]. BRAF mutation is an activating mutation that causes over-proliferation and prevention of apoptosis [8]. BRAF mutation is seen most commonly and could potentially be used as a biomarker for colon adenocarcinoma, melanoma, lung adenocarcinoma and thyroid gland papilloma [9].

In colorectal cancer (CRC), BRAF mutation status is associated with poor prognosis - with those positive for BRAF-mutant CRC having an overall survival of 10.4 months compared to 34.7 months for BRAF wild-type patients [10]. As a predictive biomarker, there is no association between the presence of BRAF mutation and chemotherapy, whilst the evidence regarding its predictive role for anti-EGFR agents is also still debated [11]. However, diagnostically, BRAF mutations assist with diagnostic differentiation between Lynch Syndrome (BRAF negative) and sporadic microsatellite instability tumours (BRAF mutation in 40-50%) [12].

BRAF mutated melanoma appears more in younger patients and is associated with poorer survival than patients with wild-type melanoma at diagnosis and pre-treatment [11]. However, BRAF inhibitors Vemurafenib and Dabrafenib have shown great clinical efficacy against unresectable BRAF mutated melanoma, serving BRAF as an important predictive biomarker [13]. The development of BRAF inhibitors has essentially improved the overall survival of patients with BRAF mutated melanomas, and those with treatment seem to have an overall more positive outcome than wild-type BRAF melanomas [13].

In thyroid papilloma cancer, BRAF V600E mutations occurred on the mRNA level of papilloma cancers in 56.3% of patients. In the context of a diagnostic biomarker, a study by Tran *et al.* found that by utilising BRAF mutations, a detection assay for thyroid cancers improved by 28% and the specificity improved to 100% [14]. The prognostic relevance of BRAF V600E is still controversial in literature but can help with the determination for eligibility for targeted BRAF inhibitor therapy such as with Lenvatinib, Vemurafenib or Sorafenib [15]. BRAF may also be used as diagnostic biomarker in pilocytic astrocytomas in children [16].

Breast Cancer Gene 1 and 2 (BRCA 1 and 2)

BRCA1 and 2 are tumour suppressor genes. Mutation of these genes can lead to the decreased expression of BRCA1 and 2 proteins, resulting in a reduction in DNA repair and increased risk of breast, ovarian and prostate cancer [17]. The BRCA gene mutation is more often used as a prognostic, predictive and diagnostic biomarker rather than the decreased expression of its protein. The lifetime risk for individuals with a mutated BRCA1 or BRCA 2 is 40-80% for breast cancer, 45-60% for ovarian cancer and up to 40% for prostate cancer [18].

In terms of prognosis, the overall survivability of any BRCA mutation compared to those with sporadic breast cancer was very similar at 2 years (97% and 96.6%, respectively, 5 years (83.8% and 85%, respectively) and 10 years (73.4% and 70.1%, respectively) [19].

As a predictive biomarker, clinical studies have suggested an increased response to DNA-targeted chemotherapy for patients with BRCA1 mutations [20].

In patients with ovarian cancer, the prognosis of BRCA1/2 mutation-related cancers mainly depends on the stage of cancer when the patient was diagnosed [21]. There have been some studies that have investigated the prognostic value of BRCA1/2 mutation-positive ovarian cancer patients *versus* controls. It was shown that those with BRCA mutation carriers have a more favourable prognosis than non-carriers [22]. Furthermore, some studies have shown that heterozygous ovarian cancer patients showed more favourable overall survivability [23]. However, there has also been clinical evidence that has shown the opposite [24]. In comparing BRCA 1 and BRCA 2, patients with just the BRCA 2 mutation seem to have a better prognosis than BRCA 1 [24].

As a predictive biomarker, BRCA mutation-positive ovarian cancer patients have been associated with greater response to chemotherapy, namely alkylating drugs, platinum compounds, pegylated liposomal doxorubicin, and trabectedin. These patients seem to also express a longer disease-free interval after chemotherapy treatment [25]. BRCA 1 and 2 mutations may also lead to an increase in fallopian tube cancer, melanoma, endometrial cancer, pancreatic, prostate and CRC [18].

Calretinin

Calretinin (CR) is a calcium (Ca^{2+}) binding protein that functions on the cellular level to buffer and monitor Ca^{2+} levels whilst modulating neuronal excitability [26]. Originally found in neurons, these proteins are also interestingly located on mesothelial cells and over-expressed in the epithelioid-type malignant pleural mesothelioma (MM) [27]. CR, consequently, is considered to be a significant marker of MM [28], with preliminary studies suggesting it has a 71% sensitivity at a specificity of 95% when distinguishing patients with mesothelioma from those who are asbestos-exposed [29]. The epithelioid subtype has a better prognosis over the sarcomatoid or biphasic variants and makes up 60% of MM prevalence [30]. Only this subtype is said to benefit from surgery with curative intent [31]. Considering CR's specificity to epithelial type MM, its utility as a diagnostic tool with further research on its value as a screening tool could improve prognosis through early detection of epithelioid MM and early surgical intervention.

CD117

Approximately 95% of gastrointestinal stromal tumours (GIST) are CD117 (also known as KIT) positive, whilst 80% of them have CD117 mutations [32]. Mutation of CD117 essentially leads to pro-oncogenic function resulting in increased cell growth and survival [33]. These mutations often occur on exons 11 and 9, with an incidence rate of 70% and 15%, respectively [33]. Clinical significance of the mutation site correlates with treatment effectiveness. Imatinib, a tyrosine kinase inhibitor (TKI), blocks signal transduction by binding to CD117 and has clinically significant therapeutic effects for patients with CD117 positive GIST, in particular, mutations on CD117 exon 11 [32, 34, 35]. The prognostic value of utilising CD117 as a biomarker in high-risk GIST populations or amongst GIST patients is not well established, but identifying CD117-positive

GIST can initiate TKI therapy early and with a good response rate [36]. It is important to identify CD117 exon mutation status as alternative sites of mutation in GIST patients can have an increased likelihood of treatment resistance [37]. CD117's prognostic value as a biomarker is also currently examined in ovarian cancer [38] and non-small cell lung cancer [39].

CD20

CD20 antigen is commonly used as a B cell marker and is found in higher than normal amounts in patients with B-cell lymphomas and leukemias [40]. There are limited studies regarding its use as a diagnostic biomarker, but it may help as a predictive factor towards the prognosis of undergoing cancer treatments.

As a prognostic biomarker, in classical Hodgkin's lymphoma, patients that had Reed-Sternberg or Hodgkin cells that expressed CD20 saw a more positive trend for overall survival [41]. Furthermore, in patients with Adult B-cell acute lymphoblastic leukemia, the overall survivability was greater for CD20 negative patients [42]. Here, higher relapse was seen in acute lymphoblastic leukemia patients that were CD20 positive [43]. However, the development of cancer treatments over the last few decades has reduced this prognostic difference between CD20 positive and negative acute lymphoblastic leukemia patients [42].

As a predictive biomarker, patients with B cell lymphomas who have a higher expression of CD20 seem to have a better response to Rituximab therapy than CD20 negative cancers [44].

Other cancers that have positive immunohistochemical staining of CD20 include spindle cell thymomas and T cell lymphomas. The value of CD20 as a clinically important prognostic biomarker for these cancers is still to be investigated [45].

CD30

CD30 is expressed in classical Hodgkin's lymphoma and can be used as a diagnostic biomarker [46]. It is also often used to differentiate between nodular lymphocyte predominant Hodgkin's lymphoma (CD30 negative) from classical Hodgkin's lymphoma (CD30 positive) [47]. Prognostically, soluble CD30 has been demonstrated to be an indicator of disease activity, in turn correlating with clinical outcomes for Hodgkin's lymphoma. Elevated soluble CD30 correlates with patients who have a poor 5-year survival rate (less than 50%), whilst patients with a lower soluble CD30 saw a more favourable 5-year survival [48].

Similar to Hodgkins Lymphoma, soluble CD30 also is a biological serum diagnostic tumour biomarker for anaplastic large cell lymphoma [49]. However, there currently seems to be little to no studies regarding the prognostic value of CD30 in patients with this cancer.

The identification of CD30 has significant value therapeutically as it can help positively determining the efficacy of CD30-directed therapies, such as Brentuximab Vedotin, for classical Hodgkin's and large anaplastic cell lymphomas [50].

Chromogranin A

Chromogranin A (CgA) is an acidic protein that is expressed by several normal and neoplastic cells of neuroendocrine or endocrine origin [51]. CgA elevation can be related to a number of different benign or malignant conditions, including acute coronary syndrome, pancreatitis and even with the use of corticosteroids [52], each with ranging sensitivities and specificities. Pathologically high levels, however, are considered to be linked to neuroendocrine tumours (NET), although this is an area of debate in literature [52]. Some studies have shown the prognostic value of CgA for NET patients. CgA >75mmol/L has a 22% five-year overall survival (OS) *versus* 63% with NET patients where CgA <75mmol/L [53]. CgA's sensitivity and specificity for NETs are often considered to be high, depending on the primary site and degree of differentiation [54], although there are numerous factors that limit its use in clinical application, including large daily variability, interference in levels from food intake [55], its interaction with medications such as proton pump inhibitors [56] and risk of increased false-positives from benign conditions [52]. Such fall-backs make it difficult to establish a recognised standard for a clinically acceptable CgA biomarker cut-off limit.

Cytokeratin (TPA, TPS & CYFRA 21.1)

Tissue polypeptide antigen (TPA), tissue polypeptide-specific antigen (TPS) and serum cytokeratin fragment 21.1 (Cyfra 21.1) are expressed globally in all tissues and play a central role in cancer formation and progression. Cyfra 21.1 has an established role in lung cancer (with the exception of small cell lung cancer). It is routinely used in biomarker panels, with an average sensitivity of 61% [57]. Cyfra 21.1 was also studied in its use in patients with squamous cell carcinoma of the oesophagus, obtaining a low sensitivity but a high specificity, proving valuable as a future diagnostic marker [58]. For bladder cancer, it demonstrated value as a cancer detection marker than a diagnostic tool, although this requires further analysis [59]. TPA (above 255 IU/l) and TPS (above 200 IU/l) have a landmark role in the detection of distant metastasis in breast cancer or CRC patients, helping to improve early diagnosis rates and imaging intervention [60]. TPS, TPA and cyfra 21.1 are associated with other cancers, but their prognostic roles are more obscure, outdated and less reliable.

Desmin

Desmin is commonly known as an intermediate filament protein contained in smooth muscle cells and, more importantly, in tumour desmoplastic stroma [61]. Desmin's role as a protein biomarker is ambiguous and still being investigated. Preliminary studies have shown an over-expression of desmin in CRC, especially that of stage 3 [62]. Desmin's link with carcinogenic angiogenesis is an explanation of the protein being significantly elevated in patients with mature tumours [63]. Its elevated expression in advanced stage CRC correlated with increased severity and decreased survival rates for patients [64]. As a biomarker, desmin shows promising signs of having predictive and staging value for CRC, but studies are in the early stages, and the results have little consistency. Desmin is also a highly sensitive marker for tumour invasiveness in GIST [65] and embryonal sarcomas [66]. Interestingly, it is also down-regulated in gall bladder cancer (GBC) [67]. However, large-scale study and new data are required for desmin to be a reliable marker for the above cancers.

Epidermal Growth Factor Receptor (EGFR)

EGFR missense mutations, deletions and insertions are seen most commonly in lung adenocarcinoma, glioblastoma multiforme (GBM), breast invasive ductal carcinoma and colon adenocarcinoma [68]. In patients with lung adenocarcinoma, EGFR mutation testing is important, as a positive mutation is a strong predictive biomarker for the commencement of potential therapeutic response towards EGFR, namely, targeted tyrosine kinase inhibitor (EGFR-TKI) immunotherapies (Afatinib, Osimertinib and Erlotinib) [69]. Tyrosine kinase inhibitors can often help slow the progression of lung cancer for multiple years but will unfortunately not have a curative intent [69].

Furthermore, EGFR has been found to be amplified in 40%, overexpressed in 60% and deleted or mutated in 24-67% of GBM neoplasms [70]. EGFR overexpression is characteristic of more aggressive GBM phenotypes, whilst the prognostic value of EGFR gene amplification detection is still clinically investigated [70]. Some studies present evidence towards a lack of correlation between EGFR amplification and disease progression, whilst some others describe EGFR amplification to be linked with tumourogenesis and thus a significant and unfavourable predictor for overall survival in patients younger than 60 years [71]. Furthermore, the most common EGFR mutation, EGFRΔIII, is a positive therapeutic predictive factor for Cetuximab treatment, a monoclonal antibody towards C225 [71]. In contrast, clinical trials evaluating EGFR Gefitinib, Erlotinib or Lapatinib in GBMs have demonstrated minimal clinical activity of EGFR tyrosine kinase inhibitor activity towards EGFRΔIII cancers due to insufficient Akt activation [71].

Lastly, activating EGFR mutations occurring in CRC is a positive predictive biomarker for Cetuximab therapy effectiveness, whilst those occurring in breast cancer may see effectiveness in EGFR tyrosine kinase treatment [71].

Echinoderm Microtubule-Associated Protein-Like 4 (EML4) and Anaplastic Lymphoma Kinase (ALK) Fusion (EML4-ALK Fusion)

The identification of EML4-ALK tumour protein, expressed from the EML4-ALK gene rearrangement, is an important biomarker in lung adenocarcinoma [72]. As it has only been identified in a low percentage of patients (1.6-13.5%), there are still limited studies of this protein. However, in a study by Kometani *et al.*, the 5-year survival rate of those without EML4-ALK fusion was 59.4% whilst none of the patients with the EML4-ALK rearrangement reached 5 years [73]. The study's findings also demonstrated that after a univariate analysis of factors such as age, gender and smoking history, EML4-ALK fusion showed significantly shorter survival [73]. However, after a multivariate analysis that included all variables together, the study concluded that EML4-ALK was not a significant prognostic factor overall [73].

Furthermore, a study by Liao *et al.*, concluded that the EML4-ALK fusion gene and its protein are often detected in younger patients, patients who were non or light smokers and those who did not have mutations in EGFR and RAS [74]. These patients also seemed to have a better outcome with chemotherapy cisplatin plus pemetrexed treatment [74]. However, there is still only limited information surrounding the EML4-ALK fusion protein, and as discussed earlier, further studies are required to determine its true value as a diagnostic, predictive or prognostic biomarker.

Estrogen Receptor/Progesterone Receptor (ER/PR)

Estrogen receptor (ER) and progesterone receptor (PR) may act as biomarkers for breast, endometrial and ovarian cancer [75].

For breast cancer, ER-positive tumours are generally well-differentiated, less aggressive and have a better prognosis than ER-negative tumours [76]. In general, increased disease-free survival, decreased recurrence and decreased time to treatment failure have been more positively linked to ER-positive tumours [76]. As a predictive biomarker, ER-positive tumours are able to have a more effective response than non-ER-positive tumours to endocrine therapy such as Tamoxifen or Toremidene in premenopausal patients and letrozole or anastrozole in post-menopausal patients [77]. Tamoxifen and Toremidene target estrogen receptors to suppress oestrogen signalling in breast cancers, whilst letrozole and anastrozole are aromatase inhibitors to inhibit oestrogen synthesis [77]. PR is mainly present in ER-positive tumours and rarely in ER-negative tumours [75]. PR-positive breast cancers are usually less proliferative, less aggressive and have a more favourable prognosis [75]. However, its significance as a predictive biomarker in determining the effectiveness to endocrine medical therapy is still debated [78].

Patients with triple-negative breast cancer (PR, ER and HER2 negative) have a very aggressive type of breast cancer and have a poorer prognosis, with a 77% survival rate after 5 years (90% survival on average after 5 years for those without triple negative cancer) [79]. Triple-negative breast cancer is common amongst women under 40 years old and of African-American descent [79].

For ovarian cancer, about 77% of all cases are ER-positive [75]. Under pathological reasoning, it was believed that the tumorigenic response of ovarian cancer to estrogen depended on over-expression of ER and would thus be associated with a poorer prognosis [80]. However, in terms of clinical evidence, one study found a correlation between patients with higher ER expression and those having endometrial carcinoma or high-grade serous carcinoma with peritoneal metastases [81], whereas another study concluded that overall survival was greater in patients with ER-positive ovarian cancer [82]. For PR, studies have shown that progesterone and its receptors protect against ovarian cancer [83]. Concurrently, studies have shown that the expression of PR has shown to be associated with a more favourable prognosis [80].

In endometrial cancer, PR and ER may both be positive in patients [84]. However, PR status holds more prognostic value than ER status, as there are more independent correlations between PR immunohistochemistry and clinicopathological parameters such as clinical staging and establishing tumour grade [84]. PR also mediates the growth inhibitory effects of progesterone and has been associated with improved response to progestogen treatment for endometrial cancer [85].

FIP1-like-1/Platelet-derived Growth Factor Alpha (FIP1L1-PDGFRα)

FIP1L1-PDGFRα fusion gene is the most common genetic abnormality of chronic eosinophilic leukemia (CEL) [86]. It encodes the FIP1L1-PDGFRα fusion protein, which acts as a positive predictive biomarker for clinical efficacy of treatment with imatinib, a drug that blocks the tumorigenic kinase activity of the protein [87]. FIP1L1-PDGFRα positive CEL patients have an extremely good response rate to imatinib therapy, with most achieving complete haematological and molecular remission [87].

Friend Leukaemia Integration-1 Protein (FLI-1)

FLI-1 protein is associated with proliferation and tumorigenesis [88]. FLI---positivity in an immunohistochemical panel is most suggestive of Ewing Sarcoma, with reactivity reaching 63% to 100% of tumours [89]. The protein's specificity for Ewing Sarcoma makes it of great value when differentiating between common alternative diagnoses such as small cell osteosarcoma and mesenchymal chondrosarcoma, where the protein is negative [89]. FLI-1 is also positive in vascular cancers [88] and lymphoblastic lymphomas [89]. In vascular tumours, it is both extremely sensitive (94%) and specific (100%) for both benign and malignant tumours [88]. Regardless of its clinical use as a diagnostic tool for Ewing sarcoma or vascular tumours, FLI-1's prognostic value is yet to be evaluated in a study.

Glial Fibrillary Acidic Protein (GFAP)

GFAP is produced by astrocytes and is considered a ubiquitous marker of brain injury. It has a clinically significant role in stroke [90], but its role in cancer is less clear. Studies have evaluated an elevated GFAP in cases of high-grade glioma [91] and GBM [92]. For example, GFAP was abundantly expressed and correlated linearly to tumour volume in high-grade malignant glioma patients [91]. Patients with GBM also had similar trends of GFAP in relation to volume of tumour, with a suggested level of >0.20µg/L of GFAP being highly suggestive of GBM [92]. Metastatic brain tumour has been reported of having low GFAP, which allows the protein to be a useful marker to rule out differentials of GBM [92]. However, the limitation of this finding is that if GFAP is low, it does not rule out GBM, making it a poor screening tool [92]. Due to its specificity to GBM, once a diagnosis is established, studies are investigating whether the protein can be utilised as a marker for post-operative tumour recurrence [93].

Gross Cystic Disease Fluid Protein-15 (GCDFP-15)

Gross cystic disease fluid protein-15 (GCDFP-15) is a protein that is expressed in apocrine metaplasia of the breast [94]. It has high specificity in females for metastatic breast cancer as the protein is only otherwise elevated in tumours such as prostate cancer and carcinomas of skin appendages [95]. In fact, when comparing GCDFP-15 with non-mammary malignancies, there was a specificity of 95% for breast cancers. GCDFP-15 is, therefore, clinically utilised as a specific marker for breast cancer [95]. GCDFP-15 positive tumours that are estrogen receptor-negative show a favourable prognosis for patient survival, likely due to GCDFP-15's link to androgen receptor expression, which by itself suggests a 'good-prognosis tumour' [94]. Additionally, molecular apocrine and HER-2 positive tumours that are positive for GCDFP-15 have a good prognosis [96]. GCDFP-15 has good sensitivity for tumours of breast origin, whether that be a primary tumour or nodal metastasis. Its role in specific types of breast cancer is still an area of research.

Human Epidermal Growth Factor Receptor 2 (HER2)/neu

HER2 is overexpressed in 15-20% of primary breast cancers and is usually associated with a more aggressive tumour [97]. HER2 amplification is linked to high cellular activity that stimulates excessive tumour growth [97]. As a result, HER2 expression in breast cancer correlates with a poor prognosis and is associated with higher grade tumours, lymph node invasion, recurrence and mortality [98]. Poor prognosis is also seen in patients that are HER2 positive with zero lymph node involvement [98]. Furthermore, HER2 is a predictive biomarker in response to HER2-targeted therapies such as Trastuzumab, Lapatinib and Pertuzumab [99]. Its expression also correlates with increased response to chemotherapy with anthracyclines and taxanes [75].

HER2 is also overexpressed in gastric cancer (about 30%), and although there is a lack of extensive wide clinical evidence, a positive HER2 status appears to be a poor prognostic indicator [100]. In contrast, CRC HER-2 overexpression has been seen to have little prognostic influence on patient survival [101]. Similar to breast cancer, HER2 also acts as a predictive biomarker for HER2 targeted therapy, such as with Trastuzumab, for both CRC and gastric cancer [100, 101]. Furthermore, for CRC, studies show that HER2 activation and its downstream signalling pathways have been implicated in anti-EGFR therapy resistance [102].

hPG80

Progastrin or hPG80 is the precursor of gastrin that is secreted extracellularly by tumour cells. Eighty percent of CRC patients have elevated hPG80's [103]. Even patients with adenomatous polyps, which is a precursor lesion to colorectal adenocarcinoma, have an elevated hPG80 [103]. The key advantage of this protein is that it is not present in the normal intestinal epithelium. Consequently, it has been suggested as a beneficial biomarker for CRC or CRC development, although a concentration level to diagnose a pathology needs to be established [104]. Since it is not secreted by normal tissue, it can be utilised to indicate the progression of cancer, development of cancer and post-treatment effectiveness. Anti-hPG80 antibody therapy is being investigated and has been utilised to decrease CRC progression in mice [105]. Consequently, future hPG80 cancer lines could benefit from this treatment which could result in an improved prognosis. Recent studies have also prompted hPG80's value as a ubiquitous cancer marker, demonstrating its use outside of its classical role in CRC [106]. Certain cancers such as hepatocellular carcinoma and renal cell carcinoma (RCC) [107] were studied specifically and had elevated hPG80. In fact, the study on RCC even suggested that elevated levels of hPG80 are associated with a poorer overall survival rate [107].

Human Melanoma Black 45 (HMB-45)

Human melanoma black 45 (HMB-45) is an antibody regularly found in immunohistochemical assays used for the detection of metastatic and primary melanoma. Non-melanoma human cancers do not have a reaction to HMB-45, other than a few odd rare tumours, and therefore, these proteins are considered to be highly sensitive to melanoma [108]. Sensitivities range from 75% to 95% for metastatic melanoma of conventional forms [109]. HMG-45 is, however, negative to desmoplastic or spindle cell variants [109]. The protein is also heavily studied for its use in sentinel node staining to improve sensitivity for metastatic melanoma where if positive, it represents early-stage tumour dissemination [109]. Regardless, there are insufficient studies to evaluate its prognostic value. However, since it can be considered a marker for metastasis, its detection could lead to earlier intervention and consequent improvement in prognosis. The complexity of HMB-45 lies in its ability to detect benign lesions of superficial dermal melanocytic origin, such as blue nevi [109]. However, studies have found this to be mitigated by using HMB-45 in conjunction with other serum markers [109].

Inhibin

Inhibins are growth factors (Inhibin A and B) produced primarily by ovarian follicles in women and Sertoli cells in men and play a significant role in both sexes' reproductive cycle [110]. Inhibin has been identified as a potential biomarker for ovarian cancer, especially that of the granulosa cell type and mucinous epithelial type [110]. Inhibin's advantage is that its levels are virtually insignificant in post-menopausal women. The presence of tumours, therefore, will result in an increase in inhibin levels, meaning that any elevation can be considered suspicious [110]. This is particularly important as two-thirds of ovarian cancer cases are found in post-menopausal women who also have the worst prognosis of any gynaecological malignancy, with a 5-year expectancy rate of less than 30% [110]. Its downfall is that the levels measured in premenopausal women are more difficult to interpret. Together with CA125, there is a sensitivity and specificity of 95% [110]. In terms of its prognostic significance, its effectiveness in detecting early cancerous growth is yet to be proven.

Keratin 17 and 19

There are 54 known keratins (KRs), and their activity is well known in cancer cells ranging from growth to metastasis [111]. KR-17 is the most well established in the literature for its involvement in cancer. Poor prognostic outcomes have been established with KR-17 overexpression in gastric cancer [112], breast cancer [113], epithelial ovarian cancer [114], endometrial cancer [115] and high-grade cervical cancer (HSIL) [116]. For example, in patients with HSIL, the median survival for high KR-17 expression was more than twice that of those with low KR-17 expression [115]. In bladder cancer, KR-17 has a diagnostic value with high sensitivity and specificity, although it is a poor indicator of prognosis [117].

KR-19 has also been a biomarker of investigation, especially in regards to its over-expression in highly aggressive breast cancer such as HER2 positive [118]. KR-19 expression is also a negative prognostic indicator for hepatocellular carcinoma [119]. Other keratin markers such as KR-7 are known for their involvement in CRC [120] and other cancers, but these variants will not be discussed in this chapter.

KRAS

KRAS gene encodes for the K-Ras protein, which regulates cell growth, differentiation, and apoptosis [121]. The detection of KRAS mutation is commonly used as a diagnostic biomarker for many cancers, with the most common being lung, pancreatic and colon adenocarcinoma [122]. The incidence of KRAS mutation in lung adenocarcinoma is 10 to 30%, but its prognostic significance is still being extensively investigated [122]. Many studies have indicated a lack of value in utilising a positive KRAS mutation as a prognostic biomarker for lung adenocarcinoma. Identifying Kras mutation has yet to be found beneficial in determining a positive survival time with or without the intervention of preoperative chemotherapy with Mitomycin, Ifosfamide or Cisplatin [123]. Trials have also indicated a lack of response towards EGFR-TKIs for patients with KRAS mutations, as KRAS is downstream from EGFR and thus, can activate its downstream effectors independently of upstream tyrosine kinase receptor activation [123].

In pancreatic cancer, clinical studies have demonstrated that the detection of KRAS mutation increases the sensitivity, accuracy and negative predictive value of cytopathology for the positive diagnosis of pancreatic cancer [124]. The detection of KRAS mutation in plasma often correlates with a worse prognosis [124]. Furthermore, there are often therapeutic implications, with KRAS-blocking drugs, such as Sotorasib, having a significant positive effect on pancreatic cancer patients [124, 125].

Activating KRAS mutations are found in 35% of polyps in CRC and can be negative predictors for therapeutic EGFR regimens in primary or metastatic CRC [126]. Studies have shown that only those with wild-type KRAS will have an effective clinical response to Cetuximab and Panitumumab [126].

Melanoma Antigen Recognized by T cells 1 (MART-1)

MART-1 (Melan-A) is a useful antigen for the diagnosis of metastatic melanoma [127]. The protein is expressed in almost 90% of primary melanoma, proving to be a very useful diagnostic marker [127]. Studies have found a significant relationship between the loss of MART-1 expression for patients with melanoma >1mm thickness and poorer overall survival interval [127]. Often these patients would be in an advanced stage of malignant melanoma. This is also the case in sentinel lymph node investigations, where the expression of MART-1 has been identified as contributing to a worse prognosis [128]. An additional diagnostic strength of MART-1 is its ability to stain spindle cell type melanoma which other markers such as HMB-45 do not. MART-1's main downfall is its difficulty in differentiating between malignant or benign lesions, although this is an area of contention as some recent studies have suggested that it is expressed more in malignant lesions [129].

Myogenic Differentiation 1 (MyoD1)

Myogenic Differentiation 1 (MyoD1) functions by regulating the cell cycle by promoting cell differentiation and apoptosis [130]. The dysregulated expression of MyoD1 is linked with multiple cancers, including breast cancer, CRC, gastric cancer, head and neck cancer, lung adenocarcinoma, retinoblastoma and medulloblastoma [130]. Its prognostic value in each of these cancers has yet to be established. MyoD1 was also found to have almost a 100% expression rate in rhabdomyosarcoma (RMS), consequently being recommended as a standard biomarker for this cancer [131]. In fact, the decreased expression of MyoD1 often indicated a poorer prognosis with a higher likelihood of recurrence or metastasis in those with non-alveolar type RMS [132]. Additionally, in CRC, MyoD1 hypermethylation was a significant prognostic indicator with a shorter survival time than those without hypermethylation, although it is not routinely used as a CRC biomarker [133].

Muscle-Specific Actin (MSA)

Research into muscle-specific actin (MSA) is not as well established as its common counterpart, desmin, and its prognostic value in most cancers has not been ascertained. MSA, however, is a recommended component of a routine immunohistochemical assay for patients with paediatric RMS due to its incredibly high sensitivity and specificity [134]. However, this is more of a diagnostic tool as there are only a few studies conducted on the prognostic outcome for RMS patients. It also has diagnostic value for laryngeal leiomyosarcoma, a rare tumour, although more studies are required for it to be utilised for clinical practice [135].

Neurofilament

Consisting of several different subunits that have potential in cancer research, neurofilaments (NFs) are primarily found in neurons. These proteins are valuable biomarkers for neurodegenerative diseases, but their clinical value for cancers is still being investigated. NFs, in particular the light subunit (NFL), were found to be expressed in 92.3% of breast cancers and downregulated in lymph node metastasis [136]. Consequently, a lower NFL expression was suggestive of a worse prognosis with a lower five-year disease-free survival for early-stage breast cancer patients [136]. Similar trends of low NF levels have been identified in other cancers, too, such as gastric cancer [137] and prostate cancer [138]. Although, its prognostic value still needs to be determined in these cancers. A more prolific recent finding was the relationship between NF and brain metastasis in non-small cell lung cancer patients. NF light polypeptide was significantly elevated in patients with brain metastases [139]. In fact, patients that were categorised as having low NFL levels compared to normal had double the overall survival rate when compared to those with high NFL levels [139]. Clinically this is significant as brain metastases are often fatal with poor outcomes and clinicians desperately need biomarkers for early intervention to ensure a better prognosis for patients.

Platelet-Derived Growth Factor Receptor (PDGFR)

PDGFR is detected in a variety of cancers, including ovarian, breast, GIST and more, and is primarily used as a biomarker for treatment efficacy and prognosis [140]. For example, positive immunostaining for PDGF is an adverse prognostic biomarker for those with breast cancers as it is correlated with those who have advanced stage IV cancer, less favourable clinicopathological factors and a shorter survival time [141]. Similarly, in ovarian cancer, the detection of subtype PDGFR alpha is also associated with a poor prognosis [140].

For GIST, subtype PDGFR alpha can act as a diagnostic biomarker for atypical patients that do not exhibit positive immunoreactivity for the usual diagnostic biomarkers CD117/DOG [142]. Prognostically, PDGFRA mutated GISTs tend to develop a more indolent clinical course and have a more favourable outcome post-surgery [143]. As a predictive biomarker, the most common GIST PDGFRA mutation, the exon 18 D842V substitution, results in a change in the kinase activation loop, in turn creating resistance to imatinib and thus low overall survival during imatinib or sunitinib treatment [144]. Strangely enough, those exon 18 mutations without D842V mutations are, in fact, sensitive to imatinib treatment [145]. Imatinib tyrosine kinase inhibitor therapy is currently the mainstay for unresectable or metastatic GIST [146].

Other tumours that PDGFR may have prognostic significance include pancreatic, lung adenocarcinoma, gastric tumours and melanoma [147].

Promyelocytic Leukemia Protein–Retinoic Acid Receptor alpha (PML/RARα)

PML and RAR gene rearrangement results in the expression of fusion PML/RAR alpha mRNA protein that molecularly characterises acute promyelocytic leukemia [148]. Thus, specific detection of PML/RARα protein in serum or bone marrow acts as a diagnostic tool for acute promyelocytic leukemia [148]. Monitoring PML/RARα proteins also provide the ability to monitor disease course and response to therapy [149]. A detectable increase in PML/RARα proteins can be detected 4-6 months before hematologic relapse when monitoring residual disease during follow-up [149].

S100

S100 proteins are a family of proteins that may all be associated with the progression, diagnosis and treatment of various cancers, and to name a few - melanoma, breast, lung, ovarian, colon and pancreatic cancer [150]. For example, protein S100B is an important and highly studied biomarker for melanoma in terms of treatment as well as for melanoma staging and prognostic evaluation [150]. Elevated S100B in pre-treatment patients is often correlated with worsened tumour progression, increased risk of metastatic growth, decreased efficacy of treatment and a reduction in survival rates [150]. There is also continuing development of S100B inhibitors in medical cancer intervention for melanoma [151].

Furthermore, S100A4 (Metastasin) is also another commonly studied protein in the S100 family [152]. S100A4 is associated with cellular invasion and metastasis, acting as a prognostic biomarker for many cancers, including ovarian, pancreatic, CRC and GBM. Elevated S100A4 is often seen in those patients with more aggressive tumours, more advanced staging and poorer survival [153].

S100A11 is commonly over-expressed in ovarian cancer cells and can be another important biomarker for diagnosis and treatment [154]. Furthermore, the protein can also be used to predict metastatic risk for pancreatic cancer, as S100A11 is thought to upregulate the Pi3K/AKT signalling pathway, which mediates metastasis in tumour cells [154]. Other notable proteins not covered in this chapter that act as prognostic or diagnostic biomarkers in the s100 family include S100A1-16 and S100P [150].

Synaptophysin

Synaptophysin is a broad spectrum neuroendocrine marker [155]. It is a membrane glycoprotein in neuronal presynaptic vesicles and is expressed in neuroendocrine tumours, including paragangliomas, pheochromocytomas and in neuroendocrine epithelial tumours such as islet cell, gastrointestinal tumours (GIT) and bronchial tract tumours [155]. Through immunohistochemistry, the use of monoclonal antibodies on synaptophysin can be used to identify, characterise and diagnostically differentiate between several different neuroendocrine tumours [156]. However, for some neuroendocrine tumours, synaptophysin is present in both benign and malignant lesions or may be absent in some tumours altogether. As a result, the detection of secretogranin I and II simultaneously in an immunohistochemical panel can help with developing criteria to divide neuroendocrine tumours into various subtypes [156].

Thyroid Transcription Factor 1 (TTF-1)

TTF-1 is a tissue specific transcription factor that is expressed in thyroid and lung epithelial cells [157]. As it has a narrow expression in the human body, TTF-1 is an important biomarker used in the diagnosis of a variety of tumours originating from the thyroid (papillary, follicular and medullary) or lung (adenocarcinoma, small cell or carcinoid tumours) [157].

More specifically, TTF-1 allows investigators to identify neoplasms as having a lung origin [158]. For example, for adenocarcinomas in body fluid cavities, TTF-1 can be used to differentiate adenocarcinomas originating from the lung from other carcinomas with similar morphologies, such as those from the breast, GIT and RCC [159]. The prognostic value of TTF-1 in lung carcinoma is still undetermined. Some bodies of research claim there is no association with prognosis [160], whilst some studies identified that TTF-1 expression correlated with less aggressive behaviour of stage 1 adenocarcinomas and a more favourable outcome [158].

For thyroid carcinomas, especially papillary carcinomas, patients exhibiting a normal level of TTF-1 alongside having a BRAF mutation seemed to have a lower level of disease recurrence in their prognostic outcome [161]. Conversely, those with low levels of TTF-1 and a BRAF mutation showed an approximate 1/3 disease recurrence in the same time frame [161].

Vimentin

Vimentin staining is primarily utilised as a broad diagnostic biomarker [162]. As it is an intermediate filament for mesenchymal tissue, it can confirm mesenchymal origin for tumours of soft tissue [162]. Vimentin is also overexpressed in carcinomas of the cortex, thyroid, breast, melanoma, RCC (except chromophobe RCC), central nervous system (CNS) and GIT tumours [163]. As an example of its diagnostic value as a biomarker, endocervical adenocarcinoma (Vimentin negative) and endometrial carcinoma (vimentin-positive) can be differentiated from each other using vimentin identification as part of a serum panel [164].

Its prognostic value as a biomarker varies amongst cancers. In hepatocellular carcinomas, vimentin expression was typically associated with metastasis and thus a poorer prognosis [163]. Furthermore, in NSCLC and cervical cancer, vimentin positivity was significantly associated with invasiveness of the tumours and poor prognosis [165, 166]. However, in cervical cancer, the significance of the overexpression of vimentin in prognosis is still debated as survival is still seen to be strongly influenced by age, tumour size, presence of lymph node metastases and clinical stage [166].

CONCLUDING REMARKS

Evaluating and establishing protein biomarkers is a continuing area of research and has allowed medical professionals to diagnose and treat cancers in ways that were once not possible. Understanding the varying diagnostic, prognostic and predictive value of biomarkers for their respective cancers provides a wealth of knowledge in their treatment. For example, estrogen receptor, progesterone receptor and HER2 are strongly linked to breast cancer prognosis and have revolutionised endocrinological and monoclonal antibody therapy. Furthermore, CD20 and CD30 are two notable protein biomarkers that have played a significant role in assisting in the diagnosis and prognosis of lymphoma and leukemias. Other tumour markers, such as CD117 and hPG80, show immense promise for cancer patients in future clinical practice once an established concentration level can be obtained. Table **1**, based on current literature, summarises the tumour protein antigens used as biomarkers for the different cancers that have a prognostic and diagnostic role. The myriad of protein biomarkers and their diverse roles in disease is not entirely limited to this paper, and our understanding of it is continuing to grow daily with the hopes of advancing cancer diagnosis and treatment in order to minimise its impact on the burden of illness.

CONSENT FOR PUBLICATION

Not applicable.

CONFLICT OF INTEREST

The authors declare no conflict of interest, financial or otherwise.

ACKNOWLEDGEMENTS

The authors are thankful to the Molecular and Cellular Pathology, School of Medicine and Dentistry, Griffith University, Gold Coast, Australia, for providing the technical support for the work.

REFERENCES

[1] Barlow WE, Lehman CD, Zheng Y, *et al.* Performance of diagnostic mammography for women with signs or symptoms of breast cancer. J Natl Cancer Inst 2002; 94(15): 1151-9. [http://dx.doi.org/10.1093/jnci/94.15.1151] [PMID: 12165640]

[2] Ding L, Zhang Z, Shang D, *et al.* α-Smooth muscle actin-positive myofibroblasts, in association with epithelial-mesenchymal transition and lymphogenesis, is a critical prognostic parameter in patients with oral tongue squamous cell carcinoma. J Oral Pathol Med 2014; 43(5): 335-43. [http://dx.doi.org/10.1111/jop.12143] [PMID: 24313357]

[3] Smitha A, Rao K, Umadevi HS, Smitha T, Sheethal HS, Vidya MA. Immunohistochemical study of α-smooth muscle actin expression in oral leukoplakia and oral squamous cell carcinoma. J Oral Maxillofac Pathol 2019; 23(1): 59-64. [PMID: 31110418]

[4] Lee HW, Park YM, Lee SJ, *et al.* Alpha-smooth muscle actin (ACTA2) is required for metastatic potential of human lung adenocarcinoma. Clin Cancer Res 2013; 19(21): 5879-89. [http://dx.doi.org/10.1158/1078-0432.CCR-13-1181] [PMID: 23995859]

[5] da Silva AC, Jammal MP, Etchebehere RM, Murta EFC, Nomelini RS. Role of Alpha-Smooth Muscle Actin and Fibroblast Activation Protein Alpha in Ovarian Neoplasms. Gynecol Obstet Invest 2018; 83(4): 381-7. [http://dx.doi.org/10.1159/000488088] [PMID: 29621774]

[6] Anggorowati N, Ratna Kurniasari Ch, Damayanti K, *et al.* Histochemical and Immunohistochemical Study of α-SMA, Collagen, and PCNA in Epithelial Ovarian Neoplasm. Asian Pac J Cancer Prev 2017; 18(3): 667-71. [PMID: 28440973]

[7] Barras D. *BRAF* Mutation in Colorectal Cancer: An Update. Biomark Cancer 2015; 7s1 (Suppl. 1).BIC.S25248. [http://dx.doi.org/10.4137/BIC.S25248] [PMID: 26396549]

[8] Caputo E. A Look Inside of the Complex Pathogenesis of B-RAF(V600E)-Driven Cancer. Theranostics 2017; 7(7): 2108-10. [http://dx.doi.org/10.7150/thno.20460] [PMID: 28638488]

[9] Sánchez-Torres JM, Viteri S, Molina MA, Rosell R. BRAF mutant non-small cell lung cancer and treatment with BRAF inhibitors. Transl Lung Cancer Res 2013; 2(3): 244-50. [PMID: 25806238]

[10] Tran B, Kopetz S, Tie J, *et al.* Impact of BRAF mutation and microsatellite instability on the pattern of metastatic spread and prognosis in metastatic colorectal cancer. Cancer 2011; 117(20): 4623-32. [http://dx.doi.org/10.1002/cncr.26086] [PMID: 21456008]

[11] Richman SD, Seymour MT, Chambers P, *et al.* KRAS and BRAF mutations in advanced colorectal cancer are associated with poor prognosis but do not preclude benefit from oxaliplatin or irinotecan: results from the MRC FOCUS trial. J Clin Oncol 2009; 27(35): 5931-7. [http://dx.doi.org/10.1200/JCO.2009.22.4295] [PMID: 19884549]

[12] Domingo E, Niessen RC, Oliveira C, *et al.* BRAF-V600E is not involved in the colorectal tumorigenesis of HNPCC in patients with functional MLH1 and MSH2 genes. Oncogene 2005; 24(24): 3995-8. [http://dx.doi.org/10.1038/sj.onc.1208569] [PMID: 15782118]

[13] Long GV, Menzies AM, Nagrial AM, *et al.* Prognostic and clinicopathologic associations of oncogenic BRAF in metastatic melanoma. J Clin Oncol 2011; 29(10): 1239-46. [http://dx.doi.org/10.1200/JCO.2010.32.4327] [PMID: 21343559]

[14] Tran TV, Dang KX, Pham QH, *et al.* Evaluation of the expression levels of $BRAF^{V600E}$ mRNA in primary tumors of thyroid cancer using an ultrasensitive mutation assay. BMC Cancer 2020; 20(1): 368. [http://dx.doi.org/10.1186/s12885-020-06862-w] [PMID: 32357861]

[15] Naoum GE, Morkos M, Kim B, Arafat W. Novel targeted therapies and immunotherapy for advanced thyroid cancers. Mol Cancer 2018; 17(1): 51. [http://dx.doi.org/10.1186/s12943-018-0786-0] [PMID: 29455653]

[16] Penman CL, Faulkner C, Lowis SP, Kurian KM. Current Understanding of BRAF Alterations in Diagnosis, Prognosis, and Therapeutic Targeting in Pediatric Low-Grade Gliomas. Front Oncol 2015; 5: 54. [http://dx.doi.org/10.3389/fonc.2015.00054] [PMID: 25785246]

[17] Casaubon JT, Kashyap S, Regan JP. Regan JP BRCA 1 and 2 In StatPearls, Treasure Island (FL),. 2021.

[18] Paul A, Paul S. The breast cancer susceptibility genes (BRCA) in breast and ovarian cancers. Front Biosci 2014; 19(4): 605-18. [http://dx.doi.org/10.2741/4230] [PMID: 24389207]

[19] Petrucelli N, Daly MB, Pal T. BRCA1- and BRCA2-Associated Hereditary Breast and Ovarian Cancer. In: Adam MP, Ardinger HH, Pagon RA, Eds. GeneReviews ((R)). Seattle, WA 1993; Vol. R.

[20] James CR, Quinn JE, Mullan PB, Johnston PG, Harkin DP. BRCA1, a potential predictive biomarker in the treatment of breast cancer. Oncologist 2007; 12(2): 142-50. [http://dx.doi.org/10.1634/theoncologist.12-2-142] [PMID: 17296808]

[21] Ben David Y, Chetrit A, Hirsh-Yechezkel G, *et al.* Effect of BRCA mutations on the length of survival in epithelial ovarian tumors. J Clin Oncol 2002; 20(2): 463-6. [http://dx.doi.org/10.1200/JCO.2002.20.2.463] [PMID: 11786575]

[22] Bolton KL, Chenevix-Trench G, Goh C, *et al.* Association between BRCA1 and BRCA2 mutations and survival in women with invasive epithelial ovarian cancer. JAMA 2012; 307(4): 382-90. [http://dx.doi.org/10.1001/jama.2012.20] [PMID: 22274685]

[23] Chetrit A, Hirsh-Yechezkel G, Ben-David Y, Lubin F, Friedman E, Sadetzki S. Effect of BRCA1/2 mutations on long-term survival of patients with invasive ovarian cancer: the national Israeli study of ovarian cancer. J Clin Oncol 2008; 26(1): 20-5. [http://dx.doi.org/10.1200/JCO.2007.11.6905] [PMID: 18165636]

[24] Pharoah PD, Easton DF, Stockton DL, Gayther S, Ponder BA. Survival in familial, BRCA1-associated, and BRCA2-associated epithelial ovarian cancer. Cancer Res 1999; 59(4): 868-71. [PMID: 10029077]

[25] Quinn JE, James CR, Stewart GE, *et al.* BRCA1 mRNA expression levels predict for overall survival in ovarian cancer after chemotherapy. Clin Cancer Res 2007; 13(24): 7413-20. [http://dx.doi.org/10.1158/1078-0432.CCR-07-1083] [PMID: 18094425]

[26] Link T, Passek S, Wimberger P, *et al.* Serum calretinin as an independent predictor for platinum resistance and prognosis in ovarian cancer. Int J Cancer 2020; 146(9): 2608-18. [http://dx.doi.org/10.1002/ijc.32676] [PMID: 31509615]

[27] Johnen G, Gawrych K, Raiko I, *et al.* Calretinin as a blood-based biomarker for mesothelioma. BMC Cancer 2017; 17(1): 386. [http://dx.doi.org/10.1186/s12885-017-3375-5] [PMID: 28558669]

[28] Blum W, Pecze L, Rodriguez JW, Steinauer M, Schwaller B. Regulation of calretinin in malignant mesothelioma is mediated by septin 7 binding to the CALB2 promoter. BMC Cancer 2018; 18(1): 475. [http://dx.doi.org/10.1186/s12885-018-4385-7] [PMID: 29699512]

[29] Casjens S, Weber DG, Johnen G, *et al.* Assessment of potential predictors of calretinin and mesothelin to improve the diagnostic performance to detect malignant mesothelioma: results from a population-based cohort study. BMJ Open 2017; 7(10)e017104. [http://dx.doi.org/10.1136/bmjopen-2017-017104] [PMID: 29025836]

[30] Zhang YZ, Brambilla C, Molyneaux PL, *et al.* Presence of pleomorphic features but not growth patterns improves prognostic stratification of epithelioid malignant pleural mesothelioma by 2□tier nuclear grade. Histopathology 2020; 77(3): 423-36. [http://dx.doi.org/10.1111/his.14127] [PMID: 32333813]

[31] Rusch VW, Giroux D, Kennedy C, *et al.* Initial analysis of the international association for the study of lung cancer mesothelioma database. J Thorac Oncol 2012; 7(11): 1631-9. [http://dx.doi.org/10.1097/JTO.0b013e31826915f1] [PMID: 23070243]

[32] Sanchez-Hidalgo JM, Duran-Martinez M, Molero-Payan R, *et al.* Gastrointestinal stromal tumors: A multidisciplinary challenge. World J Gastroenterol 2018; 24(18): 1925-41. [http://dx.doi.org/10.3748/wjg.v24.i18.1925] [PMID: 29760538]

[33] Corless CL, Barnett CM, Heinrich MC. Gastrointestinal stromal tumours: origin and molecular oncology. Nat Rev Cancer 2011; 11(12): 865-78. [http://dx.doi.org/10.1038/nrc3143] [PMID: 22089421]

[34] DeMatteo RP. Nanoneoadjuvant therapy of gastrointestinal stromal tumor (GIST). Ann Surg Oncol 2009; 16(4): 799-800. [http://dx.doi.org/10.1245/s10434-009-0316-9] [PMID: 19169754]

[35] Eisenberg BL. The SSG XVIII/AIO Trial. Am J Clin Oncol 2013; 36(1): 89-90. [http://dx.doi.org/10.1097/COC.0b013e31827a7f55] [PMID: 23334483]

[36] Parab TM, DeRogatis MJ, Boaz AM, *et al.* Gastrointestinal stromal tumors: a comprehensive review. J Gastrointest Oncol 2018; 10(1): 144-54. [http://dx.doi.org/10.21037/jgo.2018.08.20] [PMID: 30788170]

[37] Cassier PA, Fumagalli E, Rutkowski P, *et al.* Outcome of patients with platelet-derived growth factor receptor alpha-mutated gastrointestinal stromal tumors in the tyrosine kinase inhibitor era. Clin Cancer Res 2012; 18(16): 4458-64. [http://dx.doi.org/10.1158/1078-0432.CCR-11-3025] [PMID: 22718859]

[38] Yang B, Yan X, Liu L, Jiang C, Hou S. Overexpression of the cancer stem cell marker CD117 predicts poor prognosis in epithelial ovarian cancer patients: evidence from meta-analysis. OncoTargets Ther 2017; 10: 2951-61. [http://dx.doi.org/10.2147/OTT.S136549] [PMID: 28652777]

[39] Sakabe T, Azumi J, Haruki T, Umekita Y, Nakamura H, Shiota G. CD117 expression is a predictive marker for poor prognosis in patients with non-small cell lung cancer. Oncol Lett 2017; 13(5): 3703-8. [http://dx.doi.org/10.3892/ol.2017.5925] [PMID: 28521472]

[40] Pavlasova G, Mraz M. The regulation and function of CD20: an "enigma" of B-cell biology and targeted therapy. Haematologica 2020; 105(6): 1494-506. [http://dx.doi.org/10.3324/haematol.2019.243543] [PMID: 32482755]

[41] Tzankov A, Krugmann J, Fend F, Fischhofer M, Greil R, Dirnhofer S. Prognostic significance of CD20 expression in classical Hodgkin lymphoma: a clinicopathological study of 119 cases. Clin Cancer Res 2003; 9(4): 1381-6. [PMID: 12684408]

[42] Esteban RE, Christianne B, Alvaro A, Demichelis-Gómez R. Prognostic Effect of CD20 Expression in Adult B-cell Acute Lymphoblastic Leukemia. Clin Lymphoma Myeloma Leuk 2018; 18(5): 361-7. [http://dx.doi.org/10.1016/j.clml.2018.02.013] [PMID: 29544762]

[43] Solano-Genesta M, Tarín-Arzaga L, Velasco-Ruiz I, *et al.* CD20 expression in B-cell precursor acute lymphoblastic leukemia is common in Mexican patients and lacks a prognostic value. Hematology 2012; 17(2): 66-70. [http://dx.doi.org/10.1179/102453312X13221316477741] [PMID: 22664043]

[44] Horvat M, Kloboves Prevodnik V, Lavrencak J, Jezersek Novakovic B. Predictive significance of the cut-off value of CD20 expression in patients with B-cell lymphoma. Oncol Rep 2010; 24(4): 1101-7. [PMID: 20811695]

[45] Bellizzi AM. An Algorithmic Immunohistochemical Approach to Define Tumor Type and Assign Site of Origin. Adv Anat Pathol 2020; 27(3): 114-63. [http://dx.doi.org/10.1097/PAP.0000000000000256] [PMID: 32205473]

[46] Döring C, Hansmann ML, Agostinelli C, *et al.* A novel immunohistochemical classifier to distinguish Hodgkin lymphoma from ALK anaplastic large cell lymphoma. Mod Pathol 2014; 27(10): 1345-54. [http://dx.doi.org/10.1038/modpathol.2014.44] [PMID: 24633193]

[47] Hartmann S, Cogliatti S, Hansmann ML. Noduläres lymphozytenprädominantes Hodgkin-Lymphom und seine Differenzialdiagnosen. Pathologe 2013; 34(3): 233-43. [http://dx.doi.org/10.1007/s00292-013-1747-4] [PMID: 23494280]

[48] Visco C, Nadali G, Vassilakopoulos TP, *et al.* Very high levels of soluble CD30 recognize the patients with classical Hodgkin's lymphoma retaining a very poor prognosis. Eur J Haematol 2006; 77(5): 387-94. [http://dx.doi.org/10.1111/j.1600-0609.2006.00725.x] [PMID: 16879607]

[49] Nadali G, Vinante F, Stein H, *et al.* Serum levels of the soluble form of CD30 molecule as a tumor marker in CD30+ anaplastic large-cell lymphoma. J Clin Oncol 1995; 13(6): 1355-60. [http://dx.doi.org/10.1200/JCO.1995.13.6.1355] [PMID: 7751879]

[50] van der Weyden CA, Pileri SA, Feldman AL, Whisstock J, Prince HM. Understanding CD30 biology and therapeutic targeting: a historical perspective providing insight into future directions. Blood Cancer J 2017; 7(9)e603. [http://dx.doi.org/10.1038/bcj.2017.85] [PMID: 28885612]

[51] D'amico MA, Ghinassi B, Izzicupo P, Manzoli L, Di Baldassarre A. Biological function and clinical relevance of chromogranin A and derived peptides. Endocr Connect 2014; 3(2): R45-54. [http://dx.doi.org/10.1530/EC-14-0027] [PMID: 24671122]

[52] Gkolfinopoulos S, Tsapakidis K, Papadimitriou K, Papamichael D, Kountourakis P. Chromogranin A as a valid marker in oncology: Clinical application or false hopes? World J Methodol 2017; 7(1): 9-15. [http://dx.doi.org/10.5662/wjm.v7.i1.9] [PMID: 28396845]

[53] Ardill JES, Erikkson B. The importance of the measurement of circulating markers in patients with neuroendocrine tumours of the pancreas and gut. Endocr Relat Cancer 2003; 10(4): 459-62. [http://dx.doi.org/10.1677/erc.0.0100459] [PMID: 14713258]

[54] Kanakis G, Kaltsas G. Biochemical markers for gastroenteropancreatic neuroendocrine tumours (GEP-NETs). Best Pract Res Clin Gastroenterol 2012; 26(6): 791-802.

[http://dx.doi.org/10.1016/j.bpg.2012.12.006] [PMID: 23582919]

[55] Granberg D, Stridsberg M, Seensalu R, *et al.* Plasma chromogranin A in patients with multiple endocrine neoplasia type 1. J Clin Endocrinol Metab 1999; 84(8): 2712-7. [http://dx.doi.org/10.1210/jcem.84.8.5938] [PMID: 10443665]

[56] Fossmark R, Jianu CS, Martinsen TC, Qvigstad G, Syversen U, Waldum HL. Serum gastrin and chromogranin A levels in patients with fundic gland polyps caused by long-term proton-pump inhibition. Scand J Gastroenterol 2008; 43(1): 20-4. [http://dx.doi.org/10.1080/00365520701561959] [PMID: 18938772]

[57] Stieber P, Dienemann H, Hasholzner U, *et al.* Comparison of cytokeratin fragment 19 (CYFRA 21-1), tissue polypeptide antigen (TPA) and tissue polypeptide specific antigen (TPS) as tumour markers in lung cancer. Clin Chem Lab Med 1993; 31(10): 689-94. [http://dx.doi.org/10.1515/cclm.1993.31.10.689] [PMID: 7507359]

[58] Brockmann JG, St Nottberg H, Glodny B, Heinecke A, Senninger NJ. CYFRA 21-1 serum analysis in patients with esophageal cancer. Clin Cancer Res 2000; 6(11): 4249-52. [PMID: 11106239]

[59] Huang YL, Chen J, Yan W, Zang D, Qin Q, Deng AM. Diagnostic accuracy of cytokeratin-19 fragment (CYFRA 21–1) for bladder cancer: a systematic review and meta-analysis. Tumour Biol 2015; 36(5): 3137-45. [http://dx.doi.org/10.1007/s13277-015-3352-z] [PMID: 25854170]

[60] Kucera R, Topolcan O, Fiala O, *et al.* The Role of TPS and TPA in the Diagnostics of Distant Metastases. Anticancer Res 2016; 36(2): 773-7. [PMID: 26851038]

[61] De Wever O, Demetter P, Mareel M, Bracke M. Stromal myofibroblasts are drivers of invasive cancer growth. Int J Cancer 2008; 123(10): 2229-38. [http://dx.doi.org/10.1002/ijc.23925] [PMID: 18777559]

[62] Arentz G, Chataway T, Price TJ, *et al.* Desmin expression in colorectal cancer stroma correlates with advanced stage disease and marks angiogenic microvessels. Clin Proteomics 2011; 8(1): 16. [http://dx.doi.org/10.1186/1559-0275-8-16] [PMID: 22141345]

[63] Nehls V, Denzer K, Drenckhahn D. Pericyte involvement in capillary sprouting during angiogenesis *in situ.* Cell Tissue Res 1992; 270(3): 469-74. [http://dx.doi.org/10.1007/BF00645048] [PMID: 1283113]

[64] Ma Y, Peng J, Liu W, *et al.* Proteomics identification of desmin as a potential oncofetal diagnostic and prognostic biomarker in colorectal cancer. Mol Cell Proteomics 2009; 8(8): 1878-90. [http://dx.doi.org/10.1074/mcp.M800541-MCP200] [PMID: 19460759]

[65] Liegl B, Hornick JL, Antonescu CR, Corless CL, Fletcher CDM. Rhabdomyosarcomatous differentiation in gastrointestinal stromal tumors after tyrosine kinase inhibitor therapy: a novel form of tumor progression. Am J Surg Pathol 2009; 33(2): 218-26. [http://dx.doi.org/10.1097/PAS.0b013e31817ec2e6] [PMID: 18830121]

[66] Dias P, Kumar P, Marsden HB, *et al.* Evaluation of desmin as a diagnostic and prognostic marker of childhood rhabdomyosarcomas and embryonal sarcomas. Br J Cancer 1987; 56(3): 361-5. [http://dx.doi.org/10.1038/bjc.1987.203] [PMID: 3311112]

[67] Tiwari PK, Bhunia S, Barbhuiya MA, Gupta S, Shrivastava BR. Epigenetic downregulation of desmin in gall bladder cancer reveals its potential role in disease progression. Indian J Med Res 2020; 151(4): 311-8. [http://dx.doi.org/10.4103/ijmr.IJMR_501_18] [PMID: 32461394]

[68] Gao Y, Vallentgoed W, French P. Finding the Right Way to Target EGFR in Glioblastomas; Lessons from Lung Adenocarcinomas. Cancers (Basel) 2018; 10(12): 489. [http://dx.doi.org/10.3390/cancers10120489] [PMID: 30518123]

[69] Harrison PT, Vyse S, Huang PH. Rare epidermal growth factor receptor (EGFR) mutations in non-small cell lung cancer. Semin Cancer Biol 2020; 61: 167-79.
[http://dx.doi.org/10.1016/j.semcancer.2019.09.015] [PMID: 31562956]

[70] Hatanpaa KJ, Burma S, Zhao D, Habib AA. Epidermal growth factor receptor in glioma: signal transduction, neuropathology, imaging, and radioresistance. Neoplasia 2010; 12(9): 675-84.
[http://dx.doi.org/10.1593/neo.10688] [PMID: 20824044]

[71] Xu H, Zong H, Ma C, *et al.* Epidermal growth factor receptor in glioblastoma. Oncol Lett 2017; 14(1): 512-6.
[http://dx.doi.org/10.3892/ol.2017.6221] [PMID: 28693199]

[72] Wen M, Wang X, Sun Y, *et al.* Detection of EML4-ALK fusion gene and features associated with EGFR mutations in Chinese patients with non-small-cell lung cancer. OncoTargets Ther 2016; 9: 1989-95.
[http://dx.doi.org/10.2147/OTT.S100303] [PMID: 27103824]

[73] Kometani T, Sugio K, Osoegawa A, Seto T, Ichinose Y. Clinicopathological features of younger (aged ≤ 50 years) lung adenocarcinoma patients harboring the *EML4-ALK* fusion gene. Thorac Cancer 2018; 9(5): 563-70.
[http://dx.doi.org/10.1111/1759-7714.12616] [PMID: 29517858]

[74] Liao BC, Lin CC, Shih JY, Yang JCH. Treating patients with *ALK* -positive non-small cell lung cancer: latest evidence and management strategy. Ther Adv Med Oncol 2015; 7(5): 274-90.
[http://dx.doi.org/10.1177/1758834015590593] [PMID: 26327925]

[75] Patani N, Martin LA, Dowsett M. Biomarkers for the clinical management of breast cancer: International perspective. Int J Cancer 2013; 133(1): 1-13.
[http://dx.doi.org/10.1002/ijc.27997] [PMID: 23280579]

[76] Hammond MEH, Hayes DF, Dowsett M, *et al.* American Society of Clinical Oncology/College Of American Pathologists guideline recommendations for immunohistochemical testing of estrogen and progesterone receptors in breast cancer. J Clin Oncol 2010; 28(16): 2784-95.
[http://dx.doi.org/10.1200/JCO.2009.25.6529] [PMID: 20404251]

[77] De Abreu FB, Schwartz GN, Wells WA, Tsongalis GJ. Personalized therapy for breast cancer. Clin Genet 2014; 86(1): 62-7.
[http://dx.doi.org/10.1111/cge.12381] [PMID: 24635704]

[78] Davies C, Godwin J, Gray R, *et al.* Relevance of breast cancer hormone receptors and other factors to the efficacy of adjuvant tamoxifen: patient-level meta-analysis of randomised trials. Lancet 2011; 378(9793): 771-84.
[http://dx.doi.org/10.1016/S0140-6736(11)60993-8] [PMID: 21802721]

[79] Ovcaricek T, Frkovic S, Matos E, Mozina B, Borstnar S. Triple negative breast cancer - prognostic factors and survival. Radiol Oncol 2011; 45(1): 46-52.
[http://dx.doi.org/10.2478/v10019-010-0054-4] [PMID: 22933934]

[80] Lee P, Rosen DG, Zhu C, Silva EG, Liu J. Expression of progesterone receptor is a favorable prognostic marker in ovarian cancer. Gynecol Oncol 2005; 96(3): 671-7.
[http://dx.doi.org/10.1016/j.ygyno.2004.11.010] [PMID: 15721410]

[81] Chen S, Dai X, Gao Y, Shen F, Ding J, Chen Q. The positivity of estrogen receptor and progesterone receptor may not be associated with metastasis and recurrence in epithelial ovarian cancer. Sci Rep 2017; 7(1): 16922.
[http://dx.doi.org/10.1038/s41598-017-17265-6] [PMID: 29208958]

[82] Shen Z, Luo H, Li S, *et al.* Correlation between estrogen receptor expression and prognosis in epithelial ovarian cancer: a meta-analysis. Oncotarget 2017; 8(37): 62400-13.
[http://dx.doi.org/10.18632/oncotarget.18253] [PMID: 28977954]

[83] Ho SM. Estrogen, progesterone and epithelial ovarian cancer. Reprod Biol Endocrinol 2003; 1(1): 73.

[http://dx.doi.org/10.1186/1477-7827-1-73] [PMID: 14577831]

[84] Fukuda K, Mori M, Uchiyama M, Iwai K, Iwasaka T, Sugimori H. Prognostic significance of progesterone receptor immunohistochemistry in endometrial carcinoma. Gynecol Oncol 1998; 69(3): 220-5.
[http://dx.doi.org/10.1006/gyno.1998.5023] [PMID: 9648591]

[85] Sieh W, Köbel M, Longacre TA, *et al.* Hormone-receptor expression and ovarian cancer survival: an Ovarian Tumor Tissue Analysis consortium study. Lancet Oncol 2013; 14(9): 853-62.
[http://dx.doi.org/10.1016/S1470-2045(13)70253-5] [PMID: 23845225]

[86] Cools J. FIP1L1-PDGFR alpha, a therapeutic target for the treatment of chronic eosinophilic leukemia. Verh K Acad Geneeskd Belg 2005; 67(3): 169-76.
[PMID: 16089297]

[87] Qu SQ, Qin TJ, Xu ZF, *et al.* Long-term outcomes of imatinib in patients with FIP1L1/PDGFRA associated chronic eosinophilic leukemia: experience of a single center in China. Oncotarget 2016; 7(22): 33229-36.
[http://dx.doi.org/10.18632/oncotarget.8906] [PMID: 27120808]

[88] Folpe AL, Chand EM, Goldblum JR, Weiss SW. Expression of Fli-1, a nuclear transcription factor, distinguishes vascular neoplasms from potential mimics. Am J Surg Pathol 2001; 25(8): 1061-6.
[http://dx.doi.org/10.1097/00000478-200108000-00011] [PMID: 11474291]

[89] Lee AF, Hayes MM, LeBrun D, *et al.* FLI-1 distinguishes Ewing sarcoma from small cell osteosarcoma and mesenchymal chondrosarcoma. Appl Immunohistochem Mol Morphol 2011; 19(3): 233-8.
[http://dx.doi.org/10.1097/PAI.0b013e3181fd6697] [PMID: 21084965]

[90] Wunderlich MT, Wallesch CW, Goertler M. Release of glial fibrillary acidic protein is related to the neurovascular status in acute ischemic stroke. Eur J Neurol 2006; 13(10): 1118-23.
[http://dx.doi.org/10.1111/j.1468-1331.2006.01435.x] [PMID: 16987165]

[91] Brommeland T, Rosengren L, Fridlund S, Hennig R, Isaksen V. Serum levels of glial fibrillary acidic protein correlate to tumour volume of high-grade gliomas. Acta Neurol Scand 2007; 116(6): 380-4.
[http://dx.doi.org/10.1111/j.1600-0404.2007.00889.x] [PMID: 17986096]

[92] Tichy J, Spechtmeyer S, Mittelbronn M, *et al.* Prospective evaluation of serum glial fibrillary acidic protein (GFAP) as a diagnostic marker for glioblastoma. J Neurooncol 201 6 126 (2): 361-9

[93] Husain H, Savage W, Grossman SA, *et al.* Pre- and post-operative plasma glial fibrillary acidic protein levels in patients with newly diagnosed gliomas. J Neurooncol 2012; 109(1): 123-7.
[http://dx.doi.org/10.1007/s11060-012-0874-8] [PMID: 22492246]

[94] Darb-Esfahani S, von Minckwitz G, Denkert C, *et al.* Gross cystic disease fluid protein 15 (GCDFP-15) expression in breast cancer subtypes. BMC Cancer 2014; 14(1): 546.
[http://dx.doi.org/10.1186/1471-2407-14-546] [PMID: 25070172]

[95] Wick MR, Lillemoe TJ, Copland GT, Swanson PE, Manivel JC, Kiang DT. Gross cystic disease fluid protein-15 as a marker for breast cancer: Immunohistochemical analysis of 690 human neoplasms and comparison with alpha-lactalbumin. Hum Pathol 1989; 20(3): 281-7.
[http://dx.doi.org/10.1016/0046-8177(89)90137-8] [PMID: 2542151]

[96] Ni YB, Tsang JYS, Chan SK, Tse GM. GATA-binding protein 3, gross cystic disease fluid protein-15 and mammaglobin have distinct prognostic implications in different invasive breast carcinoma subgroups. Histopathology 2015; 67(1): 96-105.
[http://dx.doi.org/10.1111/his.12625] [PMID: 25425335]

[97] Slamon DJ, Clark GM, Wong SG, Levin WJ, Ullrich A, McGuire WL. Human breast cancer: correlation of relapse and survival with amplification of the HER-2/neu oncogene. Science 1987; 235(4785): 177-82.
[http://dx.doi.org/10.1126/science.3798106] [PMID: 3798106]

[98] Payne SJL, Bowen RL, Jones JL, Wells CA. Predictive markers in breast cancer - the present. Histopathology 2008; 52(1): 82-90.
[http://dx.doi.org/10.1111/j.1365-2559.2007.02897.x] [PMID: 18171419]

[99] Kreutzfeldt J, Rozeboom B, Dey N, De P. The trastuzumab era: current and upcoming targeted HER2+ breast cancer therapies. Am J Cancer Res 2020; 10(4): 1045-67.
[PMID: 32368385]

[100] Rüschoff J, Hanna W, Bilous M, *et al.* HER2 testing in gastric cancer: a practical approach. Mod Pathol 2012; 25(5): 637-50.
[http://dx.doi.org/10.1038/modpathol.2011.198] [PMID: 22222640]

[101] De Cuyper A, Van Den Eynde M, Machiels JP. HER2 as a Predictive Biomarker and Treatment Target in Colorectal Cancer. Clin Colorectal Cancer 2020; 19(2): 65-72.
[http://dx.doi.org/10.1016/j.clcc.2020.02.007] [PMID: 32229076]

[102] Seshacharyulu P, Ponnusamy MP, Haridas D, Jain M, Ganti AK, Batra SK. Targeting the EGFR signaling pathway in cancer therapy. Expert Opin Ther Targets 2012; 16(1): 15-31.
[http://dx.doi.org/10.1517/14728222.2011.648617] [PMID: 22239438]

[103] Najib S, Kowalski-Chauvel A, Do C, Roche S, Cohen-Jonathan-Moyal E, Seva C. Progastrin a new pro-angiogenic factor in colorectal cancer. Oncogene 2015; 34(24): 3120-30.
[http://dx.doi.org/10.1038/onc.2014.255] [PMID: 25109333]

[104] Konturek PC, Bielanski W, Konturek SJ, *et al.* Progastrin and cyclooxygenase-2 in colorectal cancer. Dig Dis Sci 2002; 47(9): 1984-91.
[http://dx.doi.org/10.1023/A:1019652224424] [PMID: 12353842]

[105] Koh TJ, Bulitta CJ, Fleming JV, Dockray GJ, Varro A, Wang TC. Gastrin is a target of the β-catenin/TCF-4 growth-signaling pathway in a model of intestinal polyposis. J Clin Invest 2000; 106(4): 533-9.
[http://dx.doi.org/10.1172/JCI9476] [PMID: 10953028]

[106] You B, Mercier F, Assenat E, *et al.* The oncogenic and druggable hPG80 (Progastrin) is overexpressed in multiple cancers and detected in the blood of patients. EBioMedicine 2020; 51102574.
[http://dx.doi.org/10.1016/j.ebiom.2019.11.035] [PMID: 31877416]

[107] Kohli M, Tan W, Vire B, *et al.* Prognostic Value of Plasma hPG_{80} (Circulating Progastrin) in Metastatic Renal Cell Carcinoma. Cancers (Basel) 2021; 13(3): 375.
[http://dx.doi.org/10.3390/cancers13030375] [PMID: 33498444]

[108] Mahmood MN, Lee MW, Linden MD, Nathanson SD, Hornyak TJ, Zarbo RJ. Diagnostic value of HMB-45 and anti-Melan A staining of sentinel lymph nodes with isolated positive cells. Mod Pathol 2002; 15(12): 1288-93.
[http://dx.doi.org/10.1097/01.MP.0000037313.33138.DF] [PMID: 12481009]

[109] Baisden BL, Askin FB, Lange JR, Westra WH. HMB-45 immunohistochemical staining of sentinel lymph nodes: a specific method for enhancing detection of micrometastases in patients with melanoma. Am J Surg Pathol 2000; 24(8): 1140-6.
[http://dx.doi.org/10.1097/00000478-200008000-00012] [PMID: 10935655]

[110] Robertson DM, Pruysers E, Jobling T. Inhibin as a diagnostic marker for ovarian cancer. Cancer Lett 2007; 249(1): 14-7.
[http://dx.doi.org/10.1016/j.canlet.2006.12.017] [PMID: 17320281]

[111] Zhang N, Zhang R, Zou K, *et al.* Keratin 23 promotes telomerase reverse transcriptase expression and human colorectal cancer growth. Cell Death Dis 2017; 8(7)e2961.
[http://dx.doi.org/10.1038/cddis.2017.339] [PMID: 28749462]

[112] Ide M, Kato T, Ogata K, Mochiki E, Kuwano H, Oyama T. Keratin 17 expression correlates with tumor progression and poor prognosis in gastric adenocarcinoma. Ann Surg Oncol 2012; 19(11): 3506-14.

[http://dx.doi.org/10.1245/s10434-012-2437-9] [PMID: 22695933]

[113] Merkin RD, Vanner EA, Romeiser JL, *et al.* Keratin 17 is overexpressed and predicts poor survival in estrogen receptor–negative/human epidermal growth factor receptor-2–negative breast cancer. Hum Pathol 2017; 62: 23-32.
[http://dx.doi.org/10.1016/j.humpath.2016.10.006] [PMID: 27816721]

[114] Wang YF, Lang HY, Yuan J, *et al.* Overexpression of keratin 17 is associated with poor prognosis in epithelial ovarian cancer. Tumour Biol 2013; 34(3): 1685-9.
[http://dx.doi.org/10.1007/s13277-013-0703-5] [PMID: 23430585]

[115] Bai JDK, Babu S, Roa-Peña L, *et al.* Keratin 17 is a negative prognostic biomarker in high-grade endometrial carcinomas. Hum Pathol 2019; 94: 40-50.
[http://dx.doi.org/10.1016/j.humpath.2019.09.005] [PMID: 31655172]

[116] Escobar-Hoyos LF, Yang J, Zhu J, *et al.* Keratin 17 in premalignant and malignant squamous lesions of the cervix: proteomic discovery and immunohistochemical validation as a diagnostic and prognostic biomarker. Mod Pathol 2014; 27(4): 621-30.
[http://dx.doi.org/10.1038/modpathol.2013.166] [PMID: 24051697]

[117] Babu S, Mockler DC, Roa-Peña L, *et al.* Keratin 17 is a sensitive and specific biomarker of urothelial neoplasia. Mod Pathol 2019; 32(5): 717-24.
[http://dx.doi.org/10.1038/s41379-018-0177-5] [PMID: 30443013]

[118] Kabir NN, Rönnstrand L, Kazi JU. Keratin 19 expression correlates with poor prognosis in breast cancer. Mol Biol Rep 2014; 41(12): 7729-35.
[http://dx.doi.org/10.1007/s11033-014-3684-6] [PMID: 25156534]

[119] Kawai T, Yasuchika K, Ishii T, *et al.* Keratin 19, a Cancer Stem Cell Marker in Human Hepatocellular Carcinoma. Clin Cancer Res 2015; 21(13): 3081-91.
[http://dx.doi.org/10.1158/1078-0432.CCR-14-1936] [PMID: 25820415]

[120] Harbaum L, Pollheimer MJ, Kornprat P, *et al.* Keratin 7 expression in colorectal cancer - freak of nature or significant finding? Histopathology 2011; 59(2): 225-34.
[http://dx.doi.org/10.1111/j.1365-2559.2011.03694.x] [PMID: 21884201]

[121] D'Arcangelo M, Cappuzzo F. K-Ras Mutations in Non-Small-Cell Lung Cancer: Prognostic and Predictive Value. ISRN Mol Biol 2012; 2012: 1-8.
[http://dx.doi.org/10.5402/2012/837306] [PMID: 27398239]

[122] Jančík S, Drábek J, Radzioch D, Hajdúch M. Clinical relevance of KRAS in human cancers. J Biomed Biotechnol 2010; 2010: 1-13.
[http://dx.doi.org/10.1155/2010/150960] [PMID: 20617134]

[123] Martin P, Leighl NB, Tsao MS, Shepherd FA. KRAS mutations as prognostic and predictive markers in non-small cell lung cancer. J Thorac Oncol 2013; 8(5): 530-42.
[http://dx.doi.org/10.1097/JTO.0b013e318283d958] [PMID: 23524403]

[124] Buscail L, Bournet B, Cordelier P. Role of oncogenic KRAS in the diagnosis, prognosis and treatment of pancreatic cancer. Nat Rev Gastroenterol Hepatol 2020; 17(3): 153-68.
[http://dx.doi.org/10.1038/s41575-019-0245-4] [PMID: 32005945]

[125] Hong DS, Fakih MG, Strickler JH, *et al.* KRAS ^{G12C} Inhibition with Sotorasib in Advanced Solid Tumors. N Engl J Med 2020; 383(13): 1207-17.
[http://dx.doi.org/10.1056/NEJMoa1917239] [PMID: 32955176]

[126] Harbison CT, Horak CE, Ledeine JM, *et al.* Validation of companion diagnostic for detection of mutations in codons 12 and 13 of the KRAS gene in patients with metastatic colorectal cancer: analysis of the NCIC CTG CO.17 trial. Arch Pathol Lab Med 2013; 137(6): 820-7.
[http://dx.doi.org/10.5858/arpa.2012-0367-OA] [PMID: 23030695]

[127] Berset M, Cerottini JP, Guggisberg D, *et al.* Expression of melan-a/MART-1 antigen as a prognostic factor in primary cutaneous melanoma. Int J Cancer 2001; 95(1): 73-7.

[http://dx.doi.org/10.1002/1097-0215(20010120)95:1<73::AID-IJC1013>3.0.CO;2-S] [PMID: 11241315]

[128] Hochberg M, Lotem M, Gimon Z, Shiloni E, Enk CD. Expression of tyrosinase, MIA and MART-1 in sentinel lymph nodes of patients with malignant melanoma. Br J Dermatol 2002; 146(2): 244-9. [http://dx.doi.org/10.1046/j.1365-2133.2002.04579.x] [PMID: 11903234]

[129] Nazarian RM, Prieto VG, Elder DE, Duncan LM. Melanoma biomarker expression in melanocytic tumor progression: a tissue microarray study. J Cutan Pathol 2010; 37(s1) (Suppl. 1): 41-7. [http://dx.doi.org/10.1111/j.1600-0560.2010.01505.x] [PMID: 20482674]

[130] Wu F, Qin Y, Jiang Q, *et al.* MyoD1 suppresses cell migration and invasion by inhibiting FUT4 transcription in human gastric cancer cells. Cancer Gene Ther 2020; 27(10-11): 773-84. [http://dx.doi.org/10.1038/s41417-019-0153-3] [PMID: 31831855]

[131] Folpe AL. MyoD1 and myogenin expression in human neoplasia: a review and update. Adv Anat Pathol 2002; 9(3): 198-203. [http://dx.doi.org/10.1097/00125480-200205000-00003] [PMID: 11981115]

[132] Ahmed AA, Habeebu S, Farooqi MS, *et al.* MYOD1 as a prognostic indicator in rhabdomyosarcoma. Pediatr Blood Cancer 2021; 68(9)e29085. [http://dx.doi.org/10.1002/pbc.29085] [PMID: 33913590]

[133] Hiranuma C, Kawakami K, Oyama K, Ota N, Omura K, Watanabe G. Hypermethylation of the MYOD1 gene is a novel prognostic factor in patients with colorectal cancer. Int J Mol Med 2004; 13(3): 413-7. [http://dx.doi.org/10.3892/ijmm.13.3.413] [PMID: 14767572]

[134] Rangdaeng S, Truong LD. Comparative immunohistochemical staining for desmin and muscle-specific actin. A study of 576 cases. Am J Clin Pathol 1991; 96(1): 32-45. [http://dx.doi.org/10.1093/ajcp/96.1.32] [PMID: 1712542]

[135] Marioni G, Staffieri C, Marino F, Staffieri A. Leiomyosarcoma of the larynx: Critical analysis of the diagnostic role played by immunohistochemistry. Am J Otolaryngol 2005; 26(3): 201-6. [http://dx.doi.org/10.1016/j.amjoto.2004.11.007] [PMID: 15858778]

[136] Li XQ, Li L, Xiao CH, Feng YM. NEFL mRNA expression level is a prognostic factor for early-stage breast cancer patients. PLoS One 2012; 7(2)e31146. [http://dx.doi.org/10.1371/journal.pone.0031146] [PMID: 22319610]

[137] Liu S, Huang Z, Zhang L, *et al.* Plasma Neurofilament Light Chain May Be a Biomarker for the Inverse Association Between Cancers and Neurodegenerative Diseases. Front Aging Neurosci 2020; 12: 10. [http://dx.doi.org/10.3389/fnagi.2020.00010] [PMID: 32082140]

[138] Schleicher RL, Hunter SB, Zhang M, *et al.* Neurofilament heavy chain-like messenger RNA and protein are present in benign prostate and down-regulated in prostatic carcinoma. Cancer Res 1997; 57(16): 3532-6. [PMID: 9270025]

[139] Winther-Larsen A, Hviid CVB, Meldgaard P, Sorensen BS, Sandfeld-Paulsen B. Neurofilament Light Chain as A Biomarker for Brain Metastases. Cancers (Basel) 2020; 12(10): 2852. [http://dx.doi.org/10.3390/cancers12102852] [PMID: 33023150]

[140] Appiah-Kubi K, Wang Y, Qian H, *et al.* Platelet-derived growth factor receptor/platelet-derived growth factor (PDGFR/PDGF) system is a prognostic and treatment response biomarker with multifarious therapeutic targets in cancers. Tumour Biol 2016; 37(8): 10053-66. [http://dx.doi.org/10.1007/s13277-016-5069-z] [PMID: 27193823]

[141] Seymour L, Bezwoda WR. Positive immunostaining for platelet derived growth factor (PDGF) is an adverse prognostic factor in patients with advanced breast cancer. Breast Cancer Res Treat 1994; 32(2): 229-33.

[http://dx.doi.org/10.1007/BF00665774] [PMID: 7865852]

[142] Wu CE, Tzen CY, Wang SY, Yeh CN. Clinical Diagnosis of Gastrointestinal Stromal Tumor (GIST): From the Molecular Genetic Point of View. Cancers (Basel) 2019; 11(5): 679. [http://dx.doi.org/10.3390/cancers11050679] [PMID: 31100836]

[143] Szucs Z, Thway K, Fisher C, *et al.* Molecular subtypes of gastrointestinal stromal tumors and their prognostic and therapeutic implications. Future Oncol 2017; 13(1): 93-107. [http://dx.doi.org/10.2217/fon-2016-0192] [PMID: 27600498]

[144] Heinrich MC, Owzar K, Corless CL, *et al.* Correlation of kinase genotype and clinical outcome in the North American Intergroup Phase III Trial of imatinib mesylate for treatment of advanced gastrointestinal stromal tumor: CALGB 150105 Study by Cancer and Leukemia Group B and Southwest Oncology Group. J Clin Oncol 2008; 26(33): 5360-7. [http://dx.doi.org/10.1200/JCO.2008.17.4284] [PMID: 18955451]

[145] Corless CL, Schroeder A, Griffith D, *et al.* PDGFRA mutations in gastrointestinal stromal tumors: frequency, spectrum and *in vitro* sensitivity to imatinib. J Clin Oncol 2005; 23(23): 5357-64. [http://dx.doi.org/10.1200/JCO.2005.14.068] [PMID: 15928335]

[146] Blanke CD, Rankin C, Demetri GD, *et al.* Phase III randomized, intergroup trial assessing imatinib mesylate at two dose levels in patients with unresectable or metastatic gastrointestinal stromal tumors expressing the kit receptor tyrosine kinase: S0033. J Clin Oncol 2008; 26(4): 626-32. [http://dx.doi.org/10.1200/JCO.2007.13.4452] [PMID: 18235122]

[147] Raica M, Cimpean AM. Platelet-Derived Growth Factor (PDGF)/PDGF Receptors (PDGFR) Axis as Target for Antitumor and Antiangiogenic Therapy. Pharmaceuticals (Basel) 2010; 3(3): 572-99. [http://dx.doi.org/10.3390/ph3030572] [PMID: 27713269]

[148] Diverio D, Riccioni R, Mandelli F, Lo Coco F. The PML/RAR alpha fusion gene in the diagnosis and monitoring of acute promyelocytic leukemia. Haematologica 1995; 80(2): 155-60. [PMID: 7628753]

[149] Applegate TL, Iland HJ, Mokany E, Todd AV. Diagnosis and molecular monitoring of acute promyelocytic leukemia using DzyNA reverse transcription-PCR to quantify PML/RARalpha fusion transcripts. Clin Chem 2002; 48(8): 1338-43. [http://dx.doi.org/10.1093/clinchem/48.8.1338] [PMID: 12142392]

[150] Harpio R, Einarsson R. S100 proteins as cancer biomarkers with focus on S100B in malignant melanoma. Clin Biochem 2004; 37(7): 512-8. [http://dx.doi.org/10.1016/j.clinbiochem.2004.05.012] [PMID: 15234232]

[151] Hartman KG, McKnight LE, Liriano MA, Weber DJ. The evolution of S100B inhibitors for the treatment of malignant melanoma. Future Med Chem 2013; 5(1): 97-109. [http://dx.doi.org/10.4155/fmc.12.191] [PMID: 23256816]

[152] Ikenaga N, Ohuchida K, Mizumoto K, *et al.* S100A4 mRNA is a diagnostic and prognostic marker in pancreatic carcinoma. J Gastrointest Surg 2009; 13(10): 1852-8. [http://dx.doi.org/10.1007/s11605-009-0978-4] [PMID: 19653048]

[153] Lv Y, Niu Z, Guo X, Yuan F, Liu Y. Serum S100 calcium binding protein A4 (S100A4, metatasin) as a diagnostic and prognostic biomarker in epithelial ovarian cancer. Br J Biomed Sci 2018; 75(2): 88-91. [http://dx.doi.org/10.1080/09674845.2017.1394052] [PMID: 29421955]

[154] Li W, Cui Z, Kong Y, Liu X, Wang X. Serum Levels of S100A11 and MMP-9 in Patients with Epithelial Ovarian Cancer and Their Clinical Significance. BioMed Res Int 2021; 2021: 1-5. [http://dx.doi.org/10.1155/2021/7341247] [PMID: 33763485]

[155] Gould VE, Wiedenmann B, Lee I, *et al.* Synaptophysin expression in neuroendocrine neoplasms as determined by immunocytochemistry. Am J Pathol 1987; 126(2): 243-57. [PMID: 3103452]

[156] Wiedenmann B, Franke WW, Kuhn C, Moll R, Gould VE. Synaptophysin: a marker protein for neuroendocrine cells and neoplasms. Proc Natl Acad Sci USA 1986; 83(10): 3500-4. [http://dx.doi.org/10.1073/pnas.83.10.3500] [PMID: 3010302]

[157] Ordóñez NG. Thyroid transcription factor-1 is a marker of lung and thyroid carcinomas. Adv Anat Pathol 2000; 7(2): 123-7. [http://dx.doi.org/10.1097/00125480-200007020-00007] [PMID: 10721419]

[158] Anagnostou VK, Syrigos KN, Bepler G, Homer RJ, Rimm DL. Thyroid transcription factor 1 is an independent prognostic factor for patients with stage I lung adenocarcinoma. J Clin Oncol 2009; 27(2): 271-8. [http://dx.doi.org/10.1200/JCO.2008.17.0043] [PMID: 19064983]

[159] Gomez-Fernandez C, Jorda M, Delgado PI, Ganjei-Azar P. Thyroid transcription factor 1. Cancer 2002; 96(5): 289-93. [http://dx.doi.org/10.1002/cncr.10743] [PMID: 12378596]

[160] Oktay E, Oflazoglu U, Varol Y, *et al.* The prognostic role of thyroid transcription factor-1 in lung adenocarcinoma. J Cancer Res Ther 2020; 16(4): 737-44. [http://dx.doi.org/10.4103/jcrt.JCRT_1404_16] [PMID: 32930112]

[161] Lopez-Campistrous A, Thiesen A, Gill AJ, Ghosh S, McMullen TPW. Loss of nuclear localization of thyroid transcription factor 1 and adverse outcomes in papillary thyroid cancer. Hum Pathol 2019; 91: 36-42. [http://dx.doi.org/10.1016/j.humpath.2019.06.002] [PMID: 31229486]

[162] Wong KF, Luk JM. Discovery of lamin B1 and vimentin as circulating biomarkers for early hepatocellular carcinoma. Methods Mol Biol 2012; 909: 295-310. [http://dx.doi.org/10.1007/978-1-61779-959-4_19] [PMID: 22903723]

[163] Dmello C, Sawant S, Alam H, *et al.* Vimentin regulates differentiation switch *via* modulation of keratin 14 levels and their expression together correlates with poor prognosis in oral cancer patients. PLoS One 2017; 12(2)e0172559. [http://dx.doi.org/10.1371/journal.pone.0172559] [PMID: 28225793]

[164] Kong CS, Beck AH, Longacre TA. A panel of 3 markers including p16, ProExC, or HPV ISH is optimal for distinguishing between primary endometrial and endocervical adenocarcinomas. Am J Surg Pathol 2010; 34(7): 915-26. [http://dx.doi.org/10.1097/PAS.0b013e3181e3291e] [PMID: 20534993]

[165] Tadokoro A, Kanaji N, Liu D, *et al.* Vimentin Regulates Invasiveness and Is a Poor Prognostic Marker in Non-small Cell Lung Cancer. Anticancer Res 2016; 36(4): 1545-51. [PMID: 27069130]

[166] Gilles C, Polette M, Piette J, *et al.* Vimentin expression in cervical carcinomas: association with invasive and migratory potential. J Pathol 1996; 180(2): 175-80. [http://dx.doi.org/10.1002/(SICI)1096-9896(199610)180:2<175::AID-PATH630>3.0.CO;2-G] [PMID: 8976877]

CHAPTER 9

Enzymes: Tumour Associated Biomarker

Farhadul Islam[1,*]

[1] *Department of Biochemistry and Molecular Biology, University of Rajshahi, Rajshahi-6205, Bangladesh*

Abstract: Enzymes catalyse biochemical reactions and tightly regulate biophysical and metabolic pathways to maintain cellular homeostasis. However, the unregulated activity of these enzymes results in metabolic disorders and genetic diseases, including cancer. In cancer, significant alteration of enzyme levels and/or activity can be detected during malignant transformation, thus, it can be used as a potential biomarker in clinical applications. For example, serum levels of lactate dehydrogenase (LDH), neuron-specific enolase (NSE) and thymidine kinase 1(TK1), alkaline phosphatases (ALPs), tumour M2-PK, hexokinase (HK), *etc*., significantly increased in patients with various cancers, such as metastatic breast cancer, intracranial germ cell tumours, ovarian serous carcinomas, oesophagus, cervical, gastrointestinal, prostate, renal cell carcinoma, head and neck and lung cancers. Also, they are associated with various clinicopathological factors, such as stage, grade, lymph node metastasis, distant metastasis, *etc*. In addition, overexpression of carbonic anhydrase XII (CAXII), matrix metalloproteinases (MMPs) and aldehyde dehydrogenase 1 (ALDH1), in cancer tissues, is associated with the presence of several cancers and correlated with the progression of the diseases. Therefore, screening of these enzymes at the point-of-care settings could facilitate better management of patients with cancer. This chapter summarizes the roles of cancer associated-enzymes, especially emphasizing their clinical significance in patients with various cancers.

Keywords: Alkaline phosphatase, Aldehyde dehydrogenase 1, Biosynthesis, Carbonic anhydrase XII, Cancer bioenergetics, Cancer metabolism, Ghrelin O-Acyl Transferase, Glucose-6-phosphate dehydrogenase, Hexokinase, Lactate dehydrogenase, Matrix metalloproteinases, Metabolic enzymes, Neuron-specific enolase, Receptor-interacting protein kinase, Thymidine kinase, Tumour M2-PK, Urokinase-type plasminogen activator, Warburg effects.

* **Corresponding author Farhadul Islam:** Department of Biochemistry and Molecular Biology, University of Rajshahi, Rajshahi-6205, Bangladesh; Email: farhad_bio83@ru.ac.bd

INTRODUCTION

Enzymes are biocatalysts, accelerating the biochemical reactions in almost all metabolic processes in the cells at a rate fast enough to sustain life [1]. Individual steps of metabolic pathways are catalysed and regulated by enzymes in cells, thus, tight control of enzymatic activity is essential for cellular homeostasis. Any malfunction, such as mutations, overproduction, underproduction or deletion *etc.*, of a single critical enzyme, can lead to metabolic, such as Tay-Sachs disease and genetic diseases, including cancers [2, 3]. For example, malfunction of enzymes involved in DNA repair causes cancers due to less capability to repair mutations in their genome, thereby slowing the accumulation of genetic alterations, resulting in cancer development [4].

Altered metabolism, such as altered bioenergetics (aerobic glycolysis, reduced oxidative phosphorylation), increased biosynthesis (production of biosynthetic pathways intermediates), redox balance, *etc.*, are evident in cancer cells in comparison to most normal tissue cells. These changes support the acquisition and maintenance of malignant properties known as cancer metabolism. In cancer, these reprogrammed activities improve cellular fitness to provide selective advantages during tumour formation either by supporting cell survival under stressful microenvironment or by allowing uncontrolled growth and proliferation [5].

Metabolic reprogramming (enhanced or suppressed metabolic activity) and oncometabolite (metabolites increased significantly in cancer) are two key phenomena in cancer as a consequence of malfunction of metabolic enzymes due to tumorigenic mutations and /or other factors [6]. Aerobic glycolysis, or Warburg effect- constitutive glucose uptake and production of lactate regardless of oxygen availability, is a prominent example of metabolic reprogramming in cancer [7]. Enhanced glycolytic flux in cancer cells produces increased glycolytic intermediates, which provide the metabolic demands of other pathways in proliferating cells. Also, the increased flux of tricarboxylic acid (TCA) cycle intermediates is used as the precursor for macromolecule synthesis in cancer cells [8]. Thus, metabolic reprogramming of cancer cells allows increased biosynthesis of biomolecules for uncontrolled proliferating cells. In addition, alteration of metabolic enzymes generates oncometabolite, such as D-2-hydroxyglutarate, citrate, *etc.*, which in turn stabilize hypoxia-inducible factor 1, nuclear factor-like 2, thus, can inhibit p53, prolyl hydroxylase 3 along with regulation of DNA/histone methylation [9]. These activities induce cellular growth and proliferation by activating cell growth signalling. Also, the oncometabolite promote glutaminolysis, glycolysis and generation of reactive oxygen species (ROS), resulting in increased cellular growth and proliferation. Furthermore, epigenetic and genetic alterations of metabolic enzymes are associated with increased fatty acid β-oxidation, which can induce epithelial-mesenchymal transition (EMT). Thus, alterations of metabolic enzymes stimulate carcinogenesis by activating cell proliferation and survival signalling.

Additionally, the detachment of cancer cells from the extracellular matrix (ECM), a step in cancer metastasis (the main reason for cancer-related mortality), is critically regulated by enzymatic activity [10]. Altered cellular metabolism can induce the death of detached cells by elevated production of ROS due to low glucose influx during ECM detachment. Importantly, the metabolic enzyme receptor-interacting protein kinase (RIPK) family induces necrosis of ECM-detached cells by mitophagy (selective degradation of mitochondria by autophagy)-mediated increased ROS production [10]. Also, suppression of RIPK1-mediated mitophagy stimulates *in vivo* tumour growth. In addition, RIPK1 higher expression is associated with improved survival of patients with lung cancer [10].

Enzymes play crucial roles in cancer pathogenesis and distant metastasis in various cancers. Thus, the implications of enzymes as cancer biomarkers hold promise for the better management of patients with cancers. Hence, this chapter discusses the clinical significance and biomarker roles of cancer-associated enzymes in disease diagnostic, prognostics and predictive perspective.

Enzyme Biomarkers in Cancer

Enzymes have the potential to be used as biochemical markers for cancer screening, detection, prognosis, and therapeutic response predictions, as the alterations of gene expression encoding enzymes during malignant transformation can be detected in resulting cancers. Although, a single cancer-specific enzyme with clinical applications for all tumours is yet to be identified, however, alterations of enzymes activity and/or levels in cancer compared to the normal tissues may have the potential for cancer screening, prognosis, monitoring treatment response and clinical stratifications of patients with cancers. The enzymes that have biomarker implications in various cancers are summarized in Table 1. In the following sections, we discuss the biomarker roles of important enzymes in cancer.

Table 1. Enzymes with cancer biomarker significance.

Enzymes	Clinical Significance	References
GOAT	Diagnostic and predictive marker for biological aggressiveness of cancer in patients prostate cancer	12-14

(Table 1) cont.....

Enzymes	Clinical Significance	References
LDH	Prognostic and therapy response biomarker for breast, lung, and hypo-pharyngeal cancer	16-20
NSE	Identification of small-cell carcinomas and has potential for screening and prognosis of neuroendocrine tumours, neuroblastoma, melanoma, renal cell carcinoma, seminoma, carcinoid tumours, Merkel cell tumour, dysgerminomas, immature teratoma and malignant phaeochromocytomas.	22-24
ALPs	Diagnostic and prognostic roles in intracranial germ cell tumour, seminoma, penial region tumours. Early detection biomarker for ovarian serous carcinoma and predictive biomarker for intracranial germ cell tumour recurrence.	26-29
TK1	Screening, stratification of tumour stages, monitoring of therapy response and prognosis of patients with breast, oesophagus, cervical, gastrointestinal, prostate, renal cell carcinoma, head and neck and lung cancers.	31
Tumour M2-PK	Screening and prognosis of patients with lung, breast, renal, gastrointestinal, cervical, bladder, pancreatic and skin cancers.	35, 37-39
uPA	Diagnostic, prognostic and metastatic biomarkers for the patients with breast, prostate and cholangiocarcinomas.	43-45
CAXII	Screening and prognosis of patients with lung and brain cancers. Also, predicts the recurrence of breast cancer.	47-48, 50
ALDH1	Predictive biomarker for therapy resistance in ovarian cancer, a prognostic marker for early-stage lung cancer.	52-53
MMPs	Predictive markers for biological aggressiveness of various cancer such as prostate cancer, cholangiocarcinomas, ovarian cancer, and cervical and lung cancers. Also, a prognostic marker for ovarian cancer.	56-57
HK	Therapy resistance predictive biomarker for non-small cell lung carcinomas. Prognostic marker for cervical and ovarian cancers.	61-63
G6PD	Predictive marker for recurrent metastasis and progression free-survival of breast carcinomas. Also, predictive marker for invasion and metastasis of gastric cancer.	65-66

Ghrelin O-Acyl Transferase (GOAT)

The enzyme GOAT, also known as membrane-bound O-acyltransferase domain containing 4, is encoded by the *MBOAT4* gene, mediates octanoylation of ghrelin at Ser-3 residue and regulates the ghrelin activity [11]. In patients with prostate cancer, urine and plasma levels of GOAT significantly elevated in comparison to healthy individuals. Urine GOAT levels were associated with the tumour grading (Gleason score) and the biological aggressiveness of cancer [12]. Another study noted that plasma/urine GOAT levels were correlated with cancer aggressiveness and metabolic conditions such as diabetes in patients with prostate cancer. Also, plasma GOAT levels showed higher specificity and sensitivity to detect prostate cancer in comparison to other biomarkers, such as prostate-specific antigen

(PSA), especially in non-diabetic patients [13]. Additionally, plasma GOAT levels were higher in prostate cancer patients when compared to the controls. The high plasma GOAT levels were associated with the Gleason score and the presence of metastasis in patients with prostate cancer [14]. Thus, GOAT could be used as a diagnostic and predictive marker for the aggressiveness of patients with prostate cancer.

Lactate Dehydrogenase (LDH)

Lactate dehydrogenase (LDH) catalyzes the final step of glycolysis (conversion of pyruvate to lactate), and it plays a critical role in cancer metabolism. LDH levels provide intracellular metabolic characteristics (*i. e.* aerobic or anaerobic metabolism) of cancer cells [15]. Importantly, increased plasma LDH levels were associated with poor prognosis of patients with various cancers. For example, high plasma LDH levels act as an independent prognostic marker for metastatic breast cancer and elevated LDH levels are associated with poorer survival of patients with metastatic breast cancer [16]. Also, high serum LDH levels correlated with advanced pathological tumour stages, poor prognosis and clinical outcome of patients with breast cancer [17]. In addition, high LDH in patients with advanced non-small cell lung cancer (NSCLC) pretreated with platinum-based chemotherapy is significantly associated with lower overall survival, indicating the therapy response predictive implication of LHD in cancer patients [18]. Salivary LDH levels were significantly increased in patients with oral cancer when compared to control, and the elevated LDH was associated with higher histological tumour grade [19]. Furthermore, elevated serum LDH levels in patients with hypo-pharyngeal cancer undergoing pre-treatment (surgery) act as an independent prognostic factor with unfavourable clinical outcomes [20]. Thus, routine analysis of LDH in point-of-care settings such as in clinics and hospitals could provide information for better management of patients with cancers.

Neuron Specific Enolase (NSE)

Neuron-specific enolase (NSE), also known as enolase 2 or Gamma-enolase, is encoded by the *ENO2* gene [21]. The expression of NSE can be used to identify neuronal cells and cells originating from neuroendocrine. Small-cell carcinomas originated from neuroendocrine origin produce NSE, thus, it is used to distinguish small-cell carcinomas from other cancers [22]. Also, NSE, along with other biomarkers such as chromogranin A, carcinoembryonic antigen and urinary 5-hydroxyindol-3-acetic acid, is used for the screening, prognosis and follow-up of patients with neuroendocrine tumours [23]. In addition, NSE is useful for the diagnosis of gastroenteropancreatic-neuroendocrine tumours, and elevated levels of NSE have been noted in patients with neuroblastoma [24]. Furthermore, higher levels of serum NSE have been noted in patients with melanoma, renal cell carcinoma, seminoma, carcinoid tumours, Merkel cell tumour, dysgerminomas, immature teratoma and malignant phaeochromocytomas [24]. Therefore, NSE could act as a clinical marker for various cancers, especially cancers of neuroendocrine origin.

Alkaline Phosphatases (ALPs)

Alkaline phosphatase (ALP) catalyses the hydrolysis of monoester in alkaline conditions, resulting in the dephosphorylation of biomolecules. The enzyme has different isozymes, and in humans, it has four isozymes, *i. e.* germ cell (GALP), tissue nonspecific (LALP), intestinal (IALP), and placental (PALP), which are predominant [25]. ALPs play crucial roles in the vital cellular process, including cell growth, migration and apoptosis, by regulating phosphorylation/dephosphorylation, and abnormal expression of APLs has been associated with various cancers. For example, higher levels of cerebrospinal fluid (CSF) PALP were associated with intracranial germ cell tumours and had the potential to be used as a biomarker for initial diagnosis of intracranial germ cell tumours and recurrence of the disease [26]. Increment of serum PALP levels associated with the patients of seminoma and monitoring the serum levels of PALP provide important information on disease progression [27]. Also, PLAP in CSF could act as a biomarker for optimizing surgical treatment strategies in patients with penial region germ cell tumours [28]. Furthermore, the expression of PALP in tissue samples acts as a marker for early detection of ovarian serous carcinoma and its expression is associated with prognosis [29]. Thus, the levels or activity of ALP, especially PLAP, has the potential to be used as a biomarker for various cancers, however, their clinical applications need to be established.

Thymidine Kinase 1 (TK1)

Thymidine kinase (TK) is a phosphotransferase enzyme with two isoforms (TK1 and TK1) in human cells. TK1 is a cell-cycle-dependent form and is upregulated during the S phase, thereby known as a proliferating biomarker [30]. Since, TK1 is involved in the proliferation of cells, and its aberrant expression is associated with various human malignancies. Its serum concentration is a useful biomarker for screening to detect potential malignancy along with identification of early-stage tumours, monitoring therapy response and prognosis for various cancers, including breast, oesophagus, cervical, gastrointestinal, prostate, renal cell carcinoma, head & neck and lung cancers [31]. For instance, a significantly higher level of TK1 was noted in patients with lung cancer compared to the control. Also, the detection of TK1 with CEA, NSE and CYFRA21-1 improved the diagnostic value for patients with lung squamous cell carcinoma, adenocarcinoma and small cell lung cancer [32]. Another study reported that TK1 significantly overexpressed in patients with lung, colorectal and breast cancers in comparison to that of healthy control. In addition, TK1 could be a potential clinical biomarker for the treatment of patients with lung, breast and colorectal cancers [33].

Tumour M2-PK

Tumour M2-PK is the synonym for a dimeric form of pyruvate kinase isozyme type M2. It is the key enzyme involved in tumour metabolism, especially aerobic glycolysis and its aberrant expression is associated with various cancers [34]. The levels of plasma and stool tumour M2-PK can act as a biomarker for the metabolic status of tumours. Enzyme-linked immunosorbent assay (ELISA) measurement of tumour M2-PK in human plasma and faecal (stool) level is used to follow up patients with various cancers, including lung, breast, renal, gastrointestinal, cervical, and skin cancers.

Clinical studies noted that serum and faecal tumour M2-PK levels of patients were significantly higher in patients with colorectal cancer compared to that of healthy individuals [35, 36]. Another study reviewed the diagnostic and prognostic significance of tumour M2-PK in gastrointestinal malignancies and reported that stool and plasma tumour M2-PK levels elevated significantly in cancer patients, especially pancreatobiliary and colorectal cancers. Tumour M2-PK can be used adjunctive detection biomarker for pancreatobiliary cancer along with CA 19-9 in clinical settings [37]. Also, elevated levels of tumour M2-PK are associated with poorer prognosis in patients with pancreatic cancer [38]. In addition, tumour M2-PK levels in urine samples were significantly increased in patients with bladder cancers and elevated levels of tumour M2-PK correlated with the presence of bladder cancers [39]. Thus, tumour M2-PK has the potential to be used as a cancer biomarker for screening and prognosis in patients with various cancers, especially gastrointestinal malignancies.

Urokinase-Type Plasminogen Activator (uPA)

Urokinase-type plasminogen activator (uPA), also known as Urokinase, encoded by the *PLAU* gene, is a serene protease [40]. uPA acts on plasminogen (an inactive form of plasmin), activating plasmin, which triggers a proteolytic cascade associated with extracellular matrix degradation. The degradation of the extracellular matrix promotes cancer cell proliferation, invasion and migration, resulting in distance metastasis [41]. Aberrant expression of uPA is associated with tumour progression in a number of malignancies [42]. For example, elevated expression of uPA in patients with breast cancers is associated with poor prognosis and can be used as the diagnostic marker for breast cancer patients [43]. uPA and its receptor uPAR are significantly overexpressed in patients with prostate cancer in comparison to the control. Therefore, they can be used as a diagnostic marker and therapeutic targets for therapy development [44]. Furthermore, overexpression of uPA was noted in patients with cholangiocarcinomas, and higher expression of uPA was associated with lymph node invasion and distance metastasis in patients with cholangiocarcinomas [45]. Thus, elevated expression of uPA can be used as a cancer biomarker, especially for metastatic cancers.

Carbonic Anhydrase XII (CAXII)

This enzyme is a membrane-associated isoform of carbonic anhydrase, encoded by the *CA-12* gene and catalyses the reversible hydration of carbon dioxide [46]. An elevated level of CAXII has been noted in several cancers and is associated with clinicopathological factors. For instance, elevated serum CAXII levels were found in patients with lung cancer when compared with healthy control and the higher levels were associated with poor histological tumour grade [47]. Also, elevated expression of CAXII was noted in brain tumours, and expression levels increased with the advancement of malignancy. Moreover, overexpression is associated with the metastasis of the disease [48]. However, a study noted the better prognostic significance of CAXII in patients with non-small cell carcinomas [49]. Higher expression of CAXII is associated with lower tumour grade and histological type and better survival of patients with cancers [49]. Another study reported that expression of CAXII correlated with lower histological grade of tumour in patients with breast cancer. Also, expression of CAXII is associated with a lower rate of cancer recurrence and better survival of patients with breast cancer [50]. Thus, the implication of CAXII as a cancer biomarker needs to be validated by incorporating large-scale cohort studies for clinical application.

Aldehyde Dehydrogenase 1 (ALDH1)

The enzyme aldehyde dehydrogenase 1 (ALDH1) catalyses the oxidation of intracellular aldehyde and converts retinol to retinoic acid, which in turn is involved in stem cell differentiation [51]. Expression of ALDH1A1, a member of the ALDH1 family protein (enzyme) associated with chemotherapy resistance and poor clinical outcome in patients with ovarian cancer [52]. Also, expression of ALDH1 correlated with tumour grade and pathological stages and poor prognosis of patients with lung cancer, especially early-stage lung cancers [53]. In addition, elevated level of ALDH1 activity has been noted in several other cancers, including breast, brain, acute myeloid leukaemia, and multiple myelomas [54]. Therefore, ALDH1 detection could have the potential to be used as a prognostic cancer biomarker.

Matrix Metalloproteinases (MMPs)

Matrix metalloproteinases (MMPs) are a family of calcium-dependent zinc-containing endopeptidases that degrade extracellular matrix by breaking down basement membrane components such as collagen, elastin, fibronectin, laminin and proteoglycans [55]. In cancer, MMPs activity triggers angiogenesis, migration and invasion, thereby promoting distance metastasis of cancer cells. The diagnostic and prognostic significance of MMPs is also reported in various cancers, including prostate cancer, cholangiocarcinomas, ovarian cancer, and cervical and lung cancers. For example, MMPs expression is associated with the neural invasion of patients with cholangiocarcinomas [56]. Elevated expression of MMPs was associated with the aggressiveness of ovarian cancer, and higher expression of MMP-2 in cancer cells in peritoneal implants predicts significant risk of death of patients (*i. e.* poor prognosis) by the disease [57]. In addition, higher MMP-9 expression is associated with biological aggressiveness, *e. g.* poor differentiation and higher grade of tumour in patients with non-small cell lung carcinomas [58]. Thus, analysis of MMPs expression in cancer samples may predict the biological aggressiveness of the disease and could assist the physician in therapy selection.

Hexokinase (HK)

Hexokinase (HK) catalyses the conversion of hexose (glucose) to hexose--phosphate (glucose-6-phosphate), the first rate-limiting step of glycolysis. In addition, HK, especially HKII (isoform of HK) capable of binding to the voltage-dependent anion channel (VDAC) on the mitochondrial outer membrane [59]. This interaction of HKII and VDAC enhances glycolytic flux in cancer cells. Also, HKII binding to VDAC stabilizes the mitochondrial membrane, thereby limiting the release of pro-apoptotic factors, such as cytochrome C and AIF, from the mitochondrial intermembrane space, resulting in increased cell survival by escaping apoptosis [60].

Additionally, preclinical and clinical studies reported the biomarker roles of HK in various cancers. For example, circulating tumour cells (CTCs) expressing higher HK and cytokeratin are associated with cancer metastasis and therapy resistance in patients with non-small cell lung carcinomas [61]. Higher HKII and cytokeratin expressing CTCs in the peripheral blood of these patients had poor therapy response and shorter progression-free survival [61]. Another study found that HK1 (another isoform of HK) expression was significantly higher in ovarian cancer when compared to that of control. Overexpression of HK1 may act as an independent prognostic biomarker as its overexpression is associated with a poor survival rate in patients with ovarian cancers [62]. A gene expression profiling interactive analysis (GEPIA) and clinical sample analysis study noted that HK2 is highly overexpressed in patients with cervical cancer in comparison to that of control. Also, higher HK2 expression correlated with larger tumour size, higher pathological grade and poor prognosis of patients with cervical cancers [63]. Therefore, HK has the potential to be used as a prognostic indicator in various cancer for clinical applications.

Glocuse-6-Phosphate Dehydrogenase (G6PD)

Glucose-6-phosphate dehydrogenase (G6PD) catalyses the conversion of D-glucose-6-phospahte to 6-phospho-D-glucono-1, 5-lactone, a rate-limiting step in pentose phosphate pathway [64]. Studies noted that G6PD activity is involved in cell growth and proliferation. Aberrant activity of this enzyme has been noted in various cancers, including breast, ovarian, cervical, prostate and bladder cancers [54, 64]. Overexpression of G6PD was noted in patients with primary breast carcinomas. The higher G6PF expression predicts a higher risk of recurrent metastasis and progression-free survival in patients with breast carcinomas [65]. Another study noted that G6PD significantly overexpressed in patients with gastric cancer when compared to that of control. Higher expression of G6PD correlated with clinicopathological factors such as tumour size, invasion, lymph node metastasis, and distant metastasis in patients with gastric cancer. Also, the G6PD expression level could act as an independent prognostic factor for patients followed by radical resection of the tumours [66]. Thus, G6PD might be regarded as a potential prognostic marker for several cancers in clinical settings.

CONCLUDING REMARKS

Metabolic reprogramming, such as altered bioenergetics, increased biosynthesis and redox balance, are the major hallmarks of cancer development. These metabolic alterations in cancer cells could be attributed to enzymes involved in different metabolic and biophysical pathways, and aberrant activation and/or levels of these enzymes are associated with cancer initiation and progression. Thus, the altered levels of these enzymes during malignant transformation can provide the promising potential to be used as a diagnostic, prognostic and predictive cancer biomarker in clinical applications. However, cancer-specific single-enzyme-based biomarkers for cancer are yet to be established. Also, the levels of a single enzyme alone cannot be clinically useful for screening, prognosis, monitoring therapy response, early-stage detection *etc.*, for all types of cancer. Although, an imbalance of these enzyme activities has been used to assist clinical evaluations of cancer patients.

CONSENT FOR PUBLICATION

Not applicable.

CONFLICT OF INTEREST

The author declares no conflict of interest, financial or otherwise.

ACKNOWLEDGEMENT

The author acknowledged the University of Rajshahi, Bangladesh, for providing technical support.

REFERENCES

[1] Berg JM, Tymoczko JL, Stryer L. Biochemistry. New York: W H Freeman 2002. https://www.ncbi.nlm.nih.gov/books/NBK21154/

[2] Okada S, O'Brien JS. Tay-Sachs disease: generalized absence of a beta-D-N-acetylhexosaminidase component. Science 1969; 165(3894): 698-700. [http://dx.doi.org/10.1126/science.165.3894.698] [PMID: 5793973]

[3] Cleaver JE. Defective repair replication of DNA in xeroderma pigmentosum. Nature 1968; 218(5142): 652-6. [http://dx.doi.org/10.1038/218652a0] [PMID: 5655953]

[4] Bartkova J, Hořejší Z, Koed K, *et al.* DNA damage response as a candidate anti-cancer barrier in early human tumorigenesis. Nature 2005; 434(7035): 864-70. [http://dx.doi.org/10.1038/nature03482] [PMID: 15829956]

[5] DeBerardinis RJ, Chandel NS. Fundamentals of cancer metabolism. Sci Adv 2016; 2(5): e1600200. [http://dx.doi.org/10.1126/sciadv.1600200] [PMID: 27386546]

[6] Ward PS, Thompson CB. Metabolic reprogramming: a cancer hallmark even warburg did not anticipate. Cancer Cell 2012; 21(3): 297-308. [http://dx.doi.org/10.1016/j.ccr.2012.02.014] [PMID: 22439925]

[7] Koppenol WH, Bounds PL, Dang CV. Otto Warburg's contributions to current concepts of cancer metabolism. Nat Rev Cancer 2011; 11(5): 325-37. [http://dx.doi.org/10.1038/nrc3038] [PMID: 21508971]

[8] Ahn CS, Metallo CM. Mitochondria as biosynthetic factories for cancer proliferation. Cancer Metab 2015; 3(1): 1. [http://dx.doi.org/10.1186/s40170-015-0128-2] [PMID: 25621173]

[9] Sajnani K, Islam F, Smith RA, Gopalan V, Lam AKY. Genetic alterations in Krebs cycle and its impact on cancer pathogenesis. Biochimie 2017; 135: 164-72. [http://dx.doi.org/10.1016/j.biochi.2017.02.008] [PMID: 28219702]

[10] Hawk MA, Gorsuch CL, Fagan P, *et al.* RIPK1-mediated induction of mitophagy compromises the viability of extracellular-matrix-detached cells. Nat Cell Biol 2018; 20(3): 272-84. [http://dx.doi.org/10.1038/s41556-018-0034-2] [PMID: 29459781]

[11] Gutierrez JA, Solenberg PJ, Perkins DR, *et al.* Ghrelin octanoylation mediated by an orphan lipid transferase. Proc Natl Acad Sci USA 2008; 105(17): 6320-5. [http://dx.doi.org/10.1073/pnas.0800708105] [PMID: 18443287]

[12] Jiménez-Vacas JM, Gómez-Gómez E, Montero-Hidalgo AJ, *et al.* Clinical Utility of Ghrelin--Acyltransferase (GOAT) Enzyme as a Diagnostic Tool and Potential Therapeutic Target in Prostate

Cancer. J Clin Med 2019; 8(12): 2056.
[http://dx.doi.org/10.3390/jcm8122056] [PMID: 31766715]

[13] Hormaechea-Agulla D, Gómez-Gómez E, Ibáñez-Costa A, *et al.* Ghrelin O-acyltransferase (GOAT) enzyme is overexpressed in prostate cancer, and its levels are associated with patient's metabolic status: Potential value as a non-invasive biomarker. Cancer Lett 2016; 383(1): 125-34.
[http://dx.doi.org/10.1016/j.canlet.2016.09.022] [PMID: 27693462]

[14] Gómez-Gómez E, Jiménez-Vacas JM, Carrasco-Valiente J, *et al.* Plasma ghrelin *O*-acyltransferase (GOAT) enzyme levels: A novel non-invasive diagnosis tool for patients with significant prostate cancer. J Cell Mol Med 2018; 22(11): 5688-97.
[http://dx.doi.org/10.1111/jcmm.13845] [PMID: 30256519]

[15] Jurisic V, Radenkovic S, Konjevic G. The Actual Role of LDH as Tumor Marker, Biochemical and Clinical Aspects. Adv Exp Med Biol 2015; 867: 115-24.
[http://dx.doi.org/10.1007/978-94-017-7215-0_8] [PMID: 26530363]

[16] Pelizzari G, Basile D, Zago S, *et al.* Lactate Dehydrogenase (LDH) Response to First-Line Treatment Predicts Survival in Metastatic Breast Cancer: First Clues for A Cost-Effective and Dynamic Biomarker. Cancers (Basel) 2019; 11(9): 1243.
[http://dx.doi.org/10.3390/cancers11091243] [PMID: 31450641]

[17] Agrawal A, Gandhe MB, Gupta D, Reddy MV. Preliminary Study on Serum Lactate Dehydrogenase (LDH)-Prognostic Biomarker in Carcinoma Breast. J Clin Diagn Res 2016; 10(3): BC06-8.
[http://dx.doi.org/10.7860/JCDR/2016/17111.7364] [PMID: 27134855]

[18] Jong C, Deneer VHM, Kelder JC, Ruven H, Egberts TCG, Herder GJM. Association between serum biomarkers CEA and LDH and response in advanced non□small cell lung cancer patients treated with platinum□based chemotherapy. Thorac Cancer 2020; 11(7): 1790-800.
[http://dx.doi.org/10.1111/1759-7714.13449] [PMID: 32383328]

[19] Lokesh K, Kannabiran J, Rao MD. Salivary Lactate Dehydrogenase (LDH)- A Novel Technique in Oral Cancer Detection and Diagnosis. J Clin Diagn Res 2016; 10(2): ZC34-7.
[http://dx.doi.org/10.7860/JCDR/2016/16243.7223] [PMID: 27042582]

[20] Wu J, You K, Chen C, *et al.* High Pretreatment LDH Predicts Poor Prognosis in Hypopharyngeal Cancer. Front Oncol 2021; 11: 641682.
[http://dx.doi.org/10.3389/fonc.2021.641682] [PMID: 33777804]

[21] Liu C, Wang H, Wang W, *et al.* ENO2 Promotes Cell Proliferation, Glycolysis, and Glucocorticoid-Resistance in Acute Lymphoblastic Leukemia. Cell Physiol Biochem 2018; 46(4): 1525-35.
[http://dx.doi.org/10.1159/000489196] [PMID: 29689546]

[22] Clegg N, Ferguson C, True LD, *et al.* Molecular characterization of prostatic small-cell neuroendocrine carcinoma. Prostate 2003; 55(1): 55-64.
[http://dx.doi.org/10.1002/pros.10217] [PMID: 12640661]

[23] Bajetta E, Ferrari L, Martinetti A, *et al.* Chromogranin A, neuron specific enolase, carcinoembryonic antigen, and hydroxyindole acetic acid evaluation in patients with neuroendocrine tumors. Cancer 1999; 86(5): 858-65.
[http://dx.doi.org/10.1002/(SICI)1097-0142(19990901)86:5<858::AID-CNCR23>3.0.CO;2-8] [PMID: 10463986]

[24] Isgrò MA, Bottoni P, Scatena R. Neuron-Specific Enolase as a Biomarker: Biochemical and Clinical Aspects. Adv Exp Med Biol 2015; 867: 125-43.
[http://dx.doi.org/10.1007/978-94-017-7215-0_9] [PMID: 26530364]

[25] Millán JL. Alkaline Phosphatases. Purinergic Signal 2006; 2(2): 335-41.
[http://dx.doi.org/10.1007/s11302-005-5435-6] [PMID: 18404473]

[26] Okamoto M, Yamaguchi S, Ishi Y, *et al.* Diagnostic Capability of Cerebrospinal Fluid-Placental Alkaline Phosphatase Value in Intracranial Germ Cell Tumor. Oncology 2021; 99(1): 23-31.

[http://dx.doi.org/10.1159/000509395] [PMID: 32906115]

[27] Koshida K, Uchibayashi T, Yamamoto H, Hirano K. Significance of placental alkaline phosphatase (PLAP) in the monitoring of patients with seminoma. Br J Urol 1996; 77(1): 138-42. [http://dx.doi.org/10.1046/j.1464-410X.1996.74324.x] [PMID: 8653285]

[28] Chiba K, Aihara Y, Komori T, Kawamata T. Placental alkaline phosphatase in cerebrospinal fluid as a biomarker for optimizing surgical treatment strategies for pineal region germ cell tumors. Brain Tumor Pathol 2020; 37(2): 60-8. [http://dx.doi.org/10.1007/s10014-020-00364-0] [PMID: 32367333]

[29] Orsaria M, Londero AP, Marzinotto S, Di Loreto C, Marchesoni D, Mariuzzi L. Placental type alkaline phosphatase tissue expression in ovarian serous carcinoma. Cancer Biomark 2017; 17(4): 479-86. [http://dx.doi.org/10.3233/CBM-160665] [PMID: 27802199]

[30] Jagarlamudi KK, Shaw M. Thymidine kinase 1 as a tumor biomarker: technical advances offer new potential to an old biomarker. Biomarkers Med 2018; 12(9): 1035-48. [http://dx.doi.org/10.2217/bmm-2018-0157] [PMID: 30039979]

[31] Zhou J, He E, Skog S. The proliferation marker thymidine kinase 1 in clinical use. Mol Clin Oncol 2013; 1(1): 18-28. [http://dx.doi.org/10.3892/mco.2012.19] [PMID: 24649117]

[32] Jiang ZF, Wang M, Xu JL. Thymidine kinase 1 combined with CEA, CYFRA21-1 and NSE improved its diagnostic value for lung cancer. Life Sci 2018; 194: 1-6. [http://dx.doi.org/10.1016/j.lfs.2017.12.020] [PMID: 29247745]

[33] Weagel EG, Burrup W, Kovtun R, *et al.* Membrane expression of thymidine kinase 1 and potential clinical relevance in lung, breast, and colorectal malignancies. Cancer Cell Int 2018; 18(1): 135. [http://dx.doi.org/10.1186/s12935-018-0633-9] [PMID: 30214377]

[34] Liu VM, Vander Heiden MG. The Role of Pyruvate Kinase M2 in Cancer Metabolism. Brain Pathol 2015; 25(6): 781-3. [http://dx.doi.org/10.1111/bpa.12311] [PMID: 26526946]

[35] Tonus C, Neupert G, Sellinger M. Colorectal cancer screening by non-invasive metabolic biomarker fecal tumor M2-PK. World J Gastroenterol 2006; 12(43): 7007-11. [http://dx.doi.org/10.3748/wjg.v12.i43.7007] [PMID: 17109496]

[36] Meng W, Zhu HH, Xu ZF, *et al.* Serum M2-pyruvate kinase: A promising non-invasive biomarker for colorectal cancer mass screening. World J Gastrointest Oncol 2012; 4(6): 145-51. [http://dx.doi.org/10.4251/wjgo.v4.i6.145] [PMID: 22737276]

[37] Hathurusinghe HR, Goonetilleke KS, Siriwardena AK. Current status of tumor M2 pyruvate kinase (tumor M2-PK) as a biomarker of gastrointestinal malignancy. Ann Surg Oncol 2007; 14(10): 2714-20. [http://dx.doi.org/10.1245/s10434-007-9481-x] [PMID: 17602267]

[38] Bandara IA, Baltatzis M, Sanyal S, Siriwardena AK. Evaluation of tumor M2-pyruvate kinase (Tumor M2-PK) as a biomarker for pancreatic cancer. World J Surg Oncol 2018; 16(1): 56. [http://dx.doi.org/10.1186/s12957-018-1360-3] [PMID: 29540198]

[39] Liu W, Woolbright BL, Pirani K, *et al.* Tumor M2-PK: A novel urine marker of bladder cancer. PLoS One 2019; 14(6): e0218737. [http://dx.doi.org/10.1371/journal.pone.0218737] [PMID: 31246990]

[40] Masanori N, Ryuji H, Teruo K, *et al.* Molecular cloning of cDNA coding for human preprourokinase. Gene 1985; 36(1-2): 183-8. [http://dx.doi.org/10.1016/0378-1119(85)90084-8] [PMID: 2415429]

[41] Tang L, Han X. The urokinase plasminogen activator system in breast cancer invasion and metastasis. Biomed Pharmacother 2013; 67(2): 179-82.

[http://dx.doi.org/10.1016/j.biopha.2012.10.003] [PMID: 23201006]

[42] Madunić J. The Urokinase Plasminogen Activator System in Human Cancers: An Overview of Its Prognostic and Predictive Role. Thromb Haemost 2018; 118(12): 2020-36. [http://dx.doi.org/10.1055/s-0038-1675399] [PMID: 30419600]

[43] Mahmood N, Mihalcioiu C, Rabbani SA. Multifaceted Role of the Urokinase-Type Plasminogen Activator (uPA) and Its Receptor (uPAR): Diagnostic, Prognostic, and Therapeutic Applications. Front Oncol 2018; 8: 24. [http://dx.doi.org/10.3389/fonc.2018.00024] [PMID: 29484286]

[44] Li Y, Cozzi PJ. Targeting uPA/uPAR in prostate cancer. Cancer Treat Rev 2007; 33(6): 521-7. [http://dx.doi.org/10.1016/j.ctrv.2007.06.003] [PMID: 17658220]

[45] Thummarati P, Wijitburaphat S, Prasopthum A, *et al.* High level of urokinase plasminogen activator contributes to cholangiocarcinoma invasion and metastasis. World J Gastroenterol 2012; 18(3): 244-50. [http://dx.doi.org/10.3748/wjg.v18.i3.244] [PMID: 22294827]

[46] Türeci Ö, Sahin U, Vollmar E, *et al.* Human carbonic anhydrase XII: cDNA cloning, expression, and chromosomal localization of a carbonic anhydrase gene that is overexpressed in some renal cell cancers. Proc Natl Acad Sci USA 1998; 95(13): 7608-13. [http://dx.doi.org/10.1073/pnas.95.13.7608] [PMID: 9636197]

[47] Kobayashi M, Matsumoto T, Ryuge S, *et al.* CAXII Is a sero-diagnostic marker for lung cancer. PLoS One 2012; 7(3): e33952. [http://dx.doi.org/10.1371/journal.pone.0033952] [PMID: 22439015]

[48] Proescholdt MA, Mayer C, Kubitza M, *et al.* Expression of hypoxia-inducible carbonic anhydrases in brain tumors. Neuro-oncol 2005; 7(4): 465-75. [http://dx.doi.org/10.1215/S1152851705000025] [PMID: 16212811]

[49] Ilie MI, Hofman V, Ortholan C, *et al.* Overexpression of carbonic anhydrase XII in tissues from resectable non-small cell lung cancers is a biomarker of good prognosis. Int J Cancer 2011; 128(7): 1614-23. [http://dx.doi.org/10.1002/ijc.25491] [PMID: 20521252]

[50] Watson PH, Chia SK, Wykoff CC, *et al.* Carbonic anhydrase XII is a marker of good prognosis in invasive breast carcinoma. Br J Cancer 2003; 88(7): 1065-70. [http://dx.doi.org/10.1038/sj.bjc.6600796] [PMID: 12671706]

[51] Yoshida A, Hsu LC, Davé V. Retinal oxidation activity and biological role of human cytosolic aldehyde dehydrogenase. Enzyme 1992; 46(4-5): 239-44. [http://dx.doi.org/10.1159/000468794] [PMID: 1292933]

[52] Wang YC, Yo YT, Lee HY, *et al.* ALDH1-bright epithelial ovarian cancer cells are associated with CD44 expression, drug resistance, and poor clinical outcome. Am J Pathol 2012; 180(3): 1159-69. [http://dx.doi.org/10.1016/j.ajpath.2011.11.015] [PMID: 22222226]

[53] Jiang F, Qiu Q, Khanna A, *et al.* Aldehyde dehydrogenase 1 is a tumor stem cell-associated marker in lung cancer. Mol Cancer Res 2009; 7(3): 330-8. [http://dx.doi.org/10.1158/1541-7786.MCR-08-0393] [PMID: 19276181]

[54] Baig MH, Adil M, Khan R, *et al.* Enzyme targeting strategies for prevention and treatment of cancer: Implications for cancer therapy. Semin Cancer Biol 2019; 56: 1-11. [http://dx.doi.org/10.1016/j.semcancer.2017.12.003] [PMID: 29248538]

[55] Deryugina EI, Quigley JP. Matrix metalloproteinases and tumor metastasis. Cancer Metastasis Rev 2006; 25(1): 9-34. [http://dx.doi.org/10.1007/s10555-006-7886-9] [PMID: 16680569]

[56] Kirimlioğlu H, Türkmen I, Başsüllü N, Dirican A, Karadağ N, Kirimlioğlu V. The expression of matrix metalloproteinases in intrahepatic cholangiocarcinoma, hilar (Klatskin tumor), middle and

distal extrahepatic cholangiocarcinoma, gallbladder cancer, and ampullary carcinoma: role of matrix metalloproteinases in tumor progression and prognosis. Turk J Gastroenterol 2009; 20(1): 41-7. [PMID: 19330734]

[57] Périgny M, Bairati I, Harvey I, *et al.* Role of immunohistochemical overexpression of matrix metalloproteinases MMP-2 and MMP-11 in the prognosis of death by ovarian cancer. Am J Clin Pathol 2008; 129(2): 226-31. [http://dx.doi.org/10.1309/49LA9XCBGWJ8F2KM] [PMID: 18208802]

[58] Leinonen T, Pirinen R, Böhm J, Johansson R, Ropponen K, Kosma VM. Expression of matrix metalloproteinases 7 and 9 in non-small cell lung cancer. Lung Cancer 2006; 51(3): 313-21. [http://dx.doi.org/10.1016/j.lungcan.2005.11.002] [PMID: 16423426]

[59] Fan Y, Zong WX. Hacking hexokinase halts tumor growth. Cancer Biol Ther 2008; 7(7): 1136-8. [http://dx.doi.org/10.4161/cbt.7.7.6536] [PMID: 18698161]

[60] Sun L, Shukair S, Naik TJ, Moazed F, Ardehali H. Glucose phosphorylation and mitochondrial binding are required for the protective effects of hexokinases I and II. Mol Cell Biol 2008; 28(3): 1007-17. [http://dx.doi.org/10.1128/MCB.00224-07] [PMID: 18039843]

[61] Yang L, Yan X, Chen J, *et al.* Hexokinase 2 discerns a novel circulating tumor cell population associated with poor prognosis in lung cancer patients. Proc Natl Acad Sci USA 2021; 118(11): e2012228118. [http://dx.doi.org/10.1073/pnas.2012228118] [PMID: 33836566]

[62] Li Y, Tian H, Luo H, Fu J, Jiao Y, Li Y. Prognostic Significance and Related Mechanisms of Hexokinase 1 in Ovarian Cancer. OncoTargets Ther 2020; 13: 11583-94. [http://dx.doi.org/10.2147/OTT.S270688] [PMID: 33204111]

[63] Liu C, Wang X, Zhang Y. The Roles of HK2 on Tumorigenesis of Cervical Cancer. Technol Cancer Res Treat 2019; 18 [http://dx.doi.org/10.1177/1533033819871306] [PMID: 31530094]

[64] Kuo W, Lin J, Tang TK. Human glucose-6-phosphate dehydrogenase (G6PD) gene transforms NIH 3T3 cells and induces tumors in nude mice. Int J Cancer 2000; 85(6): 857-64. [http://dx.doi.org/10.1002/(SICI)1097-0215(20000315)85:6<857::AID-IJC20>3.0.CO;2-U] [PMID: 10709108]

[65] Pu H, Zhang Q, Zhao C, *et al.* Overexpression of G6PD is associated with high risks of recurrent metastasis and poor progression-free survival in primary breast carcinoma. World J Surg Oncol 2015; 13(1): 323. [http://dx.doi.org/10.1186/s12957-015-0733-0] [PMID: 26607846]

[66] Wang J, Yuan W, Chen Z, *et al.* Overexpression of G6PD is associated with poor clinical outcome in gastric cancer. Tumour Biol 2012; 33(1): 95-101. [http://dx.doi.org/10.1007/s13277-011-0251-9] [PMID: 22012600]

CHAPTER 10

Glycoproteins and Cancer Biomarkers

Md Abedul Haque[1,*]

[1] *The University of Texas MD Anderson Cancer Center, Houston, Texas-77033, USA*

Abstract: Glycoproteins or glycosylated proteins are carbohydrates (oligosaccharide chains or glycan's) linked proteins and execute important functions in the biological systems, such as embryonic development, cell-to-cell recognition, adhesion, pathogen identification and immune functions. It is evident that the alteration of glycoproteins in cells are associated with a number of human diseases, including cancer, rheumatoid arthritis, inflammatory diseases as well as immunodeficiency diseases. Recent advances in modern technologies in cancer treatment are promising. However, researchers and clinicians are still searching for appropriate biomarkers for the early detection and management of patients with cancer. Altered glycoprotein levels are associated with critical events in cancer pathogenesis and progression. Also, abnormal glycosylation of protein is a common regulatory event in carcinogenesis, therefore, aberrant glycosylation could act as a promising resource in identifying a cancer biomarker for diagnosis and monitoring of the progression of patients with cancers. This chapter summarizes the major clinically approved glycoproteins utilized for screening, diagnosis, and monitoring of the treatment response of patients with cancers.

Keywords: α-fetoprotein, Biomarkers, Breast Cancer, Cancer antigen, Carbohydrates, Cancer Diagnosis Glycoprotein, Cell, Colon cancer, Glycosylation, Glycan, Lung cancer, Microenvironment, Mucins, Neoplasia, N-Glycosylation, Ovarian Cancer, O-glycosylation, Proteins, Prostate cancer, Prostate-specific antibody, Targeting therapy.

INTRODUCTION

Cancer is one of the major public health concerns and leading causes of death worldwide [1]. Besides health concerns, the economic burden of medical costs for cancer treatments is also expected to increase significantly in the future due to less improvements in overall survival rate, changes in treatment patterns and other related medical costs following a cancer diagnosis. Still, the management of cancers is posing the greatest threat and challenge to the modern medical sciences, thus, the development of correct screening and diagnosis strategies and treatment

* **Corresponding author Md. Abedul haque:** The University of Texas MD Anderson Cancer Center, Houston, Texas-77033, USA; Email: MHaque@mdanderson.org

and monitoring approaches for cancers remain a major field of biomedical research throughout the world. The advances in ongoing cancer treatment, including surgical resection, chemo-radiotherapy, hormonal therapy, immune therapy and targeted therapy, are appreciable, however, the overall disease-free survival rate and complete recovery are still disappointed due to heterogeneity of tumor population and acquired drug resistance [2]. Therefore, proper management of patients with cancer-specific biomarkers, molecularly targeting therapy and effective medication plan to prolong disease-free survival is a promising approach to save millions of lives as well as billions of dollars.

Previous studies indicated that neoplastic transformation results from a series of cellular events, which in turn could alter the cellular growth, development, proliferation, survival and general physiology of the affected tissues or organs. Traditionally, genetic mutations are believed to be strongly related to the pathogenesis of neoplastic disease development, however, changes in non-genetic materials, such as epigenetic alterations, could also significantly contribute to the neoplastic transformations. Epigenetic changes such as acetylation, methylation, and histone glycosylated proteins act as key regulatory components of neoplastic-transformation and progression in many cancers [3]. Glycoproteins are a group of post-translationally modified proteins in which oligosaccharide chains or glycans are covalently liked to amino acid side chains. Glycoproteins are ubiquitously distributed and play an important role in various biological processes, including cell signalling, cell-cell interaction, immune recognition, cell proliferation, and differentiation [4, 5]. Therefore, altered levels of glycoproteins possess a close relationship with the progression of many diseases, such as autoimmune disease, rheumatoid arthritis, inflammatory diseases, Alzheimer's disease, and cancers [6, 7]. Proteins are glycosylated in cancer cells either in benign or malignant conditions, and induce cancer development, progression and metastasis [5, 8]. So, glycoproteins represent promising biomarkers to detect, diagnose, and manage various cancer types [9].

Aberrant glycoproteins levels are observed in several human cancers, such as prostate, colorectal, breast, and hepatocellular carcinoma (HCC) [10 - 14]. Identification of the changes of glycoproteins at early stages of cancers is helpful for clinicians in treatments plan that can enhance survival rates. This chapter summarizes the major clinically approved glycoproteins, which are not only aberrantly expressed in different stages of cancers but also create potential opportunities for researchers and clinicians to use these aberrant glycoproteins as a biomarker for screening, diagnosis and monitoring tools for cancer treatments.

Protein Glycosylation in Cancer

During neoplastic transformation, abnormal glycosylation of proteins is one of the epigenetic (or post-translational) modifications of proteins that manipulate the biological activity and appear to regulate cellular growth and proliferation, survival, as well as mediate metastasis in several cancers [3, 15]. The protein glycosylation required a coordinated presence of a complex array of enzymes, organelles, and other factors, *i. e.,* factors for post-translational modifications. The complex process can enzymatically add sugar molecules to the protein either as a linkage of monosaccharides or as whole oligosaccharides (glycans)] to the specific residue (amino acids) of the glycoprotein. Approximately 50% of amino acids in a protein (*e.g.,* 9 out of 20) can be modified either by a single monosaccharide or a glycan chain with oligosaccharides. In the case of mammals, the most frequent glycan's consist of 10 monosaccharides building blocks—Glc (Glucose), Gal (Galactose), GlcNAc (N-acetylglucosamine), GalNAc (N-acetylgalactosamine), Fuc (Fucose) Fuc, Man (Mannose), Xyl (Xylose), GlcA (Glucuronic acid), IdoA (Iduronic acid), and Neu5Ac (5-N-acetylneuraminic acid or sialic acid). They are derivatives of glucose found in all cells (Fig. **1**) [16].

In mammalian cells, two types of protein glycosylation are mainly observed, such as N -Glycosylation and O -Glycosylation. Both types of glycosylation often coexist in the same protein. N-glycosylation involves the attachment of glycan's ranging in complexity to select asparagine (or less commonly, arginine) residues. The addition of N-glycan`s initiated in the endoplasmic reticulum (ER) and further diversified in the Golgi apparatus [17]. While in O-glycosylation, single sugars (N- acetylglucosamine) or glycan's are added to serine, threonine, and, less often, to tyrosine or other hydroxyl-containing residues. O-glycosylation of proteins is primed in ER and Golgi-apparatus or cytosol by stepwise enzymatic transfer of monosaccharides [18]. Increased N-glycosylation rate is associated with cancer growth and metastasis. For example, β1, 6 N-acetyl glucosaminyl transferase V (GnT-V; MGAT5) is one of the most relevant glycosyl transferases associated with the migration, invasion, and metastasis of cancer. On the other hand, the expression of β1–6 branched oligosaccharides regulated by GnT-V serves as a marker for tumor progression, metastasis, and poor prognosis in breast and colorectal cancers [19, 20]. Similarly, aberrant O- glycosylation's correlated with the pathogenesis of lung and pancreatic cancers. For instance, the expression of N-acetyl galactosaminyl transferase (GALNT) 3 is a potential diagnostic and prognostic marker for lung and pancreatic cancers [21, 22]. In addition, GALNT6 can glycosylate and stabilize onco-protein MUC1 (mucin 1), thereby contributing to mammary carcinogenesis by disruption of β-catenin and E-cadherin. Also, GALNT6-fibronectin signalling is an important component for the development and procreation of breast cancers [23, 24].

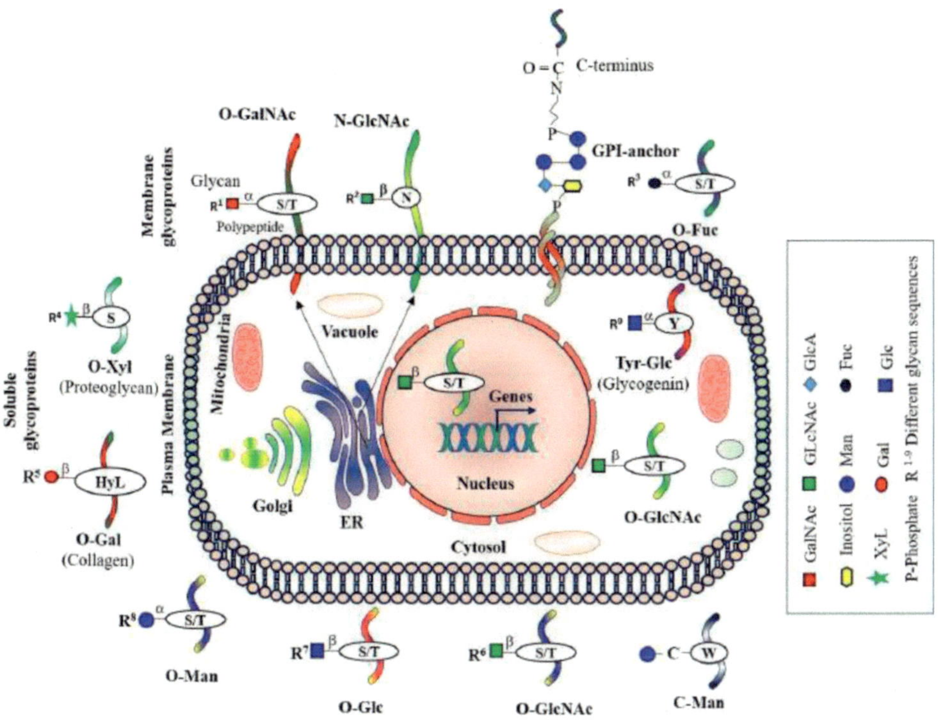

Fig. (1). Glycoproteins and modification of amino acids by specific glycan structures in animal cells. Cellular components involved in secretory pathways, such as endoplasmic reticulum (ER) and Golgi apparatus, can lead to membrane localization and secretion of glycoproteins. Various forms of glycan's are linked to glycoproteins in the cytoplasm, nucleus, and mitochondria. Some glycan's linked proteins can also be extended (R groups indicated) with many additional sugar molecules to form oligosaccharides or polysaccharides. Also, *O*-GlcNAc may be added to glycoproteins in the cytoplasm, nucleus, and mitochondria. This single GlcNAc residue is not extended but can be reversibly added and removed. The multiple other types of glycan linkages to proteins can be extended (R groups indicated) with many additional sugar molecules to form oligosaccharides or polysaccharides, all termed glycans. The common mono-saccharides that makeup animal glycans are indicated: *N*-acetylglucosamine (GlcNAc), *N*-acetylgalactosamine (GalNAc), fucose (Fuc), galactose (Gal), glucose (Glc), glucuronic acid (GlcA), mannose (Man), and xylose (Xyl). Other abbreviations: ER, endoplasmic reticulum; GPI, glycosylphosphatidylinositol; HyL, hydroxylated lysine.

Glycoproteins as Cancer Biomarkers

Biomarker-specific molecularly targeting therapy is one of the medical advances of recent cancer treatments. In patients with cancers, the survival rates are significantly associated with the pathological stages of cancer at which they are diagnosed, thus, early detection with minimally invasive strategies/approaches could have wider acceptance and would improve the survival rates along with the quality of life of patients. However, the asymptomatic nature of cancer at an early stage, patient's economic burden, health unconsciousness and reluctance to seek medical advice lead to the diagnosis of many cases at a relatively advanced stage. Nevertheless, the advancement of modern biomedical technology and the development of computational algorithms help in the identification of cancer biomarkers, which help physicians to manage cancer patients with an effective treatment plan. To date, the approved biomarkers for cancer used in clinical settings have the utmost implications in diagnosis and treatment for widespread cancer patients. However, it is evident that a single biomarker is an effective and specific screening and/or diagnostic tool yet to be developed for most cancers [25]. This is possibly due to several epidemiological factors, mutation and inter- and intra-tumors heterogeneity intensify the possibility that an individual could have various tumors, thereby different stages in the same patient [26].

An aberrant level of glycoproteins or irregular protein glycosylation is an important cancer hallmark, which provides crucial information for the diagnosis of the disease [3, 27]. However, in mammals, the biosynthesis of oligosaccharides is not template-dependent like proteins or nucleic acids biosynthesis, thus, their structural complexity reinforces multiple roles in cellular functionality such as cell-to-cell recognition, cell-to-matrix interactions, which in turn modulate cancer growth and progression *via* regulation of cellular adhesion, anchoring and trafficking in tumour microenvironment [28, 29]. The fact is that majority of human serum proteins (proteome) are glycoproteins [30], and they enter into the circulating system by active secretion or leakage such as necrosis and apoptosis from tissues or blood cells. Therefore, the complex structure of carbohydrate varies in response to multiple stimuli implying the pathophysiological status of the organisms. In addition, most of the glycoproteins levels increased in benign diseases, whereas some of them are not detectable at the early stages of cancer. Importantly, a higher level of aberrant glycosylation has been associated with poor prognosis of patients with cancers, which in turn, could provide critical information to the physicians to get an idea about a more effective therapeutic regimen for better management of the patients [25]. Therefore, regardless of the shortcomings, a number of glycoproteins are being used in clinical settings as cancer-specific markers for diagnosis and monitoring of disease progression before and after treatment of various cancers (Table **1**) [31]. In the following sections of this chapter, the major clinically approved glycoproteins, which are utilized as biomarkers for cancers are described.

Glycoproteins in Liver Cancer

Liver cancer or hepatocellular carcinoma (HCC), is the most common type of primary liver cancer. The highly risk groups for this disease are the individuals with chronic liver diseases, *e.g.,* liver cirrhosis due to viral infection (hepatitis B or C). The other risk factors for HCC include chronic alcohol abuse, diabetes,

Non-Alcoholic Fatty liver disease, obesity along with afla-toxin exposure [32 - 34]. Besides the epidemiological factors, several genetic alterations, such as genetic instability, recurrent gene mutations and unregulated growth-inducing networking, also contribute to the growth and progression of HCC [34]. Management of patients with HCC remains a major challenge in clinical settings for lacking effective tools for screening and diagnosis at early stages. Consequently, the overall survival rate of HCC patients is very poor (~18%) despite the advancement of surgical resection and chemo-radiotherapies [35]. Therefore, a deeper understanding of the molecular mechanisms, proper screening as well as identification of effective markers for early-stage diagnosis are critical for better management of patients.

Table 1. Glycoproteins used as a cancer biomarker in clinical settings (FDA-approved).

Markers/Tests	Elaboration	Glycosylation Type	Cancers	Type of Detection	Implications	Year of Approval (FDA)	Markers/Tests
AFP	□-Fetoprotein	N-glycosylation	Liver, Brain, pancreas	Concentration of protein, core fucosylation (for AFP-L3)	Diagnosis, staging, detecting recurrence, and therapy monitoring	1992, 2008	AFP
PSA, Pro2-PSA	Prostate-specific antigen	N-glycosylation	Prostate	Concentration of protein	Screening and diagnosis	1986, 1994, 2012	PSA, Pro2-PSA
CA125 (MUC16)	Cancer antigen 125	O-glycosylation	Ovarian	Concentration of protein	Therapy response monitoring and detection of recurrence	1997, 2011	CA125 (MUC16)
HE4 (WFDC2)	Human epididymis protein 4	N-glycosylation	Ovarian	Concentration of protein	Therapy response monitoring and detection of recurrence	2008	HE4 (WFDC2)
OVA1 test (multiple proteins)	□-2 Microglobulin + CA 125II (up), apolipoprotein A1 + prealbumin + transferrin (down)	n/a	Ovarian	Protein concentrations	Prediction	2009	OVA1 test (multiple proteins)
ROMA test	HE4 + CA125	n/a	Ovarian	Protein concentrations	Prediction	2011	ROMA test
CA15-3 (MUC1)	Cancer antigen 15-3	O-Glycosylation	Breast	Sialylated *O*-linked oligosaccharide on MUC1	Therapy response monitoring	1997	CA15-3 (MUC1)
CA27-29	Cancer antigen 27-29		Breast	MUC1 protein levels	Therapy response monitoring	2002	CA27-29

(Table 1) cont.....

Markers/Tests	Elaboration	Glycosylation Type	Cancers	Type of Detection	Implications	Year of Approval (FDA)	Markers/Tests
CEA	Carcino-embryonic antigen	N-glycosylation	Colon, gastric, pancreatic, lung, and breast	Concentration of protein	Therapy response monitoring and detection of recurrence	1985	CEA
HER2/neu	Human epidermal growth factor receptor 2	N-glycosylation	Breast	Concentration of protein	Selection of therapeutic regimen	1998	HER2/neu
Tg	Thyroglobulin	N-glycosylation	Thyroid	Concentration of protein	Therapy response monitoring	1997	Tg
hCG	Human chorionic gonadotropin	N & O-Glycosylation	Testicular, ovarian	Concentration of protein	Diagnosis of disease, identification of stages, recurrence of disease, and therapy response monitoring	Not approved	hCG

α-fetoprotein (AFP)

α-fetoprotein (AFP) is encoded by **the***AFP*gene [36]. Structurally, AFP is a glycoprotein (~70 kDa), first identified in 1956 in human fetus serum [37]. Generally, it is produced by the fetus liver and yolk sac, however, during pregnancy, increased levels of AFP are also recorded. Clinically, AFP measurement is routinely used for the screening of certain abnormal development, such as aneuploidy in pregnant women. Besides this, increased AFP expression followed by higher levels of AFP in the serum was noted in several pathophysiological conditions, including HCC, germ cells tumour of testis, brain tumours, and pancreatic and gastrointestinal carcinomas [38]. Evidences from research and clinical data indicated that α-AFP is the most effective and specific biomarker (serological) for patients with HCC.

Serum α-AFP, a widely used HCC surveillance biomarker, was included in the international guidelines for monitoring patients' surveillance of patients with HCC [39 - 41]. Structurally, in cancer α-AFP, has a single *N*-linked oligosaccharide along with altered core–fucosylation, which can be detected by *Lens culinaris* agglutinin (LCA)-reactive assay. It was noted that elevated levels of fucosylation are associated with the progression of HCC [42]. The ratio of LCA-reactive α-AFP (AFP-L3) and total α-AFP has shown improved clinical specificity and effectiveness in HCC management [43, 44]. The level of AFP increased persistently or in a time-dependent manner in the subsets of HCC-free patients

[45, 46]. However, the elevation of AFP levels is correlated to a higher risk of HCC development [47].

Sialyl Lewis A antigen (CA19-9)

Sialyl Lewis A antigen, also known as CA19-9, is expressed in cancer as an O-linked glycoprotein and glycolipid [48]. Its levels in serum could be elevated in benign cancers of pancreatic, gastric, biliary, colonic and esophageal cancers [49, 50]. CA19-9 has been used as a prognostic biomarker for patients with HCC and post-operative cholangiocarcinoma. Higher levels (100 U/mL) of CA19-9 in serum of patients with HCC acts as an independent predictor for poorer overall survival rate, whereas in patients with cholangiocarcinoma, CA19-9 level (150 U/mL) in serum is correlated with a poor survival rate [51, 52].

Glycoproteins in Prostate Cancer

Prostate cancer (PC) is the most common cancer in men and the fifth cause of cancer-related death in the world [53, 54]. The incidence and mortality of PC are significantly associated with age, *i. e.* mostly seen in aged men (more than 65 years of age). Like most common cancer, the prevention of PC is unavailable; though, the risk of PC can be minimized by adopting a lifestyle, such as avoiding high-fat foods, taking more fruits and vegetables, and doing more physical exercise and workouts [55]. In addition, screening for individuals with a family history and African American origin at the age 45 is highly recommended for early detection of the disease.

Prostate-Specific Antigen (PSA)

Prostate-specific antigen (PSA), also known as gamma-semino-protein, is a 28.4 kDa glycoprotein produced by the prostate gland. It has a single *N*-linked glycosylation site. This protein can be categorized into glycosylated (such as gp28, gp22, gp18, and gp12) and non-glycosylated (such as p26-full length non-glycosylated PSA, or p20, p16, p10, and p6) peptides based on its glycosylation [56]. The majority of PSA is noted in semen, however, a small fraction of total PSA is noted in blood. PSA is a well-known biomarker for prostate cancer and is widely used in screening prostate cancer in clinical applications. The levels of PSA in benign prostatic hyperplasia, and prostate cancer increased significantly as these conditions cause inflammation of prostatic epithelium, followed by disruption of the epithelium, thereby diffusion PSA to the blood stream. Accordingly, the probability of the presence of prostate cancer is high with higher levels of PSA, however, a specific cutoff value of PSA level for the presence or absence of prostate cancer is not available. A number of physicians suggest a PSA cutoff level of 4 ng/mL or higher, whereas other physician uses much lower concentrations, such as 2.5 or 3 ng/mL, in deciding if an individual might need further testing for disease diagnosis. However, individuals with PSA levels 4-10 ng/mL are often known as “borderline range” and have a high risk (~025%) of prostate cancer positive, while PSA levels higher than10 ng/mL indicate the presence of prostate cancer chance more than 50%.

Although, PSA has a diagnostic implication, however, its low specificity limits its clinical applications. Thus, screening of serum PSA along with a digital rectal exam (DRE) and Gleason scoring of prostate biopsy samples provided significantly improved clinical utility, thereby having been approved by the FDA for detection of prostate cancer at early stages [57, 58]. Nonetheless, to improve the clinical utility of serum PSA test, a number of promising approaches are under investigation, including determination of each type of PSA, such as proPSA, benign PSA, and intact PSA or kallikreins other than PSA. Also, measuring the ratio of total PSA complexes with α1- chymotrypsin and α2-macroglobulin (tPSA) in comparison to that of free PSA (fPSA) and analysing PSA levels with other biomarkers such as prostate cancer antigen 3 (PCA3) *etc* [59]. Furthermore, altered modifications of PSA, such as a different form of glycosylation and fucosylation, have been observed in prostate cancer patient’s compared to healthy individuals. Therefore, the nature of glycosylation of PSA has a crucial implication in specifying along with sensitizing PSA tests for prostate cancer patients in early or advance stage diagnosis [60 - 64].

Glycoproteins in Ovarian Cancer

Ovarian cancer is a common gynaecological cancer and one of the leading cancer-related mortality cause in women, which accounts for 295,000 new cases and 185,000 deaths annually worldwide [65]. The asymptomatic nature and lack of effective screening tools lead to the diagnosis of the disease at late stages, thereby challenging the treatment modalities [66]. At the beginning of the therapeutic regimen, the current conventional therapies, including surgical resection along with chemo (platinum+taxane)-radiotherapy, is correlated with a higher response rate, however, the overall disease-free survival rate is still disappointing, and most of the patients died due to therapy-resistance of the disease [67]. Thus, to increase the survival rates of patients with ovarian cancer, novel strategies for specific biomarkers at early detection and therapeutics against treatment-refractory disease are urgently needed. A number of glycoproteins have been clinically approved for screening, diagnosis and monitoring disease-progression, staging of ovarian cancer and therapeutic responses (Table **1**).

CA125 (Cancer Antigen 125)

CA125, also known as MUC16 encoded by the *MUC16* gene, is a membrane protein having intracellular and trans-membrane domains. It is expressed by epithelial cells of various organs such as corneal, bronchial, ovarian and endometrial. The extracellular domain of CA125 sheds into the bloodstream and is used as a non-invasive biomarker for screening, diagnosis and progression of ovarian cancer [68]. In addition, it is reported that an elevation of soluble CA125 could occur in other malignancies, including gastric cancer, breast cancer, mesothelioma, non-Hodgkin lymphoma, leiomyoma and leiomyosarcoma of gastrointestinal origin *etc* [69 - 75]. Also, increased levels of CA125 was noted in benign conditions [76, 77] along with some other pathophysiological state such as during endometriosis [78], pregnancy [79], ovulatory cycles [80], liver diseases, congestive heart failure [81, 82], and in infectious disease like tuberculosis [83, 84]. Thus, it is nonspecific and unreliable for early-stage diagnosis of ovarian cancer, however, measuring serum CA125 along with ultrasonography is a standard and reliable tool for the detection of ovarian cancer in clinical settings [85]. In addition, CA125 glycoforms have the potential to distinguish between endometriosis and ovarian cancer as well as evaluation of pathological staging, grading, and histological type of ovarian cancers [86].

Human Epidermis Protein 4 (WFDC2)

HE4 (Human epididymis protein 4), also known as WFDC2, is a secretory protein of 23-27 kDa molecular weight, having a consensus site for *N*-linked glycosylation at 15 amino acid residues. Gene expression data revealed that expression of *HE4* is most frequently overexpressed in epithelial ovarian cancers [87, 88]. In ovarian cancer cells, HE4 is overexpressed and secreted as a glycoprotein [89].

Enzyme immunoassay test kit for HE4 developed by Fujirebio Diagnostics (Sweden) in June 2008. Whereas ARCHITECT HE4 automated test was developed by Abbott Diagnostics (UK) in March 2010. FDA approved these tests as supplementary and equivalent to CA125 for ovarian cancer screening and diagnosis. A recent study noted that HE4 exhibited a significantly higher specificity than that of CA125 (93% *versus* 78%) in diagnosis patients with ovarian cancer at early stages [90]. Accordingly, FDA approved the combination of the HE4 and CA125 tests in the Risk of Ovarian Malignancy Algorithm (ROMA) test, to identify the risk of developing ovarian cancer in premenopausal or postmenopausal women having an ovarian adnexal mass in September 2011 [91, 92]. It was reported that the ROMA test outperforms the individual HE4 and CA125 biomarkers in detecting ovarian cancers both at early and late stages [93].

Furthermore, HE4 glycoforms could provide insights regarding the occurrence, development, or migration of cancerous cells, which in turn, could facilitate early detection or target identification for therapeutic intervention for patients with ovarian cancer. In addition, detection of CA125 and HE4, OVA1 test (test of multiples proteins such as □-2 microglobulin, CA125II, apo-lipoprotein A1, pre-albumin and transferrin), measurement glycoprotein cancer antigen 19-9 (CA19-9), human chorionic gonadotropin (hCG) also used in diagnosis, prediction and monitoring of therapy response in patients with ovarian cancer in clinical settings [94].

Glycoproteins in Breast Cancer

Breast cancer is the leading cause of cancer-related mortality in women, with an incidence of 1.2 million cases annually in the world [95]. Although satisfactory progress at early detection, diagnosis and efficient treatment approach, including surgery, radiotherapy, hormonal therapy and chemotherapy, however, the disease still remains a significant global health burden due to less recovery rate of recurrent breast cancer (<5%) and declining response rates to therapy due to multidrug resistance (MDR) [96 - 101]. Specific and sensitive markers for proper diagnosis and prognosis could improve better management of patients with breast cancers [102]. Thus, identifying and developing effective non-invasive markers for breast cancer has a critical implication in clinical outcomes. Altered glycosylation of proteins in serum is correlated with the progression of breast cancer, thus, it has been explored as a diagnostic indicator for the disease [103, 104]. The approved glycoproteins usage in clinics for diagnosis and monitoring breast cancer progression are described below.

Mucin 1 (MUC1)

MUC1, also called cancer antigen 15-3 (CA15-3), MAM6, milk mucin antigen, CA27.29, *etc.*, is a trans-membrane O-linked oligosaccharides glycoprotein [105]. It is mostly expressed by glandular epithelial cells at a low level, especially at the apical surface of the epithelial cells in the pancreas, lung, breast, and gastrointestinal tract [106]. In cancer, MUC1 up-regulation followed by treatment associated with proliferation, invasion and survival of cancer cells *via* reducing cell-extracellular matrix adhesion along with cell-cell adhesion [107 - 109]. In addition, it is linked to the EGFRs (epidermal growth factor receptors), β-catenin, and NF-κb (nuclear factor -κb) signaling networks, thus, regulating the progression of the disease [110, 111]. Also, abnormal over-expression of MUC1 correlated with metastasis by promoting angiogenesis and chemo-resistance in patients with breast cancer [112, 113]. Therefore, MUC1 has potential roles modulating cancer initiation, progression, metastasis and therapy resistance, thus, it could be used as a prognostic biomarker.

MUC1 is aberrantly overexpressed in over 90% of breast tumors [114], and MUC1 is a well-known, routinely used biomarker for breast cancer diagnosis in combination with other serum biomarkers [115, 116]. Also, aberrant glycosylation MUC1 has the potential to be used as a biomarker for early detection of breast cancer. MUC1 is hyper-glycosylated in breast cancer samples compared to healthy tissues. The highly *O*-linked oligosaccharides glycosylated MUC1 are then diffused into the blood stream in patients with breast cancers [117]. Since, the MUC1 protein is highly overexpressed and then glycosylated aberrantly in cancers, thus, these tumor-associated glyco-peptides, especially the epitopes, are masked in non-cancerous cells and can be identified as targets for developing cancer immunotherapies and immuno-diagnostics [118 - 120].

Human Epidermal Growth Factor Receptor 2 (HER2)

HER2 is a glycoprotein, also known as cluster of differentiation 340 (CD340) or proto-oncogene Neu (185 kDa), encoded by the *ERBB2* gene. This glycoprotein has three domains: an extracellular domain, a trans-membrane lipophilic domain, and an intra-cellular tyrosine kinase domain. The extracellular domain can be cleavage, released and shed into blood [121]. HER2 is a growth-promoting protein, and over-expression was noted in 20–30% of breast cancers, and these subtypes of breast cancers showed biological aggressive phenotypes with poorer survival rates [122, 123]. The prognostic significance of HER2 in combination with MUC1 protein for the detection of breast cancer high-risk groups has been reported [124]. The combination analysis of these indicators identifies the patients who need intensive therapies [124]. Also, serum levels of HER2 indicate the response of chemotherapies in patients with breast cancers [125].

Carcinoembryonic Antigen (CEA)

CEA is a set of cell surface glycoproteins associated with cell adhesion. CEA levels are elevated in many pathophysiological conditions, including colorectal, gastric, pancreatic, non-small cell lung, and breast carcinomas [126]. Studies demonstrated that CEA levels correlated with the presence of breast cancer and the increased levels are associated with the stages of breast cancers [127 - 132]. Thus, reduction or increments of serum CEA levels could imply the disease progression or state [133 - 136]. Therefore, CEA levels might be a useful tool in the management of postsurgical follow-up in patients with breast cancer to monitor recurrence or relapse of the disease [137 - 139], along with treatment response [140 - 142].

Glycoproteins in Colon Cancer

Cancer in the colon and rectum is the third leading cause of cancer and cancer-related dead worldwide [143, 144]. The 5-year survival rate of patients with colorectal cancer is about 64% due to the improvement of current therapies, including immunotherapy, chemotherapy and surgery [144 - 146]. To improve clinical outcomes further and for more optimization of clinical management, more effective biomarkers are needed for early detection and monitoring of the disease progression.

CEA

CEA is a glycoprotein anchored to the cell surface *via* Glycosyl-phosphatidy--inositol. It generally expresses mucosal cells of gastrointestinal cells during fetal development [147]. Serum levels of CEA are elevated in heavy smokers and in some pathophysiological conditions such as gastric, colorectal, pancreatic, breast and non-small cell lung carcinomas [126].

In colorectal cancer, CEA is widely used as a prognostic and disease recurrence biomarker. The American Society of Clinical Oncology and European Group on Tumor Markers approved CEA as a recurrent biomarker following curative resection in patients with colorectal cancers [148, 149]. In addition, altered glycosylation of CEA is colorectal cancer is noted as the molecular mass of CEA in cancer is different from the normal [150, 151]. It is noted that CEA presence in colon carcinomas is intensively substituted by fucosylated and sialylated [152]. The altered glycosylated CEA could contribute to cancer metastatic spread [152]. Nevertheless, additional studies are imperative to conclude that altered CEA or its glycosylation potentially has enhanced diagnostic or prognostic significance in patients with colorectal carcinomas.

Carbohydrate Antigen 19-9 (CA19-9)

Serum CA19-9 has been used as a colon cancer biomarker for a long period in the clinical setting [153]. However, a recent study indicates that serum CA19-9 is not recommended for routine analysis such as screening, staging, and treatment monitoring of colon cancer due to a lack of validation with sufficient clinical data and less sensitivity [149]. On the other hand, the measurement of CA19-9 in combination with CEA in serum could give more insightful and powerful information in predicting the disease prognosis and guide the therapy selection. For example, it is evident that patients with elevated CEA and CA19-9 can be benefited from adjuvant-chemotherapy [154].

Glycoproteins in Lung Cancer

Lung cancer is the leading cause of cancer-related mortality due to low survival rates and the high prevalence of patients with advanced-stages during diagnosis [155]. Cigarette smoking, life-style behaviours and exposure to environmental pollutants are the causes of lung cancers [156, 157]. Among its subtypes, non-small cell lung cancer (NSCLC) is the most common subtype, accounting for about 85% of all lung cancers. This subtype exhibits stronger chemo-radiotherapy resistant. The comorbid illness, cancer heterogeneity along with lack of effective screening and diagnostic tools caused the management of lung cancer to be challenging [158]. The five-year survival rate of patients with localized lung cancer is ~56%, however, only 16% of patients with lung cancer cases are diagnosed at early stages. On the other hand, the five-year survival rate for patients with metastatic disease is only 5% [159]. Characterizing genetic and epigenetic heterogeneity in lung cancer is important for improving disease prevention and detection at early stages, along with personalized therapy and prognosis. It is noted that a number of changed glycosylation happened in lung cancers, including aberrant production of glycosylated mucins, altered branched N-glycans, and the presence of increased sialic acid on glycolipids and proteins [160]. The following sections describe the major glycoproteins associated with lung cancers.

Mucins

Mucins, a family of large glycoproteins, are expressed on the luminal epithelial surface of cells harboring an extensive *O*-linked glycosylation of proline, threonine and serine (PTS) domain [161]. They protect mucous epithelia by providing a physical and biological barrier. In addition, the trans-membrane mucins play important roles in signal transduction for growth, and survival by maintaining epithelial layer integrity. Abnormal overexpression of mucins promoted lung cancer cells growth, proliferation, survival and metastasis *via* modulating other signaling and kinases [161]. In addition, the expression MUC1, a type of mucin, is correlated with cancer stage stratification and poor prognosis [161]. Therefore, mucins could be an emerging target for the development of novel therapeutics against lung cancers. A number of strategies targeting mucins, which are overexpressed in lung cancers, are currently being investigated to develop drugs to better manage patients with lung cancers [161].

In NSCLC, overexpressed mucins could be used as a suitable prognostic biomarker [162 - 169]. For example, expression of MUC1 and MUC5AC correlated with lung cancer progression [170]. Also, it was noted that MUC1 significantly overexpressed in adenocarcinoma in comparison to that of squamous cell carcinoma (86.3 *versus* 39.1%) [170], thereby, expression of mucins could be used as a non-invasive marker for subtyping lung cancers. In addition, expression MUC4 is associated with histological grade of lung cancers [165, 171 - 173]. Additionally, expression of MUC5AC and MUC6 was noted in the cases of mucin-filled glandular and cystic lung adenocarcinomas [174], while the overexpression of MUC5AC has been associated with adenocarcinomas when compared to that of squamous cell carcinomas [175]. Furthermore, overexpression of MUC5AC is significantly associated with patients' gender, histology of the tumour, risk of distance metastasis development, poor survival and non-smoking history of patients with lung cancers [176]. Therefore, the potential of the clinical utility of mucins in lung cancer screening, diagnosis and prognosis biomarkers is emerging; however, there is no conclusive evidence for their clinical applications in clinics.

Epidermal Growth Factor Receptor (EGFR)

EGFR is a trans-membrane glycoprotein encoded by the *EGFR* gene. It has an extracellular epidermal growth factor (EGF) binding domain, a trans-membrane domain and an intra-cellular tyrosine kinase domain, which regulates signalling cascades, thereby controlling cellular proliferation and survival of cells. Genetic and epigenetic changes and abnormal expression of EGFR are associated with the pathogenesis of a number of human cancers, including NSCLC [177 - 179]. Overexpression of EGFR is noted in 62% of NSCLCs, and the overexpression is correlated with the poor prognosis of lung cancer [180]. In the USA, ~10% lung adenocarcinoma patients harbor *EGFR* mutations, whereas 30-50% Asian patients with lung cancers had shown *EGFR* mutations [180]. Mutated EGFR triggers ligand-independent tyrosine kinase activation, which leads to activation of downstream anti-apoptotic, growth-promoting and survival signaling pathways [181]. Thus, aberrant overexpression or altered activation of EGFR is characterized as a biomarker for the treatment and management of patients with lung cancers. Thus, the therapeutics targeting tyrosine kinase, *i. e.* tyrosine kinase inhibitors (TKIs), such as gefitinib, erlotinib and afatinib, in patients having *EGFR*-mutant tumors had shown significantly high responses resulting in improved progression-free survival [182]. Though, the majority of these patients develop resistance, thereby recurrence of cancer is seen due to the development of new mutations [183], thus, further research is needed to identify novel targets and develop therapies for sustainable improvement for patients with cancers.

CEA

Along with EGFR, mucins, CEA is another glycoprotein widely used biomarker for cancers [184, 185]. In lung cancer, the use of CEA as a biomarker is still debatable, however, lower cost, non-invasive nature, and lack of other reliable biomarkers make CEA a substantial alternative option in lung cancer care [186 - 191]. CEA analysis before and after surgery provides insightful information for disease progression, prediction, and in choosing the adjuvant therapy at early stages of patients with lung cancers [188, 189]. Also, CEA could act as an EGFR-TKI treatment response predictor in patients developing resistance against TKIs. Serum CEA levels correlated with EGFR-TKI treatment outcomes, thus, the presence of higher CEA levels followed by EGFR-TKI treatment indicates poorer survival in patients with EGFR-mutant lung cancers [192, 193]. However, it was also noted that CEA levels do not associate with tumor progression during EGFR-TKI treatments [194, 195]. In addition, treating lung cancer with EGFR-TKI could affect the clonality of heterogeneous lung cancers, thereby modulating the expression of CEA [196].

Glycoproteins in Pancreatic Cancer

Pancreatic adenocarcinoma is the most aggressive human malignancy with the worst prognosis (less than 5% five-year survival rate) [197]. Lack of effective tools for early detection, higher potency of metastasis and resistance to therapies contributed to the poor prognosis of the disease [198, 199]. Also, the asymptomatic nature of early stage-disease and similarities in clinical parameters between benign and malignant conditions causes it difficult to properly diagnosis the disease [200]. Therefore, it is urgently needed to identify and develop effective biomarkers for early detection and potential therapeutics for better management of patients with pancreatic cancers. Glycosylated proteins play important roles, such as protecting and lubricating the pancreatic ducts in a normal physiological state [201]. Deregulation of glycoproteins has been reported, and aberrant expression/production of glycoproteins is correlated with cancer progression along with the worst prognosis of patients with pancreatic cancers.

Cancer Antigen 19-9 (CA 19-9)

CA 19-9 also called sialyl Lewis A (sLe^A), a Lewis family member of blood group antigen, most commonly used serum biomarker for the management of patients with pancreatic cancers [202 - 204]. The level of sLe^A is low in general tissues, however, higher levels are noted in embryonic tissue [205]. Overexpression is noted in cancers of epithelia origin [206]. In healthy physiological condition, sLe^A is found on the epithelial surfaces of the ducts, while in pancreatic cancers, sLe^A is noted in the lumen of proliferating ducts and secreted into the bloodstream in high concentrations [207]. In practice, CA 19-9 is commonly used for monitoring the therapy response of patients with pancreatic cancers, however, lack of specificity and sensitivity limits its applications for diagnosis and screening in clinical settings for the management of patients with pancreatic cancers [208 - 212].

CEA

CEA is a glycoprotein identified in colon cancer tissue and overexpressed in a number of human malignancies such as colon, breast, lung, thyroid and pancreatic cancers [213 - 217]. In pancreatic cancer, 30-60% of patients had shown CEA over expression, thereby being used as a tumour biomarker [218]. However, CA19-9 could exhibit limited specificity and sensitivity in some patients, especially patients with metastasis of jaundice [219]. Also, in the cases of individuals lacking sialylated Lewis antigen expression (5-10% population), there is no use of CA19-9 as a biomarker as there is no or too little expression of CA19-9; serum CEA level was used as a potential marker for diagnosis and prognosis of patients with pancreatic cancers [220 - 222]. Therefore, an increased level of CEA could be used as an independent predictor of poor survival of patients with pancreatic cancers.

CONCLUSION

Glycoproteins are ubiquitous macromolecules that function in the secretory processes, cell surfaces and transport systems of cells, and play critical roles in a number of biological/physiological processes, including cellular growth, development, proliferation, differentiation and survival by modulating cell-signaling, cell-cell interaction and immune recognition. Also, altered glycoproteins levels are involved in the pathogenesis of many human diseases, including cancers. Accumulating information suggested that the cancer-specific alterations in glycosylation of serum glycoproteins could give us a number of promising and novel biomarkers, which in turn, could be used for screening, diagnosis, prognosis and monitoring therapy response in patients with various cancers with greater specificity and sensitivity in comparison to that of currently used biomarkers in clinical applications [223 - 225]. Furthermore, clinic-pathological results indicated that analysis of serum glycome could potentially distinguish cancer and non-cancer patients or patients with benign conditions, thus, it has the potential to diagnose the disease at earlier stages than the biomarkers currently used in clinics [226, 227]. Therefore, modern biomedical technologies provide a strong possibility of the diagnostic power of serum glycoproteins, *i.e.,* serum glycome analysis, thus, glycoproteins-based biomarkers discovery and development for cancer management is one of the most promising areas of current biomarker discovery research.

CONSENT FOR PUBLICATION

Not applicable.

CONFLICT OF INTEREST

The author declares no conflict of interest, financial or otherwise.

ACKNOWLEDGEMENT

The author is thankful to the University of Texas MD Anderson Cancer Center, Houston, Texas-77033, USA, for providing technical support to the work.

REFERENCES

[1] Siegel RL, Miller KD, Jemal A. Cancer statistics, 2020. CA Cancer J Clin 2020; 70(1): 7-30. [http://dx.doi.org/10.3322/caac.21590] [PMID: 31912902]

[2] Vasan N, Baselga J, Hyman DM. A view on drug resistance in cancer. Nature 2019; 575(7782): 299-309. [http://dx.doi.org/10.1038/s41586-019-1730-1] [PMID: 31723286]

[3] Stowell SR, Ju T, Cummings RD. Protein glycosylation in cancer. Annu Rev Pathol 2015; 10(1): 473-510. [http://dx.doi.org/10.1146/annurev-pathol-012414-040438] [PMID: 25621663]

[4] Pan S, Brentnall TA, Chen R. Glycoproteins and glycoproteomics in pancreatic cancer. World J Gastroenterol 2016; 22(42): 9288-99. [http://dx.doi.org/10.3748/wjg.v22.i42.9288] [PMID: 27895417]

[5] Crumpton MJ. Glycoproteins in relation to cell differentiation and malignancy. Prog Clin Biol Res 1982; 102 pt A: 359-70. [PMID: 7167446]

[6] Connelly MA, Gruppen EG, Otvos JD, Dullaart RPF. Inflammatory glycoproteins in cardiometabolic disorders, autoimmune diseases and cancer. Clin Chim Acta 2016; 459: 177-86. [http://dx.doi.org/10.1016/j.cca.2016.06.012] [PMID: 27312321]

[7] Regan P, McClean PL, Smyth T, Doherty M. Early Stage Glycosylation Biomarkers in Alzheimer's Disease. Medicines (Basel) 2019; 6(3): 92. [http://dx.doi.org/10.3390/medicines6030092] [PMID: 31484367]

[8] Park DD, Phoomak C, Xu G, *et al.* Metastasis of cholangiocarcinoma is promoted by extended high-mannose glycans. Proc Natl Acad Sci USA 2020; 117(14): 7633-44. [http://dx.doi.org/10.1073/pnas.1916498117] [PMID: 32213588]

[9] Yang S, Wang PG. Method development of glycoprotein biomarkers for cancers. Bioanalysis 2017; 9(12): 903-6. [http://dx.doi.org/10.4155/bio-2017-0077] [PMID: 28644045]

[10] Peracaula R, Tabarés G, Royle L, *et al.* Altered glycosylation pattern allows the distinction between prostate-specific antigen (PSA) from normal and tumor origins. Glycobiology 2003; 13(6): 457-70. [http://dx.doi.org/10.1093/glycob/cwg041] [PMID: 12626390]

[11] Kasbaoui L, Harb J, Bernard S, Meflah K. Differences in glycosylation state of fibronectin from two rat colon carcinoma cell lines in relation to tumoral progressiveness. Cancer Res 1989; 49(19): 5317-22. [PMID: 2766300]

[12] Kellokumpu S, Sormunen R, Kellokumpu I. Abnormal glycosylation and altered Golgi structure in colorectal cancer: dependence on intra-Golgi pH. FEBS Lett 2002; 516(1-3): 217-24. [http://dx.doi.org/10.1016/S0014-5793(02)02535-8] [PMID: 11959136]

[13] Ng RCY, Roberts AN, Wilson RG, Latner AL, Turner GA. Analyses of protein extracts of human breast cancers: changes in glycoprotein content linked to the malignant phenotype. Br J Cancer 1987; 55(3): 249-54. [http://dx.doi.org/10.1038/bjc.1987.48] [PMID: 2436644]

[14] Mehta A, Herrera H, Block T. Glycosylation and liver cancer. Adv Cancer Res 2015; 126: 257-79. [http://dx.doi.org/10.1016/bs.acr.2014.11.005] [PMID: 25727150]

[15] Fuster MM, Esko JD. The sweet and sour of cancer: glycans as novel therapeutic targets. Nat Rev Cancer 2005; 5(7): 526-42. [http://dx.doi.org/10.1038/nrc1649] [PMID: 16069816]

[16] Cummings RD, Pierce JM. The challenge and promise of glycomics. Chem Biol 2014; 21(1): 1-15. [http://dx.doi.org/10.1016/j.chembiol.2013.12.010] [PMID: 24439204]

[17] Reis CA, Osorio H, Silva L, Gomes C, David L. Alterations in glycosylation as biomarkers for cancer detection. J Clin Pathol 2010; 63(4): 322-9. [http://dx.doi.org/10.1136/jcp.2009.071035] [PMID: 20354203]

[18] Ho WL, Hsu WM, Huang MC, Kadomatsu K, Nakagawara A. Protein glycosylation in cancers and its potential therapeutic applications in neuroblastoma. J Hematol Oncol 2016; 9(1): 100. [http://dx.doi.org/10.1186/s13045-016-0334-6] [PMID: 27686492]

[19] Fernandes B, Sagman U, Auger M, Demetrio M, Dennis JW. Beta 1-6 branched oligosaccharides as a marker of tumor progression in human breast and colon neoplasia. Cancer Res 1991; 51(2): 718-23. [PMID: 1985789]

[20] Murata K, Miyoshi E, Kameyama M, *et al.* Expression of N-acetylglucosaminyltransferase V in colorectal cancer correlates with metastasis and poor prognosis. Clin Cancer Res 2000; 6(5): 1772-7. [PMID: 10815896]

[21] Dosaka-Akita H, Kinoshita I, Yamazaki K, *et al.* N-acetylgalactosaminyl transferase-3 is a potential new marker for non-small cell lung cancers. Br J Cancer 2002; 87(7): 751-5. [http://dx.doi.org/10.1038/sj.bjc.6600536] [PMID: 12232759]

[22] Yamamoto S, Nakamori S, Tsujie M, *et al.* Expression of uridine diphosphate N-acetyl-alph--D-galactosamine: polypeptide N-acetylgalactosaminyl transferase 3 in adenocarcinoma of the pancreas. Pathobiology 2004; 71(1): 12-8. [http://dx.doi.org/10.1159/000072957] [PMID: 14555840]

[23] Park JH, Nishidate T, Kijima K, *et al.* Critical roles of mucin 1 glycosylation by transactivated polypeptide N-acetylgalactosaminyltransferase 6 in mammary carcinogenesis. Cancer Res 2010; 70(7): 2759-69. [http://dx.doi.org/10.1158/0008-5472.CAN-09-3911] [PMID: 20215525]

[24] Park JH, Katagiri T, Chung S, Kijima K, Nakamura Y. Polypeptide N-acetylgalactosaminyltransferase 6 disrupts mammary acinar morphogenesis through O-glycosylation of fibronectin. Neoplasia 2011; 13(4): 320-IN10. [http://dx.doi.org/10.1593/neo.101440] [PMID: 21472136]

[25] Ludwig JA, Weinstein JN. Biomarkers in cancer staging, prognosis and treatment selection. Nat Rev Cancer 2005; 5(11): 845-56. [http://dx.doi.org/10.1038/nrc1739] [PMID: 16239904]

[26] Hanash SM, Pitteri SJ, Faca VM. Mining the plasma proteome for cancer biomarkers. Nature 2008; 452(7187): 571-9. [http://dx.doi.org/10.1038/nature06916] [PMID: 18385731]

[27] Christiansen MN, Chik J, Lee L, Anugraham M, Abrahams JL, Packer NH. Cell surface protein glycosylation in cancer. Proteomics 2014; 14(4-5): 525-46. [http://dx.doi.org/10.1002/pmic.201300387] [PMID: 24339177]

[28] Spiro RG. Protein glycosylation: nature, distribution, enzymatic formation, and disease implications of glycopeptide bonds. Glycobiology 2002; 12(4): 43R-56R. [http://dx.doi.org/10.1093/glycob/12.4.43R] [PMID: 12042244]

[29] Glavey SV, Huynh D, Reagan MR, *et al.* The cancer glycome: Carbohydrates as mediators of metastasis. Blood Rev 2015; 29(4): 269-79. [http://dx.doi.org/10.1016/j.blre.2015.01.003] [PMID: 25636501]

[30] Anderson NL, Anderson NG. The human plasma proteome: history, character, and diagnostic prospects. Mol Cell Proteomics 2002; 1(11): 845-67. [http://dx.doi.org/10.1074/mcp.R200007-MCP200] [PMID: 12488461]

[31] Yotsukura S, Mamitsuka H. Evaluation of serum-based cancer biomarkers: A brief review from a clinical and computational viewpoint. Crit Rev Oncol Hematol 2015; 93(2): 103-15. [http://dx.doi.org/10.1016/j.critrevonc.2014.10.002] [PMID: 25459666]

[32] Villanueva A. Hepatocellular Carcinoma. N Engl J Med. 2019; 380(1): 450-62.

[33] Younossi Z, Stepanova M, Ong JP, *et al.* Nonalcoholic steatohepatitis is thefastest growing cause of hepatocellular carcinoma in liver transplant candidates. Clin Gastroenterol Hepatol 2019; 17(4): 748-755.e3. [http://dx.doi.org/10.1016/j.cgh.2018.05.057] [PMID: 29908364]

[34] Niu ZS, Niu XJ, Wang WH. Genetic alterations in hepatocellular carcinoma: An update. World J Gastroenterol 2016; 22(41): 9069-95. [http://dx.doi.org/10.3748/wjg.v22.i41.9069] [PMID: 27895396]

[35] Kulik LM, Chokechanachaisakul A. Evaluation and management of hepatocellular carcinoma. Clin Liver Dis 2015; 19(1): 23-43. [http://dx.doi.org/10.1016/j.cld.2014.09.002] [PMID: 25454295]

[36] Harper ME, Dugaiczyk A. Linkage of the evolutionarily-related serum albumin and alpha-fetoprotein genes within q11-22 of human chromosome 4. Am J Hum Genet 1983; 35(4): 565-72. [PMID: 6192711]

[37] Bergstrand CG, Czar B. Demonstration of a new protein fraction in serum from the human fetus. Scand J Clin Lab Invest 1956; 8(2): 174. [http://dx.doi.org/10.3109/00365515609049266] [PMID: 13351554]

[38] Saito S, Ojima H, Ichikawa H, Hirohashi S, Kondo T. Molecular background of α-fetoprotein in liver cancer cells as revealed by global RNA expression analysis. Cancer Sci 2008; 99(12): 2402-9. [http://dx.doi.org/10.1111/j.1349-7006.2008.00973.x] [PMID: 19038010]

[39] Bruix J, Sherman M. Management of hepatocellular carcinoma. Hepatology 2005; 42(5): 1208-36. [http://dx.doi.org/10.1002/hep.20933] [PMID: 16250051]

[40] Bruix J, Sherman M. Management of hepatocellular carcinoma: An update. Hepatology 2011; 53(3): 1020-2. [http://dx.doi.org/10.1002/hep.24199] [PMID: 21374666]

[41] EASL-EORTC clinical practice guidelines: management of hepatocellular carcinoma. J Hepatol 2012; 56(4): 908-43. [http://dx.doi.org/10.1016/j.jhep.2011.12.001] [PMID: 22424438]

[42] Kobayashi M, Kuroiwa T, Suda T, *et al.* Fucosylated fraction of alpha-fetoprotein, L3, as a useful prognostic factor in patients with hepatocellular carcinoma with special reference to low concentrations of serum alpha-fetoprotein. Hepatol Res 2007; 37(11): 914-22. [http://dx.doi.org/10.1111/j.1872-034X.2007.00147.x] [PMID: 17610501]

[43] Shiraki K, Takase K, Tameda Y, Hamada M, Kosaka Y, Nakano T. A clinical study of lectin-reactive alpha-fetoprotein as an early indicator of hepatocellular carcinoma in the follow-up of cirrhotic patients. Hepatology 1995; 22(3): 802-7.
[http://dx.doi.org/10.1002/hep.1840220317] [PMID: 7544756]

[44] Nakagawa T, Miyoshi E, Yakushijin T, *et al.* Glycomic analysis of alpha-fetoprotein L3 in hepatoma cell lines and hepatocellular carcinoma patients. J Proteome Res 2008; 7(6): 2222-33.
[http://dx.doi.org/10.1021/pr700841q] [PMID: 18479159]

[45] Lok AS, Sterling RK, Everhart JE, *et al.* Des-gamma-carboxy prothrombin and alpha-fetoprotein as biomarkers for the early detection of hepatocellular carcinoma. Gastroenterology 2010; 138(2): 493-502.
[http://dx.doi.org/10.1053/j.gastro.2009.10.031] [PMID: 19852963]

[46] Biselli M, Conti F, Gramenzi A, *et al.* A new approach to the use of α-fetoprotein as surveillance test for hepatocellular carcinoma in patients with cirrhosis. Br J Cancer 2015; 112(1): 69-76.
[http://dx.doi.org/10.1038/bjc.2014.536] [PMID: 25314061]

[47] Bruce MG, Bruden D, McMahon BJ, *et al.* Clinical significance of elevated alpha-fetoprotein in Alaskan Native patients with chronic hepatitis C. J Viral Hepat 2008; 15(3): 179-87.
[http://dx.doi.org/10.1111/j.1365-2893.2007.00928.x] [PMID: 18233991]

[48] Ballehaninna UK, Chamberlain RS. The clinical utility of serum CA 19-9 in the diagnosis, prognosis and management of pancreatic adenocarcinoma: An evidence based appraisal. J Gastrointest Oncol 2012; 3(2): 105-19.
[PMID: 22811878]

[49] Marrelli D, Caruso S, Pedrazzani C, *et al.* CA19-9 serum levels in obstructive jaundice: clinical value in benign and malignant conditions. Am J Surg 2009; 198(3): 333-9.
[http://dx.doi.org/10.1016/j.amjsurg.2008.12.031] [PMID: 19375064]

[50] Basso D, Meggiato T, Fabris C, *et al.* Extra-hepatic cholestasis determines a reversible increase of glycoproteic tumour markers in benign and malignant diseases. Eur J Clin Invest 1992; 22(12): 800-4.
[http://dx.doi.org/10.1111/j.1365-2362.1992.tb01449.x] [PMID: 1478251]

[51] Hsu CC, Goyal A, Iuga A, *et al.* Elevated CA19-9 is associated with increased mortality in a prospective cohort of hepatocellular carcinoma patients. Clin Transl Gastroenterol 2015; 6(2): e74.
[http://dx.doi.org/10.1038/ctg.2014.22] [PMID: 25651978]

[52] Cai WK, Lin JJ, He GH, Wang H, Lu JH, Yang GS. Preoperative serum CA19-9 levels is an independent prognostic factor in patients with resected hilar cholangiocarcinoma. Int J Clin Exp Pathol 2014; 7(11): 7890-8.
[PMID: 25550829]

[53] Bray F, Ferlay J, Soerjomataram I, Siegel RL, Torre LA, Jemal A. Global cancer statistics 2018: GLOBOCAN estimates of incidence and mortality worldwide for 36 cancers in 185 countries. CA Cancer J Clin 2018; 68(6): 394-424.
[http://dx.doi.org/10.3322/caac.21492] [PMID: 30207593]

[54] Ferlay JEM, Lam F, Colombet M, *et al.* Global cancer observatory: cancer today 2019. https://gco.iarc.fr/today

[55] Rawla P. Epidemiology of Prostate Cancer. World J Oncol 2019; 10(2): 63-89.
[http://dx.doi.org/10.14740/wjon1191] [PMID: 31068988]

[56] Isono T, Tanaka T, Kageyama S, Yoshiki T. Structural diversity of cancer-related and non-cance--related prostate-specific antigen. Clin Chem 2002; 48(12): 2187-94.
[http://dx.doi.org/10.1093/clinchem/48.12.2187] [PMID: 12446475]

[57] Catalona WJ, Smith DS, Ratliff TL, *et al.* Measurement of prostate-specific antigen in serum as a screening test for prostate cancer. N Engl J Med 1991; 324(17): 1156-61.
[http://dx.doi.org/10.1056/NEJM199104253241702] [PMID: 1707140]

[58] Carter HB, Albertsen PC, Barry MJ, *et al.* Early detection of prostate cancer: AUA Guideline. J Urol 2013; 190(2): 419-26. [http://dx.doi.org/10.1016/j.juro.2013.04.119] [PMID: 23659877]

[59] Bussemakers MJG, van Bokhoven A, Verhaegh GW, *et al.* DD3: a new prostate-specific gene, highly overexpressed in prostate cancer. Cancer Res 1999; 59(23): 5975-9. [PMID: 10606244]

[60] Tajiri M, Ohyama C, Wada Y. Oligosaccharide profiles of the prostate specific antigen in free and complexed forms from the prostate cancer patient serum and in seminal plasma: a glycopeptide approach. Glycobiology 2008; 18(1): 2-8. [http://dx.doi.org/10.1093/glycob/cwm117] [PMID: 17956937]

[61] Sarrats A, Comet J, Tabarés G, *et al.* Differential percentage of serum prostate-specific antigen subforms suggests a new way to improve prostate cancer diagnosis. Prostate 2010; 70(1): 1-9. [http://dx.doi.org/10.1002/pros.21031] [PMID: 19670261]

[62] Saldova R, Fan Y, Fitzpatrick JM, Watson RWG, Rudd PM. Core fucosylation and 2-3 sialylation in serum N-glycome is significantly increased in prostate cancer comparing to benign prostate hyperplasia. Glycobiology 2011; 21(2): 195-205. [http://dx.doi.org/10.1093/glycob/cwq147] [PMID: 20861084]

[63] Kyselova Z, Mechref Y, Al Bataineh MM, *et al.* Alterations in the serum glycome due to metastatic prostate cancer. J Proteome Res 2007; 6(5): 1822-32. [http://dx.doi.org/10.1021/pr060664t] [PMID: 17432893]

[64] Peracaula R, Barrabés S, Sarrats A, Rudd PM, de Llorens R. Altered glycosylation in tumours focused to cancer diagnosis. Dis Markers 2008; 25(4-5): 207-18. [http://dx.doi.org/10.1155/2008/797629] [PMID: 19126965]

[65] Ferlay J, Colombet M, Soerjomataram I, *et al.* Estimating the global cancer incidence and mortality in 2018: GLOBOCAN sources and methods. Int J Cancer 2019; 144(8): 1941-53. [http://dx.doi.org/10.1002/ijc.31937] [PMID: 30350310]

[66] Matulonis UA, Sood AK, Fallowfield L, Howitt BE, Sehouli J, Karlan BY. Ovarian cancer. Nat Rev Dis Primers 2016; 2(1): 16061. [http://dx.doi.org/10.1038/nrdp.2016.61] [PMID: 27558151]

[67] Pitman M, Oehler MK, Pitson SM. Sphingolipids as multifaceted mediators in ovarian cancer. Cell Signal 2021; 81: 109949. [http://dx.doi.org/10.1016/j.cellsig.2021.109949] [PMID: 33571664]

[68] Bast RC Jr, Klug TL, John ES, *et al.* A radioimmunoassay using a monoclonal antibody to monitor the course of epithelial ovarian cancer. N Engl J Med 1983; 309(15): 883-7. [http://dx.doi.org/10.1056/NEJM198310133091503] [PMID: 6310399]

[69] Berruti A, Tampellini M, Torta M, Buniva T, Gorzegno G, Dogliotti L. Prognostic value in predicting overall survival of two mucinous markers: CA 15-3 and CA 125 in breast cancer patients at first relapse of disease. Eur J Cancer 1994; 30(14): 2082-4. [http://dx.doi.org/10.1016/0959-8049(94)00356-A] [PMID: 7857707]

[70] Norum LF, Erikstein B, Nustad K. Elevated CA125 in breast cancer--A sign of advanced disease. Tumour Biol 2001; 22(4): 223-8. [http://dx.doi.org/10.1159/000050620] [PMID: 11399947]

[71] Hedman M, Arnberg H, Wernlund J, Riska H, Brodin O. Tissue polypeptide antigen (TPA), hyaluronan and CA 125 as serum markers in malignant mesothelioma. Anticancer Res 2003; 23(1B): 531-6. [PMID: 12680141]

[72] Bairey O, Blickstein D, Stark P, *et al.* Serum CA 125 as a prognostic factor in non-Hodgkin's lymphoma. Leuk Lymphoma 2003; 44(10): 1733-8.

[http://dx.doi.org/10.1080/10428190310001040791] [PMID: 14692526]

[73] Burney IA, Siddiqui T, Siddiqui I. Serum CA 125 is of clinical value in the staging and follow-up of patients with non-Hodgkin's lymphoma. Cancer 1999; 85(3): 755-6. [http://dx.doi.org/10.1002/(SICI)1097-0142(19990201)85:3<755::AID-CNCR27>3.0.CO;2-O] [PMID: 10091750]

[74] Yamamoto M, Baba H, Toh Y, Okamura T, Maehara Y. Peritoneal lavage CEA/CA125 is a prognostic factor for gastric cancer patients. J Cancer Res Clin Oncol 2007; 133(7): 471-6. [http://dx.doi.org/10.1007/s00432-006-0189-2] [PMID: 17226046]

[75] Whiteley MS, Marshall J. Raised serum CA 125 level in leiomyoma and leiomyosarcoma of gastrointestinal origin. Br J Surg 2005; 80(12): 1551. [http://dx.doi.org/10.1002/bjs.1800801220] [PMID: 8298923]

[76] Meden H, Fattahi-Meibodi A. CA 125 in benign gynecological conditions. Int J Biol Markers 1998; 13(4): 231-7. [http://dx.doi.org/10.1177/172460089801300411] [PMID: 10228907]

[77] Ismail MA, Rotmensch J, Mercer LJ, Block BS, Salti GI, Holt JA. CA-125 in peritoneal fluid from patients with nonmalignant gynecologic disorders. J Reprod Med 1994; 39(7): 510-2. [PMID: 7966039]

[78] Cheng YM, Wang ST, Chou CY. Serum CA-125 in preoperative patients at high risk for endometriosis. Obstet Gynecol 2002; 99(3): 375-80. [PMID: 11864662]

[79] Baalbergen A, Van Der Weiden RMF, Janssen JW. CA-125 levels are related to the likelihood of pregnancy after *in vitro* fertilization and embryo transfer. Am J Reprod Immunol 2000; 43(1): 21-4. [http://dx.doi.org/10.1111/j.8755-8920.2000.430104.x] [PMID: 10698036]

[80] Bon GG, Kenemans P, Dekker JJ, *et al.* Fluctuations in CA 125 and CA 15 3 serum concentrations during spontaneous ovulatory cycles. Hum Reprod 1999; 14(2): 566-70. [http://dx.doi.org/10.1093/humrep/14.2.566] [PMID: 10100011]

[81] Crespo Valadés E, Malmierca Corral M. Elevated CA 125 in chronic liver disease with ascites. Gastroenterol Hepatol 2004; 27(9): 558. [PMID: 15544744]

[82] Kouris NT, Zacharos ID, Kontogianni DD, *et al.* The significance of CA125 levels in patients with chronic congestive heart failure. Correlation with clinical and echocardiographic parameters. Eur J Heart Fail 2005; 7(2): 199-203. [http://dx.doi.org/10.1016/j.ejheart.2004.07.015] [PMID: 15701467]

[83] Bilgin T, Karabay A, Dolar E, Develioğlu OH. Peritoneal tuberculosis with pelvic abdominal mass, ascites and elevated CA 125 mimicking advanced ovarian carcinoma: A series of 10 cases. Int J Gynecol Cancer 2001; 11(4): 290-4. [http://dx.doi.org/10.1136/ijgc-00009577-200107000-00006] [PMID: 11520367]

[84] De Quirós JFB, Telenti M, Leiva PS, *et al.* CA125 Serum levels in tubercolosis patients. Int J Biol Markers 1995; 10(3): 180-1. [http://dx.doi.org/10.1177/172460089501000309] [PMID: 8551062]

[85] Lloyd KO, Yin BWT, Kudryashov V. Isolation and characterization of ovarian cancer antigen CA 125 using a new monoclonal antibody (VK-8): identification as a mucin-type molecule. Int J Cancer 1997; 71(5): 842-50. [http://dx.doi.org/10.1002/(SICI)1097-0215(19970529)71:5<842::AID-IJC24>3.0.CO;2-8] [PMID: 9180155]

[86] Akita K, Yoshida S, Ikehara Y, *et al.* Different levels of sialyl-Tn antigen expressed on MUC16 in patients with endometriosis and ovarian cancer. Int J Gynecol Cancer 2012; 22(4): 531-8. [http://dx.doi.org/10.1097/IGC.0b013e3182473292] [PMID: 22367369]

[87] Schummer M, Ng WV, Bumgarner RE, *et al.* Comparative hybridization of an array of 21 500 ovarian cDNAs for the discovery of genes overexpressed in ovarian carcinomas. Gene 1999; 238(2): 375-85. [http://dx.doi.org/10.1016/S0378-1119(99)00342-X] [PMID: 10570965]

[88] Hough CD, Sherman-Baust CA, Pizer ES, *et al.* Large-scale serial analysis of gene expression reveals genes differentially expressed in ovarian cancer. Cancer Res 2000; 60(22): 6281-7. [PMID: 11103784]

[89] Drapkin R, von Horsten HH, Lin Y, *et al.* Human epididymis protein 4 (HE4) is a secreted glycoprotein that is overexpressed by serous and endometrioid ovarian carcinomas. Cancer Res 2005; 65(6): 2162-9. [http://dx.doi.org/10.1158/0008-5472.CAN-04-3924] [PMID: 15781627]

[90] Ferraro S, Braga F, Lanzoni M, Boracchi P, Biganzoli EM, Panteghini M. Serum human epididymis protein 4 *vs* carbohydrate antigen 125 for ovarian cancer diagnosis: a systematic review. J Clin Pathol 2013; 66(4): 273-81. [http://dx.doi.org/10.1136/jclinpath-2012-201031] [PMID: 23426716]

[91] Montagnana M, Danese E, Ruzzenente O, *et al.* The ROMA (Risk of Ovarian Malignancy Algorithm) for estimating the risk of epithelial ovarian cancer in women presenting with pelvic mass: is it really useful? Clin Chem Lab Med 2011; 49(3): 521-5. [http://dx.doi.org/10.1515/CCLM.2011.075] [PMID: 21288178]

[92] Karlsen MA, Sandhu N, Høgdall C, *et al.* Evaluation of HE4, CA125, risk of ovarian malignancy algorithm (ROMA) and risk of malignancy index (RMI) as diagnostic tools of epithelial ovarian cancer in patients with a pelvic mass. Gynecol Oncol 2012; 127(2): 379-83. [http://dx.doi.org/10.1016/j.ygyno.2012.07.106] [PMID: 22835718]

[93] Sandri MT, Bottari F, Franchi D, *et al.* Comparison of HE4, CA125 and ROMA algorithm in women with a pelvic mass: Correlation with pathological outcome. Gynecol Oncol 2013; 128(2): 233-8. [http://dx.doi.org/10.1016/j.ygyno.2012.11.026] [PMID: 23200911]

[94] Kirwan A, Utratna M, O'Dwyer ME, Joshi L, Kilcoyne M. Glycosylation-Based Serum Biomarkers for Cancer Diagnostics and Prognostics. BioMed Res Int 2015; 2015: 1-16. [http://dx.doi.org/10.1155/2015/490531] [PMID: 26509158]

[95] Cornejo KM, Kandil D, Khan A, Cosar EF. Theranostic and molecular classification of breast cancer. Arch Pathol Lab Med 2014; 138(1): 44-56. [http://dx.doi.org/10.5858/arpa.2012-0442-RA] [PMID: 24377811]

[96] DeSantis C, Ma J, Bryan L, Jemal A. Breast cancer statistics, 2013. CA Cancer J Clin 2014; 64(1): 52-62. [http://dx.doi.org/10.3322/caac.21203] [PMID: 24114568]

[97] Qiu N, He Y, Zhang S, Hu X, Chen M, Li H. Cullin 7 is a predictor of poor prognosis in breast cancer patients and is involved in the proliferation and invasion of breast cancer cells by regulating the cell cycle and microtubule stability. Oncol Rep 2018; 39(2): 603-10. [PMID: 29207184]

[98] Breast cancer facts & figures 2017–2018. Am. Cancer Soc 2017.

[99] DeSantis CE, Ma J, Goding Sauer A, Newman LA, Jemal A. Breast cancer statistics, 2017, racial disparity in mortality by state. CA Cancer J Clin 2017; 67(6): 439-48. [http://dx.doi.org/10.3322/caac.21412] [PMID: 28972651]

[100] Untch M, Konecny GE, Paepke S, von Minckwitz G. Current and future role of neoadjuvant therapy for breast cancer. Breast 2014; 23(5): 526-37. [http://dx.doi.org/10.1016/j.breast.2014.06.004] [PMID: 25034931]

[101] Park J, Park J, Castanares MA, Collins DS, Yeo Y. Magnetophoretic Delivery of a Tumor-Priming Agent for Chemotherapy of Metastatic Murine Breast Cancer. Mol Pharm 2019; 16(5): 1864-73. [http://dx.doi.org/10.1021/acs.molpharmaceut.8b01148] [PMID: 30916974]

[102] Zhang X, Rice M, Tworoger SS, *et al.* Addition of a polygenic risk score, mammographic density, and endogenous hormones to existing breast cancer risk prediction models: A nested case–control study. PLoS Med 2018; 15(9): e1002644. [http://dx.doi.org/10.1371/journal.pmed.1002644] [PMID: 30180161]

[103] Kyselova Z, Mechref Y, Kang P, *et al.* Breast cancer diagnosis and prognosis through quantitative measurements of serum glycan profiles. Clin Chem 2008; 54(7): 1166-75. [http://dx.doi.org/10.1373/clinchem.2007.087148] [PMID: 18487288]

[104] Potapenko IO, Haakensen VD, Lüders T, *et al.* Glycan gene expression signatures in normal and malignant breast tissue; possible role in diagnosis and progression. Mol Oncol 2010; 4(2): 98-118. [http://dx.doi.org/10.1016/j.molonc.2009.12.001] [PMID: 20060370]

[105] Nath S, Mukherjee P. MUC1: a multifaceted oncoprotein with a key role in cancer progression. Trends Mol Med 2014; 20(6): 332-42. [http://dx.doi.org/10.1016/j.molmed.2014.02.007] [PMID: 24667139]

[106] Zhou D, Xu L, Huang W, Tonn T. Epitopes of MUC1 tandem repeats in cancer as revealed by antibody crystallography: Toward glycopeptide signature-guided therapy. Molecules 2018; 23(6): 1326. [http://dx.doi.org/10.3390/molecules23061326] [PMID: 29857542]

[107] Patriarca C, Colombo P, Pio Taronna A, *et al.* Cell discohesion and multifocality of carcinoma *in situ* of the bladder: new insight from the adhesion molecule profile (e-cadherin, Ep-CAM, and MUC1). Int J Surg Pathol 2009; 17(2): 99-106. [http://dx.doi.org/10.1177/1066896908326918] [PMID: 19019843]

[108] Wesseling J, van der Valk SW, Vos HL, Sonnenberg A, Hilkens J. Episialin (MUC1) overexpression inhibits integrin-mediated cell adhesion to extracellular matrix components. J Cell Biol 1995; 129(1): 255-65. [http://dx.doi.org/10.1083/jcb.129.1.255] [PMID: 7698991]

[109] Suwa T, Hinoda Y, Makiguchi Y, *et al.* Increased invasiveness ofMUCI1 cDNA-transfected human gastric cancer MKN74 cells. Int J Cancer 1998; 76(3): 377-82. [http://dx.doi.org/10.1002/(SICI)1097-0215(19980504)76:3<377::AID-IJC15>3.0.CO;2-8] [PMID: 9579575]

[110] Bernier AJ, Zhang J, Lillehoj E, Shaw ARE, Gunasekara N, Hugh JC. Non-cysteine linked MUC1 cytoplasmic dimers are required for Src recruitment and ICAM-1 binding induced cell invasion. Mol Cancer 2011; 10(1): 93. [http://dx.doi.org/10.1186/1476-4598-10-93] [PMID: 21798038]

[111] Mansouri N, Movafagh A, Soleimani S, *et al.* Overexpression of the MUC1 gene in iranian women with breast cancer micrometastasis. Asian Pac J Cancer Prev 2016; 17(sup3): 275-8. [http://dx.doi.org/10.7314/APJCP.2016.17.S3.275] [PMID: 27165238]

[112] Pillai K, Pourgholami MH, Chua TC, Morris DL. MUC1 as a potential target in anticancer therapies. Am J Clin Oncol 2015; 38(1): 108-18. [http://dx.doi.org/10.1097/COC.0b013e31828f5a07] [PMID: 23608828]

[113] Apostolopoulos V, Stojanovska L, Gargosky SE. MUC1 (CD227): a multi-tasked molecule. Cell Mol Life Sci 2015; 72(23): 4475-500. [http://dx.doi.org/10.1007/s00018-015-2014-z] [PMID: 26294353]

[114] Rakha EA, Boyce RWG, Abd El-Rehim D, *et al.* Expression of mucins (MUC1, MUC2, MUC3, MUC4, MUC5AC and MUC6) and their prognostic significance in human breast cancer. Mod Pathol 2005; 18(10): 1295-304. [http://dx.doi.org/10.1038/modpathol.3800445] [PMID: 15976813]

[115] Baldus SE, Engelmann K, Hanisch FG. MUC1 and the MUCs: a family of human mucins with impact in cancer biology. Crit Rev Clin Lab Sci 2004; 41(2): 189-231.

[http://dx.doi.org/10.1080/10408360490452040] [PMID: 15270554]

[116] Park JH, Nishidate T, Kijima K, *et al.* Critical roles of mucin 1 glycosylation by transactivated polypeptide N-acetylgalactosaminyltransferase 6 in mammary carcinogenesis. Cancer Res 2010; 70(7): 2759-69.
[http://dx.doi.org/10.1158/0008-5472.CAN-09-3911] [PMID: 20215525]

[117] Storr SJ, Royle L, Chapman CJ, *et al.* The O-linked glycosylation of secretory/shed MUC1 from an advanced breast cancer patient's serum. Glycobiology 2008; 18(6): 456-62.
[http://dx.doi.org/10.1093/glycob/cwn022] [PMID: 18332077]

[118] Westerlind U, Hobel A, Gaidzik N, Schmitt E, Kunz H. Synthetic vaccines consisting of tumor-associated MUC1 glycopeptide antigens and a T-cell epitope for the induction of a highly specific humoral immune response. Angew Chem Int Ed 2008; 47(39): 7551-6.
[http://dx.doi.org/10.1002/anie.200802102] [PMID: 18704911]

[119] Gaidzik N, Westerlind U, Kunz H. The development of synthetic antitumour vaccines from mucin glycopeptide antigens. Chem Soc Rev 2013; 42(10): 4421-42.
[http://dx.doi.org/10.1039/c3cs35470a] [PMID: 23440054]

[120] Kaiser A, Gaidzik N, Westerlind U, *et al.* A synthetic vaccine consisting of a tumor-associated sialyl-T(N)-MUC1 tandem-repeat glycopeptide and tetanus toxoid: induction of a strong and highly selective immune response. Angew Chem Int Ed 2009; 48(41): 7551-5.
[http://dx.doi.org/10.1002/anie.200902564] [PMID: 19685547]

[121] Ludovini V, Gori S, Colozza M, *et al.* Evaluation of serum HER2 extracellular domain in early breast cancer patients: correlation with clinicopathological parameters and survival. Ann Oncol 2008; 19(5): 883-90.
[http://dx.doi.org/10.1093/annonc/mdm585] [PMID: 18187484]

[122] Gusterson BA. Identification and interpretation of epidermal growth factor and c-erbB-2 overexpression. Eur J Cancer 1992; 28(1): 263-7.
[http://dx.doi.org/10.1016/0959-8049(92)90429-6] [PMID: 1348953]

[123] Wolff AC, Hammond MEH, Schwartz JN, *et al.* American Society of Clinical Oncology/College of American Pathologists guideline recommendations for human epidermal growth factor receptor 2 testing in breast cancer. Arch Pathol Lab Med 2007; 131(1): 18-43.
[http://dx.doi.org/10.5858/2007-131-18-ASOCCO] [PMID: 19548375]

[124] Di Gioia D, Dresse M, Mayr D, Nagel D, Heinemann V, Stieber P. Serum HER2 in combination with CA 15-3 as a parameter for prognosis in patients with early breast cancer. Clin Chim Acta 2015; 440: 16-22.
[http://dx.doi.org/10.1016/j.cca.2014.11.001] [PMID: 25444743]

[125] Oyama K, Fushida S, Tsukada T, *et al.* Evaluation of serum HER2-ECD levels in patients with gastric cancer. J Gastroenterol 2015; 50(1): 41-5.
[http://dx.doi.org/10.1007/s00535-014-0941-3] [PMID: 24557054]

[126] Ni XG, Bai XF, Mao YL, *et al.* The clinical value of serum CEA, CA19-9, and CA242 in the diagnosis and prognosis of pancreatic cancer. Eur J Surg Oncol 2005; 31(2): 164-9.
[http://dx.doi.org/10.1016/j.ejso.2004.09.007] [PMID: 15698733]

[127] Lang BA, Kocent A, Nekulová M, Hlávková J. Three-year follow-up of carcinoembryonal antigen levels in the serum of patients with breast cancer. Neoplasma 1984; 31(1): 79-87.
[PMID: 6700798]

[128] Gaglia P, Caldarola B, Bussone R, *et al.* Prognostic value of CEA and ferritin assay in breast cancer: A multivariate analysis. Eur J Cancer Clin Oncol 1988; 24(7): 1151-5.
[http://dx.doi.org/10.1016/0277-5379(88)90121-6] [PMID: 3416899]

[129] Molina R, Jo J, Filella X, *et al.* c-erbB-2 oncoprotein, CEA, and CA 15.3 in patients with breast cancer: prognostic value. Breast Cancer Res Treat 1998; 51(2): 109-19.

[http://dx.doi.org/10.1023/A:1005734429304] [PMID: 9879773]

[130] Safi F, Kohler I, Röttinger E, Suhr P, Beger HG. Comparison of CA 15-3 and CEA in diagnosis and monitoring of breast cancer. Int J Biol Markers 1989; 4(4): 207-14. [http://dx.doi.org/10.1177/172460088900400405] [PMID: 2628501]

[131] Dnistrian AM, Schwartz MK, Greenberg EJ, Smith CA, Schwartz DC. Evaluation of CA M26, CA M29, CA 15-3 and CEA as circulating tumor markers in breast cancer patients. Tumour Biol 1991; 12(2): 82-90. [http://dx.doi.org/10.1159/000217692] [PMID: 2028182]

[132] Pavesi F, Lotzniker M, Scarabelli M, *et al.* Circulating CA 549 and other associated antigens in breast cancer patients. Oncology 1994; 51(1): 18-21. [http://dx.doi.org/10.1159/000227303] [PMID: 8265097]

[133] Tormey DC, Waalkes TP, Snyder JJ, Simon RM. Biological markers in breast carcinoma:III. Clinical correlations with carcinoembryonic antigen. Cancer 1977; 39(6): 2397-404. [http://dx.doi.org/10.1002/1097-0142(197706)39:6<2397::AID-CNCR2820390614>3.0.CO;2-N] [PMID: 872038]

[134] Falkson HC, van der Watt JJ, Portugal MA, Pitout MJ, Falkson G. Carcinoembryonic antigen in patients with breast cancer.An adjunctive tool to monitor response and therapy. Cancer 1978; 42(3): 1308-13. [http://dx.doi.org/10.1002/1097-0142(197809)42:3<1308::AID-CNCR2820420341>3.0.CO;2-N] [PMID: 698917]

[135] Haagensen DE Jr, Kister SJ, Vandevoorde JP, *et al.* Evaluation of carcinoembryonic antigen as a plasma monitor for human breast carcinoma. Cancer 1978; 42(S3) (Suppl.): 1512-9. [http://dx.doi.org/10.1002/1097-0142(197809)42:3+<1512::AID-CNCR2820420824>3.0.CO;2-6] [PMID: 709523]

[136] Lokich JJ, Zamcheck N, Lowenstein MW. Sequential carcinoembryonic antigen levels in the therapy of metastatic breast cancer: a predictor and monitor of response and relapse. Ann Intern Med 1978; 89(6): 902-6. [http://dx.doi.org/10.7326/0003-4819-89-6-902] [PMID: 717986]

[137] al-Jarallah MA, Behbehani AE, el-Nass SA, *et al.* Serum CA-15.3 and CEA patterns in postsurgical follow-up, and in monitoring clinical course of metastatic cancer in patients with breast carcinoma. Eur J Surg Oncol 1993; 19(1): 74-9. [PMID: 8436243]

[138] Molina R, Zanón G, Filella X, *et al.* Use of serial carcinoembryonic antigen and CA 15.3 assays in detecting relapses in breast cancer patients. Breast Cancer Res Treat 1995; 36(1): 41-8. [http://dx.doi.org/10.1007/BF00690183] [PMID: 7579505]

[139] Jäger W, Krämer S, Palapelas V, Norbert L. Breast cancer and clinical utility of CA 15—3 and CEA. Scand J Clin Lab Invest 1995; 55(sup221): 87-92. [http://dx.doi.org/10.3109/00365519509090570] [PMID: 7652494]

[140] Dnistrian AM, Schwartz MK, Greenberg EJ, Smith CA, Schwartz DC. CA 15-3 and carcinoembryonic antigen in the clinical evaluation of breast cancer. Clin Chim Acta 1991; 200(2-3): 81-93. [http://dx.doi.org/10.1016/0009-8981(91)90080-V] [PMID: 1777973]

[141] Jezeršek B, Červek J, Rudolf Z, Novaković S. Clinical evaluation of potential usefulness of CEA, CA 15-3, and MCA in follow-up of breast cancer patients. Cancer Lett 1996; 110(1-2): 137-44. [http://dx.doi.org/10.1016/S0304-3835(96)04473-4] [PMID: 9018092]

[142] Robertson JFR, Jaeger W, Syzmendera JJ, *et al.* The objective measurement of remission and progression in metastatic breast cancer by use of serum tumour markers. Eur J Cancer 1999; 35(1): 47-53. [http://dx.doi.org/10.1016/S0959-8049(98)00297-4] [PMID: 10211087]

[143] Siegel RL, Miller KD, Fuchs HE, Jemal A. Cancer Statistics, 2021. CA Cancer J Clin 2021; 71(1): 7-33.
[http://dx.doi.org/10.3322/caac.21654] [PMID: 33433946]

[144] Miller KD, Nogueira L, Mariotto AB, *et al.* Cancer treatment and survivorship statistics, 2019. CA Cancer J Clin 2019; 69(5): 363-85.
[http://dx.doi.org/10.3322/caac.21565] [PMID: 31184787]

[145] O'Keefe SJD. Diet, microorganisms and their metabolites, and colon cancer. Nat Rev Gastroenterol Hepatol 2016; 13(12): 691-706.
[http://dx.doi.org/10.1038/nrgastro.2016.165] [PMID: 27848961]

[146] van der Pool AEM, Damhuis RA, IJzermans JNM, *et al.* Trends in incidence, treatment and survival of patients with stage IV colorectal cancer: a population-based series. Colorectal Dis 2012; 14(1): 56-61.
[http://dx.doi.org/10.1111/j.1463-1318.2010.02539.x] [PMID: 21176063]

[147] Gadler H, Bremme K, Wahren B, Hammarström S. Cea and nca in amniotic fluid of normal and abnormal pregnancies. Cancer 1978; 42(S3) (Suppl.): 1579-84.
[http://dx.doi.org/10.1002/1097-0142(197809)42:3+<1579::AID-CNCR2820420834>3.0.CO;2-F] [PMID: 81709]

[148] Locker GY, Hamilton S, Harris J, *et al.* ASCO 2006 update of recommendations for the use of tumor markers in gastrointestinal cancer. J Clin Oncol 2006; 24(33): 5313-27.
[http://dx.doi.org/10.1200/JCO.2006.08.2644] [PMID: 17060676]

[149] Duffy MJ, van Dalen A, Haglund C, *et al.* Tumour markers in colorectal cancer: European Group on Tumour Markers (EGTM) guidelines for clinical use. Eur J Cancer 2007; 43(9): 1348-60.
[http://dx.doi.org/10.1016/j.ejca.2007.03.021] [PMID: 17512720]

[150] Paxton RJ, Mooser G, Pande H, Lee TD, Shively JE. Sequence analysis of carcinoembryonic antigen: identification of glycosylation sites and homology with the immunoglobulin supergene family. Proc Natl Acad Sci USA 1987; 84(4): 920-4.
[http://dx.doi.org/10.1073/pnas.84.4.920] [PMID: 3469650]

[151] Garcia M, Seigner C, Bastid C, Choux R, Payan MJ, Reggio H. Carcinoembryonic antigen has a different molecular weight in normal colon and in cancer cells due to N-glycosylation differences. Cancer Res 1991; 51(20): 5679-86.
[PMID: 1717152]

[152] Thomas SN, Zhu F, Schnaar RL, Alves CS, Konstantopoulos K. Carcinoembryonic antigen and CD44 variant isoforms cooperate to mediate colon carcinoma cell adhesion to E- and L-selectin in shear flow. J Biol Chem 2008; 283(23): 15647-55.
[http://dx.doi.org/10.1074/jbc.M800543200] [PMID: 18375392]

[153] Koprowski H, Herlyn M, Steplewski Z, Sears HF. Specific antigen in serum of patients with colon carcinoma. Science 1981; 212(4490): 53-5.
[http://dx.doi.org/10.1126/science.6163212] [PMID: 6163212]

[154] Zhang LN, OuYang PY, Xiao WW, *et al.* Elevated CA19-9 as the Most Significant Prognostic Factor in Locally Advanced Rectal Cancer Following Neoadjuvant Chemoradiotherapy. Medicine (Baltimore) 2015; 94(45): e1793.
[http://dx.doi.org/10.1097/MD.0000000000001793] [PMID: 26559251]

[155] Roeland E, Loprinzi C, Moynihan TJ, Smith TJ, Temel J. In chemotherapy for lung cancer, sometimes less is more. J Natl Compr Canc Netw 2013; 11(3): 232-5.
[http://dx.doi.org/10.6004/jnccn.2013.0034] [PMID: 23486449]

[156] Hecht SS. Tobacco smoke carcinogens and lung cancer. J Natl Cancer Inst 1999; 91(14): 1194-210.
[http://dx.doi.org/10.1093/jnci/91.14.1194] [PMID: 10413421]

[157] Ancuceanu RV, Istudor V. Pharmacologically active natural compounds for lung cancer. Altern Med Rev 2004; 9(4): 402-19.

[PMID: 15656712]

[158] Ramalingam S, Belani C. Systemic chemotherapy for advanced non-small cell lung cancer: recent advances and future directions. Oncologist 2008; 13(S1) (Suppl. 1): 5-13. [http://dx.doi.org/10.1634/theoncologist.13-S1-5] [PMID: 18263769]

[159] U.S. National Institute of Health, National Cancer Institute.

[160] Lemjabbar-Alaoui H, McKinney A, Yang YW, Tran VM, Phillips JJ. Glycosylation alterations in lung and brain cancer. Adv Cancer Res 2015; 126: 305-44. [http://dx.doi.org/10.1016/bs.acr.2014.11.007] [PMID: 25727152]

[161] Lakshmanan I, Ponnusamy MP, Macha MA, *et al.* Mucins in lung cancer: diagnostic, prognostic, and therapeutic implications. J Thorac Oncol 2015; 10(1): 19-27. [http://dx.doi.org/10.1097/JTO.0000000000000404] [PMID: 25319180]

[162] Awaya H, Takeshima Y, Yamasaki M, Inai K. Expression of MUC1, MUC2, MUC5AC, and MUC6 in atypical adenomatous hyperplasia, bronchioloalveolar carcinoma, adenocarcinoma with mixed subtypes, and mucinous bronchioloalveolar carcinoma of the lung. Am J Clin Pathol 2004; 121(5): 644-53. [http://dx.doi.org/10.1309/U4WGE9EBFJN6CM8R] [PMID: 15151204]

[163] Nguyen PL, Niehans GA, Cherwitz DL, Kim YS, Ho SB. Membrane-bound (MUC1) and secretory (MUC2, MUC3, and MUC4) mucin gene expression in human lung cancer. Tumour Biol 1996; 17(3): 176-92. [http://dx.doi.org/10.1159/000217980] [PMID: 8638091]

[164] Kaira K, Okumura T, Nakagawa K, *et al.* MUC1 expression in pulmonary metastatic tumors: a comparison of primary lung cancer. Pathol Oncol Res 2012; 18(2): 439-47. [http://dx.doi.org/10.1007/s12253-011-9465-9] [PMID: 21964914]

[165] Kwon KY, Ro JY, Singhal N, *et al.* MUC4 expression in non-small cell lung carcinomas: relationship to tumor histology and patient survival. Arch Pathol Lab Med 2007; 131(4): 593-8. [http://dx.doi.org/10.5858/2007-131-593-MEINCL] [PMID: 17425390]

[166] Hollingsworth MA, Swanson BJ. Mucins in cancer: protection and control of the cell surface. Nat Rev Cancer 2004; 4(1): 45-60. [http://dx.doi.org/10.1038/nrc1251] [PMID: 14681689]

[167] Gao J, McConnell MJ, Yu B, *et al.* MUC1 is a downstream target of STAT3 and regulates lung cancer cell survival and invasion. Int J Oncol 2009; 35(2): 337-45. [PMID: 19578748]

[168] Kim KC, Lillehoj EP. MUC1 Mucin. Am J Respir Cell Mol Biol 2008; 39(6): 644-7. [http://dx.doi.org/10.1165/rcmb.2008-0169TR] [PMID: 18617677]

[169] Lakshmanan I, Ponnusamy MP, Das S, *et al.* MUC16 induced rapid G2/M transition *via* interactions with JAK2 for increased proliferation and anti-apoptosis in breast cancer cells. Oncogene 2012; 31(7): 805-17. [http://dx.doi.org/10.1038/onc.2011.297] [PMID: 21785467]

[170] Situ D, Wang J, Ma Y, *et al.* Expression and prognostic relevance of MUC1 in stage IB non-small cell lung cancer. Med Oncol 2011; 28(S1) (Suppl. 1): 596-604. [http://dx.doi.org/10.1007/s12032-010-9752-4] [PMID: 21116877]

[171] Hanaoka J, Kontani K, Sawai S, *et al.* Analysis of MUC4 mucin expression in lung carcinoma cells and its immunogenicity. Cancer 2001; 92(8): 2148-57. [http://dx.doi.org/10.1002/1097-0142(20011015)92:8<2148::AID-CNCR1557>3.0.CO;2-6] [PMID: 11596032]

[172] Llinares K, Escande F, Aubert S, *et al.* Diagnostic value of MUC4 immunostaining in distinguishing epithelial mesothelioma and lung adenocarcinoma. Mod Pathol 2004; 17(2): 150-7. [http://dx.doi.org/10.1038/modpathol.3800027] [PMID: 14657954]

[173] Kargı A, Dinç ZA, Başok O, Üçvet A. MUC4 expression and its relation to ErbB2 expression, apoptosis, proliferation, differentiation, and tumor stage in non-small cell lung cancer (NSCLC). Pathol Res Pract 2006; 202(8): 577-83.
[http://dx.doi.org/10.1016/j.prp.2006.04.002] [PMID: 16814944]

[174] Hishida T, Ishii G, Kodama T, *et al.* Centrally located adenocarcinoma with endobronchial polypoid growth: Clinicopathological analysis of five cases. Pathol Int 2011; 61(2): 73-9.
[http://dx.doi.org/10.1111/j.1440-1827.2010.02619.x] [PMID: 21255183]

[175] Copin MC, Devisme L, Buisine MP, *et al.* From normal respiratory mucosa to epidermoid carcinoma: Expression of human mucin genes. Int J Cancer 2000; 86(2): 162-8.
[http://dx.doi.org/10.1002/(SICI)1097-0215(20000415)86:2<162::AID-IJC3>3.0.CO;2-R] [PMID: 10738241]

[176] Yu CJ, Shih JY, Lee YC, Shun CT, Yuan A, Yang PC. Sialyl Lewis antigens: association with MUC5AC protein and correlation with post-operative recurrence of non-small cell lung cancer. Lung Cancer 2005; 47(1): 59-67.
[http://dx.doi.org/10.1016/j.lungcan.2004.05.018] [PMID: 15603855]

[177] Inamura K, Ninomiya H, Ishikawa Y, Matsubara O. Is the epidermal growth factor receptor status in lung cancers reflected in clinicopathologic features? Arch Pathol Lab Med 2010; 134(1): 66-72.
[http://dx.doi.org/10.5858/2008-0586-RAR1.1] [PMID: 20073607]

[178] Ohsaki Y, Tanno S, Fujita Y, *et al.* Epidermal growth factor receptor expression correlates with poor prognosis in non-small cell lung cancer patients with p53 overexpression. Oncol Rep 2000; 7(3): 603-7.
[http://dx.doi.org/10.3892/or.7.3.603] [PMID: 10767376]

[179] Kerr KM, Bubendorf L, Edelman MJ, *et al.* Second ESMO consensus conference on lung cancer: pathology and molecular biomarkers for non-small-cell lung cancer. Ann Oncol 2014; 25(9): 1681-90.
[http://dx.doi.org/10.1093/annonc/mdu145] [PMID: 24718890]

[180] Sharma SV, Bell DW, Settleman J, Haber DA. Epidermal growth factor receptor mutations in lung cancer. Nat Rev Cancer 2007; 7(3): 169-81.
[http://dx.doi.org/10.1038/nrc2088] [PMID: 17318210]

[181] Sholl LM. Biomarkers in lung adenocarcinoma: a decade of progress. Arch Pathol Lab Med 2015; 139(4): 469-80.
[http://dx.doi.org/10.5858/arpa.2014-0128-RA] [PMID: 25255293]

[182] Mok TSK. Personalized medicine in lung cancer: what we need to know. Nat Rev Clin Oncol 2011; 8(11): 661-8.
[http://dx.doi.org/10.1038/nrclinonc.2011.126] [PMID: 21862980]

[183] Fujimoto J, Wistuba II. Current concepts on the molecular pathology of non-small cell lung carcinoma. Semin Diagn Pathol 2014; 31(4): 306-13.
[http://dx.doi.org/10.1053/j.semdp.2014.06.008] [PMID: 25239274]

[184] Gold P, Freedman SO. Specific carcinoembryonic antigens of the human digestive system. J Exp Med 1965; 122(3): 467-81.
[http://dx.doi.org/10.1084/jem.122.3.467] [PMID: 4953873]

[185] Chevinsky AH. CEA in tumors of other than colorectal origin. Semin Surg Oncol 1991; 7(3): 162-6.
[http://dx.doi.org/10.1002/ssu.2980070309] [PMID: 2068450]

[186] Ishiguro F, Fukui T, Mori S, *et al.* Serum carcinoembryonic antigen level as a surrogate marker for the evaluation of tumor response to chemotherapy in nonsmall cell lung cancer. Ann Thorac Cardiovasc Surg 2010; 16(4): 242-7.
[PMID: 21057440]

[187] Arrieta O, Villarreal-Garza C, Martínez-Barrera L, *et al.* Usefulness of Serum Carcinoembryonic Antigen (CEA) in evaluating response to chemotherapy in patients with advanced non small-cell lung

cancer: a prospective cohort study. BMC Cancer 2013; 13(1): 254. [http://dx.doi.org/10.1186/1471-2407-13-254] [PMID: 23697613]

[188] Okada M, Nishio W, Sakamoto T, *et al.* Prognostic significance of perioperative serum carcinoembryonic antigen in non-small cell lung cancer: analysis of 1,000 consecutive resections for clinical stage I disease. Ann Thorac Surg 2004; 78(1): 216-21. [http://dx.doi.org/10.1016/j.athoracsur.2004.02.009] [PMID: 15223432]

[189] Kozu Y, Maniwa T, Takahashi S, Isaka M, Ohde Y, Nakajima T. Prognostic significance of postoperative serum carcinoembryonic antigen levels in patients with completely resected pathological-stage I non-small cell lung cancer. J Cardiothorac Surg 2013; 8(1): 106. [http://dx.doi.org/10.1186/1749-8090-8-106] [PMID: 23607757]

[190] Kobayashi S, Boggon TJ, Dayaram T, *et al.* EGFR mutation and resistance of non-small-cell lung cancer to gefitinib. N Engl J Med 2005; 352(8): 786-92. [http://dx.doi.org/10.1056/NEJMoa044238] [PMID: 15728811]

[191] Sequist LV, Waltman BA, Dias-Santagata D, *et al.* Genotypic and histological evolution of lung cancers acquiring resistance to EGFR inhibitors. Sci Transl Med 2011; 3(75): 75ra26. [http://dx.doi.org/10.1126/scitranslmed.3002003] [PMID: 21430269]

[192] Gao Y, Song P, Li H, Jia H, Zhang B. Elevated serum CEA levels are associated with the explosive progression of lung adenocarcinoma harboring EGFR mutations. BMC Cancer 2017; 17(1): 484. [http://dx.doi.org/10.1186/s12885-017-3474-3] [PMID: 28705152]

[193] Taniguchi Y, Horiuchi H, Morikawa T, Usui K. Small-Cell Carcinoma Transformation of Pulmonary Adenocarcinoma after Osimertinib Treatment: A Case Report. Case Rep Oncol 2018; 11(2): 323-9. [http://dx.doi.org/10.1159/000489603] [PMID: 29928211]

[194] Facchinetti F, Aldigeri R, Aloe R, Bortesi B, Ardizzoni A, Tiseo M. CEA serum level as early predictive marker of outcome during EGFR-TKI therapy in advanced NSCLC patients. Tumour Biol 2015; 36(8): 5943-51. [http://dx.doi.org/10.1007/s13277-015-3269-6] [PMID: 25731731]

[195] Fang L, He J, Xia J, *et al.* Resistance to epithelial growth factor receptor tyrosine kinase inhibitors in a patient with transformation from lung adenocarcinoma to small cell lung cancer: A case report. Oncol Lett 2017; 14(1): 593-8. [http://dx.doi.org/10.3892/ol.2017.6229] [PMID: 28693210]

[196] Hashimoto N, Imaizumi K, Honda T, *et al.* Successful re-treatment with gefitinib for carcinomatous meningitis as disease recurrence of non-small-cell lung cancer. Lung Cancer 2006; 53(3): 387-90. [http://dx.doi.org/10.1016/j.lungcan.2006.05.016] [PMID: 16824645]

[197] Siegel RL, Miller KD, Jemal A. Cancer statistics, 2018. CA Cancer J Clin 2018; 68(1): 7-30. [http://dx.doi.org/10.3322/caac.21442] [PMID: 29313949]

[198] Garrido-Laguna I, Hidalgo M. Pancreatic cancer: from state-of-the-art treatments to promising novel therapies. Nat Rev Clin Oncol 2015; 12(6): 319-34. [http://dx.doi.org/10.1038/nrclinonc.2015.53] [PMID: 25824606]

[199] Maitra A, Hruban RH. Pancreatic Cancer. Annu Rev Pathol 2008; 3(1): 157-88. [http://dx.doi.org/10.1146/annurev.pathmechdis.3.121806.154305] [PMID: 18039136]

[200] Klöppel G, Adsay NV. Chronic pancreatitis and the differential diagnosis *versus* pancreatic cancer. Arch Pathol Lab Med 2009; 133(3): 382-7. [http://dx.doi.org/10.5858/133.3.382] [PMID: 19260744]

[201] Moniaux N, Andrianifahanana M, Brand RE, Batra SK. Multiple roles of mucins in pancreatic cancer, a lethal and challenging malignancy. Br J Cancer 2004; 91(9): 1633-8. [http://dx.doi.org/10.1038/sj.bjc.6602163] [PMID: 15494719]

[202] Magnani JL, Nilsson B, Brockhaus M, *et al.* A monoclonal antibody-defined antigen associated with gastrointestinal cancer is a ganglioside containing sialylated lacto-N-fucopentaose II. J Biol Chem

1982; 257(23): 14365-9.
[http://dx.doi.org/10.1016/S0021-9258(19)45389-1] [PMID: 7142214]

[203] Herlyn M, Sears HF, Steplewski Z, Koprowski H. Monoclonal antibody detection of a circulating tumor-associated antigen. I. Presence of antigen in sera of patients with colorectal, gastric, and pancreatic carcinoma. J Clin Immunol 1982; 2(2): 135-40.
[http://dx.doi.org/10.1007/BF00916897] [PMID: 7068815]

[204] Yue T, Partyka K, Maupin KA, *et al.* Identification of blood-protein carriers of the CA 19-9 antigen and characterization of prevalence in pancreatic diseases. Proteomics 2011; 11(18): 3665-74.
[http://dx.doi.org/10.1002/pmic.201000827] [PMID: 21751362]

[205] Lahdenne P, Pitkänen S, Rajantie J, *et al.* Tumor markers CA 125 and CA 19-9 in cord blood and during infancy: developmental changes and use in pediatric germ cell tumors. Pediatr Res 1995; 38(5): 797-801.
[http://dx.doi.org/10.1203/00006450-199511000-00026] [PMID: 8552451]

[206] Goonetilleke KS, Siriwardena AK. Systematic review of carbohydrate antigen (CA 19-9) as a biochemical marker in the diagnosis of pancreatic cancer. Eur J Surg Oncol 2007; 33(3): 266-70.
[http://dx.doi.org/10.1016/j.ejso.2006.10.004] [PMID: 17097848]

[207] Kalthoff H, Kreiker C, Schmiegel WH, Greten H, Thiele HG. Characterization of CA 19-9 bearing mucins as physiological exocrine pancreatic secretion products. Cancer Res 1986; 46(7): 3605-7.
[PMID: 3708591]

[208] Shah UA, Saif MW. Tumor markers in pancreatic cancer: 2013. JOP 2013; 14(4): 318-21.
[PMID: 23846917]

[209] Barton JG, Bois JP, Sarr MG, *et al.* Predictive and prognostic value of CA 19-9 in resected pancreatic adenocarcinoma. J Gastrointest Surg 2009; 13(11): 2050-8.
[http://dx.doi.org/10.1007/s11605-009-0849-z] [PMID: 19756875]

[210] Galli C, Basso D, Plebani M. CA 19-9: handle with care. Clin Chem Lab Med 2013; 51(7): 1369-83.
[http://dx.doi.org/10.1515/cclm-2012-0744] [PMID: 23370912]

[211] Yue T, Maupin KA, Fallon B, *et al.* Enhanced discrimination of malignant from benign pancreatic disease by measuring the CA 19-9 antigen on specific protein carriers. PLoS One 2011; 6(12): e29180.
[http://dx.doi.org/10.1371/journal.pone.0029180] [PMID: 22220206]

[212] Tempero MA, Uchida E, Takasaki H, Burnett DA, Steplewski Z, Pour PM. Relationship of carbohydrate antigen 19-9 and Lewis antigens in pancreatic cancer. Cancer Res 1987; 47(20): 5501-3.
[PMID: 3308077]

[213] Kamholz SL. Immunologic diagnosis of human digestive tract cancer. Carcinoembryonic antigens. Am J Gastroenterol 1973; 59(3): 233-43.
[PMID: 4121819]

[214] Molina R, Barak V, van Dalen A, *et al.* Tumor markers in breast cancer- European Group on Tumor Markers recommendations. Tumour Biol 2005; 26(6): 281-93.
[http://dx.doi.org/10.1159/000089260] [PMID: 16254457]

[215] Grunnet M, Sorensen JB. Carcinoembryonic antigen (CEA) as tumor marker in lung cancer. Lung Cancer 2012; 76(2): 138-43.
[http://dx.doi.org/10.1016/j.lungcan.2011.11.012] [PMID: 22153832]

[216] Juweid M, Sharkey RM, Behr T, *et al.* Improved detection of medullary thyroid cancer with radiolabeled antibodies to carcinoembryonic antigen. J Clin Oncol 1996; 14(4): 1209-17.
[http://dx.doi.org/10.1200/JCO.1996.14.4.1209] [PMID: 8648376]

[217] Meng Q, Shi S, Liang C, *et al.* Diagnostic and prognostic value of carcinoembryonic antigen in pancreatic cancer: a systematic review and meta-analysis. OncoTargets Ther 2017; 10: 4591-8.
[http://dx.doi.org/10.2147/OTT.S145708] [PMID: 28979147]

[218] Nazli O, Bozdag AD, Tansug T, Kir R, Kaymak E. The diagnostic importance of CEA and CA 19-9 for the early diagnosis of pancreatic carcinoma. Hepatogastroenterology 2000; 47(36): 1750-2. [PMID: 11149048]

[219] Hata S, Sakamoto Y, Yamamoto Y, *et al.* Prognostic impact of postoperative serum CA 19-9 levels in patients with resectable pancreatic cancer. Ann Surg Oncol 2012; 19(2): 636-41. [http://dx.doi.org/10.1245/s10434-011-2020-9] [PMID: 21863360]

[220] Hamanaka Y, Hamanaka S, Suzuki M. Sialyl Lewis(a) ganglioside in pancreatic cancer tissue correlates with the serum CA 19-9 level. Pancreas 1996; 13(2): 160-5. [http://dx.doi.org/10.1097/00006676-199608000-00007] [PMID: 8829184]

[221] Takasaki H, Uchida E, Tempero MA, Burnett DA, Metzgar RS, Pour PM. Correlative study on expression of CA 19-9 and DU-PAN-2 in tumor tissue and in serum of pancreatic cancer patients. Cancer Res 1988; 48(6): 1435-8. [PMID: 3162196]

[222] Imaoka H, Mizuno N, Hara K, *et al.* Prognostic impact of carcinoembryonic antigen (CEA) on patients with metastatic pancreatic cancer: A retrospective cohort study. Pancreatology 2016; 16(5): 859-64. [http://dx.doi.org/10.1016/j.pan.2016.05.007] [PMID: 27256641]

[223] Zhang S, Jiang K, Zhang Q, Guo K, Liu Y. Serum fucosylated paraoxonase 1 as a potential glycobiomarker for clinical diagnosis of early hepatocellular carcinoma using ELISA Index. Glycoconj J 2015; 32(3-4): 119-25. [http://dx.doi.org/10.1007/s10719-015-9576-8] [PMID: 25702281]

[224] Vermassen T, Speeckaert MM, Lumen N, Rottey S, Delanghe JR. Glycosylation of prostate specific antigen and its potential diagnostic applications. Clin Chim Acta 2012; 413(19-20): 1500-5. [http://dx.doi.org/10.1016/j.cca.2012.06.007] [PMID: 22722018]

[225] Rho J, Mead JR, Wright WS, *et al.* Discovery of sialyl Lewis A and Lewis X modified protein cancer biomarkers using high density antibody arrays. J Proteomics 2014; 96: 291-9. [http://dx.doi.org/10.1016/j.jprot.2013.10.030] [PMID: 24185138]

[226] Ozcan S, Barkauskas DA, Renee Ruhaak L, *et al.* Serum glycan signatures of gastric cancer. Cancer Prev Res (Phila) 2014; 7(2): 226-35. [http://dx.doi.org/10.1158/1940-6207.CAPR-13-0235] [PMID: 24327722]

[227] Kim JH, Park CW, Unmet D, *et al.* Mass spectrometric screening of ovarian cancer with serum glycans. Disease Markers, 2014, 634289: 9 2014.

Part 4: Hormone & Small Molecular Biomarkers

CHAPTER 11

Hormones as Cancer Biomarkers

Plabon Kumar Das[1,2] and **Farhadul Islam**[1,2,*]

[1] *Department of Biochemistry and Molecular Biology, University of Rajshahi, Rajshahi-6205, Bangladesh*

[2] *Institute for Glycomics, Griffith University, Gold Coast, QLD-4222, Australia*

Abstract: Among all the cancer biomarkers, hormones are less discussed despite having the ability to be used as potential biomarkers in the diagnosis and prognosis of various cancers. When a tissue, normally produces hormones in lesser quantity, produces a hormone in excess levels, then hormones can be used as tumour biomarkers. Sometimes it is also seen that a hormone is produced by the tissue, which is not normally associated with the secretion of that hormone. For example, calcitonin, a protein hormone produced by the thyroid gland, is reported to be increased in production in thyroid carcinoma. Another protein hormone, namely human chorionic gonadotropin (hCG), is used as a biomarker in choriocarcinoma, testicular tumors, *etc.* On the other hand, a lower level of testosterone hormone is found in prostate cancer, indicating its role in prostate cancer prognosis. There are other peptidase and steroid hormones, such as insulin, glucagon, estrogen and progesterone which significantly contribute to various tumours and are used as valuable biomarkers in the diagnosis and prognosis. Taken into consideration, in this chapter, we discuss the roles of multiple peptides and steroid hormones in the diagnosis and prognosis of various cancer types.

Keywords: Hormones, Biomarkers, Breast cancer, Cancers, Calcitonin, Choriocarcinoma, Diagnosis, Estrogen, Gastrin, Glucagon, Gonadotropin, Human chorionic gonadotrophin, Insulin, Prognosis, Peptide hormones, Progesterone, Prolactin, Steroid hormone, Thyroid cancer, Thyroid stimulating hormone, *etc.*

INTRODUCTION

Tumour biomarkers are biomolecules produced by tumours or noncancerous tissues in response to the presence of tumours [1]. Those biomolecules are altered genetic, epigenetic material, proteins and hormones. Hormones are the chemical messengers that regulate crucial functions. For example, they maintain energy metabolism, growth, stress and reproduction. They bind to the receptors on plasma membrane and initiate the signalling cascade for the cellular process [2].

* **Corresponding author Farhadul Islam:** Department of Biochemistry and Molecular Biology, University of Rajshahi, Rajshahi-6205, Bangladesh; Email: farhad_bio83@ru.ac.bd

Their actions are very wide and can maintain growth either positively or negatively.

In cancer, they can regulate apoptosis and immune response in patients, thus can contribute to the development and progression of various cancers either positively or negatively. Levels of hormones, such as estrogen, progesterone may act as the risk factor of some common cancers, including breast cancer and prostate cancer [3]. A hormone can act as tumour biomarker when it is produced in excess by diseased tissue compared to normal tissue, or even when ectopically produced by other tissues which are not normally involved in the production of that hormone [1]. For example, calcitonin, a hormone produced by the parafollicular cells (also kwon as C-cells) of thyroid gland, has been observed to produce in excess in medullary thyroid carcinomas [4]. Human chorionic gonadotropin (hCG), a placental hormone primarily produced by syncytiotropoblastic cells during pregnancy, however, can be generated in testicular cancers, thereby can be o used as a maker of testicular cancers as a panel of alpha-phetoprotein, lactate dehydrogenase and hCG [5]. In addition, changes of hormonal level was noted in major types of cancers, such as breast, prostate, endometrial and thyroid cancers [6]. For example, Luteinizing hormone (LH) was reported to be upregulated in breast, prostate, endometrial and thyroid cancers, whereas thyroid stimulating hormone (TSH) and prolactin is upregulated in ovarian, pancreatic and endometrial cancers [7 - 9]. Moreover, another hormone known as adrenocorticotropic hormone (ACTH) was upregulated in ovarian and endometrial cancers [2]. Thus, a number of hormones could have the potential to be used as the biomarkers for various cancers (Table **1**). Therefore, measuring the level of these hormones in cancer tissue or nearby normal tissue will help us to diagnose cancer early and determine the prognosis effectively. In this chapter, we describe the roles of various hormones as potential biomarkers and their clinical application in the diagnosis as well as in monitoring the disease process.

Table 1. Hormones as tumour biomarkers.

Hormones	Types	Function as Biomarkers	References
Calcitonin	Peptide	Aids in the diagnosis of medullary thyroid cancer	[13, 14]
hCG	Peptide	Diagnosis of choriocarcinoma, testicular tumors, and ovarian germ cell tumors (GCTs)	[18]
Insulin	Peptide	Helps in the diagnosis of insulinoma	[26]
Gastrin	Peptide	Aids in the diagnosis of Gastrinoma	[30, 31]
Glucagon	Peptide	Diagnosis of glucagonomas	[36]
Prolactin	Peptide	Aids in the diagnosis of ovarian cancer	[38]
TSH	Peptide	Aids in the diagnosis of thyroid cancer and breast cancer	[44]

(Table 1) cont.....

Hormones	Types	Function as Biomarkers	References
Estrogen	Steroid	Higher level is seen in breast, endometrial, prostate and ovarian and thyroid cancers and laryngeal squamous cell carcinoma	[46 - 50]
Progesterone	Steroid	Increases cancer stem cell characteristics in breast cancer	[54, 55]
Testosterone	Steroid	Lower level is seen in prostate cancer	[62 - 64]

HORMONES AS BIOMARKERS IN VARIOUS CANCERS

Peptide Hormones as Cancer Biomarkers

Peptide hormones, made of amino acids, are water soluble and act on the surface of target cells *via* second messenger [10]. After releasing into the circulation, these hormones interact with receptors on plasma membrane of target cells (Fig. **1**). This interaction initiates intracellular signalling pathways involved in the regulation of various physiological processes, including energy metabolism, growth, stress, and reproduction [10]. These hormones are a vital component in many cellular processes, however, excessive amount of circulating peptide hormones is often associated with various tumours, such as pancreatic cancer, medullary thyroid cancer, *etc*. Thus, these hormones could have potentially be used as a tumour biomarker for the specified types of cancers. The roles of various peptide hormones as biomarkers in cancers will be discussed in the following sections.

Calcitonin

Calcitonin, a linear peptide consisting of 32 amino acids, is released from the parafollicular cell, also known as C-cells of the thyroid gland. Circulating calcium drives the secretion of calcitonin and regulates calcium homeostasis [11, 12]. Excessive calcitonin is seen in medullary thyroid cancer, a predominant thyroid malignancy in United States, accounting for 1%–2% of thyroid malignancies [13]. It was noted that serum calcitonin concentration was associated with tumour size inpatients with medullary thyroid cancer [14]. However, the level of serum calcitonin is not recommended as a diagnostic tool for medullary thyroid cancer due to the fact that calcitonin concentrations could also be associated with other conditions, such as acute and chronic renal failure, hypercalcemia, pulmonary disease, and other malignancies [11, 15]. Thus, the level of serum calcitonin could have the potential to be used as a prognostic marker to monitor therapy response in patients with medullary thyroid cancer.

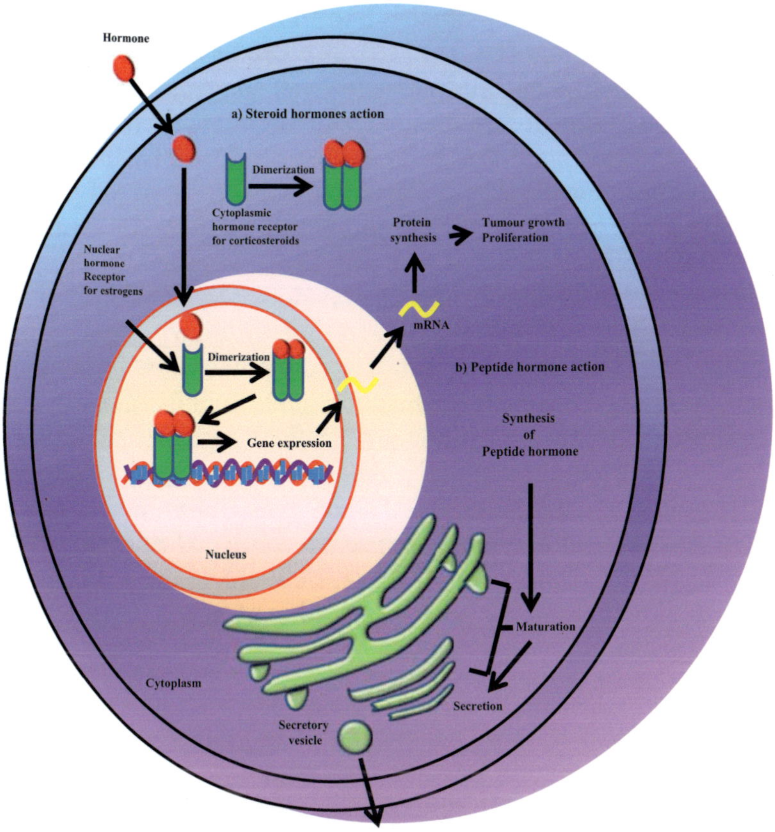

Fig. (1). Overview of peptide and steroid hormonal action in cells. a) Action of steroid hormone: Steroid hormones after entering into plasma membrane bind with either cytoplasmic receptors (glucocorticoids hormones) or nuclear hormone receptors (estrogen hormones). The receptors dimerize with each other followed by hormone binding, and dimerized receptors then act as transcription factor to regulate the expressions of target genes, therebyactivate the growth and survival signaling. **b)** Action of peptide hormone: Peptide hormones are synthesized and matured in the endoplasmic reticulum. After releasing of mature peptide hormones into circulation from tumour cells, they interact with receptors located on the plasma membrane of target cells to trigger a cascade of intracellular signalling.

Human Chorionic Gonadotropin (hCG)

Human chorionic gonadotropin (hCG), is one of the most important hormone biomarkers used in cancer due to its indispensable role in human malignancies, including cell transformation, angiogenesis, metastatization, and immune escape. hCG is expressed by both trophoblastic and non-trophoblastic human cancers [16]. Therefore, for example, hCG testing is often used for the clinical management of placental trophoblastic malignancies and germ cell tumors of the testis and the ovary [16]. hCG is synthesized mainly by trophoblast cells of the placenta but a small amount is also produced in the pituitary of non-pregnant women and men [17]. Determining the level of hCG in serum has been used as a diagnostic tool to identify various cancers like choriocarcinoma, testicular tumors, and ovarian germ cell tumors (GCTs) [18]. A close association between tumour growth and hCG levels in these malignancies was suggested, and hCG levels are used to identify the stage in the clinical management of those tumours [18]. Furthermore, it was also found that hCG can be produced by tumours which are not derived from trophoblastic tissue. Carcinomas, such as, of the pancreas, ovary and breast may have hormone (hCG) increased [19]. hCG is a heterodimer composed of beta(β) and alpha(α) subunit [20].Increased α subunit level is happened to be involved in thyrotroph- or gonadotroph-derived pituitary tumours [21], aiding the diagnosis of TSH-secreting pituitary adenomas. Almost 50%–85% of patients TSH-secreting pituitary adenomas show increased level of α subunit expression [22]. However, the use of α subunit in diagnosing gonadotroph adenomas is limited, because an increased level of serum α subunit is found in 35% of patients [23]. Most interestingly, determining the level of serum hCG and β-hCG is a prominent method with 99% of sensitivity in the screening and monitoring of patients with molar pregnancy who are at risk of developing choriocarcinoma [24]. Considering all these, new studies should be designed to search for new therapies using the prognostic value of hCG.

Insulin

Insulin is produced by β-cells of pancreas and regulates carbohydrate, fat and protein metabolism [25]. Insulin is associated with a rare type of neuroendocrine tumour called insulinoma, a small tumour of the pancreas that produces excessive amount of insulin [26]. It occurs in one to four people per million every year [26]. The disease is characterized by high levels of insulin secretion from beta cells of the pancreas in the presence of low blood sugar, leading to hypoglycemia [27]. Measurement of insulin along with plasma glucose, C-peptide, and proinsulin after a 72 hours fasting can diagnose up to 99% of insulinomas [26, 28]. Therefore, it is used as the gold standard biomarker for biochemical diagnosis of insulinoma.

Gastrin

Gastrin is secreted from gastric antrum and stimulates the secretion of gastric acid by parietal cells of the stomach to increase gastric motility [29]. The secretion of gastrin along with higher level of gastric acid is used as a diagnostic biomarker in patients with gastrinoma [30, 31]. Gastrinoma, a neuroendocrine tumour of pancreas and duodenum, secretes high level of gastrin which in turn stimulate the stomach to secrete acid and enzymes [30, 31]. Moreover, these high level of gastric acid and enzymes secretion leads peptic ulcers [32].

Glucagon

Glucagon, a 29-amino acids peptide hormone produced from α cells of the pancreas and increases blood glucose level [33]. Generally, it is secreted in the blood due to hypoglycemia, stress, and exercise. Upon secretion it increases blood glucose concentration through stimulating gluconeogenesis (synthesis of glucose) and glycogenolysis (breakdown of glycogen) of liver [33, 34]. Alteration in glucagon secretion associated with a rare tumour called glucagonomas, which is a pancreatic neuroendocrine tumour that produces excessive amount of glucagon [35]. A ten times higher level of plasma glucagon is seen in patients with glucagonoma after hours of fasting, which is used as a diagnostic tool in glucagonoma [36].

Prolactin

Prolactin, another peptide hormone produced from pituitary gland, plays important roles in the development of the mammary gland [37]. Also, prolactin is secreted from various tissues such as endometrium, myometrium, cervix, and from prostate cells, immune cells, *etc* [37]. According to recent reports prolactin can be used as a biomarker for ovarian cancer. It was found that receptors for sex hormones and prolactin hormones are co-expressed and are cross-regulated [38]. These co-expression and cross-regulation suggest a possible link among estrogen, progesterone, and prolactin in the regulation of tumour growth [38]. It was reported that prolactin plays a in the development of breast cancer in association with other multiple hormones [39]. However, a proper investigation is required to confirm the role of prolactin in breast cancer development.

Thyroid Stimulating Hormone (TSH)

Thyroid-stimulating hormone (TSH), also known as thyrotropin, is synthesized in anterior pituitary gland and controls endocrine functions of thyroid gland. Higher level of TSH associated with the development of thyroid cancer [40 - 43]. It was found that proliferation of thyroid cell largely depends on TSH secretion [42]. Thus, TSH could have the potential to be used a biomarker for the prognosis of thyroid cancer and targeting TSH could be a promising treatment option for differentiated thyroid cancer. Also, TSH may play a significant role in the development of breast cancer and may have prognostic significance in patients with breast cancer [44].

Steroid Hormones as Biomarker for Various Cancers

Steroid hormones are steroids (a biologically active organic compound) that act as hormone and control metabolism, inflammation, immune function, salt and water balance and development of sexual characteristics [45]. They act either by binding to extracellular receptors or passively cross the cell membrane and bind to the nuclear receptors. In cancer, the activation of signaling cascade following hormones bind to its receptor leads the expression of genes associated with cell proliferation, survival and tumour growth (Fig. **1**). Also, alteration of steroid hormones level is associated with in various cancers, including breast cancer, prostate cancer *etc* [46, 47]. The diagnostic and prognostic significance of these hormones as a biomarker in various cancers are given below.

Estrogen

Estrogens are a group of sex hormones responsible for the development and regulation of female reproductive system and secondary sex characteristics [45]. They are produced from adrenal cortex and ovary and are found both in male and female, however, their level is much higher in female, particularly in their reproductive age. They play a crucial role in the development of breast, endometrial, prostate, ovarian and thyroid cancers [46, 47]. For example, estrogen regulates proliferation, epithelial mesenchymal transition and cancer stem cell (CSC) pool in breast cancer [48, 49]. Furthermore, it is believed that Laryngeal squamous cell carcinoma (LSCC), like breast cancer, could be susceptible for estrogen secretion, which is fueled by the discovery of ER (estrogen receptor)-signalling in LSCC [50]. This finding certainly opens the door to use estrogen as a therapeutic target and as well as a prognostic biomarkers of patients with LSCC management. Also, the presence of ER could be an indicator of the biological aggressiveness of the tumour in patients with LSCC [50]. However, further investigation is required to explore the versatile role of estrogen and ER in LSCC progression. Moreover, in non-small cell lung cancer (NSCLC), expression level of estrogens along with carcinoembryonic antigen (CEA), Neuron-specific enolase (NSE), and CYFRA21- is used as a prognostic marker [51]. It was found that expression of estrogen and CEA, NSE and CYFRA21-1was higher in patients with NSCLC when compared to that of healthy individuals [51]. This positive correlation of estrogen with other well-known tumour biomarkers can significantly increase the implications of tumour biomarkers in the diagnosis and prognosis of NSCLC.

Progesterone

Progesterone is secreted from the corpus luteum and involved in the menstrual cycle, pregnancy and embryogenesis [52, 53]. It acts on various organs such as brain, breast, uterus, ovary, and cervix [52]. Progesterone stimulates the proliferation, expansion and epithelial-mesenchymal transition of breast cancer stem cells [54, 55]. Despite the absence of estrogen and progesterone receptors in breast cancer CSCs, it was found that both estrogen and progesterone play a significant role in the development of breast CSCs [54, 55]. Considering the immense role of progesterone in the development of cancers, we suggest a significant amount of studies should need be done to identify the diagnostic and prognostic value of progesterone.

Testosterone

Testosterone is primarily produced by testicles and plays a function in a male's appearance and sexual development [56]. Though the role of testosterone in the development of prostate cancer remains controversial, several studies underpin the association of testosterone and prostate cancer [56 - 58]. In 1996, Morgentaler *et al.* first proposed that a higher prevalence of prostate cancer is noted in men with a low level of total or free testosterone levels [59]. However, other studies reported conflicting results on the association between testosterone level and prostate cancer [60, 61]. Furthermore, a plethora of evidence reported that low testosterone level contributes to higher tumour grade, more biological aggressive cancers, and poorer survival of patients with prostate cancer [62 - 64]. For example, a prospective analysis of samples (n=137) unveils a reverse relationship ($p<0.01$) between testosterone level and prostate cancer [62]. Another study found a link between lower testosterone level and higher prostate cancer risk [63]. They reported that biopsy sample of 21% patients shows a testosterone level ≤ 250 ng/dL and only 12% patients with a level > 250 ng/dL ($p = 0.04$) . Another study comprising a large cohort of patients suggested similar results [64]. In this study, they collected biopsy samples(n=568) and was divided into high and low testosterone groups with a threshold testosterone level of 3.85 ng/ml. A higher rate of prostate cancer was noted in the low testosterone group (38.9 *vs*. 29.5%, $p = 0.018$) [64]. However, the level of testosterone was not correlated with disease in the grade of patients with prostate cancer [64].Thus, the prognostic significance of testosterone in patients with cancer, especially prostate cancer needs to be validated using further studies comprising larger cohort of samples.

CONCLUSION AND PERSPECTIVE

Measurement of hormone levels is useful in the diagnosis, prognosis and in the assessment of treatment response in patients with cancers. With the advent of modern technologies, it has become easier to measure the level of hormones in the body fluids of suspected cancer patients. Determining the level of hormone level on one hand, has the potential to be used as a diagnostic and prognostic tool, on the other hand, the secretion of hormones could be used as a therapeutic target in various cancers. However, several hormones are often secreted in diseases other than cancers. Thus, before using hormones as a biomarker in the diagnosis and prognosis of cancer, further studies are required.

CONSENT FOR PUBLICATION

Not applicable.

CONFLICT OF INTEREST

The authors declare no conflict of interest, financial or otherwise.

ACKNOWLEDGEMENT

The authors are thankful to the Department of Biochemistry and Molecular Biology, University of Rajshahi, Rajshahi-6205, Bangladesh, for supporting the work.

REFERENCES

[1] Faria SC, Sagebiel T, Patnana M, *et al.* Tumor markers: myths and facts unfolded. Abdom Radiol (NY) 2019; 44(4): 1575-600.
[http://dx.doi.org/10.1007/s00261-018-1845-0] [PMID: 30498924]

[2] Linkov F, Yurkovetsky Z, Lokshin A. Hormones as biomarkers: practical guide to utilizing luminex technologies for biomarker research. Methods Mol Biol 2009; 520: 129-41.
[http://dx.doi.org/10.1007/978-1-60327-811-9_9] [PMID: 19381951]

[3] Sun Q, Zhao Z. Peptide Hormones as Tumor Markers in Clinical Practice. Enzymes 2017; 42: 65-79.
[http://dx.doi.org/10.1016/bs.enz.2017.09.001] [PMID: 29054271]

[4] Cohen R, Campos JM, Salaün C, *et al.* Preoperative calcitonin levels are predictive of tumor size and postoperative calcitonin normalization in medullary thyroid carcinoma. Groupe d'Etudes des Tumeurs a Calcitonine (GETC). J Clin Endocrinol Metab 2000; 85(2): 919-22.
[http://dx.doi.org/10.1210/jcem.85.2.6556] [PMID: 10690910]

[5] Gilligan TD, Seidenfeld J, Basch EM, *et al.* American Society of Clinical Oncology Clinical Practice Guideline on uses of serum tumor markers in adult males with germ cell tumors. J Clin Oncol 2010; 28(20): 3388-404.
[http://dx.doi.org/10.1200/JCO.2009.26.4481] [PMID: 20530278]

[6] Portier CJ. Endocrine dismodulation and cancer. Neuroendocrinol Lett 2002; 23 (Suppl. 2): 43-7.
[PMID: 12163847]

[7] Cramer DW, Barbieri RL, Muto MG, Kelly A, Brucks JP, Harlow BL. Characteristics of Women with a family history of ovarian cancer. II. Follicular phase hormone levels. Cancer 1994; 74(4): 1318-22.
[http://dx.doi.org/10.1002/1097-0142(19940815)74:4<1318::AID-CNCR2820740422>3.0.CO;2-V] [PMID: 8055454]

[8] Biondi B, Filetti S, Schlumberger M. Thyroid-hormone therapy and thyroid cancer: a reassessment. Nat Clin Pract Endocrinol Metab 2005; 1(1): 32-40.
[http://dx.doi.org/10.1038/ncpendmet0020] [PMID: 16929364]

[9] Chia SY, Milas M, Reddy SK, *et al.* Thyroid-stimulating hormone receptor messenger ribonucleic acid measurement in blood as a marker for circulating thyroid cancer cells and its role in the preoperative diagnosis of thyroid cancer. J Clin Endocrinol Metab 2007; 92(2): 468-75.
[http://dx.doi.org/10.1210/jc.2006-2088] [PMID: 17118994]

[10] Kaplan LA, Pesce AJ, Wu AH. Clinical Chemistry: Theory, Analysis, Correlation. Clin Chem 1997; 43(4): 700.

[11] Fraser W. Bone and mineral metabolism Tietz textbook of clinical chemistry and molecular diagnostics-e-book. Elsevier Health Sciences 2016; p. xviii.

[12] Baregamian N, Solórzano CC. The physiology of serum calcitonin and carcinoembryonic antigen in medullary thyroid cancer.Medullary Thyroid Cancer. Cham: Springer 2016; pp. 25-31. [http://dx.doi.org/10.1007/978-3-319-39412-1_3]

[13] Wells SA Jr, Asa SL, Dralle H, *et al.* Revised American Thyroid Association guidelines for the management of medullary thyroid carcinoma. Thyroid 2015; 25(6): 567-610. [http://dx.doi.org/10.1089/thy.2014.0335] [PMID: 25810047]

[14] Costante G, Meringolo D, Durante C, *et al.* Predictive value of serum calcitonin levels for preoperative diagnosis of medullary thyroid carcinoma in a cohort of 5817 consecutive patients with thyroid nodules. J Clin Endocrinol Metab 2007; 92(2): 450-5. [http://dx.doi.org/10.1210/jc.2006-1590] [PMID: 17119000]

[15] Costante G, Filetti S. Early diagnosis of medullary thyroid carcinoma: is systematic calcitonin screening appropriate in patients with nodular thyroid disease? Oncologist 2011; 16(1): 49-52. [http://dx.doi.org/10.1634/theoncologist.2010-0344] [PMID: 21212427]

[16] Sisinni L, Landriscina M. The Role of Human Chorionic Gonadotropin as Tumor Marker: Biochemical and Clinical Aspects. Adv Exp Med Biol 2015; 867: 159-76. [http://dx.doi.org/10.1007/978-94-017-7215-0_11] [PMID: 26530366]

[17] Rehfeld JF, Bardram L, Blanke S, *et al.* The expression of peptide hormones in normal cells and tumour cells. Acta Oncol 1991; 30(4): 429-33. [http://dx.doi.org/10.3109/02841869109092397] [PMID: 1854500]

[18] Sturgenon C. Tumor markers Tietz Textbook of Clinical Chemistry and Molecular Diagnostics. St. Louis, MO: Elsevier 2016; p. xviii.

[19] Muller CY, Cole LA. The quagmire of hCG and hCG testing in gynecologic oncology. Gynecol Oncol 2009; 112(3): 663-72. [http://dx.doi.org/10.1016/j.ygyno.2008.09.030] [PMID: 19007977]

[20] Khoo NKS, Bechberger JF, Shepherd T, *et al.* SV40 Tag transformation of the normal invasive trophoblast results in a premalignant phenotype. I. Mechanisms responsible for hyperinvasivess and resistance to anti-invasive action of TGFβ. Int J Cancer 1998; 77(3): 429-39. [http://dx.doi.org/10.1002/(SICI)1097-0215(19980729)77:3<429::AID-IJC20>3.0.CO;2-1] [PMID: 9663607]

[21] Butler SA, Staite EM, Iles RK. Reduction of bladder cancer cell growth in response to hCGbeta CTP37 vaccinated mouse serum. Oncol Res 2003; 14(2): 93-100. [http://dx.doi.org/10.3727/000000003108748649] [PMID: 14649543]

[22] Elliott MM, Kardana A, Lustbader JW, Cole LA. Carbohydrate and peptide structure of the α- and β-subunits of human chorionic gonadotropin from normal and aberrant pregnancy and choriocarcinoma. Endocr J 1997; 7(1): 15-32. [http://dx.doi.org/10.1007/BF02778058] [PMID: 9449027]

[23] Hoshina M, Boime I, Mochizuki M. Cytological localization of hPL, hCG, and mRNA in chorionic tissue using *in situ* hybridization. Nippon Sanka Fujinka Gakkai Zasshi 1984; 36(3): 397-404. [PMID: 6715923]

[24] Wu H, Lustbader JW, Liu Y, Canfield RE, Hendrickson WA. Structure of human chorionic gonadotropin at 2.6 å resolution from MAD analysis of the selenomethionyl protein. Structure 1994; 2(6): 545-58. [http://dx.doi.org/10.1016/S0969-2126(00)00054-X] [PMID: 7922031]

[25] Sacks D. Diabetes mellitus Tietz Textbook of Clinical Chemistry and Molecular Diagnostics. St. Louis, MO: Elsevier 2016; p. xviii.

[26] Okabayashi T, Shima Y, Sumiyoshi T, *et al.* Diagnosis and management of insulinoma. World J Gastroenterol 2013; 19(6): 829-37.
[http://dx.doi.org/10.3748/wjg.v19.i6.829] [PMID: 23430217]

[27] Minn AH, Kayton M, Lorang D, *et al.* Insulinomas and expression of an insulin splice variant. Lancet 2004; 363(9406): 363-7.
[http://dx.doi.org/10.1016/S0140-6736(04)15438-X] [PMID: 15070567]

[28] Service FJ, Natt N. The prolonged fast. J Clin Endocrinol Metab 2000; 85(11): 3973-4.
[http://dx.doi.org/10.1210/jcem.85.11.6934] [PMID: 11095416]

[29] Sherwood RA, Walsham NE, Bjarnason I. Gastric, pancreatic, and intestinal function Tietz Textbook of Clinical Chemistry and Molecular Diagnostics, Elsevier, St Louis, MO,. 2016; p. xviii. 2238.

[30] Berna MJ, Hoffmann KM, Serrano J, Gibril F, Jensen RT. Serum gastrin in Zollinger-Ellison syndrome: I. Prospective study of fasting serum gastrin in 309 patients from the National Institutes of Health and comparison with 2229 cases from the literature. Medicine (Baltimore) 2006; 85(6): 295-330.
[http://dx.doi.org/10.1097/01.md.0000236956.74128.76] [PMID: 17108778]

[31] Norton JA. Neuroendocrine tumors of the pancreas and duodenum. Curr Probl Surg 1994; 31(2): 89-156.
[http://dx.doi.org/10.1016/0011-3840(94)90079-5] [PMID: 7904550]

[32] Ellison EC, Johnson JA. The Zollinger-Ellison syndrome: a comprehensive review of historical, scientific, and clinical considerations. Curr Probl Surg 2009; 46(1): 13-106.
[http://dx.doi.org/10.1067/j.cpsurg.2008.09.001] [PMID: 19059523]

[33] Kleinert M, Sachs S, Habegger KM, Hofmann SM, Müller TD. Glucagon Regulation of Energy Expenditure. Int J Mol Sci 2019; 20(21): 5407.
[http://dx.doi.org/10.3390/ijms20215407] [PMID: 31671603]

[34] Jiang G, Zhang BB. Glucagon and regulation of glucose metabolism. Am J Physiol Endocrinol Metab 2003; 284(4): E671-8.
[http://dx.doi.org/10.1152/ajpendo.00492.2002] [PMID: 12626323]

[35] van Beek AP, de Haas ER, van Vloten WA, Lips CJ, Roijers JF, Canninga-van Dijk MR. The glucagonoma syndrome and necrolytic migratory erythema: a clinical review. Eur J Endocrinol 2004; 151(5): 531-7.
[http://dx.doi.org/10.1530/eje.0.1510531] [PMID: 15538929]

[36] Wermers RA, Fatourechi V, Wynne AG, Kvols LK, Lloyd RV. The glucagonoma syndrome. Clinical and pathologic features in 21 patients. Medicine (Baltimore) 1996; 75(2): 53-63.
[http://dx.doi.org/10.1097/00005792-199603000-00002] [PMID: 8606627]

[37] Ormandy CJ, Camus A, Barra J, *et al.* Null mutation of the prolactin receptor gene produces multiple reproductive defects in the mouse. Genes Dev 1997; 11(2): 167-78.
[http://dx.doi.org/10.1101/gad.11.2.167] [PMID: 9009200]

[38] Ormandy CJ, Hall RE, Manning DL, *et al.* Coexpression and cross-regulation of the prolactin receptor and sex steroid hormone receptors in breast cancer. J Clin Endocrinol Metab 1997; 82(11): 3692-9.
[http://dx.doi.org/10.1210/jc.82.11.3692] [PMID: 9360527]

[39] Hankinson SE. Endogenous hormones and risk of breast cancer in postmenopausal women. Breast Dis 2006-2006-2006; 24(1): 3-15.
[http://dx.doi.org/10.3233/BD-2006-24102] [PMID: 16917136]

[40] Hoffmann J, Sommer A. Steroidhormone receptors as targets for the therapy of breast and prostate cancer—recent advances, mechanisms of resistance, and new approaches. J Steroid Biochem Mol Biol

2005; 93(2-5): 191-200.
[http://dx.doi.org/10.1016/j.jsbmb.2004.12.002] [PMID: 15860262]

[41] Hargadine JR, Lowenstein JM, Greenspan FS. Elevated serum TSH in human thyroid cancer. Oncology 1970; 24(3): 172-80.
[http://dx.doi.org/10.1159/000224517] [PMID: 4907361]

[42] Sailer B, Mehl U, Hörmann R, Moser E, Mann K. Highly sensitive determination of TSH in the follow-up of TSH-suppressive therapy of patients with differentiated thyroid cancer. Nucl Med (Stuttg) 1988; 27(1): 24-8.
[http://dx.doi.org/10.1055/s-0038-1628906] [PMID: 3368333]

[43] Huang H, Rusiecki J, Zhao N, *et al.* Thyroid-Stimulating Hormone, Thyroid Hormones, and Risk of Papillary Thyroid Cancer: A Nested Case–Control Study. Cancer Epidemiol Biomarkers Prev 2017; 26(8): 1209-18.
[http://dx.doi.org/10.1158/1055-9965.EPI-16-0845] [PMID: 28377419]

[44] Tarquini B, Benvenuti M, Legnaioli M, Bazzani M, Cagnoni M, Halberg F. Mammary cancer risk: circulating TSH and prolactin, fibrocystic breast disease in chronoepidemiologic perspective. Cancer Detect Prev 1981; 4(1-4): 525-34.
[PMID: 7349819]

[45] Ascenzi P, Bocedi A, Marino M. Structure–function relationship of estrogen receptor α and β: Impact on human health. Mol Aspects Med 2006; 27(4): 299-402.
[http://dx.doi.org/10.1016/j.mam.2006.07.001] [PMID: 16914190]

[46] Pearce ST, Jordan VC. The biological role of estrogen receptors α and β in cancer. Crit Rev Oncol Hematol 2004; 50(1): 3-22.
[http://dx.doi.org/10.1016/j.critrevonc.2003.09.003] [PMID: 15094156]

[47] Ruggiero RJ, Likis FE. Estrogen: physiology, pharmacology, and formulations for replacement therapy. J Midwifery Womens Health 2002; 47(3): 130-8.
[http://dx.doi.org/10.1016/S1526-9523(02)00233-7] [PMID: 12071379]

[48] Fillmore CM, Gupta PB, Rudnick JA, *et al.* Estrogen expands breast cancer stem-like cells through paracrine FGF/Tbx3 signaling. Proc Natl Acad Sci USA 2010; 107(50): 21737-42.
[http://dx.doi.org/10.1073/pnas.1007863107] [PMID: 21098263]

[49] Palafox M, Ferrer I, Pellegrini P, *et al.* RANK induces epithelial-mesenchymal transition and stemness in human mammary epithelial cells and promotes tumorigenesis and metastasis. Cancer Res 2012; 72(11). 2879-88.
[http://dx.doi.org/10.1158/0008-5472.CAN-12-0044] [PMID: 22496457]

[50] Verma A, Schwartz N, Cohen DJ, Boyan BD, Schwartz Z. Estrogen signaling and estrogen receptors as prognostic indicators in laryngeal cancer. Steroids 2019; 152: 108498.
[http://dx.doi.org/10.1016/j.steroids.2019.108498] [PMID: 31539535]

[51] Bai Y, Shen W, Zhu M, *et al.* Combined detection of estrogen and tumor markers is an important reference factor in the diagnosis and prognosis of lung cancer. J Cell Biochem 2019; 120(1): 105-14.
[http://dx.doi.org/10.1002/jcb.27130] [PMID: 30216488]

[52] Kim JJ, Kurita T, Bulun SE. Progesterone action in endometrial cancer, endometriosis, uterine fibroids, and breast cancer. Endocr Rev 2013; 34(1): 130-62.
[http://dx.doi.org/10.1210/er.2012-1043] [PMID: 23303565]

[53] Lee K, Jeong J, Tsai MJ, Tsai S, Lydon JP, DeMayo FJ. Molecular mechanisms involved in progesterone receptor regulation of uterine function. J Steroid Biochem Mol Biol 2006; 102(1-5): 41-50.
[http://dx.doi.org/10.1016/j.jsbmb.2006.09.006] [PMID: 17067792]

[54] Eblaghie MC, Song SJ, Kim JY, Akita K, Tickle C, Jung HS. Interactions between FGF and Wnt signals and Tbx3 gene expression in mammary gland initiation in mouse embryos. J Anat 2004;

205(1): 1-13.
[http://dx.doi.org/10.1111/j.0021-8782.2004.00309.x] [PMID: 15255957]

[55] Simões BM, Alferez DG, Howell SJ, Clarke RB. The role of steroid hormones in breast cancer stem cells. Endocr Relat Cancer 2015; 22(6): T177-86.
[http://dx.doi.org/10.1530/ERC-15-0350] [PMID: 26381288]

[56] Rodriguez KM, Pastuszak AW, Khera M. The Role of Testosterone Therapy in the Setting of Prostate Cancer. Curr Urol Rep 2018; 19(8): 67.
[http://dx.doi.org/10.1007/s11934-018-0812-1] [PMID: 29961247]

[57] Watts EL, Appleby PN, Perez-Cornago A, *et al.* Low Free Testosterone and Prostate Cancer Risk: A Collaborative Analysis of 20 Prospective Studies. Eur Urol 2018; 74(5): 585-94.
[http://dx.doi.org/10.1016/j.eururo.2018.07.024] [PMID: 30077399]

[58] Yassin A, AlRumaihi K, Alzubaidi R, Alkadhi S, Al Ansari A. Testosterone, testosterone therapy and prostate cancer. Aging Male 2019; 22(4): 219-27.
[http://dx.doi.org/10.1080/13685538.2018.1524456] [PMID: 30614347]

[59] Morgentaler A, Bruning CO III, DeWolf WC. Occult prostate cancer in men with low serum testosterone levels. JAMA 1996; 276(23): 1904-6.
[http://dx.doi.org/10.1001/jama.1996.03540230054035] [PMID: 8968017]

[60] Klap J, Schmid M, Loughlin KR. The relationship between total testosterone levels and prostate cancer: a review of the continuing controversy. J Urol 2015; 193(2): 403-14.
[http://dx.doi.org/10.1016/j.juro.2014.07.123] [PMID: 25260832]

[61] Khera M, Crawford D, Morales A, Salonia A, Morgentaler A. A new era of testosterone and prostate cancer: from physiology to clinical implications. Eur Urol 2014; 65(1): 115-23.
[http://dx.doi.org/10.1016/j.eururo.2013.08.015] [PMID: 24011426]

[62] Lei K, Chen L, Georgiou EX, *et al.* Progesterone acts *via* the nuclear glucocorticoid receptor to suppress IL-1β-induced COX-2 expression in human term myometrial cells. PLoS One 2012; 7(11): e50167.
[http://dx.doi.org/10.1371/journal.pone.0050167] [PMID: 23209664]

[63] Morgentaler A, Rhoden EL. Prevalence of prostate cancer among hypogonadal men with prostate-specific antigen levels of 4.0 ng/mL or less. Urology 2006; 68(6): 1263-7.
[http://dx.doi.org/10.1016/j.urology.2006.08.1058] [PMID: 17169647]

[64] Wu GS, Song YL, Yin ZQ, *et al.* Ganoderiol A-enriched extract suppresses migration and adhesion of MDA-MB-231 cells by inhibiting FAK-SRC-paxillin cascade pathway. PLoS One 2013; 8(10): e76620.
[http://dx.doi.org/10.1371/journal.pone.0076620] [PMID: 24204647]

CHAPTER 12

miRNAs as Epigenetic Cancer Biomarker

Afraa Mamoori[1,*]

[1] *Department of Pathology and Forensic Medicine, School of Medicine, University of Babylon, Hillah, Iraq*

Abstract: Despite the fact that the mortality rate of many types of cancer has decreased in the last decades, cancer remains one of the most challenging diseases in the world. The number of newly diagnosed cases with advanced stages in different types of cancer is still high because available tests are not efficient enough to be used for screening. In addition, the available diagnostic tests failed to diagnose certain types of cancer until late presentation. Furthermore, therapeutic agents currently in clinical use to treat a certain type of malignant tumours still show a high rate of resistance in some patients. Many types of available cancer biomarkers failed to manage and resolve this problem because of the lack of both sensitivity and specificity of these markers. Advanced researches in epigenetics highlight the importance of certain non-coding genes in diagnosing and follow-up of patients with different types of cancer. One of these substances is microRNAs (miRNAs) which showed high sensitivity and specificity as cancer biomarkers. miRNAs are highly stable and expressed in different types of human body samples; some of them are tissue specific. These features make them available as cancer biomarkers, and they are started to be in clinical use recently.

Keywords: Biomarkers, Cancer, Diagnosis, Prognosis, Epigenetic, Clinical, Facts, Specificity, Sensitivity, Non-coding RNAs, Fluid, Sample, Tissue, Commercialized miRNAs, miRview test, miRNAs, Therapeutic resistance, Epithelial-mesenchymal transition.

INTRODUCTION

Cancer biomarkers can simply describe as substances like DNA, RNA, protein and peptides present in the human body and its products, which have the ability to identify cancer development, cancer progression and response to the therapeutic agents. These substances become extremely important in clinical practice after the increase in genomic profiling and molecular target therapy technology. Cancer biomarkers can be classified into three types depending on their clinical use [1]. The first type is called diagnostic biomarkers, which are used to identify certain

* **Corresponding author Afraa Mamoori:** Department of Pathology and Forensic Medicine, School of Medicine, University of Babylon, Hillah, Iraq; E-mail: afraajawad@yahoo.com

types of cancer. The second type is named prognostic biomarkers, which are clinically used to determine the risk and recurrence of cancer. The last type is the predictive biomarkers, which are used to predict the usefulness of drugs in the treatment of various types of cancer [2, 3].

The usual cancer biomarkers which are in clinical practice for several years show limitations for the use as diagnostic, prognostic and predictive biomarkers because they are low in both specificity and sensitivity towards certain types of cancer. For example, Prostate Specific Antigen (PSA), which has been in clinical use as a prognostic and diagnostic biomarker for prostate cancer for many decades, is being increasingly criticised for its false positive diagnostic rate [4]. Moreover, CA19-9, which is the only biomarker approved to use in clinical practice for pancreatic cancer diagnosis and prognosis, showed only 79% sensitivity and 82% specificity with poor predictive value in the symptomatic patients reaching only 0.5-0.9% [5].

High throughput sequencing in epigenetic researches raises the opportunity of using the microRNAs as cancer biomarkers with more sensitivity and specificity than the old cancer biomarkers. Thus, this chapter will discuss the importance of using these molecules in different types of cancer as diagnostic and prognostic markers. Herein, we will identify the important research findings in the field and show the miRNAs introduced to clinical practice recently.

MiRNAs and Epigenetics

The term "Epigenetics" can be defined as heritable alterations in gene expression without changes to the DNA bases sequence; they play an integral part in genomic stability and gene transcription [6]. Epigenetics is composed of 3 components, *i.e.* DNA methylation, Histone modifications, and Non-coding RNAs [7]. The term "non-coding RNAs" (ncRNAs) can be defined as the species of RNAs which are not coding for proteins; various forms of them are essential for the regulation of cellular processes, including target genes transcriptions and translations and thereby controlled cellular proliferation, differentiation, aging, longevity and so on [8]. Non-coding RNAs can be divided into two main categories (long non-coding RNAs and short non-coding RNAs) depending on the nucleotide's sequence length of their mature form. Short non-coding RNAs include (PIWI-interacting RNAs (piRNAs), circular RNAs (circRNAs), transfer RNAs (tRNAs)-derived small RNAs (ts RNAs), small nucleolar RNAs (snoRNAs) and micro RNAs (miRNAs).

Micro RNAs (miRNAs) are short non-coding RNAs. In their mature form, they are 20-24 nucleotides in length. Since their initial discovery, it has been demonstrated that this class of non-coding RNA is involved in regulating many biological pathways in a variety of multicellular organisms, including humans [9]. In relation to cancer, miRNAs can act as oncogenes or tumour suppressor genes, depending on their regulatory targets [10]. Also, miRNAs have been implicated as robust regulators in both normal and cancer stem cells (CSCs). Cancer stem cells are suggested to be responsible for the initiation and promotion of cancers as well as for enabling resistance to chemotherapeutic treatments [11 - 13].

Mode of Action of MicroRNAs

miRNAs act by post-transcriptional repression and target mRNA degradation, through a complex process. Following their transcription in pri-miRNA form, they are converted into pre-miRNAs consisting of a stem-loop structure and finally processed into the mature form of a short, double-stranded RNA of about 20 nucleotides. After this process of biogenesis, the mature miRNAs are rendered single-stranded and assembled into ribonucleoprotein complexes called (miRNAPs) or miRNA-induced silencing complex (miRISC) in association with a protein family called argonaute (AGO) [14, 15]. There are four types of AGO protein in mammals (AGO1 to AGO4), and they are mainly involved in the gene expression-repression process mediated by miRNA [16, 17]. During the process of repression, miRNAs bind to the 3' UTR of target mRNA to form base pairing in a 2-8 nucleotide long sequence (the seed region), which facilitates the complete miRNA-mRNA association [18]. miRNA binding sites are available in multiple copies which are necessary for effective repression processes [19, 20]. In addition, the degree of miRNA-mRNA complementarity is crucial for the strength of the regulatory mechanism. A perfect miRNA-mRNA complementarity will result in the destruction of the mRNA strand by AGO, while central mismatches in the miRNA sequence will promote repression of mRNA translation by strand cleavage processes [21]. This process of post-transcriptional repression of mRNAs can be achieved at either translation initiation or at a post-translational stage.

Targets Selection by MicroRNAs

Single miRNAs can regulate the function of hundreds of target genes, and one target gene can also be regulated by several miRNAs. The process of target selection for a miRNA is mainly driven by seed sequence complementarities between the miRNA and its target mRNAs [22, 23]. It is understood that there are also other factors that may participate effectively in the process of target selection, factors which we are beginning to elucidate. Titration of miRNA from its target gene *via* a phenomenon called competing endogenous RNA (ceRNA) is one of the controlling factors in determining target selection [24 - 25]. An example of such titration in cancer would be through the expression of pseudogenes to decoy a tumour suppressor miRNA from the functional transcript, and indeed an expression of several pseudogenes of cancer-related genes has been implicated in the process of target selection [26]. In addition, long non-coding RNAs (lncRNAs) are involved in the process of miRNA sequestration [27]. Recently, the presence of methylation of the N6 position of adenosine residues at specific sites within mRNAs targeted by miRNA has been identified as a potential modifier of miRNA target selection [28, 29]. Thus, it is clear that the process of target selection in miRNAs is a complex process that does not depend only on the degree of seed complementarity.

MiRNAs and Clinical Facts

miRNAs have some important features that make them clinically very important structures. They have essential roles in different types of diseases, including cancer. Clinically important facts are discussed below:

Over 60% of Human Protein-coding Genes are Controlled by miRNA

Nearly, 2300 true mature miRNAs have been discovered in the human genome till now [30]. Over 60% of human protein-coding genes are predicted to contain miRNA-binding sites in their 3′-untranslated region (3′-UTR) [31]. This finding makes them very robust regulators of different cellular processes, including cancer development and metastasis. Approximately, 12,738 protein-coding genes are predicted to have interacted with miRNAs in the human genome; from them, there are 7439 with strong evident interaction [32]. Some protein coding genes predicted as a direct or indirect target of the miRNAs are well-known genes and play important roles in different types of human cancer. For example, in colorectal cancer, KRAS and MIF were predicted as direct targets of miR-193a-3p and miR-451, respectively [33].

Tissue-specific miRNAs

The tissue-specific pattern of miRNAs plays an integral role in tissue signature, differentiation and function. They are implicated in the pathogenesis of different human diseases like cardiovascular, diabetes and cancer [34 - 36]. A high concordance of tissue-specific miRNAs between humans and rodents was determined by different scientists [37, 38]. Tissue-specific miRNAs were identified first by Landgraf *et al.*, 2007 [37]. The authors detect tissue specific expression of miR-122 in liver, of miR-9, miR-124 and miR 128a/b in the brain, of miR-7, miR-375, miR-141 and miR200a in the pituitary gland and of miR-142, miR-144, miR150, miR-155 and miR-223 in hematopoietic cells [37]. These data were confirmed later by Ludwig *et al.*, 2016 [38]. miR-124–3p was identified in different areas of brain tissue, and it was not isolated from any other organ [38].

Furthermore, high expression of miR-144 was identified in normal thyroid glands and downregulated in thyroid papillary carcinoma [38, 39]. Some types of miRNAs which were isolated from specific organs or tissues acquired the names of these organs or tissues. For example, "myomRs" was given to the miRNAs, which were isolated at a high level in myocardium and other types of muscles and play essential roles in regulation of genes that required for muscle development. These miRNAs include miR-1–3p, miR-133a-3p, miR-133b and miR-206 [38, 40, 41]. Knowing the tissue-specific miRNAs is important to understand the normal development and the diseases that arise from that tissue. Also, they can be used as tissue-specific biomarkers for some diseases that arise from these tissues. The miRNAs which are identified as tissue-specific are summarized in Table **1**. These miRNAs are used to identify the cancer of unknown primary origin (CUP).

Table 1. Tissues specific miRNAs. Each set of miRNAs identifies a specific type of tissue of origin.

MiRNAs	Tissue of origin
miR-122a, miR-200c	Liver
miR-372	Testis
miR-142-3p, miR-509	Lymph node, Melanocyte
miR-92b, miR-9*, miR-124a	Brain
miR-152, miR130a	Meninges
miR-205	Thymus (Type B2)
miR-194, miR-382, miR-210	Lung-pleura, Kidney
miR-187, miR-29b	Gastrointestinal tract, Stroma
miR-21, let-7e	Lung (carcinoid)
Let-7i, miR-29a	Colon
miR-214, miR-19b, let-7	Stomach, Pancreas
miR-27b, let-7i, miR-181b	Breast, Prostate,
miR-106b, let-7i, miR-138	Thyroid
miR-205, miR-152	Lung, Bladder
miR-345, miR-29c, miR-182	Endometrium, Ovary
miR-192, miR-345	Thymus (type B3)
miR-182, miR-34a, miR-148b	Lung (squamous), Head and Neck

miRNAs Expressed in Different types of Body Fluid, and They are Highly Stable in Human Samples

In addition to their expression in tissue samples, miRNAs were identified in different types of human samples, including saliva, blood, blood cells, serum, plasma, urine, pleural effusion, bronchial wash, ascetic fluid, cerebrospinal fluid, amniotic fluid, tears, breast milk [42 - 46]. According to the data collected for approximately 20 years, MiRNAs show high stability in different types of body samples and can persist with good quality for long time storage. In human tissue sample, miRNAs are isolated from different types of cancers and benign tumors, including colorectal, breast, lung, esophageal, brain, renal, and skin [47 - 53]. Both fresh frozen human tissue and Formalin fixed paraffin embedded tissue samples can be used to detect the miRNAs by using Real-time PCR and Taqman Array [54, 55].

Circulating miRNAs isolated from the whole blood and the blood products seem to be a promising noninvasive biomarker for cancer detection and follow-up. MiRNAs originating from different types of human tissues, are carried out into the circulation by extracellular vesicles called exosomes. The term exosomal miRNAs are applied to these types of miRNAs [56]. In addition, the amount and the composition of exosomal miRNAs are different between a healthy individual and a patient with malignancy [56]. Moreover, they reflect the tissue of their origin, which can be determined by the presence of specific surface markers [56]. Indeed, miRNAs were isolated from blood samples of different types of human malignancies, including gastric cancer, colorectal cancer, esophageal cancer, prostate cancer and non-small cell lung cancer (NSCLC) [56]. Circulating miRNAs withstand an extreme change in the pH level, freeze-thawing procedures and storage at room temperature [57]. Also, they were isolated from dried human serum samples, giving them an extra technical advantage [58, 59]. The best method that can be used to isolate miRNAs from different types of blood samples till now is the next generation sequencing (NGS) because it can detect the low concentration of circulating miRNAs, a cheap and high throughput procedure [59].

Saliva expressed a wide range of miRNAs associated with human cancers. MiR-21 was the first miRNA found to be deregulated in the saliva of human colorectal cancer; the high sensitivity and specificity detection method for salivary miR-21 in colorectal cancer raised its suitability as a diagnostic test for colorectal cancer [60]. MiR-139-5p was significantly downregulated in the saliva of patients with oral squamous cell carcinoma [61]. Furthermore, in the saliva of patients with pancreatic cancer, miR-23a and miR-23b were detected to be upregulated with a sensitivity of 85.7% and specificity of 100% [62]. Moreover, some types of cancers identified a positive correlation in the level of miRNAs between saliva and blood samples. For example, miR-21 showed significant upregulation in saliva supernatant and plasma sample of patients with esophageal cancer [63]. Saliva has more advantages than blood as a liquid biopsy because its collection is not invasive and cost-effective. Quantitative real-time PCR was the most used method to assess the level of salivary miRNAs in patients with different types of cancer.

The stability of miRNAs in different human body samples was attributed to different ways, either miRNAs incorporated themselves in to the microvesicles (MVs) or presented as a complex with some circulating proteins. Active secretion of miRNAs into the membranous enclosed microvesicles is managed by two types of vesicles (shedding vesicles and exosomes) under different pathologic alterations [64]. The mechanism by which specific miRNAs are released by shedding vesicles is still unknown, however, the ceramide-dependent and endosomal sorting complex required for transport (ESCRT) independent pathway regulates the load and release of exosomal miRNAs [65, 66].

Transport of miRNAs *via* microvesicles independent mechanism is carried out by attachment of these miRNAs to the RNAs binding proteins and high-density lipoprotein (HDL). The mechanism by which the HDL forms complex with specific miRNAs and transport them in circulation still in the primitive stage. However, the divalent cation bridging in the connection between the miRNAs and HDL leads to the protection of the associated miRNAs from degradation by external RNases [67]. In the context of comparing the exosomal and non-exosomal source of circulating miRNAs relevant as a cancer biomarker, the research found that the circulating miRNAs derived from exosomes are a better cancer biomarker than the none one [68]. Despite the fact that the number of research was done exclusively on the non-exosomal circulating miRNAs to measure their performance as a cancer biomarker were very few when compared to the exosomal type, Researchers found that exosomal miRNAs are more efficient than non-exosomal miRNAs in terms of quality, quantity and stability [68].

miRNAs are Relevant Biomarkers in Cancer Diagnosis and Prognosis

miRNAs have emerged as very promising cancer biomarkers in recent years. In addition to their stability in different human body samples and ability to withstand the stressful conditions of preservation and recovery, miRNAs are considered better diagnostic and prognostic cancer biomarkers than previous ones. For examples, combination of miR-200a-3p, miR-766-3p, miR-26a-5p, miR-142-3p, let-7d-5p, miR-130b-3p and miR-328-3p are better than cancer antigen-125 (CA-125) as biomarker in diagnosis of early stages ovarian cancer [69]. It is well known that CA-125 is increased in other types of cancers like pancreatic and colorectal cancers. Also, it is elevated in some benign conditions like pelvic inflammatory disease and pregnancy. Thus, this marker has low specificity and sensitivity for diagnosis and follow-up patients with ovarian cancer. miRNAs show the ability to diagnose different histopathologic subtypes of ovarian cancer with high sensitivity and specificity. 0.761 (95% CI, 0.674-0.849), 0.759 and 0.698, respectively, for serous type ovarian cancer, 0.745 (95% CI, 0.622-0.870), 0.737 and 0.735, respectively, for clear-cell ovarian cancer, 0.808 (95% CI, 0.716-0.900), 0.769 and 0.754, respectively, for endometrioid ovarian cancer, and 0.822 (95% CI, 0.683-0.961), 0.727 and 0.833, respectively, for mucinous ovarian cancer [69].

miR-20b-5p, miR-28-3p, miR-192-5p, miR-223-3p, and miR-296-5p were identified as a panel for diagnosis of esophageal squamous cell carcinoma with more specificity and sensitivity than the previous biomarkers (carcinoembryonic antigen and squamous cell carcinoma antigen) which were used for diagnosis of this type of cancer [70]. It is understood that carcinoembryonic antigen and squamous cell carcinoma antigen are not effective to detect the early stages of this cancer and mostly elevated in stage III and stage IV of this disease. Furthermore, plasma level of miR-196a/b is more specific than CAE and CA19-9 in detection and follow-up the patients with gastric cancer [71].

MiRNAs as prognostic markers are proved to be a strong indicator of cancer progression and cancer outcome. Higher expression of miR-128, miR-139-5p, miR-382-5p, miR-410 and lower expression of miR-424-5p and miR-101-3p are specific biomarker for poor survival rate in the patients with hepatocellular carcinoma [72]. Currently, the fellow up of the patient with hepatocellular carcinoma which is the third most common deadly cancer is done by measuring the level of serum Alfa-fetoprotein (AFP), the biomarker with low specificity for this disease [73]. However, high level of serum miR-21 considers as potential biomarker and predictor of resistance to the docetaxel based chemotherapeutic treatment in patients with castrate resistant prostate cancer [74]. Combination of miRNAs to the validated biomarkers can increase the efficacy of these biomarkers as in case of combination of miR-141 to the PSA (prostate specific antigen) and LDH (lactate dehydrogenase) lead to increase the sensitivity of prediction the outcome of the patients with prostate cancer [75]. Moreover, patients with chronic lymphocytic leukemia and have high level of miR-21 and miR-155 are more vulnerable to die earlier than those with low level of these miRNAs [76]. Furthermore, down regulation of miR-206 and miR125a-5p and high level of miR-200c are indicator of poor prognosis in patient with gastric cancer [77, 78]. Therefore, we can infer that miRNAs in the human body samples can serve as reliable indicator for both cancer diagnosis and progression. They exceed the specificity and sensitivity of cancer markers which are currently in clinical use.

The following sections will summarize the research finding regarding the consideration of miRNAs as diagnostic and/or prognostic biomarkers in different types of cancers in the form of Table **2**. The information presented in these sections were selected from the relevant researches outcome associated with the entity [79 - 144]. The published literatures with good sample size from 100 patients and above except in some papers, which used a new sample for study like gastric juice sample, the robust techniques which were used in these paper like Quantitive Real Time PCR, research plan which involved more than one phase of study like the initiation phase and the approved phase, all are the criteria that we used to include in our discussion that will be of great value for subsequent clinical application in human cancer diagnosis and prognosis.

Table 2. The role of miRNAs as diagnostic and/ or prognostic markers in different types of cancers.

Cancers	miRmiRNAs	Samples Types	No. of Patients	References
Colorectal	miR-20-5p	FFPE	544	[79]
-	miR-155-5p	Fresh Frozen tissue	372	[80]
-	miR-19a	FFPE	275	[81]
-	miR-34a-5p	Fresh Frozen tissue	267	[82]
-	miR-139-5p	Fresh Frozen tissue	204	[83]
Breast	miR-505-5p	FFPE, Plasma	236	[84]
-	miR-96-5p	-	-	-
-	miR-93	FFPE	119	[85]
-	miR-21	FFPE	100	[86]
-	miR-142-3p	Tissue sample	101	-
-	miR-483-5p	(not specified)	-	-
-	miR-483-3p	-	-	-
Gastric	miR-16	Plasma	160	[87]
-	miR-451	-	-	-
-	miR-92a	-	-	-
-	miR-25	-	-	-
-	miR-486-5p	-	-	-
	miR-376c	Tissue sample	100	[88]
-	-	(not specified)	-	-
-	-	Plasma sample	-	-
-	-	Urine sample	-	-
-	miR-21	Tissue sample	42	[89]
-	miR-106a	(not specified)	-	-
-	-	Gastric juice sample	-	-

(Table 2) cont.....

Cancers	miRmiRNAs	Samples Types	No. of Patients	References
Esophageal	miR-34a-5p	Plasma sample	166	[90]
-	miR-148a-3p	-	-	-
-	miR-181a-5p	-	-	-
-	miR-9	Plasma sample	131	[91]
-	miR-8073	Serum Sample	566	[92]
-	miR-6820-5p	-	-	-
-	miR-6794-5p	-	-	-
-	miR-3196	-	-	-
-	miR-744-5p	-	-	-
-	miR-6799-5p	-	-	-
Liver	miR-122	Plasma Sample	400	[93]
-	miR-192	-	-	-
-	miR-21	-	-	-
-	miR-223	-	-	-
-	miR-26a	-	-	-
-	miR-27a	-	-	-
-	miR-801	-	-	-
-	miR-92a-3p	Serum Sample	115	[94]
-	miR-107	-	-	-
-	miR-3126-5p	-	-	-
-	miR-10b-5p	Tissue Sample	373	[95]
-	miR-10b-3p	-	-	-
-	miR-224-5p	-	-	-
-	miR-183-5p	-	-	-
-	miR-182-5p	-	-	-
Brain	miR-15b	Serum Sample	192	[96]
-	miR-23a	-	-	-
-	miR-133a	-	-	-
-	miR-150	-	-	-
-	miR-197	-	-	-
-	miR-497	-	-	-
-	miR-548b-5p	-	-	-
-	miR-21	CSF Sample Plasma Sample	129	[97-101]
-	miR-124	Tissue Sample	147	[102]

(Table 2) cont.....

Cancers	miRmiRNAs	Samples Types	No. of Patients	References
-	miR-9	-	-	-
-	miR-9	FFPE	100	[103]
Cervical	miR-145	Tissue Sample	251	[104]
-	miR-200c	(not specified)		
-	miR-218	-	-	-
-	miR-126-3p	Mucus Sample	230	[105]
-	miR -20b-5p	-	-	-
-	miR-451a	-	-	-
-	miR -144-3p	-	-	-
-	miR-30d-5p	Plasma Sample	301	[106]
-	miR let-7d-3p	-	-	-
-	miR-144	Tissue Sample	285	[107]
-	miR-147b	-	-	-
-	miR-218	-	-	-
-	miR-425	-	-	-
-	miR-451	-	-	-
-	miR-483	-	-	-
-	miR-486	-	-	-
Uterine	miR-4758	Tissue Sample	546	[108]
-	miR-876	-	-	-
-	miR-142	-	-	-
-	miR-190b	-	-	-
-	miR-6511b	Tissue Sample	463	[108]
-	miR-184	-	-	-
-	miR-4461	-	-	-
-	miR-205	Tissue Sample	100	[109]
Ovarian	miR-200a	Tissue Sample	100	[110]
-	miR-200b	(FFPE)		
-	miR-200c	-	-	-
-	miR-200b	Serum	163	[111]
-	miR-200c	-	-	-
-	miR-7	Serum	180	[112]
-	miR-25	-	-	-
-	miR-93	-	-	-

(Table 2) cont.....

Cancers	miRmiRNAs	Samples Types	No. of Patients	References
-	miR-429	-	-	-
-	miR-532-5p	Tissue Sample	145	[113]
Prostate	miR-21	Plasma	100	[114]
-	miR-221	-	-	-
-	miR-365a-3p	Serum	178	[115]
-	miR-4286,	-	-	-
-	miR-424-5p	-	-	-
-	miR-27a-3p	-	-	-
-	miR-29b-3p	-	-	-
-	miR-511-3p	Tissue Sample	183	[116]
-	miR-191	Tissue Sample	146	[117]
Skin	miR-16	Tissue Sample	186	[118]
-	miR-211	(FFPE)	-	-
-	miR-4487	-	-	-
-	miR-4706	Serum Sample	255	[118]
-	miR-4731	-	-	-
-	miR-509-3p	-	-	-
-	miR-514a	-	-	-
-	miR-10b	Tissue Sample	101	[119]
-	miR-200b	(FFPE)	-	-
-	miR-106b-5p	Tissue Sample	154	[120]
-	miR-148a-3p	(FFPE)	-	-
-	miR-338-3p	-	-	-
Hepatic	miR-22	Serum	108	[121]
-	miR-375	Serum	149	[122]
-	miR-10a	-	-	-
-	miR-122	-	-	-
-	miR-423	-	-	-
-	miR-21	Plasma	136	[123]
-	miR-137	Tissue Sample	110	[124]
Testicular	miR-371a-3p	Serum	106	[125]
-	miR-367-3p	-	-	-
-	miR-371a-3p	Serum	616	[126]
-	miR-519	Tissue Sample	137	[127]

(Table 2) cont.....

Cancers	miRmiRNAs	Samples Types	No. of Patients	References
-	miR-375	(Fresh Frozen)	-	-
-	miR-371a-3p	-	-	-
-	miR371	Plasma	111	[128]
-	miR-429	Bone Marrow	126	[129]
-	miR-181a-3p	Whole blood	119	[130]
-	miR-216b	Bone Marrow	115	[130]
-	miR-193b-3p	Bone Marrow	348	[131]
-	miR-155	Blood Sample	111	[132]
-	miR-532	Plasma	198	[133]
Thyroid	miR-222	Tissue sample	126	[134]
-	miR-15a	(fresh frozen)	-	-
-	miR-222	Serum	106	[135]
-	miR-221	-	-	-
-	miR-146b	-	-	-
-	miR-136	Tissue sample	267	[136]
-	miR-21	(fresh frozen	-	-
-	miR-127	FFPE	-	-
Lung	miR-22,	Serum	127	[137]
-	miR-126	-	-	-
-	miR-141	Serum	108	[138]
-	miR-22,	Serum	120	[139]
-	miR15b	-	-	-
Nasopharyngeal	-	-	-	-
-	miR-22	Serum	512	[140]
-	miR-572	-	-	-
-	miR-638	-	-	-
-	miR-1234	-	-	-
-	miR-188-5p	Whole Blood	120	[141]
-	miR-4790-3p	-	-	-
-	miR-548q	Plasma and	165	[142]
-	miR-483-5p	Tissue sample	-	-
Pancreatic	miR-10b	FNA	95	[143]
-	miR-20a	Serum	197	[144]
-	miR-21	-	-	-

(Table 2) cont.....

Cancers	miRmiRNAs	Samples Types	No. of Patients	References
-	miR-24	-	-	-
-	miR-25	-	-	-
-	miR-99a	-	-	-
-	miR-185	-	-	-
-	miR-191	-	-	-

Commercialized miRNAs, which are Currently in Clinical Practice as Diagnostic Markers

Some miRNAs enter the market in the United State of America as diagnostic biomarkers for certain types of cancers. Several diagnostic tests are developed by Rosetta Genomics, a molecular diagnostic company that uses miRNAs to diagnose different cancers [145]. The diagnostic tests which are developed by this company and currently are in clinical use, as given below:

miRview Meso Test

miRview meso test is the first test, which was started to be used by clinicians in USA in 2011 and used to differentiate Malignant Pleural Mesothelioma (MPM), a cancer connected to asbestos exposure, from other carcinomas in the lung using FFPE (Formalin Fixed Paraffin Embedded) samples [146, 147]. The importance of this test is attributed to the fact that there is no single diagnostic test that is entirely exclusive for the differentiation of MPM from other carcinomas of the lung [148]. In addition, pathologic diagnosis suffers from significant inter-observer variation [149]. In the absence of a single specific and reliable marker, mesothelioma can be difficult to identify from other cancers. miRview meso test is a highly accurate test that may assist physicians to rule out mesothelioma in patients diagnosed with adenocarcinoma in the lung which has been exposed to mesothelioma-related substances [150]. This test was developed according to the research findings, in which the authors identified that Hsa-miR-193a-3p was overexpressed in MPM, while hsa-miR-200c and hsa-miR-192 were overexpressed in peripheral lung adenocarcinoma and carcinomas that frequently metastasize to lung pleura [151]. The assay reached a sensitivity of 100% and a specificity of 94% [151].

miRview Squamous

miRview squamous is a molecular diagnostic that depends on the using a single miRNA (has-miR-205) to differentiate squamous from non-squamous Non-Small Cell Lung Cancer (NSCLC) started to commercialize in USA in 2011 by Rosetta

Genomics [152]. This test depends on the fact that has-miR-205 is a highly specific marker for squamous cell carcinoma of lung cancer, the sensitivity of this test reaches 96% and specificity of 90% [152]. The accurate diagnosis of squamous type from other types of NSCLC was challenging due to the difference in the readings among individual pathologists and the heterogeneity of this cancer [152]. In addition, immunohistochemical markers currently used for this differentiation like p63 is a sensitive marker but is not a highly specific test because 30% of adenocarcinomas and 37% of large cell undifferentiated carcinomas also express this marker [153]. Moreover, the other markers of squamous cell cancers, like cytokeratin 14, are of low sensitivity for squamous cell carcinoma of lung cancer; its sensitivity is 53% [154].

Accurate diagnosis of squamous cell carcinoma of lung cancer is important to start a suitable therapeutic treatment. Some newly developed therapies, which are currently in clinical use for the treatment of lung cancers, have potential risk in patients with such a subclass of this cancer. From these targeted therapies are tumor angiogenesis inhibitors which can cause pulmonary hemorrhage in those patients [155]. Currently, miRview squamous test can be performed before surgical resection of lung cancer and treatment of this cancer can be started before surgery because this test can perform by using Fine Needle Aspirate (FNA) biopsy and provide very accurate results [156].

miRview Lung

Lung cancer is one of the most common causes of cancer-related death. It is classified into four main types: squamous cell carcinoma and non-squamous non–small cell lung cancer, carcinoid, and small cell carcinoma. miRview lung test depends on the measurement of the expression level of eight miRNAs to diagnose all lung cancer subtypes using Quantitive-Real Time PCR [156]. Final approval of using this diagnostic test in all 50 states of the USA was approved in November 2012 [156]. Cytologic samples (fine-needle aspiration and bronchial brushing and washing) and histologic samples can be used for this assay with the same performance [157]. Thus, this test is simple, reliable and can be used preoperatively to allow the decision of therapeutic treatment as soon as possible. This test comes with an accuracy of 94% in the diagnosis of all lung cancer subtypes and resolves the discrepancy amongst the pathologist in their definitive diagnosis [157]. Studies show that the number of lung cancer cases that were classified correctly by routine examination of cytopathologists was 66% for adenocarcinoma and 53% for squamous cell carcinoma [158]. In addition, immumohistochemical test like p63 faced limitations as a diagnostic marker in lung cancer due to low specificity and sensitivity [158].

Reaching the right diagnosis and accurate identification of lung cancer subtypes is very important because of the differences in the therapeutic regime for each subtype. For example, small cell lung cancer is a very aggressive disease treated by chemotherapeutic agents. The patients do not benefit from the surgical resection, in reverse to the carcinoid subtype, which is a low-grade malignancy and can be treated by surgery [159]. Moreover, Avastin, which is used commonly in the treatment of a non-squamous type of non-small cell lung cancer, is contraindicated in patients with a squamous type of non-small cell lung cancer because of 30% mortality in those patients [160].

miRview Mets

The routine pathologic tests fail to locate the primary origin of secondary metastasis in 2%-5% of the patients, and this is called cancer of unknown primary origin (CUP) which is characterized by early and aggressive metastasis [161]. Immunohistochemistry is the available diagnostic assay for CUP, however, this assay fails to identify the origin of cancer in 30% of the patients [162]. miRview mets is a test that uses miRNAs to identify the primary origin of secondary metastasis cancer (Table **1**). The second generation of this assay entered the marketing field in USA in 2014 and depends on the measurement of 64 miRNAs to identify the primary origin of metastatic cancers [163]. The test diagnoses 42 types of cancers with sensitivity and specificity up to 90% and 99%, respectively [163]. The test was performed by using tissue samples, RNA Microarray, and Quantitative Real-Time PCR. Some miRNAs which are used in this test and the types of cancer identified are summarized in Table **1** [163].

miRview Kidney

This test identifies the four main subtypes of renal cell carcinoma (clear cell, papillary, chromophobe, and oncocytoma) with a specificity of 98% and sensitivity of 95% by using 24 different miRNAs [164]. Some of these miRNAs are shown in Table **3**. It has been in clinical use in USA since 2014. The measurement level of these miRNAs is performed on a microarray platform using FFPE samples [164]. Finding a reliable biomarker to accurately determine the four main subtypes of renal cell carcinoma is in demand because of the differences in the responses of renal cell carcinoma subtypes to the current and future targeted therapies. The four main subtypes of renal cell carcinoma and their classification using miRNAs-based assay are shown in Fig. (**1**) [164].

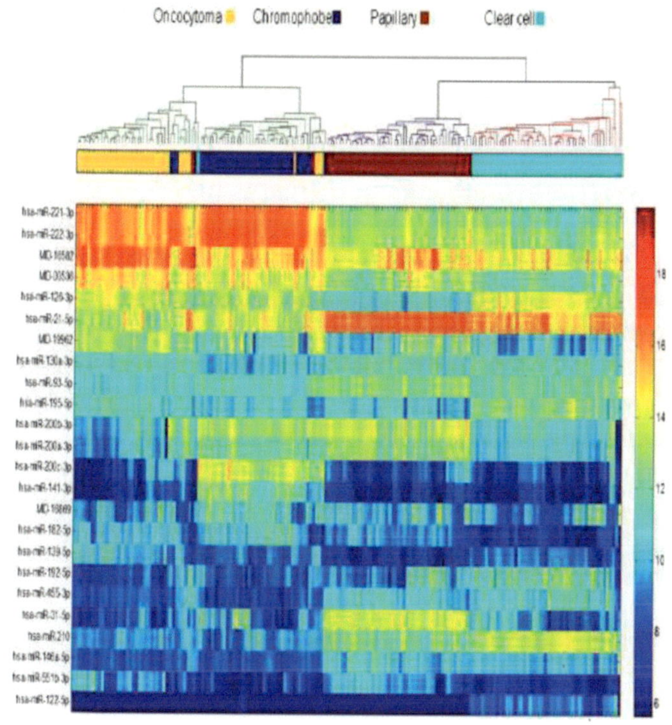

Fig. (1). miRNAs based test to sub classify renal cell carcinomas. The figure **shows** that four main types of this type of cancer (clear cell, papillary, chromophobe, and oncocytoma) can be diagnose by using 24 panels of miRNAs and giving different colors by using Agilent miRNAs microarray platform.

Table 3. miRNAs used to differentiate subtypes of renal cell carcinoma with their nucleotides sequences.

MiRNAs	Sequences
hsa-miR-106a	5′-AAAAGTGCTTACAGTGCAGGTAG-3′
hsa miR-125a-5p	5′-TCCCTGAGACCCTTTAACCTGTGA-3′
hsa-miR-129-3p	5′-AAGCCCTTACCCCAAAAAGCAT-3′
hsa-miR-205	5′-TCCTTCATTCCACCGGAGTCTG-3′
hsa-miR-21	5′-TAGCTTATCAGACTGATGTTGA-3′
hsa-miR-29b	5′-TAGCACCATTTGAAATCAGTGTT-3′
hsa-miR-375	5′-TTTGTTCGTTCGGCTCGCGTGA-3′
hsa-miR-7	5′-TGGAAGACTAGTGATTTTGTTGT-3′

Mirnas as Crucial Regulatory Marker in Epithelial-Mesenchymal Transition Process

It is well known that the epithelial-mesenchymal transition (EMT) process is a process that leads to cancer stem cell formation, cancer invasion and metastasis, and cancer resistance to chemotherapeutic treatment. The role of non-coding RNAs in EMT has been identified by demonstrating the crucial regulatory functions of several miRNAs in this complex program (Fig. **2**). miR-200 family (miR-200a, miR-200b, miR-200c, miR-141, and miR-429) and miR-205 are the first robust discovered regulatory miRNAs of EMT [165]. Expression of miR-200 family associated strongly with epithelial differentiation. In addition, there is a reciprocal feedback loop between these microRNAs and the transcriptional factors Zinc finger E-box binding family (ZEB); transcription factors of this program [166]. miR-200 family targeting *E-cadherin* (CDH1) and *vimentin* (VIM) of EMT components during the regulatory process [167]. Moreover, miR-34 family members directly control *Snail 1*(SNAI1)-dependent EMT [168, 169]. Also, miR-23a participates in FasL (Fas ligand) -induced EMT process by inhibiting E-Cadherin [170].

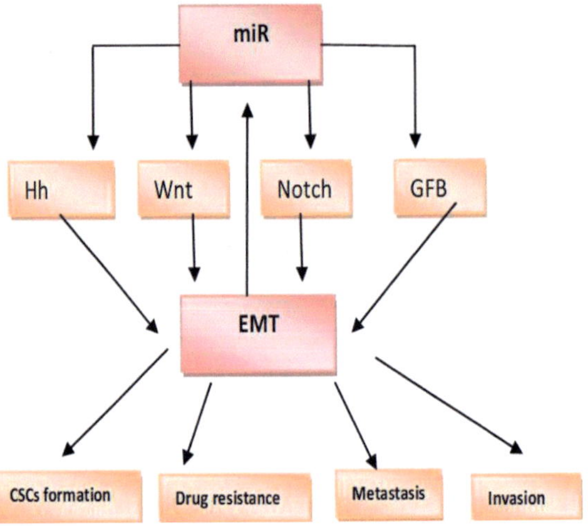

Fig. (2). Role of microRNAs in EMT. There are reciprocal regulatory functions between miRNAs and EMT inducers, miRNAs can regulate different EMT signalling pathways, inturn EMT inducers can modulate the function of these genetic molecules, which again regulate the EMT signalling pathways.

miR-21 proposed to regulate the EMT and CSCs in breast cancer; the study shows that depletion of miR-21 lead to decrease CSCs numbers by targeting *PTEN* [171]. miR-106-25 cluster was identified as a potential regulator of EMT by targeting *Smad 7* in breast cancer which ultimately led to initiate cells with stem cell characteristics [172]. Let 7d negatively regulate the EMT by targeting *Twist* and *Snail* in human oral squamous cell carcinoma; therefore, downregulation of this microRNA will enhance cancer invasiveness and resistance to chemotherapy [173]. To maintain a proper number of stem cells that are required to ensure the self-renewal of normal stem cells, Asymmetrical cell division (ACD) is necessary, and this is achieved by several EMT inducers [174].

In colonic cancer, *Snail*, considered an inducer of EMT, is responsible for shifting the ACD to symmetrical cell division (SCD) and acquiring colon CSCs characters [174]. *Snail* initiates the expression of miR-146a through the B-catenin-TCF4 (transcription factor 4) complex; this miRNA, in turn, targets *Numb* to stabilize B-catenin and maintain Wnt and SCD activity [174]. Additionally, the level of Snail expression in CD44+ cells of human colonic cancer HCT-15 and HCT-116 is high and correlates inversely with the level of miR-203 [175]. In the same study, the authors express the mechanism of regulation EMT, which is dependent on the interaction of EMT initiator with the miR-203 promoter region [175]. *Snail* suppressed the activity of the miR-203 promoter. In addition to that, E-box elements, which are located upstream of the transcription start site of miR-203, are crucial for *Snail*-mediated repression of miR-203 promoter activity [175]. Deregulation of miRNAs expressions play a role in initiating and maintaining the stemness features through the EMT process by involving several regulatory signals.

CONCLUSION

Short non-coding RNAs (miRNAs) play essential roles in cancer development and progression. The availability of these substances in different types of human body samples and the stability of them in these samples make these structures very promising for cancer detection and follow-up. Some of these molecules started to be used clinically in some countries, showing high sensitivity and specificity in cancer diagnosis and prognosis.

CONSENT FOR PUBLICATION

Not applicable.

CONFLICT OF INTEREST

The author declares no conflict of interest, financial or otherwise.

ACKNOWLEDGEMENT

The author thanks the Department of Pathology and Forensic Medicine, School of Medicine, University of Babylon, Iraq, for providing the technical facilities of the work.

REFERENCES

[1] Goossens N, Nakagawa S, Sun X, Hoshida Y. Cancer biomarker discovery and validation. Transl Cancer Res 2015; 4(3): 256-69.
[PMID: 26213686]

[2] Slamon DJ, Leyland-Jones B, Shak S, *et al.* Use of chemotherapy plus a monoclonal antibody against HER2 for metastatic breast cancer that overexpresses HER2. N Engl J Med 2001; 344(11): 783-92.
[http://dx.doi.org/10.1056/NEJM200103153441101] [PMID: 11248153]

[3] Piccart-Gebhart MJ, Procter M, Leyland-Jones B, *et al.* Trastuzumab after adjuvant chemotherapy in HER2-positive breast cancer. N Engl J Med 2005; 353(16): 1659-72.
[http://dx.doi.org/10.1056/NEJMoa052306] [PMID: 16236737]

[4] Adhyam M, Gupta AK. A Review on the Clinical Utility of PSA in Cancer Prostate. Indian J Surg Oncol 2012; 3(2): 120-9.
[http://dx.doi.org/10.1007/s13193-012-0142-6] [PMID: 23730101]

[5] Hasan S, Jacob R, Manne U, Paluri R. Advances in pancreatic cancer biomarkers. Oncol Rev 2019; 13(1): 410.
[http://dx.doi.org/10.4081/oncol.2019.410] [PMID: 31044028]

[6] Bird A. Perceptions of epigenetics. Nature 2007; 447(7143): 396-8.
[http://dx.doi.org/10.1038/nature05913] [PMID: 17522671]

[7] Mazzone R, Zwergel C, Artico M, *et al.* The emerging role of epigenetics in human autoimmune disorders Clin Epigenetics 2019; 26: 11:34.
[http://dx.doi.org/10.1186/s13148-019-0632-2]

[8] Kim SS, Lee SV. Non-Coding RNAs in *Caenorhabditis elegans* Aging. Mol Cells 2019; 42(5): 379-85.
[PMID: 31094164]

[9] Jansson MD, Lund AH. MicroRNA and cancer. Mol Oncol 2012; 6(6): 590-610.
[http://dx.doi.org/10.1016/j.molonc.2012.09.006] [PMID: 23102669]

[10] Maroof H, Salajegheh A, Smith RA, Lam AKY. Role of microRNA-34 family in cancer with particular reference to cancer angiogenesis. Exp Mol Pathol 2014; 97(2): 298-304.
[http://dx.doi.org/10.1016/j.yexmp.2014.08.002] [PMID: 25102298]

[11] Liu C, Tang DG. MicroRNA regulation of cancer stem cells. Cancer Res 2011; 71(18): 5950-4.
[http://dx.doi.org/10.1158/0008-5472.CAN-11-1035] [PMID: 21917736]

[12] Zhou N, Mo YY. Roles of microRNAs in cancer stem cells. Front Biosci (Schol Ed) 2012; 4(3): 810-8.
[PMID: 22202092]

[13] Takahashi R, Miyazaki H, Ochiya T. The role of microRNAs in the regulation of cancer stem cells. Front Genet 2014; 4: 295.
[http://dx.doi.org/10.3389/fgene.2013.00295] [PMID: 24427168]

[14] Filipowicz W, Bhattacharyya SN, Sonenberg N. Mechanisms of post-transcriptional regulation by microRNAs: are the answers in sight? Nat Rev Genet 2008; 9(2): 102-14.
[http://dx.doi.org/10.1038/nrg2290] [PMID: 18197166]

[15] Mamoori A, Gopalan V, Smith RA, Lam AKY. Modulatory roles of microRNAs in the regulation of different signalling pathways in large bowel cancer stem cells. Biol Cell 2016; 108(3): 51-64.
[http://dx.doi.org/10.1111/boc.201500062] [PMID: 26712035]

[16] Peters L, Meister G. Argonaute proteins: mediators of RNA silencing. Mol Cell 2007; 26(5): 611-23.
[http://dx.doi.org/10.1016/j.molcel.2007.05.001] [PMID: 17560368]

[17] Tolia NH, Joshua-Tor L. Slicer and the Argonautes. Nat Chem Biol 2007; 3(1): 36-43.
[http://dx.doi.org/10.1038/nchembio848] [PMID: 17173028]

[18] Grimson A, Farch K, Johnston WK. Garrett- Engele P, Lim LP, Bartel DP. MicroRNA Targeting Specifity in mammals: determinants beyond seed pairing. Mol Cell 2007; 27: 91-105. [http://dx.doi.org/10.1016/j.molcel.2007.06.017] [PMID: 17612493]

[19] Doench JG, Sharp PA. Specificity of microRNA target selection in translational repression. Genes Dev 2004; 18(5): 504-11. [http://dx.doi.org/10.1101/gad.1184404] [PMID: 15014042]

[20] Brennecl J, Stark A, Russell RB, Cohen SM. Principle of micro RNA-target recognition. PLoS Biol 2005; 3: 404-18.

[21] Carthew RW, Sontheimer EJ. Origins and Mechanisms of miRNAs and siRNAs. Cell 2009; 136(4): 642-55. [http://dx.doi.org/10.1016/j.cell.2009.01.035] [PMID: 19239886]

[22] Ameres SL, Zamore PD. Diversifying microRNA sequence and function. Nat Rev Mol Cell Biol 2013; 14(8): 475-88. [http://dx.doi.org/10.1038/nrm3611] [PMID: 23800994]

[23] Wilczynska A, Bushell M. The complexity of miRNA-mediated repression. Cell Death Differ 2015; 22(1): 22-33. [http://dx.doi.org/10.1038/cdd.2014.112] [PMID: 25190144]

[24] Salmena L, Poliseno L, Tay Y, Kats L, Pandolfi PP. A ceRNA hypothesis: the Rosetta Stone of a hidden RNA language? Cell 2011; 146(3): 353-8. [http://dx.doi.org/10.1016/j.cell.2011.07.014] [PMID: 21802130]

[25] Sarver AL, Subramanian S. Competing endogenous RNA database. Bioinformation 2012; 8(15): 731-3. [http://dx.doi.org/10.6026/97320630008731] [PMID: 23055620]

[26] Poliseno L, Salmena L, Zhang J, Carver B, Haveman WJ, Pandolfi PP. A coding-independent function of gene and pseudogene mRNAs regulates tumour biology. Nature 2010; 465(7301): 1033-8. [http://dx.doi.org/10.1038/nature09144] [PMID: 20577206]

[27] Wang Z, Ahmad A, Li Y, Azmi AS, Miele L, Sarkar FH. Targeting notch to eradicate pancreatic cancer stem cells for cancer therapy. Anticancer Res 2011; 31(4): 1105-13. [PMID: 21508353]

[28] Meyer KD, Saletore Y, Zumbo P, Elemento O, Mason CE, Jaffrey SR. Comprehensive analysis of mRNA methylation reveals enrichment in 3′ UTRs and near stop codons. Cell 2012; 149(7): 1635-46. [http://dx.doi.org/10.1016/j.cell.2012.05.003] [PMID: 22608085]

[29] Niu Y, Zhao X. WuYS, Li MM, Wang XJ, Yang YG. N6 methyl-adenosine(m6A) in RAN: An old modification with a novel epigenetic function. Genomics Proteomics Bioinformatics 2013; 11: 8-17. [http://dx.doi.org/10.1016/j.gpb.2012.12.002] [PMID: 23453015]

[30] Alles J, Fehlmann T, Fischer U, *et al.* An estimate of the total number of true human miRNAs. Nucleic Acids Res 2019; 47(7): 3353-64. [http://dx.doi.org/10.1093/nar/gkz097] [PMID: 30820533]

[31] Matin F, Jeet V, Clements JA, Yousef GM, Batra J. MicroRNA Theranostics in Prostate Cancer Precision Medicine. Clin Chem 2016; 62(10): 1318-33. [http://dx.doi.org/10.1373/clinchem.2015.242800] [PMID: 27540032]

[32] Leclercq M, Diallo AB, Blanchette M. Prediction of human miRNA target genes using computationally reconstructed ancestral mammalian sequences. Nucleic Acids Res. 2017; 45: 556–566. Nucleic Acids Res 2019; 2347: 3353-64.

[33] Mamoori A, Wahab R, Islam F, *et al.* Clinical and biological significance of miR-193a-3p targeted KRAS in colorectal cancer pathogenesis. Hum Pathol 2018; 71: 145-56. [http://dx.doi.org/10.1016/j.humpath.2017.10.024] [PMID: 29104111]

[34] Calin GA, Sevignani C, Dumitru CD, *et al.* Human microRNA genes are frequently located at fragile sites and genomic regions involved in cancers. Proc Natl Acad Sci USA 2004; 101(9): 2999-3004. [http://dx.doi.org/10.1073/pnas.0307323101] [PMID: 14973191]

[35] van Rooij E, Sutherland LB, Liu N, *et al.* A signature pattern of stress-responsive microRNAs that can evoke cardiac hypertrophy and heart failure. Proc Natl Acad Sci USA 2006; 103(48): 18255-60. [http://dx.doi.org/10.1073/pnas.0608791103] [PMID: 17108080]

[36] Esquela-Kerscher A, Slack FJ. Oncomirs — microRNAs with a role in cancer. Nat Rev Cancer 2006; 6(4): 259-69. [http://dx.doi.org/10.1038/nrc1840] [PMID: 16557279]

[37] Landgraf P, Rusu M, Sheridan R, *et al.* A mammalian microRNA expression atlas based on small RNA library sequencing. Cell 2007; 129(7): 1401-14. [http://dx.doi.org/10.1016/j.cell.2007.04.040] [PMID: 17604727]

[38] Ludwig N, Leidinger P, Becker K, *et al.* Distribution of miRNA expression across human tissues. Nucleic Acids Res 2016; 44(8): 3865-77. [http://dx.doi.org/10.1093/nar/gkw116] [PMID: 26921406]

[39] Swierniak M, Wojcicka A, Czetwertynska M, *et al.* In-depth characterization of the microRNA transcriptome in normal thyroid and papillary thyroid carcinoma. J Clin Endocrinol Metab 2013; 98(8): E1401-9. [http://dx.doi.org/10.1210/jc.2013-1214] [PMID: 23783103]

[40] Callis TE, Chen JF, Wang DZ. MicroRNAs in skeletal and cardiac muscle development. DNA Cell Biol 2007; 26(4): 219-25. [http://dx.doi.org/10.1089/dna.2006.0556] [PMID: 17465888]

[41] Thum T, Catalucci D, Bauersachs J. MicroRNAs: novel regulators in cardiac development and disease. Cardiovasc Res 2008; 79(4): 562-70. [http://dx.doi.org/10.1093/cvr/cvn137] [PMID: 18511432]

[42] Leidinger P, Backes C, Blatt M, *et al.* The blood-borne miRNA signature of lung cancer patients is independent of histology but influenced by metastases. Mol Cancer 2014; 13(1): 202. [http://dx.doi.org/10.1186/1476-4598-13-202] [PMID: 25175044]

[43] Ludwig N, Nourkami-Tutdibi N, Backes C, *et al.* Circulating serum miRNAs as potential biomarkers for nephroblastoma. Pediatr Blood Cancer 2015; 62(8): 1360-7. [http://dx.doi.org/10.1002/pbc.25481] [PMID: 25787821]

[44] Leidinger P, Galata V, Backes C, *et al.* Longitudinal study on circulating miRNAs in patients after lung cancer resection. Oncotarget 2015; 6(18): 16674-85. [http://dx.doi.org/10.18632/oncotarget.4322] [PMID: 26078336]

[45] Leidinger P, Backes C, Meder B, Meese E, Keller A. The human miRNA repertoire of different blood compounds. BMC Genomics 2014; 15(1): 474. [http://dx.doi.org/10.1186/1471-2164-15-474] [PMID: 24928098]

[46] Sohel MMH. Circulating microRNAs as biomarkers in cancer diagnosis. Life Sci 2020; 248: 117473. [http://dx.doi.org/10.1016/j.lfs.2020.117473] [PMID: 32114007]

[47] Mamoori A, Wahab R, Islam F, *et al.* Clinical and biological significance of miR-193a-3p targeted KRAS in colorectal cancer pathogenesis. Hum Pathol 2018; 71: 145-56. [http://dx.doi.org/10.1016/j.humpath.2017.10.024] [PMID: 29104111]

[48] Akbulut H, Ersoy YE, Coskunpinar E, *et al.* The role of miRNAs as a predictor of multicentricity in breast cancer. Mol Biol Rep 2019; 46(2): 1787-96. [http://dx.doi.org/10.1007/s11033-019-04629-6] [PMID: 30707415]

[49] Zhu Y, Li T, Chen G, *et al.* Identification of a serum microRNA expression signature for detection of lung cancer, involving miR-23b, miR-221, miR-148b and miR-423-3p. Lung Cancer 2017; 114: 6-11.

[http://dx.doi.org/10.1016/j.lungcan.2017.10.002] [PMID: 29173767]

[50] Zeng B, Zhang X, Zhao J, *et al.* The role of DNMT1/hsa-miR-124-3p/BCAT1 pathway in regulating growth and invasion of esophageal squamous cell carcinoma. BMC Cancer 2019; 19(1): 609. [http://dx.doi.org/10.1186/s12885-019-5815-x] [PMID: 31226958]

[51] Yin X, Huo Z, Yan S, *et al.* MiR-205 inhibits sporadic vestibular schwannoma cells proliferation by targeting cyclin-dependent kinase 14. World Neurosurg. 2020; S1878-8750(20): 32418-9.

[52] Liu J, Liu B, Guo Y, *et al.* Key miRNAs and target genes played roles in the development of clear cell renal cell carcinoma. Cancer Biomark 2018; 23(2): 279-90. [http://dx.doi.org/10.3233/CBM-181558] [PMID: 30198869]

[53] Wang WM, Wu C, Jin HZ. Exosomes in chronic inflammatory skin diseases and skin tumors. Exp Dermatol 2019; 28(3): 213-8. [PMID: 30537027]

[54] Peiró-Chova L, Peña-Chilet M, López-Guerrero JA, *et al.* High stability of microRNAs in tissue samples of compromised quality. Virchows Arch 2013; 463(6): 765-74. [http://dx.doi.org/10.1007/s00428-013-1485-2] [PMID: 24197449]

[55] de Biase D, Visani M, Morandi L, *et al.* miRNAs expression analysis in paired fresh/frozen and dissected formalin fixed and paraffin embedded glioblastoma using real-time pCR. PLoS One 2012; 7(4): e35596. [http://dx.doi.org/10.1371/journal.pone.0035596] [PMID: 22530056]

[56] Cui M, Wang H, Yao X, *et al.* Circulating MicroRNAs in Cancer: Potential and Challenge. Front Genet 2019; 10: 626. [http://dx.doi.org/10.3389/fgene.2019.00626] [PMID: 31379918]

[57] Arroyo JD, Chevillet JR, Kroh EM, *et al.* Argonaute2 complexes carry a population of circulating microRNAs independent of vesicles in human plasma. Proc Natl Acad Sci USA 2011; 108(12): 5003-8. [http://dx.doi.org/10.1073/pnas.1019055108] [PMID: 21383194]

[58] Diener C, Galata V, Keller A, Meese E. MicroRNA profiling from dried blood samples. Crit Rev Clin Lab Sci 2019; 56(2): 111-7. [http://dx.doi.org/10.1080/10408363.2018.1561641] [PMID: 30696311]

[59] Ponnusamy V, Kapellou O, Yip E, *et al.* A study of microRNAs from dried blood spots in newborns after perinatal asphyxia: a simple and feasible biosampling method. Pediatr Res 2016; 79(5): 799-805. [http://dx.doi.org/10.1038/pr.2015.276] [PMID: 26720606]

[60] Li BX, Yu Q, Shi ZL, Li P, Fu S. Circulating microRNAs in esophageal squamous cell carcinoma: association with locoregional staging and survival. Int J Clin Exp Med 2015; 8(5): 7241-50. [PMID: 26221263]

[61] Rapado-González Ó, Majem B, Muinelo-Romay L, *et al.* Human salivary microRNAs in Cancer. J Cancer 2018; 9(4): 638-49. [http://dx.doi.org/10.7150/jca.21180] [PMID: 29556321]

[62] Duz MB, Karatas OF, Guzel E, *et al.* Identification of miR-139-5p as a saliva biomarker for tongue squamous cell carcinoma: a pilot study. Cell Oncol (Dordr) 2016; 39(2): 187-93. [http://dx.doi.org/10.1007/s13402-015-0259-z] [PMID: 26650483]

[63] Humeau M, Vignolle-Vidoni A, Sicard F, *et al.* Salivary microRNA in pancreatic cancer patients. PLoS One 2015; 10(6): e0130996. [http://dx.doi.org/10.1371/journal.pone.0130996] [PMID: 26121640]

[64] Zhao C, Sun X, Li L. Biogenesis and function of extracellular miRNAs. ExRNA 2019; 1(1): 38. [http://dx.doi.org/10.1186/s41544-019-0039-4]

[65] Hurley JH. ESCRT complexes and the biogenesis of multivesicular bodies. Curr Opin Cell Biol 2008;

20(1): 4-11.
[http://dx.doi.org/10.1016/j.ceb.2007.12.002] [PMID: 18222686]

[66] Williams RL, Urbé S. The emerging shape of the ESCRT machinery. Nat Rev Mol Cell Biol 2007; 8(5): 355-68.
[http://dx.doi.org/10.1038/nrm2162] [PMID: 17450176]

[67] Vickers KC, Palmisano BT, Shoucri BM, Shamburek RD, Remaley AT. MicroRNAs are transported in plasma and delivered to recipient cells by high-density lipoproteins. Nat Cell Biol 2011; 13(4): 423-33.
[http://dx.doi.org/10.1038/ncb2210] [PMID: 21423178]

[68] Nik Mohamed Kamal NNSB, Shahidan WNS. Non-Exosomal and Exosomal Circulatory MicroRNAs: Which Are More Valid as Biomarkers? Front Pharmacol 2020; 10: 1500.
[http://dx.doi.org/10.3389/fphar.2019.01500] [PMID: 32038230]

[69] Yokoi A, Yoshioka Y, Hirakawa A, *et al.* A combination of circulating miRNAs for the early detection of ovarian cancer. Oncotarget 2017; 8(52): 89811-23.
[http://dx.doi.org/10.18632/oncotarget.20688] [PMID: 29163790]

[70] Huang Z, Zhang L, Zhu D, *et al.* A novel serum microRNA signature to screen esophageal squamous cell carcinoma. Cancer Med 2017; 6(1): 109-19.
[http://dx.doi.org/10.1002/cam4.973] [PMID: 28035762]

[71] Tsai MM, Wang CS, Tsai CY, *et al.* Circulating microRNA-196a/b are novel biomarkers associated with metastatic gastric cancer. Eur J Cancer 2016; 64: 137-48.
[http://dx.doi.org/10.1016/j.ejca.2016.05.007] [PMID: 27420607]

[72] Di Bisceglie AM, Sterling RK, Chung RT, *et al.* Serum alpha-fetoprotein levels in patients with advanced hepatitis C: Results from the HALT-C Trial. J Hepatol 2005; 43(3): 434-41.
[http://dx.doi.org/10.1016/j.jhep.2005.03.019] [PMID: 16136646]

[73] Mirzaei H, Sahebkar A, Mohammadi M, *et al.* Circulating microRNAs in Hepatocellular Carcinoma: Potential Diagnostic and Prognostic Biomarkers. Curr Pharm Des 2016; 22(34): 5257-69.
[http://dx.doi.org/10.2174/1381612822666160303110838] [PMID: 26935703]

[74] Mekhail SM, Yousef PG, Jackinsky SW, Pasic M, Yousef GM. miRNA in Prostate Cancer: New Prospects for Old Challenges. EJIFCC 2014; 25(1): 79-98.
[PMID: 27683458]

[75] Gonzales JC, Fink LM, Goodman OB Jr, Symanowski JT, Vogelzang NJ, Ward DC. Comparison of circulating MicroRNA 141 to circulating tumor cells, lactate dehydrogenase, and prostate-specific antigen for determining treatment response in patients with metastatic prostate cancer. Clin Genitourin Cancer 2011; 9(1): 39-45.
[http://dx.doi.org/10.1016/j.clgc.2011.05.008] [PMID: 21723797]

[76] Balatti V, Pekarky Y, Croce CM. Role of microRNA in chronic lymphocytic leukemia onset and progression. J Hematol Oncol 2015; 8(1): 12.
[http://dx.doi.org/10.1186/s13045-015-0112-x] [PMID: 25886051]

[77] Yang Q, Zhang C, Huang B, *et al.* Downregulation of microRNA-206 is a potent prognostic marker for patients with gastric cancer. Eur J Gastroenterol Hepatol 2013; 25(8): 953-7.
[http://dx.doi.org/10.1097/MEG.0b013e32835ed691] [PMID: 23751352]

[78] Nishida N, Mimori K, Fabbri M, *et al.* MicroRNA-125a-5p is an independent prognostic factor in gastric cancer and inhibits the proliferation of human gastric cancer cells in combination with trastuzumab. Clin Cancer Res 2011; 17(9): 2725-33.
[http://dx.doi.org/10.1158/1078-0432.CCR-10-2132] [PMID: 21220473]

[79] Cheng D, Zhao S, Tang H, *et al.* MicroRNA-20a-5p promotes colorectal cancer invasion and metastasis by downregulating Smad4. Oncotarget 2016; 7(29): 45199-213.
[http://dx.doi.org/10.18632/oncotarget.9900] [PMID: 27286257]

[80] Qu YL, Wang HF, Sun ZQ, *et al.* Up-regulated miR-155-5p promotes cell proliferation, invasion and metastasis in colorectal carcinoma. Int J Clin Exp Pathol 2015; 8(6): 6988-94. [PMID: 26261588]

[81] Huang L, Wang X, Wen C, *et al.* Hsa-miR-19a is associated with lymph metastasis and mediates the TNF-α induced epithelial-to-mesenchymal transition in colorectal cancer. Sci Rep 2015; 5(1): 13350. [http://dx.doi.org/10.1038/srep13350] [PMID: 26302825]

[82] Gao J, Li N, Dong Y, *et al.* miR-34a-5p suppresses colorectal cancer metastasis and predicts recurrence in patients with stage II/III colorectal cancer. Oncogene 2015; 34(31): 4142-52. [http://dx.doi.org/10.1038/onc.2014.348] [PMID: 25362853]

[83] Li Q, Liang X, Wang Y, *et al.* miR-139-5p Inhibits the Epithelial-Mesenchymal Transition and Enhances the Chemotherapeutic Sensitivity of Colorectal Cancer Cells by Downregulating BCL2. Sci Rep 2016; 6(1): 27157. [http://dx.doi.org/10.1038/srep27157] [PMID: 27244080]

[84] Matamala N, Vargas MT, González-Cámpora R, *et al.* Tumor microRNA expression profiling identifies circulating microRNAs for early breast cancer detection. Clin Chem 2015; 61(8): 1098-106. [http://dx.doi.org/10.1373/clinchem.2015.238691] [PMID: 26056355]

[85] Hu J, Xu J, Wu Y, *et al.* Identification of microRNA-93 as a functional dysregulated miRNA in triple-negative breast cancer. Tumour Biol 2015; 36(1): 251-8. [http://dx.doi.org/10.1007/s13277-014-2611-8] [PMID: 25238878]

[86] Sempere LF, Christensen M, Silahtaroglu A, *et al.* Altered MicroRNA expression confined to specific epithelial cell subpopulations in breast cancer. Cancer Res 2007; 67(24): 11612-20. [http://dx.doi.org/10.1158/0008-5472.CAN-07-5019] [PMID: 18089790]

[87] Zhu C, Ren C, Han J, *et al.* A five-microRNA panel in plasma was identified as potential biomarker for early detection of gastric cancer. Br J Cancer 2014; 110(9): 2291-9. [http://dx.doi.org/10.1038/bjc.2014.119] [PMID: 24595006]

[88] Hung PS, Chen CY, Chen WT, *et al.* miR-376c promotes carcinogenesis and serves as a plasma marker for gastric carcinoma. PLoS One 2017; 12(5): e0177346. [http://dx.doi.org/10.1371/journal.pone.0177346] [PMID: 28486502]

[89] Cui L, Zhang X, Ye G, *et al.* Gastric juice MicroRNAs as potential biomarkers for the screening of gastric cancer. Cancer 2013; 119(9): 1618-26. [http://dx.doi.org/10.1002/cncr.27903] [PMID: 23335180]

[90] Lin Z, Chen Y, Lin Y, *et al.* Potential miRNA biomarkers for the diagnosis and prognosis of esophageal cancer detected by a novel absolute quantitative RT-qPCR method. Sci Rep 2020; 10(1): 20065. [http://dx.doi.org/10.1038/s41598-020-77119-6] [PMID: 33208781]

[91] Cui Y, Xue Y, Dong S, Zhang P. Plasma microRNA-9 as a diagnostic and prognostic biomarker in patients with esophageal squamous cell carcinoma. J Int Med Res 2017; 45(4): 1310-7. [http://dx.doi.org/10.1177/0300060517709370] [PMID: 28587538]

[92] Sudo K, Kato K, Matsuzaki J, *et al.* Development and Validation of an Esophageal Squamous Cell Carcinoma Detection Model by Large-Scale MicroRNA Profiling. JAMA Netw Open 2019; 2(5): e194573. [http://dx.doi.org/10.1001/jamanetworkopen.2019.4573] [PMID: 31125107]

[93] Zhou J, Yu L, Gao X, *et al.* Plasma microRNA panel to diagnose hepatitis B virus-related hepatocellular carcinoma. J Clin Oncol 2011; 29(36): 4781-8. [http://dx.doi.org/10.1200/JCO.2011.38.2697] [PMID: 22105822]

[94] Zhang Y, Li T, Qiu Y, *et al.* Serum microRNA panel for early diagnosis of the onset of hepatocellular carcinoma. Medicine (Baltimore) 2017; 96(2): e5642. [http://dx.doi.org/10.1097/MD.0000000000005642] [PMID: 28079796]

[95] Zhao X, Dou J, Cao J, *et al.* Uncovering the potential differentially expressed miRNAs as diagnostic biomarkers for hepatocellular carcinoma based on machine learning in The Cancer Genome Atlas database. Oncol Rep 2020; 43(6): 1771-84. [http://dx.doi.org/10.3892/or.2020.7551] [PMID: 32236623]

[96] Yang C, Wang C, Chen X, *et al.* Identification of seven serum microRNAs from a genome-wide serum microRNA expression profile as potential noninvasive biomarkers for malignant astrocytomas. Int J Cancer 2013; 132(1): 116-27. [http://dx.doi.org/10.1002/ijc.27657] [PMID: 22674182]

[97] Baraniskin A, Kuhnhenn J, Schlegel U, Schmiegel W, Hahn S, Schroers R. MicroRNAs in cerebrospinal fluid as biomarker for disease course monitoring in primary central nervous system lymphoma. J Neurooncol 2012; 109(2): 239-44. [http://dx.doi.org/10.1007/s11060-012-0908-2] [PMID: 22729947]

[98] Akers JC, Ramakrishnan V, Kim R, *et al.* MicroRNAs in cerebrospinal fluid as biomarker for disease course monitoring in primary central nervous system lymphoma. PLoS One 2013; 8: e78115. [http://dx.doi.org/10.1371/journal.pone.0078115] [PMID: 24205116]

[99] Wang Q, Li P, Li A, *et al.* Plasma specific miRNAs as predictive biomarkers for diagnosis and prognosis of glioma. J Exp Clin Cancer Res 2012; 31(1): 97. [http://dx.doi.org/10.1186/1756-9966-31-97] [PMID: 23174013]

[100] Rao SAM, Santosh V, Somasundaram K. Genome-wide expression profiling identifies deregulated miRNAs in malignant astrocytoma. Mod Pathol 2010; 23(10): 1404-17. [http://dx.doi.org/10.1038/modpathol.2010.135] [PMID: 20711171]

[101] Ping Y, Xiaoying HE, Xiaogang LI. Identification of miR-128 and miR-21 in the cerebrospinal fluid as biomarker for the diagnosis of glioma. International Journal of Laboratory Medicine 2014; 18: 2464-5.

[102] Ye X, Wei W, Zhang Z, *et al.* Identification of microRNAs associated with glioma diagnosis and prognosis. Oncotarget 2017; 8(16): 26394-403. [http://dx.doi.org/10.18632/oncotarget.14445] [PMID: 28060761]

[103] Tian FX, Ma HF, Zhang Q. Identification of Mir-9 in Glioma Diagnosis and Prognosis. Clin Lab 2020; 66(07/2020.) [http://dx.doi.org/10.7754/Clin.Lab.2019.190914] [PMID: 32658431]

[104] Liang B, Li Y, Wang T. A three miRNAs signature predicts survival in cervical cancer using bioinformatics analysis. Sci Rep 2017; 7(1): 5624. [http://dx.doi.org/10.1038/s41598-017-06032-2] [PMID: 28717180]

[105] Kawai S, Fujii T, Kukimoto I, *et al.* Identification of miRNAs in cervical mucus as a novel diagnostic marker for cervical neoplasia. Sci Rep 2018; 8(1): 7070. [http://dx.doi.org/10.1038/s41598-018-25310-1] [PMID: 29728572]

[106] Zheng M, Hou L, Ma Y, *et al.* Exosomal let-7d-3p and miR-30d-5p as diagnostic biomarkers for non-invasive screening of cervical cancer and its precursors. Mol Cancer 2019; 18(1): 76. [http://dx.doi.org/10.1186/s12943-019-0999-x] [PMID: 30940131]

[107] Wu YS, Lin H, Chen D, *et al.* A four-miRNA signature as a novel biomarker for predicting survival in endometrial cancer. Gene 2019; 697: 86-93. [http://dx.doi.org/10.1016/j.gene.2019.01.046] [PMID: 30779946]

[108] Wang P, Zeng Z, Shen X, Tian X, Ye Q. Identification of a Multi-RNA-Type-Based Signature for Recurrence-Free Survival Prediction in Patients with Uterine Corpus Endometrial Carcinoma. DNA Cell Biol 2020; 39(4): 615-30. [http://dx.doi.org/10.1089/dna.2019.5148] [PMID: 32105510]

[109] Wilczynski M, Danielska J, Dzieniecka M, Szymanska B, Wojciechowski M, Malinowski A. Prognostic and Clinical Significance of miRNA-205 in Endometrioid Endometrial Cancer. PLoS One

2016; 11(10): e0164687.
[http://dx.doi.org/10.1371/journal.pone.0164687] [PMID: 27737015]

[110] Cao Q, Lu K, Dai S, Hu Y, Fan W. Clinicopathological and prognostic implications of the miR-200 family in patients with epithelial ovarian cancer. Int J Clin Exp Pathol 2014; 7(5): 2392-401.
[PMID: 24966949]

[111] Meng X, Müller V, Milde-Langosch K, Trillsch F, Pantel K, Schwarzenbach H. Diagnostic and prognostic relevance of circulating exosomal miR-373, miR-200a, miR-200b and miR-200c in patients with epithelial ovarian cancer. Oncotarget 2016; 7(13): 16923-35.
[http://dx.doi.org/10.18632/oncotarget.7850] [PMID: 26943577]

[112] Meng X, Joosse SA, Müller V, *et al.* Diagnostic and prognostic potential of serum miR-7, miR-16, miR-25, miR-93, miR-182, miR-376a and miR-429 in ovarian cancer patients. Br J Cancer 2015; 113(9): 1358-66.
[http://dx.doi.org/10.1038/bjc.2015.340] [PMID: 26393886]

[113] Wei H, Tang QL, Zhang K, Sun JJ, Ding RF. miR-532-5p is a prognostic marker and suppresses cells proliferation and invasion by targeting TWIST1 in epithelial ovarian cancer. Eur Rev Med Pharmacol Sci 2018; 22(18): 5842-50.
[PMID: 30280764]

[114] Ibrahim N, Abdellateif M, Thabet G, *et al.* Combining PHI and miRNAs as Biomarkers in Prostate Cancer Diagnosis and Prognosis. Clin Lab 2019; 65(07/2019): 65.
[http://dx.doi.org/10.7754/Clin.Lab.2019.181213] [PMID: 31307177]

[115] Lyu J, Zhao L, Wang F, *et al.* Discovery and Validation of Serum MicroRNAs as Early Diagnostic Biomarkers for Prostate Cancer in Chinese Population. BioMed Res Int 2019; 2019: 1-9.
[http://dx.doi.org/10.1155/2019/9306803] [PMID: 31534967]

[116] Zhang F, Wu Z. Significantly altered expression of miR-511-3p and its target AKT3 has negative prognostic value in human prostate cancer. Biochimie 2017; 140: 66-72.
[http://dx.doi.org/10.1016/j.biochi.2017.06.007] [PMID: 28624527]

[117] Liu J, Yan Y, Shi J, *et al.* Upregulation of microRNA-191 can serve as an independent prognostic marker for poor survival in prostate cancer. Medicine (Baltimore) 2019; 98(29): e16193.
[http://dx.doi.org/10.1097/MD.0000000000016193] [PMID: 31335671]

[118] Stark MS, Klein K, Weide B, *et al.* The Prognostic and Predictive Value of Melanoma-related MicroRNAs Using Tissue and Serum: A MicroRNA Expression Analysis. EBioMedicine 2015; 2(7): 671-80.
[http://dx.doi.org/10.1016/j.ebiom.2015.05.011] [PMID: 26288839]

[119] Lindahl LM, Besenbacher S, Rittig AH, *et al.* Prognostic miRNA classifier in early-stage mycosis fungoides: development and validation in a Danish nationwide study. Blood 2018; 131(7): 759-70.
[http://dx.doi.org/10.1182/blood-2017-06-788950] [PMID: 29208599]

[120] Zeng Z, Dong J, Li Y, *et al.* The expression level and diagnostic value of microRNA-22 in HCC patients. Artif Cells Nanomed Biotechnol 2020; 48(1): 683-6.
[http://dx.doi.org/10.1080/21691401.2019.1703723] [PMID: 32088997]

[121] An Y, Gao S, Zhao WC, *et al.* Novel serum microRNAs panel on the diagnostic and prognostic implications of hepatocellular carcinoma. World J Gastroenterol 2018; 24(24): 2596-604.
[http://dx.doi.org/10.3748/wjg.v24.i24.2596] [PMID: 29962816]

[122] Tomimaru Y, Eguchi H, Nagano H, *et al.* Circulating microRNA-21 as a novel biomarker for hepatocellular carcinoma. J Hepatol 2012; 56(1): 167-75.
[http://dx.doi.org/10.1016/j.jhep.2011.04.026] [PMID: 21749846]

[123] Sakabe T, Azumi J, Umekita Y, *et al.* Prognostic relevance of miR-137 in patients with hepatocellular carcinoma. Liver Int 2017; 37(2): 271-9.
[http://dx.doi.org/10.1111/liv.13213] [PMID: 27473646]

[124] Syring I, Bartels J, Holdenrieder S, Kristiansen G, Müller SC, Ellinger J. Circulating Serum miRNA (miR-367-3p, miR-371a-3p, miR-372-3p and miR-373-3p) as Biomarkers in Patients with Testicular Germ Cell Cancer. J Urol 2015; 193(1): 331-7. [http://dx.doi.org/10.1016/j.juro.2014.07.010] [PMID: 25046619]

[125] Dieckmann KP, Radtke A, Geczi L, *et al.* Serum Levels of MicroRNA-371a-3p (M371 Test) as a New Biomarker of Testicular Germ Cell Tumors: Results of a Prospective Multicentric Study. J Clin Oncol 2019; 37(16): 1412-23. [http://dx.doi.org/10.1200/JCO.18.01480] [PMID: 30875280]

[126] Shen H, Shih J, Hollern DP, *et al.* Integrated Molecular Characterization of Testicular Germ Cell Tumors. Cell Rep 2018; 23(11): 3392-406. [http://dx.doi.org/10.1016/j.celrep.2018.05.039] [PMID: 29898407]

[127] Nappi L, Thi M, Lum A, *et al.* Developing a Highly Specific Biomarker for Germ Cell Malignancies: Plasma miR371 Expression Across the Germ Cell Malignancy Spectrum. J Clin Oncol 2019; 37(33): 3090-8. [http://dx.doi.org/10.1200/JCO.18.02057] [PMID: 31553692]

[128] Zhang LC, Zhong C, Ma YJ, Liu M, Nong WX. [Expression of MiR-429 in Patients with Acute Lymphoblastic Leukemia and Its Prognostic Value]. Zhongguo Shi Yan Xue Ye Xue Za Zhi 2020; 28(1): 119-24. [PMID: 32027263]

[129] Ma X, Pan Q, Fang C, *et al.* MicroRNA-181a-3p as a diagnostic and prognostic biomarker for acute myeloid leukemia. Mediterr J Hematol Infect Dis 2020; 12(1): e2020012. [http://dx.doi.org/10.4084/mjhid.2020.012] [PMID: 32180907]

[130] Zhang T, Wu D, Zhou J, *et al.* Overexpression of *miR-216b* : Prognostic and predictive value in acute myeloid leukemia. J Cell Physiol 2018; 233(4): 3274-81. [http://dx.doi.org/10.1002/jcp.26171] [PMID: 28884855]

[131] Bhayadia R, Krowiorz K, Haetscher N, *et al.* Endogenous Tumor Suppressor microRNA-193b: Therapeutic and Prognostic Value in Acute Myeloid Leukemia. J Clin Oncol 2018; 36(10): 1007-16. [http://dx.doi.org/10.1200/JCO.2017.75.2204] [PMID: 29432078]

[132] Ferrajoli A, Shanafelt TD, Ivan C, *et al.* Prognostic value of miR-155 in individuals with monoclonal B-cell lymphocytosis and patients with B chronic lymphocytic leukemia. Blood 2013; 122(11): 1891-9. [http://dx.doi.org/10.1182/blood-2013-01-478222] [PMID: 23821659]

[133] Lin X, Ling Q, Lv Y, *et al.* Plasma exosome-derived microRNA-532 as a novel predictor for acute myeloid leukemia. Cancer Biomark 2020; 28(2): 151-8. [http://dx.doi.org/10.3233/CBM-191164] [PMID: 32176633]

[134] Liu X, He M, Hou Y, *et al.* Expression profiles of microRNAs and their target genes in papillary thyroid carcinoma. Oncol Rep 2013; 29(4): 1415-20. [http://dx.doi.org/10.3892/or.2013.2263] [PMID: 23380809]

[135] Zhang Y, Xu D, Pan J, *et al.* Dynamic monitoring of circulating microRNAs as a predictive biomarker for the diagnosis and recurrence of papillary thyroid carcinoma. Oncol Lett 2017; 13(6): 4252-66. [http://dx.doi.org/10.3892/ol.2017.6028] [PMID: 28599426]

[136] Park JL, Kim SK, Jeon S, Jung CK, Kim YS. MicroRNA Profile for Diagnostic and Prognostic Biomarkers in Thyroid Cancer. Cancers (Basel). 2021; 5; 13:632. [http://dx.doi.org/10.3390/cancers13040632]

[137] Shang AQ, Xie YN, Wang J, *et al.* Predicative values of serum microRNA-22 and microRNA-126 levels for non-small cell lung cancer development and metastasis: a case-control study. Neoplasma 2017; 64(3): 453-9. [http://dx.doi.org/10.4149/neo_2017_317] [PMID: 28253725]

[138] Zhao Y. The diagnostic and prognostic role of circulating miR-141 expression in non-small-cell lung cancer patients. Int J Clin Exp Pathol 2018; 11(5): 2597-604. [PMID: 31938373]

[139] Shi GL, Chen Y, Sun Y, Yin YJ, Song CX. Significance of Serum MicroRNAs in the Auxiliary Diagnosis of Non-Small Cell Lung Cancer. Clin Lab 2017; 63(01/2017): 133-40. [http://dx.doi.org/10.7754/Clin.Lab.2016.160710] [PMID: 28164492]

[140] Liu N, Cui RX, Sun Y, *et al.* A four-miRNA signature identified from genome-wide serum miRNA profiling predicts survival in patients with nasopharyngeal carcinoma. Int J Cancer 2014; 134(6): 1359-68. [http://dx.doi.org/10.1002/ijc.28468] [PMID: 23999999]

[141] Wen W, Mai SJ, Lin HX, *et al.* Identification of two microRNA signatures in whole blood as novel biomarkers for diagnosis of nasopharyngeal carcinoma. J Transl Med 2019; 17(1): 186. [http://dx.doi.org/10.1186/s12967-019-1923-2] [PMID: 31159814]

[142] Zheng XH, Cui C, Ruan HL, *et al.* Plasma microRNA profiling in nasopharyngeal carcinoma patients reveals miR-548q and miR-483-5p as potential biomarkers. Chin J Cancer 2014; 33(7): 330-8. [PMID: 24874644]

[143] Preis M, Gardner TB, Gordon SR, *et al.* MicroRNA-10b expression correlates with response to neoadjuvant therapy and survival in pancreatic ductal adenocarcinoma. Clin Cancer Res 2011; 17(17): 5812-21. [http://dx.doi.org/10.1158/1078-0432.CCR-11-0695] [PMID: 21652542]

[144] Liu R, Chen X, Du Y, *et al.* Serum microRNA expression profile as a biomarker in the diagnosis and prognosis of pancreatic cancer. Clin Chem 2012; 58(3): 610-8. [http://dx.doi.org/10.1373/clinchem.2011.172767] [PMID: 22194634]

[145] Chambers H. Isis, Alnylam Pair To Seek Disease-Fighting Drugs. San Diego Business Journal 2007.

[146] Business Wire (2010). Data Presented at ASCO 2010 by M. D. Anderson Researchers Demonstrate the ability of miRview™ mets to Identify the Most Likely Origin of Metastases in Cancer of Unknown Primary. https://www.businesswire.com/news/home/20100607006074/en/Data-Presented-AS-O-2010-M.-D.-Anderson

[147] Meleth S, Whitehead N, Evans TS, Lux L. Technology Assessment on Genetic Testing or Molecular Pathology Testing of Cancers with Unknown Primary Site to Determine Origin. Rockville (MD). US: Agency for Healthcare Research and Quality 2013 https://www.ncbi.nlm.nih.gov/books/NBK285008/

[148] Bruno R, Alì G, Fontanini G. Molecular markers and new diagnostic methods to differentiate malignant from benign mesothelial pleural proliferations: a literature review. J Thorac Dis 2018; 10(S2) (Suppl. 2): S342-52. [http://dx.doi.org/10.21037/jtd.2017.10.88] [PMID: 29507804]

[149] Schulte JJ, Husain AN. Update on the pathologic diagnosis of malignant mesothelioma. Transl Lung Cancer Res 2020; 9(3): 917-23. [http://dx.doi.org/10.21037/tlcr-19-620] [PMID: 32676357]

[150] https://www.sec.gov/Archives/edgar/data/1362959/000114420409001713/v136962_ex99-1.htm

[151] Benjamin H, Lebanony D, Rosenwald S, *et al.* A diagnostic assay based on microRNA expression accurately identifies malignant pleural mesothelioma. J Mol Diagn 2010; 12(6): 771-9. [http://dx.doi.org/10.2353/jmoldx.2010.090169] [PMID: 20864637]

[152] Lebanony D, Benjamin H, Gilad S, *et al.* Diagnostic assay based on hsa-miR-205 expression distinguishes squamous from nonsquamous non-small-cell lung carcinoma. J Clin Oncol 2009; 27(12): 2030-7. [http://dx.doi.org/10.1200/JCO.2008.19.4134] [PMID: 19273703]

[153] Au NHC, Gown AM, Cheang M, *et al.* P63 expression in lung carcinoma: a tissue microarray study of

408 cases. Appl Immunohistochem Mol Morphol 2004; 12(3): 240-7.
[http://dx.doi.org/10.1097/00129039-200409000-00010] [PMID: 15551738]

[154] Reis-Filho JS, Simpson PT, Martins A, Preto A, Gärtner F, Schmitt FC. Distribution of p63, cytokeratins 5/6 and cytokeratin 14 in 51 normal and 400 neoplastic human tissue samples using TARP-4 multi-tumor tissue microarray. Virchows Arch 2003; 443(2): 122-32.
[http://dx.doi.org/10.1007/s00428-003-0859-2] [PMID: 12884041]

[155] Piperdi B, Merla A, Perez-Soler R. Targeting angiogenesis in squamous non-small cell lung cancer. Drugs 2014; 74(4): 403-13. r
[http://dx.doi.org/10.1007/s40265-014-0182-z] [PMID: 24578213]

[156] www.rosettagenomics.com

[157] Gilad S, Lithwick-Yanai G, Barshack I, *et al.* Classification of the four main types of lung cancer using a microRNA-based diagnostic assay. J Mol Diagn 2012; 14(5): 510-7.
[http://dx.doi.org/10.1016/j.jmoldx.2012.03.004] [PMID: 22749746]

[158] Khayyata S, Yun S, Pasha T, *et al.* Value of P63 and CK5/6 in distinguishing squamous cell carcinoma from adenocarcinoma in lung fine-needle aspiration specimens. Diagn Cytopathol 2009; 37(3): 178-83.
[http://dx.doi.org/10.1002/dc.20975] [PMID: 19170169]

[159] Tanca A, Addis MF, Pagnozzi D, *et al.* Proteomic analysis of formalin-fixed, paraffin-embedded lung neuroendocrine tumor samples from hospital archives. J Proteomics 2011; 74(3): 359-70.
[http://dx.doi.org/10.1016/j.jprot.2010.12.001] [PMID: 21147281]

[160] Johnson DH, Fehrenbacher L, Novotny WF, *et al.* Randomized phase II trial comparing bevacizumab plus carboplatin and paclitaxel with carboplatin and paclitaxel alone in previously untreated locally advanced or metastatic non-small-cell lung cancer. J Clin Oncol 2004; 22(11): 2184-91.
[http://dx.doi.org/10.1200/JCO.2004.11.022] [PMID: 15169807]

[161] Pentheroudakis G, Golfinopoulos V, Pavlidis N. Switching benchmarks in cancer of unknown primary: From autopsy to microarray. Eur J Cancer 2007; 43(14): 2026-36.
[http://dx.doi.org/10.1016/j.ejca.2007.06.023] [PMID: 17698346]

[162] Anderson GG, Weiss LM. Determining tissue of origin for metastatic cancers: meta-analysis and literature review of immunohistochemistry performance. Appl Immunohistochem Mol Morphol 2010; 18(1): 3-8.
[http://dx.doi.org/10.1097/PAI.0b013e3181a75e6d] [PMID: 19550296]

[163] Meiri E, Mueller WC, Rosenwald S, *et al.* A second-generation microRNA-based assay for diagnosing tumor tissue origin. Oncologist 2012; 17(6): 801-12.
[http://dx.doi.org/10.1634/theoncologist.2011-0466] [PMID: 22618571]

[164] Spector Y, Fridman E, Rosenwald S, *et al.* Development and validation of a microRNA-based diagnostic assay for classification of renal cell carcinomas. Mol Oncol 2013; 7(3): 732-8.
[http://dx.doi.org/10.1016/j.molonc.2013.03.002] [PMID: 23587442]

[165] Gregory PA, Bert AG, Paterson EL, *et al.* The miR-200 family and miR-205 regulate epithelial to mesenchymal transition by targeting ZEB1 and SIP1. Nat Cell Biol 2008; 10(5): 593-601.
[http://dx.doi.org/10.1038/ncb1722] [PMID: 18376396]

[166] Craene BD, Berx G. Regulatory networks defining EMT during cancer initiation and progression. Nat Rev Cancer 2013; 13(2): 97-110.
[http://dx.doi.org/10.1038/nrc3447] [PMID: 23344542]

[167] Park SM, Gaur AB, Lengyel E, Peter ME. The miR-200 family determines the epithelial phenotype of cancer cells by targeting the E-cadherin repressors ZEB1 and ZEB2. Genes Dev 2008; 22(7): 894-907.
[http://dx.doi.org/10.1101/gad.1640608] [PMID: 18381893]

[168] Kim NH, Kim HS, Li XY, *et al.* A p53/miRNA-34 axis regulates Snail1-dependent cancer cell epithelial–mesenchymal transition. J Cell Biol 2011; 195(3): 417-33.

[http://dx.doi.org/10.1083/jcb.201103097] [PMID: 22024162]

[169] Siemens H, Jackstadt R, Hünten S, *et al.* miR-34 and SNAIL form a double-negative feedback loop to regulate epithelial-mesenchymal transitions. Cell Cycle 2011; 10(24): 4256-71. [http://dx.doi.org/10.4161/cc.10.24.18552] [PMID: 22134354]

[170] Zheng H, Li W, Wang Y, *et al.* miR-23a inhibits E-cadherin expression and is regulated by AP-1 and NFAT4 complex during Fas-induced EMT in gastrointestinal cancer. Carcinogenesis 2014; 35(1): 173-83. [http://dx.doi.org/10.1093/carcin/bgt274] [PMID: 23929433]

[171] Han M, Liu M, Wang Y, *et al.* Antagonism of miR-21 reverses epithelial-mesenchymal transition and cancer stem cell phenotype through AKT/ERK1/2 inactivation by targeting PTEN. PLoS One 2012; 7(6): e39520. [http://dx.doi.org/10.1371/journal.pone.0039520] [PMID: 22761812]

[172] Smith AL, Iwanaga R, Drasin DJ, *et al.* The miR-106b-25 cluster targets Smad7, activates TGF-β signaling, and induces EMT and tumor initiating cell characteristics downstream of Six1 in human breast cancer. Oncogene 2012; 31(50): 5162-71. [http://dx.doi.org/10.1038/onc.2012.11] [PMID: 22286770]

[173] Chang CJ, Hsu CC, Chang CH, *et al.* Let-7d functions as novel regulator of epithelial-mesenchymal transition and chemoresistant property in oral cancer. Oncol Rep 2011; 26(4): 1003-10. [PMID: 21725603]

[174] Hwang WL, Jiang JK, Yang SH, *et al.* MicroRNA-146a directs the symmetric division of Snail-dominant colorectal cancer stem cells. Nat Cell Biol 2014; 16(3): 268-80. [http://dx.doi.org/10.1038/ncb2910] [PMID: 24561623]

[175] Ju S-Y, Chiou S-H, Su Y. Maintenance of the stemness in CD44+ HCT-15 and HCT-116 human colon cancer cells requires miR-203 suppression. Stem Cell Res (Amst) 2014; 12(1): 86-100. [http://dx.doi.org/10.1016/j.scr.2013.09.011]

Part 5: Novel Methods for Cancer Biomarker Detection

CHAPTER 13

Electrochemical and Optical Detection of MicroRNAs as Biomarkers for Cancer Diagnosis

Riham Zayani[1], **Amira Ben Hassine**[1], **Amal Rabti**[1], **Amal Raouafi**[1] and **Noureddine Raouafi**[1,*]

[1] *Sensors and Biosensors Group, Analytical Chemistry & Electrochemistry Lab. (LR99ES15), Faculty of Science, University of Tunis El Manar, Tunis El Manar, Tunisia*

Abstract: According to the miRBase (v 22.1), released on October 2018, there are more than 1900 identified human microRNA mature sequences. MicroRNAs (aka miRNAs or miRs) are a class of short non-coding RNA sequences, which have been detected within the cells or in body fluids. They act as gene expression regulators and intervene in numerous physiologic and development processes. They post-transcriptionally/translationally regulate expression of some proteins by forming miRNA-induced silencing complex (mRISC) by binding to 3'-UTR regions of the target messenger RNA to inhibit the protein synthesis. It has been noted that up- and down-regulation of miRs are associated with the pathogenesis of several types of human cancers since their target proteins are tumor-suppressive or oncogenic ones. This chapter will present a general summary of miRNA biogenesis, their link to cancer, and biological methods for their detection. Thanks to their ease of use and high sensitivity, electrochemical and optical techniques were used to detect miRNAs with or without the assistance of amplification methods. We will review the state-of-the-art electrochemical and optical methods for their detection, emphasizing the progress achieved in the last five years (2015-2020). Finally, we will present the main advantages, challenges, and future prospects for future research on detecting miRNAs for clinical diagnosis or prognosis in cancers.

Keywords: Amperometry, Amplification, Biomarkers, Biosensors, Cancer, Detection, Diagnosis, EIS, Electrochemistry, Fluorescence, Hybridization, miRNAs, Nanodevices, Optical, Prognosis, Potentiometry, Raman, SPR, SERS, UV-visible.

INTRODUCTION

According to the International Agency for Research on Cancer (IARC) data,

* **Corresponding author Noureddine Raouafi:** Sensors and Biosensors Group, Analytical Chemistry & Electrochemistry Lab. (LR99ES15), Faculty of Science, University of Tunis El Manar, Tunis El Manar, Tunisia; E-mail: noureddine.raouafi@fst.utm.tn

Farhadul Islam (Ed.)

cancer is the second leading cause of death. In 2018, approximately 18.08 million new cases were diagnosed, and 9.55 million died from various forms of cancer.

Lung, colorectum, stomach, liver and breast cancers account for more than 50% of the death toll [1]. Breast cancer is the leading cause among female gender, while for the male population, it is lung cancer. Projections show that in 2040, the cancer incidence will rise by 63.4% (from 18.08 million in 2018 to 29.53 million in 2040), while the death toll will rise by 71.5% (from 9.55 million in 2018 to 16.83 million in 2040) (Chart **1**). This could be explained by the worldwide population growing and aging. Furthermore, seven among ten deaths are recorded in low- and middle-income countries, linking the proliferation and mortality from cancer to development issues. Fig. (**1**) shows the cancer burden and the necessary steps to reduce it.

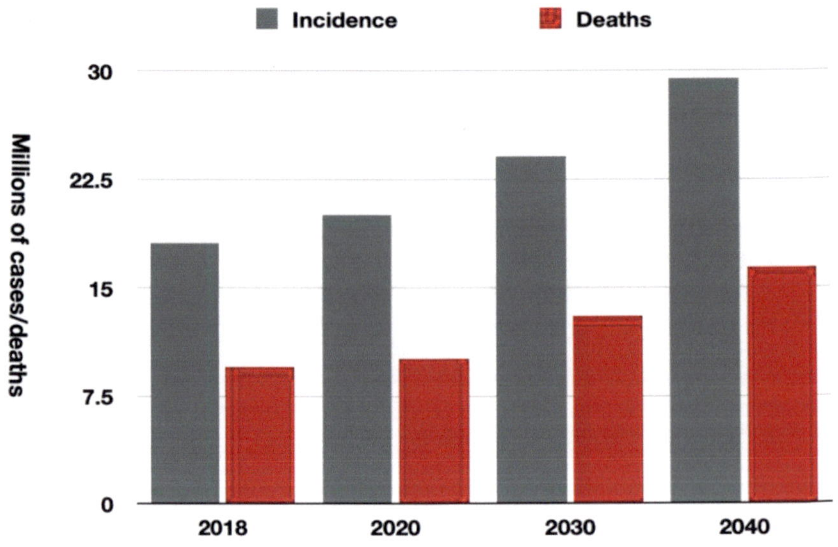

Fig. (1). Estimations of the incidence of cancer and death toll from cancer for the period 2020-2040.

The UICC identified a set of immediate actions for all stakeholders announced in the World Cancer Declaration, aiming to achieve nine concrete targets to reduce premature death from cancer and to improve the quality of life and the survival rates of patients [2]. The sixth key point was the "*Universal access to screening and early detection for cancer*", which can be easily achieved by providing non-invasive and cost-effective methods not requiring sophisticated apparatuses and/or skilled personnel. Furthermore, educating people about the cancer risk factors, such as tobacco, virus infection by human papilloma and hepatitis B viruses, environmental pollution, carcinogens and radiations, implanting early cancer screening methods in primary healthcare facilities, and the adequate management of cancer patients should also help in reducing substantially the cancer burden in low- and middle-income countries. Early diagnosis can be readily achieved through highly sensitive yet affordable tools, such as biosensors that can be used in low-resource settings and low-income countries [3].

In the last two decades, biosensors have emerged as an appealing alternative to classic analytical methods, such as HPLC, mass spectrometry, ELISA, Western Blot, *etc*. Due to their small size, biosensors can be used for rapid and on-site monitoring to provide real-time information avoiding sampling and analysis in central laboratories. Furthermore, electrochemical biosensors rapidly gained a place of choice since they fit with ASSURED criteria (affordable, sensitive, specific, user-friendly, robust/rapid, equipment-free, deliverable to end-users) for the selection of diagnosis methods [4]. These devices find use in numerous fields, such as healthcare, food safety, environmental monitoring, biosecurity, *etc* [5 - 9].

Since the discovery of CEA in 1965 to be used as the first blood serum biomarker for colon cancer [10], several others such CA 19-9 for pancreatic and colorectal cancer [11], CA 15-3 [12] and CA-125 [13] for breast and ovarian cancers [14] and the PSA as the most reliable biomarker for prostate cancer diagnosis [15]. Nowadays, several other biomarkers are used for screening and diagnostic to predict the recurrence of cancer or the response to therapy, such as HER2 occurring in 20% of breast cancer cases, which tend to be more aggressive than the other forms [16]. Several RNAs are being explored as cancer biomarkers [17], in particular short non-coding RNAs, such as circRNAs [18], miRNAs [19], and piRNAs [20]. So far, miRNAs are the most studied ones [17, 19, 21, 22].

This chapter will present an overview of miRNAs, their biogenesis, biological role and implications in cancer. Later, we will present the electrochemical and optical-based techniques used to detect these biomarkers, and we will conclude and provide some perspectives. The advantages, challenges as well as prospects in that effervescent field of analytical field will be critically discussed.

What are miRNAs?

miRNAs are short (*ca.* 18 to 22 nucleotides), single-stranded, non-coding RNA sequences lacking a polyadenylated tail and a protective group at 3'end [23]. They belong to the small interfering RNAs (RNAi) family, which post-transcriptionally regulates gene expression. They are involved in many biological functions, such as embryonic evolution, cell differentiation and metabolism [24 - 33]. They are also involved in several pathologies. For instance, they act on cell proliferation, and gene repression linking them to cancer [29, 30, 32, 34]. They regulate approximately 40% of the biological processes [30]. miRNAs are present in all eukaryotic organisms and are the most frequent group of small RNA present in mammals. According to miRBase v22.1, we count more than 1900 specific human miRNAs, and each can interact with one or several different mRNA at its 3'-UTR [35]. Furthermore, the genomes of several other species (271 in total), such as viruses, mice, rats, flies, worms and Arabidopsis, are known to encode miRNAs [36, 37].

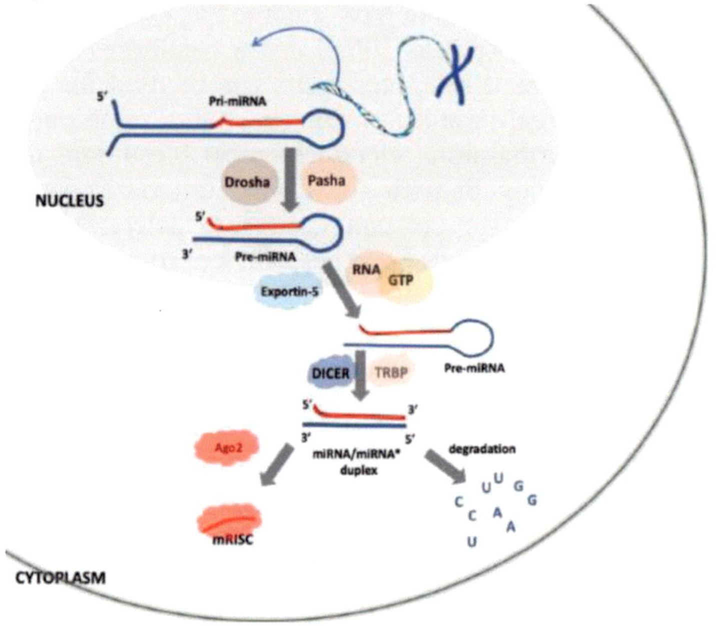

Fig. (2). Canonical pathway to miRNA biogenesis starting from gene.

Biogenesis of miRNAs

The biogenesis of miRNA gene clusters, commonly from the intergenic origin, is a multistep process (Fig. **2**). In fact, miRNAs are transcribed by RNA polymerase II to generate pri-miRNAs, which contain 500–3000 nucleotides with poly-A tail at the 3' end and a 7-methylguanosine cap at the 5' end [38]. Subsequently, the 60–110 nucleotides long pre-miRNAs, having hairpin-like structure, are formed after cleavage of pri-miRNAs by the microprocessor complex, composed of RNAase III endonuclease Drosha enzyme and DGCR8 protein [39]. These pre-miRNAs are exported to the cytoplasm by exportin-5 and Ran-GTP complex [40], and are further processed by the TRBP protein and the RNase III Dicer enzyme to produce a short (*ca.* 22-nts long) mature miRNA duplex (miRNA/miRNA*). The Ago1–4 protein family, particularly AGO2, drives the unwinding of this duplex to generate two single-stranded miRNAs, whereas the passenger strand miRNAs* are usually degraded. However, after integration into the multiprotein RNA-induced silencing complex, the mature miRNAs bind to partial or full-complementary sequences of the target messenger RNAs to regulate their expression by inducing translational repression or mRNA destabilization [41, 42].

Biological Role of miRNAs

Post-transcriptional gene regulation by mediating the degradation of mRNAs and by regulating transcription and translation through canonical and non-canonical mechanisms is the main role of miRNA [43]. When the miRISC complex containing the miRNA strand binds to full-complementary target mRNA through its 3'-untranslated region (3'-UTR), this mechanism is called canonical and is further followed by mRNA deadenylation, translation suppression and finally, degradation [44]. However, when the chains of both miRISC complex and mRNA are not entirely complementary, non-canonical mechanisms take place [45]. About 60% of the interactions between the miRISC and mRNA are non-canonical, which means that a single miRNA could potentially target numerous mRNAs (as much as 200 mRNAs) [46], while at the same time, one mRNA could contain multiple binding sites for miRNAs leading to regulation of numerous biological processes [47]. In fact, miRNAs are involved in a wide range of regulatory functions in biological processes such as cell/tissue development, differentiation, metabolism, homeostasis, proliferation and apoptosis and immune responses. Deregulation of their expression is associated with various pathological conditions, including neurological diseases, cardiovascular diseases, diabetes mellitus and cancers [44, 48 - 51]. Various factors can alter the miRNA biogenesis and functions, such as: (i) epigenetic modifications, (ii) alteration in protein activity involved in this process, (iii) single nucleotide polymorphisms (SNPs) in miRNA genes, (iv) hereditary mutations in the miRNA seed region; (v) somatic mutation in miRNA genes, and (vi) somatic copy-number variation of miRNA genes [52]. Furthermore, miRNA played a crucial role in intercellular signaling as they were detected in 12 types of human fluid such as serum, plasma, urine and saliva [53], and their expression has been characterized in 61 types of tissue [54], which make them potential biomarkers for human pathologies.

miRNAs and Cancer

Cancer is a group of potentially life-threatening diseases affecting nearly every part of the body, involving the transformation of normal cells into cancerous cells ultimately turning a pre-cancerous tissue into a malignant tumor in a multistage process. It is due to the interaction of genetic factors present in an individual with external agents such as physical and chemical carcinogens, and biological infections. Ageing and tobacco consumption constitute the major risk factors for cancer development. Generally, imaging, biopsy and a few serological cancer biomarkers are used for cancer diagnosis. However, these approaches are not always cancer type or subtype oriented in addition to the considerable risk caused by the biopsy to the patient, and the low specificity and sensitivity of blood-based biomarkers [55].

In this context, the analysis of miRNAs in cancer patient fluids as a liquid biopsy process has shown great diagnostic potential. In the last decade, extensive studies have demonstrated that the expression of miRNAs is profoundly altered in all cancers. In fact, miRNAs have a major role in the development and progression of cancer diseases by disrupting the normal function of proto-oncogenes, which is achieved through tumor suppressor miRNAs, and tumor suppressor genes, through oncomiRs, by inhibition or inducement of their function, respectively, leading to the acceleration of cell division and tumor growing [56]. Usually, the oncomiRs tend to be excessively represented, while the miRNAs with tumor suppression function are expressed insufficiently. For example, miR-21 (more precisely miRNA-21-5p), considered an oncogenic miRNA, is frequently described as being upregulated in CRC, having an active role in cell proliferation, invasion and migration through targeting genes, such as PDCD4, SPRY2 and PTEN [57]. On the other hand, miR-143 and miR-145, found to be downregulated in CRC, are considered tumor suppressor miRNAs, modulating the expression of important oncogenes such as KRAS, MYC, CD44 and BRAF, which promote chronic inflammation and neoplastic progression [57]. However, miRNAs can act both as suppressors or oncomiRs. For example, miR-155 was first considered an oncomiR for lymphoma and PC [58, 59], but later it was viewed as a tumor suppressor in the cases of OC and GC [60, 61]. One of the main reasons causing the abnormality of miRNA expression in cancer is the localization of 50% of the miRNA coding genes in genomic cancer areas that are translocated or amplified in malignancies [62]. Yet, in most cancers, miRNAs are apparently deregulated, which maybe induced by transcriptional deregulation, epigenetic alterations (DNA methylation, mutation, and DNA copy abnormalities) and problems in miRNA biogenesis pathways [63]. Moreover, cell-cycle regulation and exit (senescence), in addition to cell differentiation and proliferation, are controlled by certain families of miRNA that, if mutated, can cause abnormalities in the cells.

All the above-mentioned facts prove that miRNAs are involved in many cancer features such as invasion, angiogenesis, and metastasis, including the immune homeostasis and normal function of the innate and adaptive immune response, which make them potential biomarkers for cancer diagnosis, prognosis and treatment prediction [64]. For instance, in the case of CRC, miR-18a, miR-155 and miR-205 repress proliferation, migration and invasion of CRC cells, whereas miR-494, miR-598 and miR-17 promote the abilities of cell proliferation, migration and invasion [65]. Moreover, miR-106a and miR-7 relate to apoptosis of CRC cells or the resistance to apoptosis, while miR-221 and miR-214 reduce autophagy in CRC cells. Meanwhile, miR-192/215 and miR-19b-1 have regulatory roles in metabolic pathways. Other recent studies reported the association of several miRNAs with GC [66], chronic and acute leukemia [67], oral cancer [68], BrC [69], HCC [70], NSCLC [71], TC [72], and other human cancers (Table **1**). Sharma *et al.* have demonstrated that 728 miRNAs were dysregulated in sixteen cancer types, namely BC, BrC, CC, CRC, EC, EnC, GC, HCC, HNSCC, LC, OC, PC, PrC, RCC, SC, and TC [34]. Moreover, they identified seven miRNAs, *i.e.,* miR-18a, miR-21, miR-143/145, miR-210, miR-218 and miR-221, showing maximum dysregulation, either up- or down-regulation, in the majority of these cancers. For example, miR-18a was found to be upregulated in BC, EnC, GC, HCC, LC, OC, PC, RCC, SC and TC cancers, while it was both upregulated and downregulated in CRC and HNSCC. Moreover, miR-21 was found to be upregulated in all studied cancers.

Table 1. Dysregulated miRNAs and their association with various cancer.

Form of Cancer	miRNAs	Dysregulation	Value	Refs.
Colorectal	miR-18a, miR-155 and miR-205 miR-494, miR-598 and miR-17	miR-18a↑, miR-155↑, miR-205↑	Diagnosis	[65]
		miR-494↓, miR-598↓, miR-17↓		
Gastric	miR-20a, miR-1, miR-27a, miR-34a, mR-423, miR-185, miR-210, miR-25, miR-92b, miR-187, miR-371, miR-378, miR-195, miR-26a, miR-142, miR-148a, miR-16, and miR-19b	miR-20a↑, miR-1↑, miR-27a↑, miR-34a↑, mR-423↑, miR-185↑, miR-210↑, miR-25↑, miR-92b↑, miR-187↑, miR-371↑, miR-378↑	Diagnosis	[73]
		miR-195↓, miR-26a↓, miR-142↓, miR-148a↓, miR-16↓, miR-19b↓		
Chronic and acute leukemia	miR-29, miR-150, miR-155, miR-181b-5p, miR-210, miR-375, miR-511 up miR-222, miR-34a, miR-199a-3p, miR-223, miR-221, miR-26a, let-7d, miR-339, miR-342, let-7b, miR-523, miR-328	miR-29↑, miR-155↑, miR-181b↑, miR-210↑, miR-375↑, miR-511↑, miR-222↑, miR-34a↑, let-7b↑, miR-523↑, miR-miR-150↑↓	Diagnosis/Prognosis	[74]
		miR-199a-3p↓, miR-223↓, miR-221↓, miR-26a↓, let-7d↓, miR-339↓, miR-342↓, miR-328↓, miR-150↑↓		
Oral	miR-21, miR-23a, miR-24, miR-31, miR-31*, miR-99b, miR-155, miR-211, miR-221, miR-26a, miR-30a, miR-32, miR-99a, miR-100, miR-375	miR-21↑, miR-23a↑, miR-24↑, miR-31↑, miR-31*↑, miR-99b↑, miR-155↑, miR-211↑, miR-221↑	Prognosis	[75]
		miR-26a↓, miR-30a↓, miR-32↓, miR-99a↓, miR-100↓, miR-375↓		

(Table 1) cont.....

Form of Cancer	miRNAs	Dysregulation	Value	Refs.
Breast	miR-10b, miR-200, miR-21, miR-301, miR-335, miR-155, miR-34a, miR-205, miR20a, miR-801, miR-409-3p, miR-133a, miR-19a, miR-484, miR-365, miR-145, and miR-409-3p	miR-10b↑, miR-200↑, miR-21↑,mi--484↑, miR-365↑, miR-145↑, miR-409-3p↑, miR-801↑, miR-409-3p↑, miR-133a↑, miR20a↑↓, miR-19a↑↓	Diagnosis/Prognosis	[76]
		miR-301↓, miR-335↓, miR-155↓, miR-34a↓, miR-205↓, miR20a↑↓, miR-19a↑↓		
Hepato-cellular Carcinoma	miR-17-92, miR-21, miR-221, miR-222, miR-224, let-7, miR-200, miR-29, miR-122, miR-123, miR-199a, and miR-199b	miR-17-92↑, miR-21↑, miR-221↑, miR-222↑, miR-224↑	Diagnosis/Prognosis	[70]
		let-7↓, miR-200↓, miR-29↓, miR-122↓, miR-123↓, miR-199a↓, miR-199b↓		
Non-small-cell Lung	miR-7, miR-25, miR-193a, miR-214, and miR-483	miR-7↓, miR-25↓, miR-193a↓, miR-214↓, miR-483↓	Diagnosis	[77]
Thyroid	miR-221, miR-222, miR-34a, miR-146b, miR-21, miR-31, miR-181, and miR-138	miR-221↑, miR-222↑, miR-34a↑, miR-146b↑, miR-21↑, miR-31↑,	Diagnosis/Prognosis	[78]
		miR-181↓, miR-138↓		
Prostate	miR-21, miR-32, miR-96, miR-125b, miR-182, miR-221/222, miR-375, miR-409, miR-24, miR-141, let-7a, let-7c, miR-1, miR-15a/16, miR-26a, miR-31, miR-34a, miR-34b, miR-99a, miR-124, miR-126, miR-133b, miR-143/145, miR-185, miR-200, miR-203, miR-205, miR-320, miR-449, and miR-940	miR-21↑, miR-32↑, miR-96↑, miR-125b↑, miR-182↑, miR-221/222↑, miR-375↑, miR-409↑, miR-24↑↓, miR-141↑↓	Diagnosis/ Prognosis/ Prediction	[79]
		let-7a↓, let-7c↓, miR-1↓, miR-15a/16↓, miR-26a↓, miR-31↓, miR-34a↓, miR-34b↓, miR-99a↓, miR-124↓, miR-126↓, miR-133b↓, miR-143/145↓, miR-185↓, miR-200↓, miR-203↓, miR-205↓, miR-320↓, miR-449↓, miR-940↓, miR-24↑↓, miR-141↑↓		
Pediatric (Osteosarcoma)	miR-199a-3p, miR-143, miR-34b, miR-133b, miR-206, miR-16-5p, miR-20a-5p, miR-25-3p, miR-106a-5p, miR-139-5p, miR-425-5p, miR451a miR-205-5p, miR-21, miR-148a, miR-196a/b, and miR199a-5p	miR-21↑, miR-148a↑, miR-196a/b↑, miR199a-5p↑	Diagnosis	[80]
		miR-199a-3p↓, miR-143↓, miR-34b↓, miR-133b↓, miR-206↓, miR-16-5p↓, miR-20a-5p↓, miR-25-3p↓, miR-106a-5p↓, miR-139-5p↓, miR-425-5p↓, miR451a↓, miR-205-5p↓		

(Table 1) cont.....

Form of Cancer	miRNAs	Dysregulation	Value	Refs.
Biliary Tract	miR-21, miR-187,miR-202, miR-483-5p,miR505-3p, miR874,miR885-5p, miR-320b,miR-92b-3p,miR1275, miR1307-3p, miR-150, miR-192, miR-1281, miR-126,miR-26a, miR-30b, miR-122, miR-483-5p, miR-194, miR-191,miR-4-6-3p,miR-1274b, miR-16, miR-484, let-7a,miR-143, miR-335, miR-412, miR-640,miR-125a-3p, miR-6893-5p, miR-1537, and miR-200c	miR-21↑, miR-187↑,miR-202↑, miR-483↑,miR505-3p↑, miR874↑,miR885-5p↑, miR-320b↑,miR-92b↑,miR1275↑, miR1307↑, miR-150↑, miR-192↑, miR-1281↑, miR-126↑,miR-26a↑, miR-30b↑, miR-122↑, miR-194↑, miR-191↑,miR-486-3p↑,miR-1274b↑, miR-16↑, miR-484↑	Diagnosis/ Prognosis	[81]
		let-7a↓,miR-143↓, miR-335↓, miR-412↓, miR-640↓,miR-125a↓, miR-6893↓, miR-1537↓, miR-200c↓		
Ovarian	miR-21, miR-29a, miR-92, miR-93, miR-126, miR-127, miR-155 and miR-99b,	miR-21↑, miR-29a↑, miR-92↑, miR-93↑, miR-126↑	Diagnosis	[82]
		miR-27↓, miR-155↓, miR-99b↓		

Generally, miRNAs are considered as potential biomarkers for cancer diagnosis, prognosis and treatment outcome prediction. In fact, findings supported the association of higher expression levels of miRNA, *i.e.,* miR-92a, miR-141, let-7a, miR-1229, miR-1246, miR-150, miR-21, miR-223, miR-23a, and miR-378, as diagnostic biomarkers, while miRNAs such as miR-141, miR-320, miR-596, and miR-203, with prognosis, malignant potential, and tumor recurrence, have been validated [83]. High expression levels of miR-106a, miR-484, and miR-130b are associated with predictive biomarkers, and low expression levels of miR-106a, miR-484, and miR-130b are prognostic in nature [83]. Furthermore, the therapeutic capability of miRNAs like miR-200 family inhibiting ovarian metastasis and potentially in other cancer types make them interesting features for developing miRNAs replacement cancer therapies [79].

Compared to other diagnostic markers, miRNAs have shown better sensitivity. Indeed, miRNAs showed superior effectiveness in diagnosing pancreatic ductal adenocarcinoma than glypican-1 and CA 19-9, the only U.S. Food and Drug Administration-approved biomarker of pancreatic ductal adenocarcinoma [84]. Additionally, the sensitivity and the diagnostic efficiencies of miR-24, miR-320a and miR-423 for early-stage CRC were better than traditional CEA and CA 19-9 [85]. Nevertheless, alterations of the level of the same miRNAs in patients with different tumor types represent a major limitation for their use as cancer diagnostic tools. For example, the increased serum level of miR-21 has been found in patients with colorectal, lung, breast, prostate, liver, esophageal, and endometrial cancers [55]. Thus, using a panel combining selected miRNAs displayed greater target organ specificity and better diagnostic value than a single miRNA or well-established clinical biomarker. For instance, a serum miRNA classifier panel containing seven miRNAs, *i.e.*, miR-29a, miR-29c, miR-133a, miR-143, miR-145, miR-192, and miR-505, exhibited greater sensitivity in HCC detection, especially small size or early-stage, than a-fetoprotein [86]. Likewise, panel combining miR-15b, miR-17, miR-21, miR-26b, and miR-145 [87], or miR-1246, miR-202, miR-21, miR-1229 and miR-532 [88] have been investigated for potential detection of CRC.

OVERVIEW OF MOLECULAR BIOLOGY DETECTION METHODS

Reverse Transcription Polymerase Chain Reaction

Quantitative RT-PCR is one of the most used techniques in molecular biology for the detection of miRNAs. It is considered a reliable thermocycler technique due to its large dynamic range, high sequence specificity and high sensitivity [89]. Its principle is outlined in Fig. (**3**).

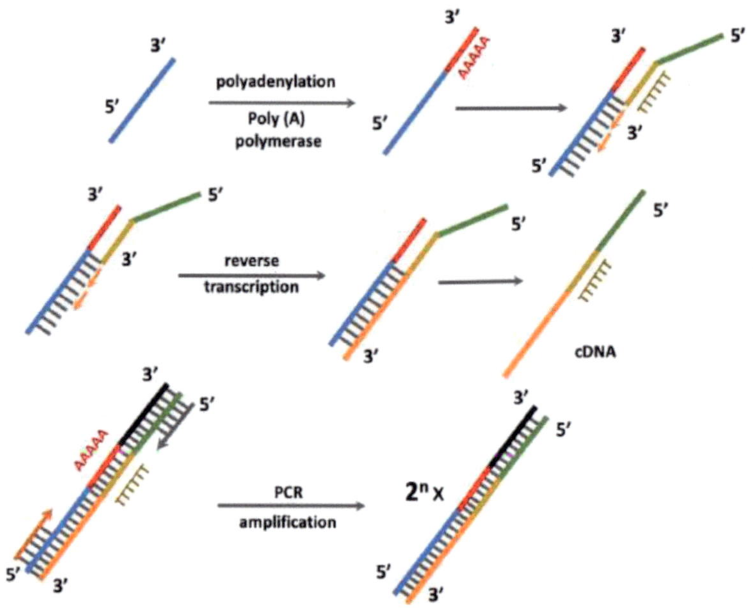

Fig. (3). Principle of RT-PCR for the detection of mature miRNAs. Details: **a)** adding a poly(A)tail to the miRNA sequences, **b)** reverse transcription with an adaptor primer using an oligo-dT with unique sequence at the 5′ end for universal reverse primer binding and **c)** cDNA is used for quantification by quantitative RT-PCR of miRNAs using specific forward and reverse primers.

Recently, Androvic *et al.* [90] reported an improved two-tailed RT-qPCR method for higher accuracy in the quantification of miRNAs. The method has a dynamic range of seven logs and is sensitive enough to detect as low as 10 copies of mature miRNA (Fig. **4**). Furthermore, it gives more reliable results than industry miRNA assays available on the market.

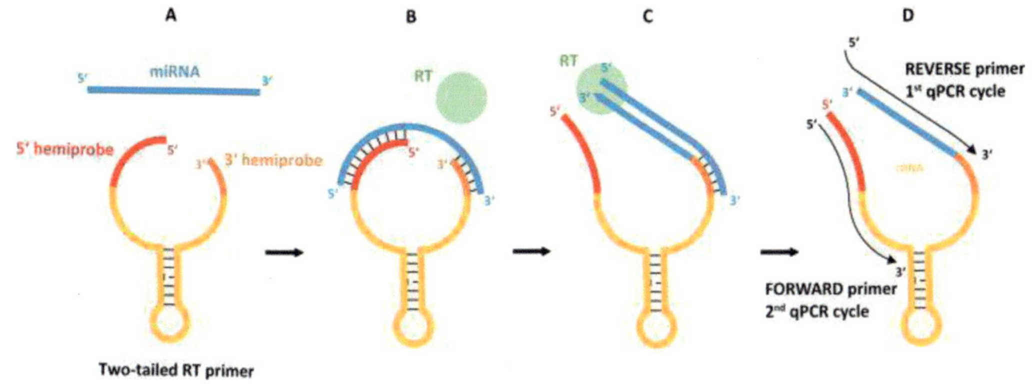

Fig. (4). Schematic illustration of two-tailed RT-qPCR. Step (A): the two-tailed RT primer has two hemiprobes which are connected to a hairpin folding sequence. Step (B): the hemiprobes bind to the ends of the target miRNA to form a stable complex. Step (C): the reverse transcriptase binds the 3'-end of the hybridized two-tailed RT primer and elongates it to form tailed cDNA. Step (D): the cDNA is amplified by qPCR using two target-specific primers.

For instance, Su *et al.* used RT-PCR for miR-199 detection as a lung cancer biomarker. They found that its overexpression can inhibit tumor cell division and metastasis. Patients with lower expression of miR-199 had higher rates of lymph node metastases and distant metastases, and their overall survival rates were lower [91]. In another study, Jia *et al.* examined the detection of miR-190, which acts as a regulator for FOXP2 genes in gastric cancer cell line SGC7901. The results showed that the miR may serve as a good target for GC diagnosis [92]. In the case of ovarian cancer, Liu *et al.* noticed that the increased expression of miR-665 suppresses the growth and migration of ovarian cancer cells. The miR-665 acts as a probe for homeobox A10 protein expressed in ovarian cancer. The RT-PCR highlights this correlation between the protein and the corresponding miRNA in the proliferation of this cancer [93]. In spite of the wide use of RT-PCR, it is time-consuming, cost-prohibitive and can lead to false positive results due to the short size and similarities between miRNAs [94].

Loop-mediated Isothermal Amplification

LAMP is an isothermal PCR showing an extensive amplification process, which makes it rapid and very sensitive. Li *et al.* used LAMP for miRNA detection, which is based on an auto-cycling strand displacement DNA synthesis. The different steps of this reaction are illustrated in Fig. (**5**). The LAMP assay uses a template DNA containing six primers: B3, B2, B1, F1c, F2c and M. The former one hybridizes with the target miR and extends in the presence of Bst DNA polymerase. The stem-loop structure can be formed after the releasing of the single-strand DNA [95].

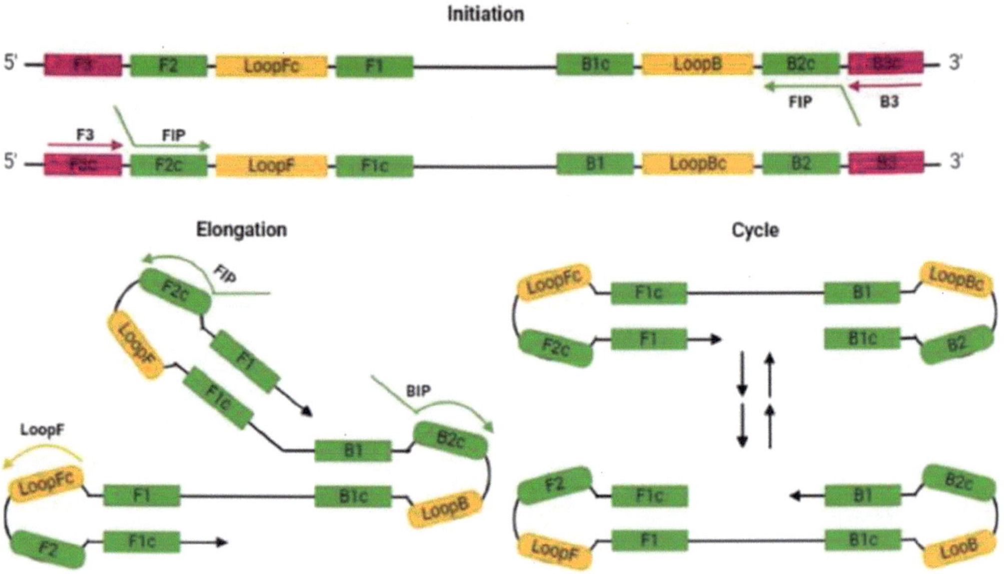

Fig. (5). Schematic representation of the LAMP principle. Reprinted with permission from [96].

In other interesting works, Sun *et al.* put forward a new one-step assay for miRNA detection based on a target-triggered LAMP (TT-LAMP). They detected down to the attomolar level of miRNAlet-7a extracted from CRC cells (HCT-116) in real samples [97]. The same miRNA has been detected by Tian *et al.* using LAMP coupled to rolling circle amplification. The RCA-LAMP exhibits much higher detection sensitivity than LAMP and offers a detection limit lowered down to 10 aM [98].

As a major drawback, LAMP is an indirect evaluation method relying on the use of fluorescent dyes, which complicate the detection of the desired products from the non-specific ones, sometimes leading to false positive results [89].

Catalytic Hairpin Assembly

CHA is an enzyme-free isothermal amplification technique, first proposed in 2008 by Yin *et al.* [99], that permits an exponential amplification of a target sequence in 15 minutes through a thermodynamically driven entropy gain process as illustrated in Fig. (**6**). Typically, CHA is a series of reactions executed in the presence of two DNA strands owing stable hairpin structures. The hairpins should successively be opened until the formation of thermodynamically favorable DNA duplexes. Thus, the products of the CHA reaction can reach 600,000-fold signal amplification [100]. However, CHA sometimes suffers from non-specific hybridization of the two hairpin probes, which causes significant background leakage. He *et al.* proposed a novel CHA integrating PDA microtube waveguide system. This heterogenous CHA exhibits better sensitivity, selectivity and low detection limit of miR-21 [101].

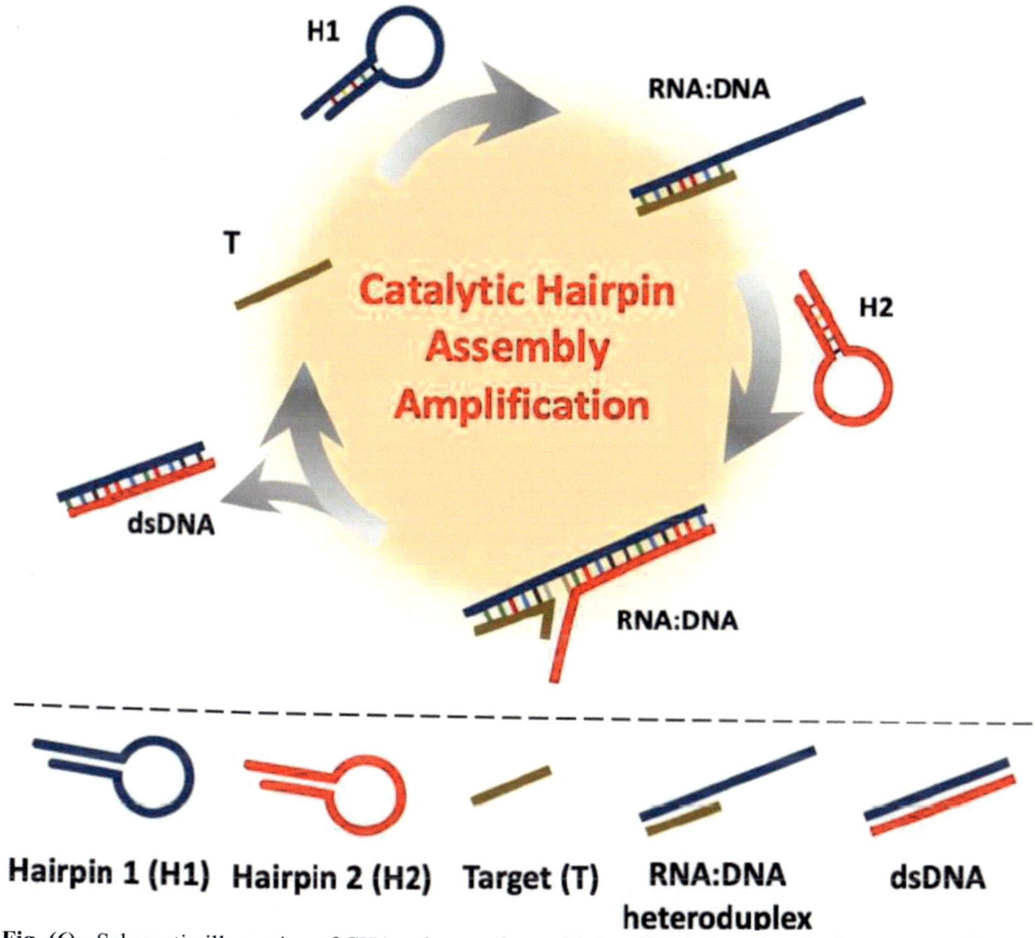

Fig. (6). Schematic illustration of CHA gel assay for multiple miRNA detection. In the presence of target miRNAs, the HDP will be unfolded to form HDP-miRNA duplexes and expose the concealed domain. Then, the corresponding HAP replaces the target miRNA to form specific HDP/HAP complexes and releases miRNA based on a thermodynamically driven entropy gain process, and the released miRNA triggers the next recycle to produce numerous corresponding HDP/HAP complexes (HDP and HAP are pair of hairpin probe). Reprinted with permission from [102].

Rolling Circle Amplification

RCA is an isothermal enzyme-assisted process, that utilizes DNA or RNA polymerases, discovered at the end of 20th century to be used as a sensitive diagnostic technique for different targets such as nucleic acids (DNA, RNA), small molecules, proteins, and cells [103]. This technique is widely used in bioassay amplification and provides long single-stranded DNA or RNA due to its simple principle and simple operation. Four essential biological reagents are needed, which are DNA polymerase, short DNA or RNA primer, a circle template and deoxynucleotide triphosphates [104]. In the presence of the DNA polymerase, the circular template has been copied hundreds to thousands of times to produce repeated units, as seen in Fig. (**7**) [105].

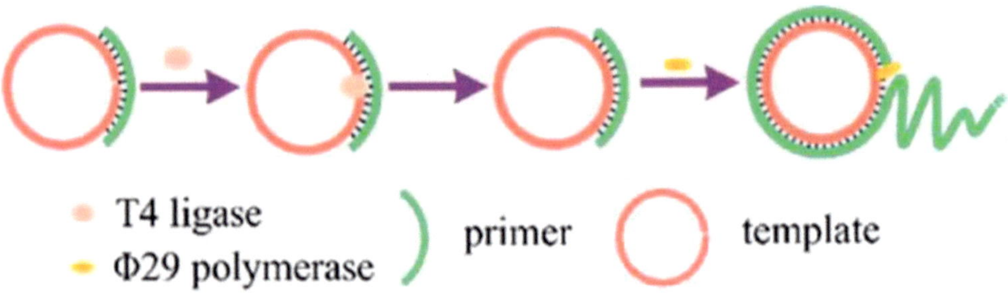

Fig. (7). Schematic illustration of rolling circle amplification strategy. Reprinted with permission from [105].

For instance, Hansen's group designed and demonstrated an automated on-chip RCA assay on a multi-chamber polymer chip platform enabling the detection of synthetic influenza targets with a limit of detection of 2 pM after 45 min of RCA [106]. In another study, Ciftci *et al.* used RCA for the indirect electrochemical detection of the Ebola virus RNA through the enzymatic catalysis of glucose by a bound GOx to the amplified nucleic acids [107].

Hybridization Chain Reaction

In 2004, Pierce and Dirks introduced for the first time a new method for nucleic acid amplification, the hybridization chain reaction (HCR). This technique is based on the presence of two stable hairpins H1 and H2, that trigger a chain reaction of hybridization once an initiator DNA is added to the mixture, as illustrated in Fig. (**8**) [108]. HCR is becoming largely used in biosensing systems such as the detection of small molecules, proteins and nucleic acids due to its excellent amplification efficiency, simple protocol, enzyme-free and isothermal nature [109].

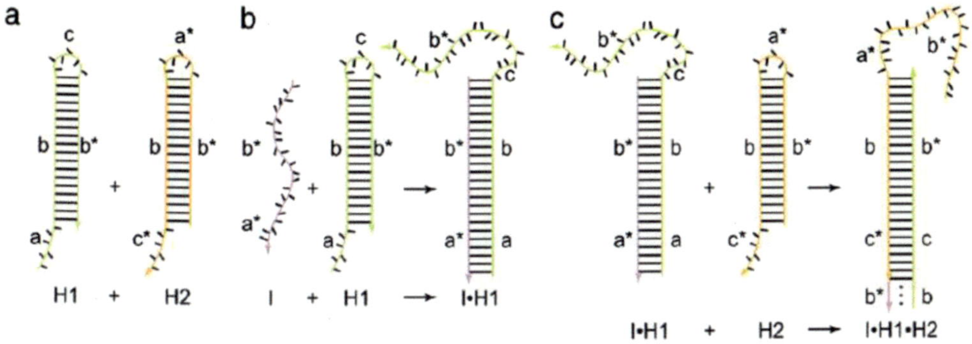

Fig. (8). Schematic representation of hybridization chain reaction using two probes [108].

Yang et al. developed a fluorescence-based biosensor using hybridization chain reaction for the detection of miRNAs. Two fluorescent hairpins are initiated with miRNAs to be hybridized and amplified. The HCR products will be anchored on the GO surface used as fluorescence signal readout. The HCR products maintain their fluorescence whereas hairpin probes can be completely quenched by GO which permits a good miRNA assay [110]. More recently, an electrochemical biosensor coupled with HCR signal amplification for exosomal microR-122 was reported by Shen's group. In the presence of the target, the hairpin probes, immobilized on the surface of gold electrode, could be opened and started the HCR. More the double helixes are long, more they capture a positively charged ruthenium complex and enhance the differential pulse voltammetry signal. This biosensor shows very good performances in terms of selectivity, specificity and sensitivity with an attomolar level detection limit [111].

ELECTROCHEMICAL DETECTION METHODS

Nowadays, electrochemical biosensors are showing attractive merits such as portability, accessibility, affordability, rapidity of response and ease, and especially compatibility with POC testing [112 - 115]. All these reasons make electrochemical biosensors an emergent alternative to conventional methods for early diagnosis and screening for many diseases like cancer.

According to IUPAC, an electrochemical biosensor is a device that can transform chemical information, relating to the expression level of a specific target, into a measurable electrical signal. This makes it possible to offer a quantitative or semi-quantitative analytical report. Usually, biosensors are made up of two elements joined in series: a receptor that represents the recognition part using a biochemical mechanism and an electrochemical transducer. Commonly, the role of the biosensor resides in its ability to measure changes occurring in the electrode or interfacial characteristics due to the presence of the target. This can be achieved through electrochemically active reporters, such as small redox molecules or enzyme-substrate pairs [115].

The urgency of rapid detection of cancer and the efficiency of electrochemical biosensors are now stimulating several groups around the world to develop increasingly efficient electrochemical biosensors. Several electrochemical techniques are currently listed for the quantification of miRNAs that are considered as relevant tumor biomarkers that link to cancer biogenesis and progress. Among these methods, voltammetry (namely cyclic voltammetry, linear scanning voltammetry, square wave voltammetry, differential pulse voltammetry, *etc.*) remains the most widely used as well as chronoamperometry and electrochemical impedance spectroscopy and capacitance.

The miRNA-based biosensors are usually based on hybridization between a single-stranded sequence immobilized on the working electrode surface and the complementary target. The detection is then conducted by a range of methodologies.

Amperometry

Among the most widely used biosensors, over names are amperometric biosensors. This is due to their flexibility, ease of design, and cost-effectiveness of the equipment. The first and most widely used example of this technique is a glucose biosensor, which uses has persisted for more than 60 years. This device is used worldwide for glucose monitoring at home emphasizing the on-site analysis. Amperometric sensing consists of cells with two or three electrodes and the application of a constant potential at the working electrode (usually carbon, platinum, and gold), *versus* a standard reference electrode such as AgCl/Ag/KCl or Hg_2Cl_2/Hg/KCl electrodes.

The electrochemical oxidation or reduction of one or more specific electroactive species, when occurred, is assessed by the measure of the current and correlated with the concentration production or consumption in the adjacent biocatalytic layer. These steady-state currents are proportional to the amount of a target analyte [116]. Thanks to its high sensitivity, this technique is favored for the detection of biomolecules at extremely low levels. Several research groups developed plenty of electrochemical biosensors for the detection of cancer-related miRNAs. For instance, Raouafi and coworkers reported a miR-21 biosensor is based on a competition between the target and its biotinylated analog in order to hybridize the immobilized probe, as shown in Fig. (**9**) [117]. The biosensor shows a good selectivity and a detection limit of 25 fM. The Determination of the mature miR-21 in RNA_t extracted from breast cells is carried out compared to those extracted from non-tumorigenic cells. The results are in agreement with the expected miRNA overexpression in cancer cells [90, 118].

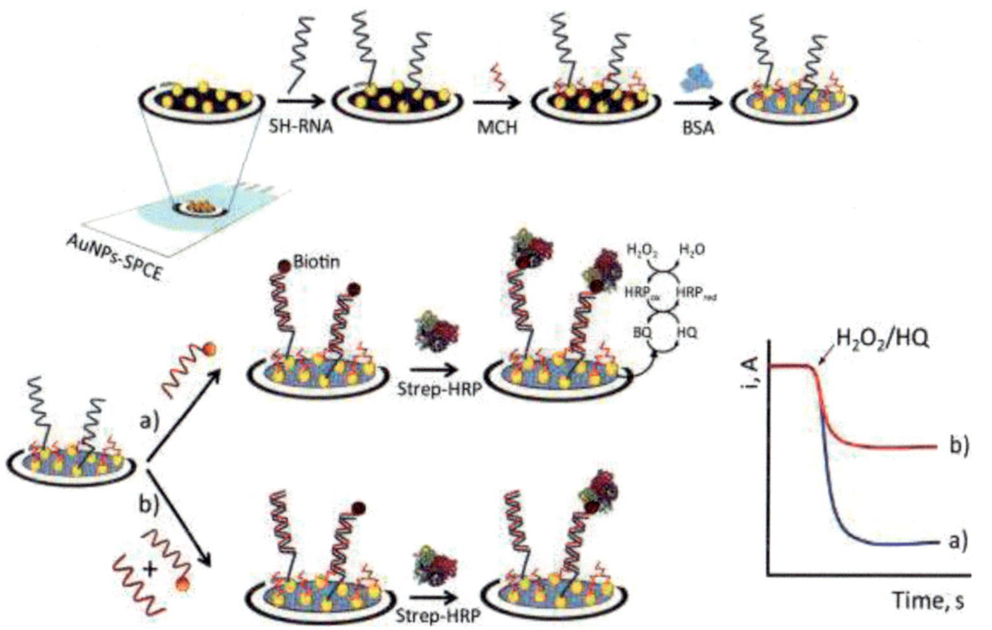

Fig. (9). Schematic illustration for the competition-based detection of miRNA using gold-modified screen-printed carbon electrodes and streptavidin/HRP for the revealing the miRNA/RNA recognition. Reprinted with permission from [117].

Campuzano *et al.* developed an amperometric magnetosensor involving the RNA-binding viral protein p19 implemented on magnetic beads [119]. The use of biotinylated anti-miR-21 allowed the formation of the HRP-labelled streptavidin-biotin complex and the amperometric readout. The biosensor allowed the detection of 0.4 fmol of a synthetic target and the analysis of a series of RNA_t samples extracted from human breast tumor specimens. The concordant results make the developed strategy potentially useful for the breast cancer diagnosis.

Overexpression of miR-21 was also proposed for other different cancer and Zhou and coworkers developed a label-free biosensor using and hemin-G-quadruplex complex for the signal amplification [120]. The approach was based on the immobilization of the thiolated hairpin structure probe on a gold electrode modified with AuNPs and the use of different DNA sequences. The calibration range was between 5 and 5000 pM with a LOD of 3.96 pM. The importance of this strategy was in its application in the target detection in the total RNA extracted from gastric, breast, hepatocarcinoma, and colon cancer cell lines. A more straightforward strategy was developed by the same group for the detection of the same target [121]. The opening of the hairpin after its hybridization with the target induces its interaction with the streptavidin-HRP bioconjugate that yields an amperometric signal. To improve the conductivity and the active surface of the electrode, the strategy used graphene and AuNPs. This assay offered a linear range between 1 and 5000 pM with a detection limit of 0.4 pM. Successful results have achieved the analysis of miR-21 expression in human HeLa cells and normal human hepatic cells.

In another interesting work, Zeng *et al.* developed a 16-channel SPGE platform for the simultaneous detection of four miRNAs linked to pancreatic carcinoma: miR-21, miR-155, miR-196a, and miR-210. A base of tetrahedral DNA nanostructures was immobilized with a fourth biotinylated ssDNA sequence at the top of this forming tetrahedron, which was complementary to the target miRNAs. Poly-HRP40 captured by the biotin catalyzed the reduction of hydrogen peroxide in the presence of TMB giving a measurable amperometric signal. The platform offered a detection limit of 10 fM and a linear range from 10 fM to 10 nM for all miRNAs. The evaluating the expression levels of these miRNAs was achieved in clinical samples resulting in 2.2-3.5-fold higher expressions of the four targets in serum samples from pancreatic cancer patients when compared to healthy donors [122]. These results were concordant with the expected overexpression of the four targets in pancreatic ductal adenocarcinoma [123]. Another strategy based on a DNA tetrahedral nanostructure with a pendant sequence was reported by Huang et *al.* [124]. The pendant hairpin can be open when recognized by the target miR-21. The released stem sequence, consisting of cMyc sequence at 3′-termini, could self-assemble with K^+ and formed the parallel G-quadruplex. This induced the construction of guanine nanowire in the presence of Mg^{2+} [125]. The oxidation of TMB was catalyzed by G-quadruplex-hemin repeat units. The detection limit was 176 fM and the logarithmic concentration ranging from 500 fM to 10 nM. Assays in direct and spiked serum samples from breast cancer patients were successfully made. Furthermore, Cheng *et al.* designed a DNA model with three functional parts for the detection of miR-21 in serum samples and based on the work of Liu *et al.* [126], which involved 5 regions. The strategy as shown in Fig. (**10**) was based on a target recognition unit, a target amplification unit, and a DNAzyme 8-7 units. The target triggered the analogs that are accompanied by a cascade of polymerase cleavage enzymes. DNAzyme was generated and mimic HRP in the presence of hemin. The amperometric response is obtained from the reduction of TMB in the presence of H_2O_2. The calibration range was from 1 aM to 100 pM, with a detection limit of 0.5 aM. The implication of four concentration of target in the recovery evaluation of serum samples showed no evident interferences allowing the developed strategy potential tool for the detection of the target miRNA in cancer-related biological samples [127].

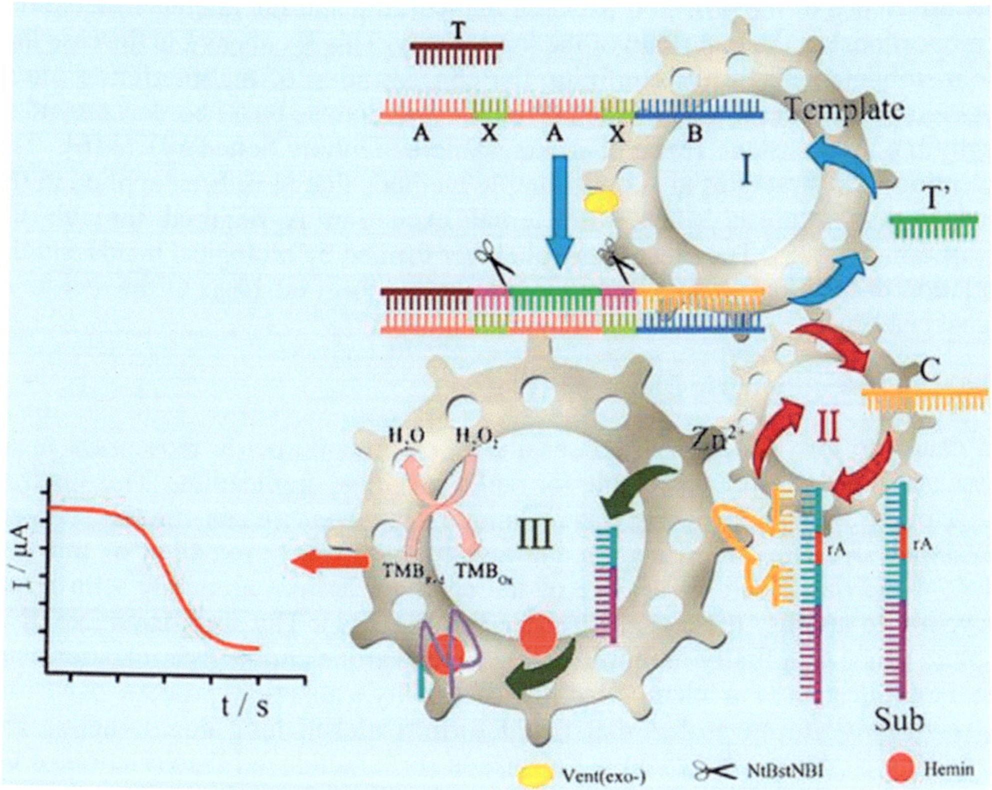

Fig. (10). Schematic illustration of the 3TICA strategy towards the miR-21. Printed with permission from [127].

Potentiometry

The potentiometric sensor operates under conditions of near-zero current flow and requires the determination of the potential variance between a working/indicator and reference electrodes. These electrodes are separated by a selective membrane in the case that no significant current flowing between them. One of the most important kinds of transducers is the ion-selective electrode, which is an electrochemical device based on recognition elements like fine films or selective membranes. The pH electrode represents the most usual device and several other ions such as fluorine, iodine or cyanide. The specificity of the selective membrane is attributed to its composition (metal salts or polymers). A bench of ion-selective electrodes is nowadays commercially available for specific detection of ions like calcium or copper. However, the gas-sensing electrode is also used and based on a gas-permeable membrane in addition to the chemically sensitive field-effect transistor, which is a semiconductor and responds to the electric gradient of the surface.

The difference of the potential between the working and the reference electrodes is proportional to the logarithm of the ion activity. This is coherent in the case that the membrane selectivity is infinite, the concentration of the interfering ion is constant or low, and if the potential differences at diverse phase borders are either negligible or constant (except at the sample-solution boundary) [116]. The potentiometric strategies area quite simple methods that have been applied in the bioanalytical interests since no external excitation is required through the measurement [128]. The electric double layer formed by biological bonds and the variation of the electric potential near the surface form the basis of the measured signal [129].

Classical Potentiometric Biosensors

To date, the low selectivity and sensitivity of potentiometric biosensors make these strategies not yet acceptable for real biomedical applications. This justifies the scarcity of works adopting this technique. However, we can cite the platform developed by Zhou and Tang for the potentiometric determination of miR-21. Their work was based on the use of the catalytic hairpin assembly with target recycling to amplify the signal illustrated in Fig. (**11**). The short-stranded DNA capture probe was firstly immobilized on the electrode and its hybridization with the target triggered a chain reaction of the hybridization process occurring between two hairpin probes that could form a nicked long double-helix. The increasing negative charges on the electrode surface-induced the variation of the electrode potential. This allowed the quantification of the target. The obtained linear range was between 0.1 pM and 10 nM with a detection limit of 43 fM. The developed biosensor showed adequate sensitivity, storage stability, and good accuracy in real sample testing [130].

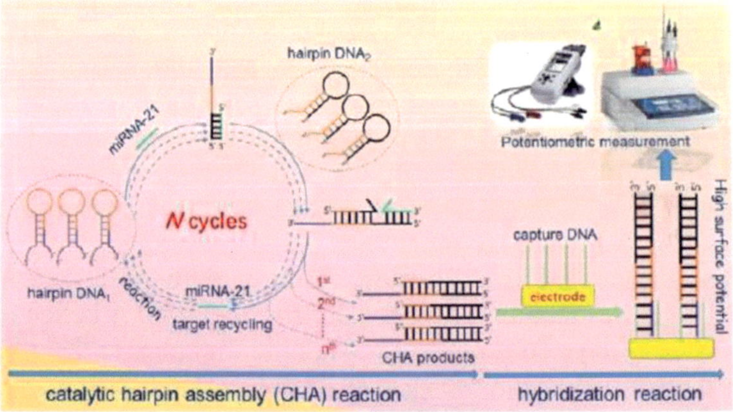

Fig. (11). Schematic illustration of CHA-mediated surface charge density on the capture DNA-modified gold electrode for the sensitive. Printed with permission from [130].

Goda *et al.* developed a platform about PCR-contained electrical readout of exosomal miR-143 and miR-146a. The platform was based on a hybridization event between the amplified cDNA and an immobilized HS–$(CH_2)_6$–DNA. A sequence of SB was also immobilized in order to reduce nonspecific adsorption by forming a thick hydration shell onto the microelectrode array. In potentiometry, the course of hybridization event is directly linked to changes that occur on the surface potential by the introduction of Coulomb charges. The developed potentiometry-based device could distinguish the target at a concentration of 420 pM with dynamic ranges of two orders of magnitude. The sensitivity for target cDNA was 6.5 mV per decade between 2 pM and 200 pM [131].

FET-Based Biosensors

As a second main electrical detection method, appears the field-effect transistor (FET) which represents a suitable option in the label-free category and can offer a miniaturized and commercialized platform especially with the assistance of nanotechnology and organic materials. The considerable recognition allocated to FET-based biosensors is due to their advantages such as high sensitivity, rapid detection, lower power demands, direct electrical readout, and manufacturing at inexpensive rates in comparison to other methods [132]. Cai *et al.* developed a graphene-based FET biosensor chip using micro manufacture processes. The process is based on the use of reduced graphene oxide, AuNPs and the hybridization event between the immobilized PNA and the target miRNA, which is monitored by the electrical measurement. The developed biosensor showed a good selectivity against one-base mismatched and non-complementary miRNA sequences. The achieved detection limit was 10 fM. Two different concentrations of miRNA were spiked in serum samples and gave a higher response than serum without target miRNA indicating the potential of this platform in further disease diagnostics [133]. The design of a semi-conducting SiNW FET biosensor array for the detection of miR-21 was achieved by Gao *et al.* The signal-stranded DNA probe was chemically tethered on SiNW surface through several steps as piranha cleaning and exposing to APTES solution followed by rinsing with absolute ethanol. A self-assembled monolayer with terminal amino group was prepared by blowing dry the surface with nitrogen and a quick heating and DNA that contained freshly prepared EDC and NHS was coupled to the surface of the nanowire. The hybridization process could be monitored in real time with this SiNW-FET sensor through the change in electrostatic potential induced by the charge accumulation at the surface. Under optimal conditions the developed sensor revealed repaid and reliable detection of 1 fM miR-21 and a specificity for SNP discrimination [134]. A crumpled graphene-based FET electrical biosensor has been developed for the detection of nucleic acids. These devices show an ultra-high sensitivity detection in buffer and human serum sample down to 600 zM and 20 aM, respectively on millimeter scale structures using adsorption and hybridization experiments of PNA and DNA with the target miRNA. The attainment of graphene in a bent and crumpled structure is made by macroscopic manipulation of the 2D layer and the resulting "nano"-sized features exhibit the superior sensing performance, good reproducibility [135]. A multiplexed electrical detection of lung cancer biomarkers was developed by using SiNW-FET devices. For a multiplexed detection of miR−126 and CEA, the SiNW nanosensor was integrated with a fluid-exchange system using PDMS with microfluidic chambers (Fig. **12**). The detection limit was 0.1 fM for miR-126 and 1 fg/mL for CEA. The specificity of the SiNW-FET biosensor was verified through the introduction of miR-125 showing no significant change of the electrical current. A differentiating between a lung cancer patient and a normal person was also achieved due to the developed device [136].

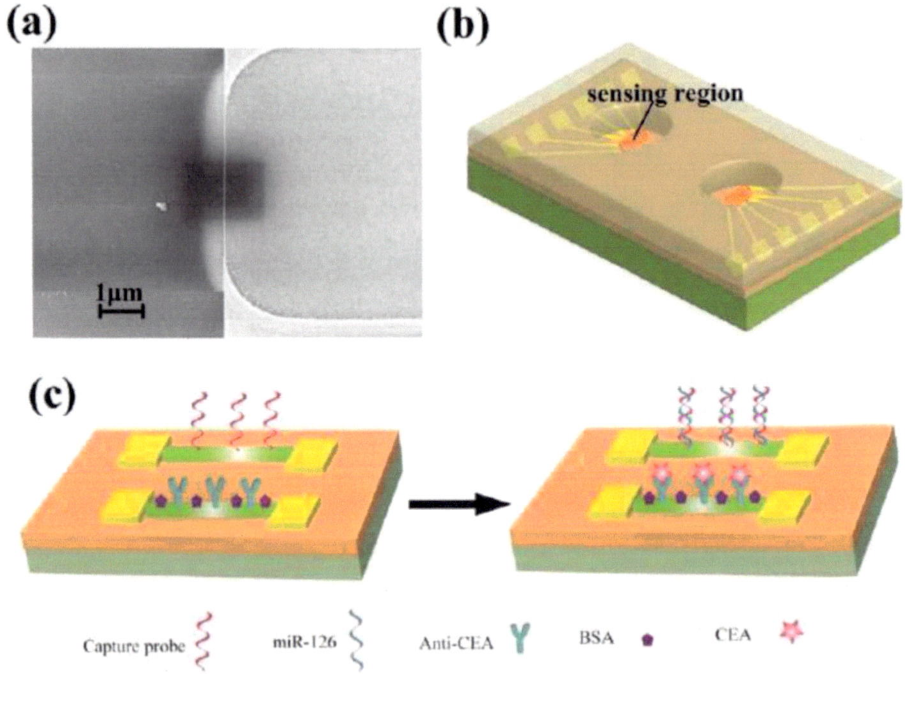

Fig. (12). (a) SEM image of the designed SiNW. **(b)** Schematic illustration of the SiNW FET integrated with PDMS chip with two macro-scale solution chambers to allow simultaneous detection. **(c)** Schematic represenetation of the multiplexed detection of CEA and miR-126.

Cyclic Voltammetry

Cyclic voltammetry, generally used to study reaction kinetics, is one of the most frequently used types of voltammetry. It is frequently used in biosensors for characterization purposes specially to follow the variation of current before and after any modification of the electrode surface [137].

Wang *et al.* designed a sensing electrode to determine the levels of miR-182 in sera of glioma patients. The strategy involved a competition between a biotinylated miRNA and a target miRNA for the hybridization of the ODN probes and then the adhesion of Fc-capped gold nanoparticle-streptavidin conjugate [138]. The high number of ferrocene tags (about 127 ± 10 tags per nanoparticle) on each gold nanoparticle represented an amplification strategy. The obtained calibration plot was between 10 fM and 2.0 pM with a 10 fM-detection limit. The biosensor was used to detect the target in serum samples without pretreatment and RNA extraction and enrichment. The miR-182 levels are be 3.1 times higher in glioma patients than in healthy donors, according to this study. This over-expression was in concordance with the results obtained from RT-qPCR measurements [139].

Fig. (**13**) illustrates a simple label-free biosensor for the detection of another cancer biomarker miR-155. The strategy used PdNPs for their electrocatalytic activity towards H_2O_2 [140] and as an adsorbent for the redox probe, the thionine. This strategy offered reverse proportionality between the peak currents and the expression level of the target with a calibration plot between 5.6 and 5.6×10^5pM, and 1.87 pM as a detection limit [141].

Labib *et al.* designed a protein-facilitated SensPEQ for the determination of miR-16, miR-21, and miR-150 signature in CLL. The biosensor was applied in human serum from healthy donors and patients at different stages of CLL in the presence of an internal standards, cel-miR-39. The strategy involved the use of a thiol-modified UIP self-assembled onto the electrode surface and two DNA strands hybridizing with the probe and the target miRNA. The DNA strands were tagged at their extremities with methylene blue giving an amplified redox signal [142].

Differential Pulse Voltammetry

Differential pulse voltammetry consists of the application of a series of regular voltage currents to the linear potential scan to significantly improve the sensitivity of the analysis over normal voltammetry methods by reducing the effect of the charging current by sampling the current just before the potential change [143]. Due to its high sensitivity, this technique is widely used for the quantification of low abundance targets [144].

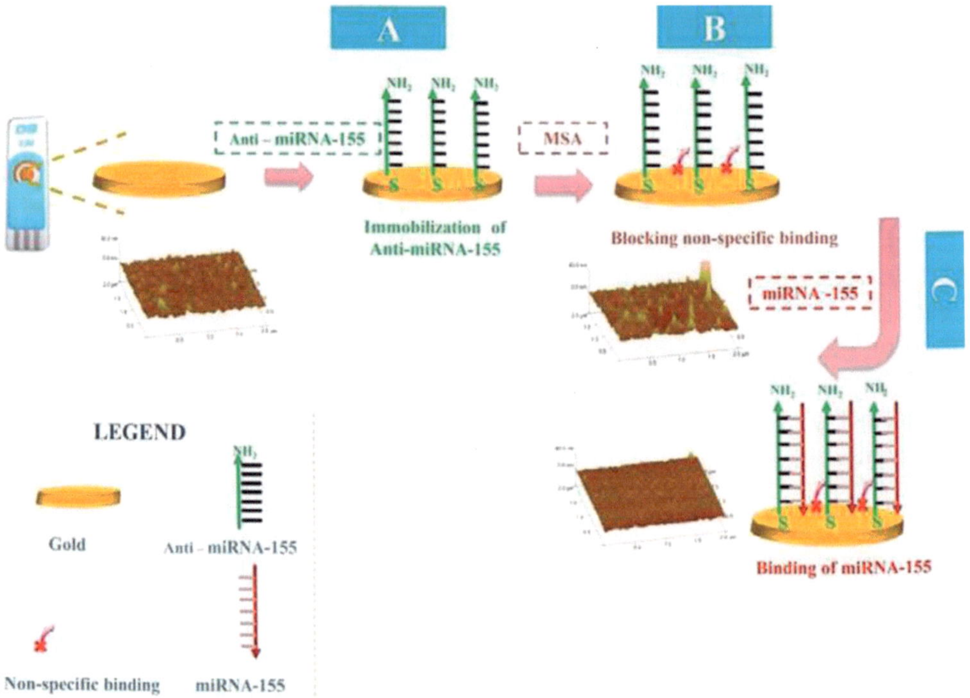

Fig. (13). Schematic illustration of electrochemical biosensor for detection of miR-155. Printed with permission from [141].

Zouari *et al.* also developed two nanomaterials-based biosensors for an amplified determination of cancer-related biomarkers. The first platform consisted of a sandwich hybridization assay involving the hybridization of the target miR-21 with an immobilized thiolated probe to the electrode surface and a biotinylated reporter. The electrodes were modified with gold nanoparticle and reduced graphene oxide and the labeling nanotracers consisted of ferrocene-capped gold nanoparticles modified with streptavidin-conjugated with a biotinylated detection probe. The ferrocene oxidation gave the DPV-measured current with a linear range from 10 fM to 2 pM and 5 fM as a detection limit. The developed biosensor was applied in the determination of miR-21 expression in sera from breast cancer patients and healthy donors. An expected overexpression of the target of about 3-4 times was obtained [145], which is in agreement with previous results reported using RT-PCR [90, 118] and HPLC–MS_2 [146].

The second report involved a disposable carbon electrode with rGO and AuNPs modified with PCA and Fc-SH, respectively. An amino-DNA was covalently immobilized on the carboxylic moicties of PCA/rGO, while Fc-SH was used as a signaling molecule. The hybridization of the amino-DNA probe with the target induced a hindrance of the electron transfer hence a decrease in the oxidation current of the ferrocene. A detection limit of 5 fM was obtained. The designed biosensor was successfully applied for the determination of the target in total RNA extracted from cells or directly in serum samples both collected from breast cancer patients [147].

A three-way junction RNA structure was developed by Mohammadniaei *et al.* for the determination of miRNA-21 in breast cancer serum samples. The strategy illustrated in Fig. (**14**) was based on a MB-modified hairpin structure that acted as the sensing moiety and two other legs that acted as the signal amplifiers subsequently to their hybridization with barcode gold nanoparticles. The opening of the hairpin structure was due to the addition of the target and followed by the hybridization with a DNA modified gold nanoflower/platinum electrode. The two MB-modified barcodes were added to engage the second detection mode and had enhanced the electrochemical signal of MB by almost 230 times. A wide linear range from 1μM down to 0.5 fM was obtained with a detection limit as low as 0.135 fM. Higher expression levels of the endogenous circulating miRNA-21 were observed in serum from breast and liver cancer samples compared with those from healthy subjects and a much higher expression was observed in breast cancer stage 3 showing a correlation between the expression levels of the studied biomarker and the progress of the disease. Furthermore, the results were in agreement with the RT-qPCR data, and the cause of the differences was ascribed to the post-treatment of the purified nucleic acids with enzymes and reagents during the RT-qPCR [148].

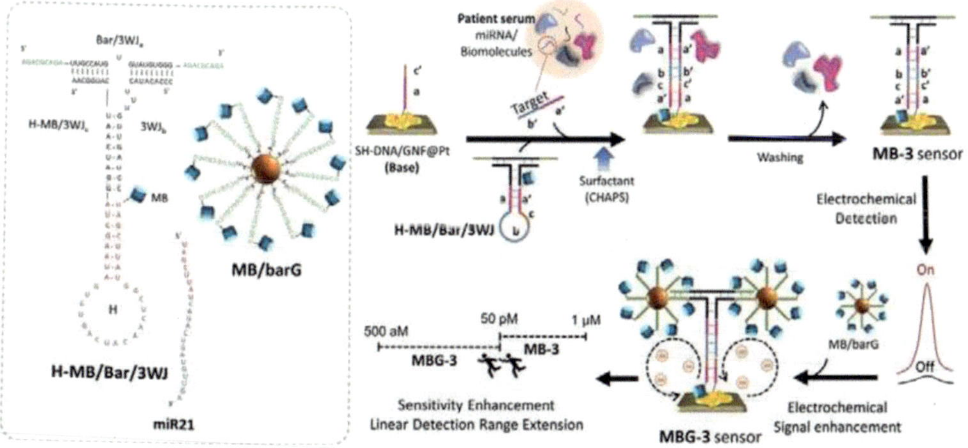

Fig. (14). Schematic diagram of the relay-race electrochemical biosensor. Left panel depicts the predicted structures and nucleic acid sequences of the H-MB/Bar/3WJ, Printed with permission from [148].

Another miRNA-21-biosensor was developed for the diagnosis of breast cancer. The platform was based on the use of hollow molybdenum disulfide microcubes and adopted an ECC redox cycling and duplex-specific nuclease strategies. The biotinylated ssDNA capture probes were first immobilized on the AuNPs/MoS_2-modified electrode followed by its hybridization with the target and the cleavage by duplex-cleavage nuclease avoiding the labeling with SA-ALP conjugates. The ECC redox cycling was then induced by ascorbic acid to produce an electrochemical response in the presence of ferrocene methanol and tris (2-carboxyethyl) phosphine. The resulting signals were inversely proportional to the target concentration and offered a dynamic range from 0.1 fM to 0.1 pM with a detection limit of 0.086 fM. Tests for the determination of the target in human serum samples from breast cancer patients were in agreement with those achieved by commercial RT-qPCR kit [149].

As well, Hong *et al.* designed likewise a simple strategy for miRNA-21 determination in serum from breast cancer patients involving an amplification by DNA concatamers illustrated in Fig. (**15**). The strategy introduced two auxiliary probes self-assembled to form one-dimensional DNA concatamers, hybridizing with the capture probe hairpin previously opened by the target. The used signal reporter was the ruthenium complex [150], which could bind to negatively charged DNA strands. The obtained linear range was between 100 aM and 100 pM and 100 aM as a detection limit. In good agreement with previously reported works [151, 152]. The developed strategy demonstrated overexpression of the target in breast cancer sera when compared to healthy samples. The obtained results were concordant with those obtained by qRT-qPCR [153].

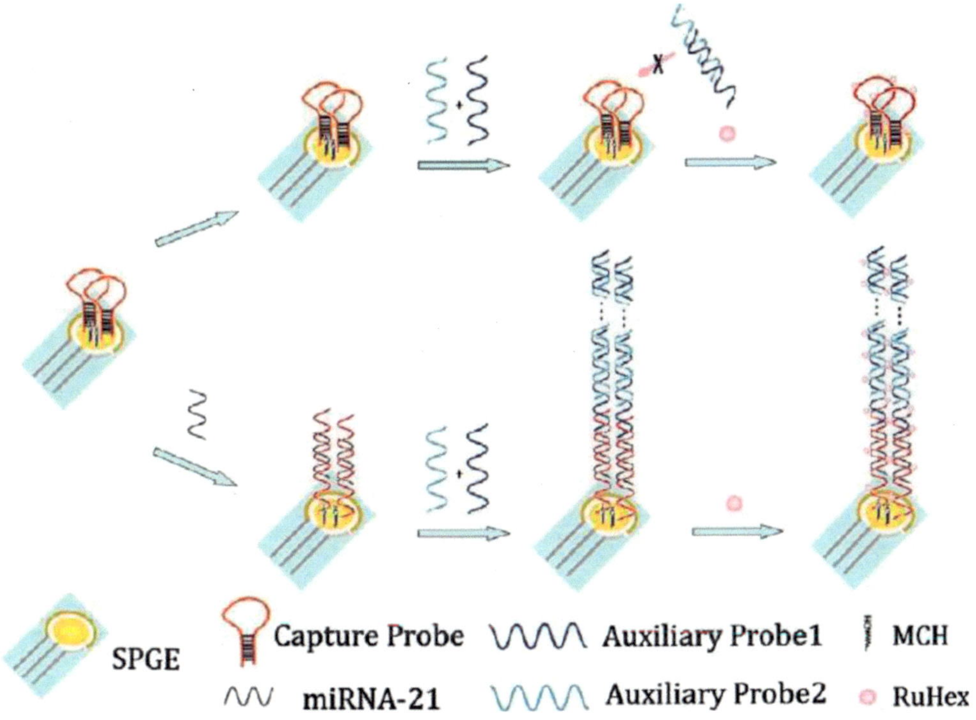

Fig. (15). Schematic representation of the concatamer-based ultrasensitive electrochemical miR biosensor to detect miR-21. Printed with permission from [153].

A label-free and amplification-free DNA origami-based platform was designed to detect miR-21. Several structural engineering capabilities and large surface area were attributed to cross-shape DNA origami nanostructures [154, 155]. Their use could increase the accessibility and the recognition efficiency of the probes. The used redox indicator was MB since it differently interacts with ssDNA and dsDNA giving different electrochemical responses [156, 157]. A linear range between 0.1 pM and 10.0 nM and a detection limit of 79.8 fM was obtained. This approach showed a good selectivity against the non-complementary miRNA but lower selectivity towards the single-base mismatched sequences at the terminal position and middle position. Good results in spiked human sera were achieved [158].

The same target biomarker was studied in the diagnosis of gastric cancer involving T4 RNA ligase 2 that initiated a specific ligation reaction and T7 exonuclease that catalyzed the first stage cyclic enzymatic amplification (CEAM). Significant amplification of the signal and hence an improvement of the detection sensitivity were due to the two-stage CEAM that are show in Fig. (**16**). The developed biosensor offered a detection range between 100 pM and 1fM and with a detection limit of 0.36 fM. The expression of target miRNA-21 was assessed in serum collected from gastric cancer patients and healthy donors revealing and overexpression of the target in cancerous subjects in agreement with results from molecular biology methods [159].

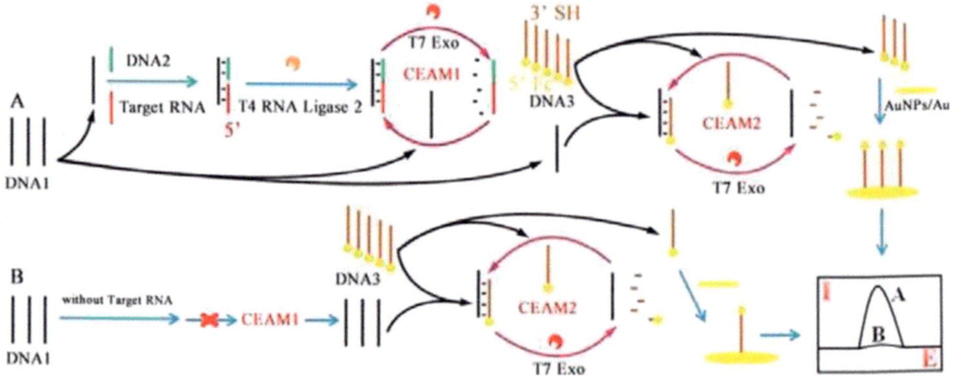

Fig. (16). A cyclic enzymatic signal amplification-based biosensor was developed for the detection of MRCA1-microRNA. Printed with permission from [159].

After the selective cleavage of the DNA from the RNA-DNA duplex, the released target could trigger a second cycle. A 3-QD@DNA NC was prepared and introduce to selectively hybridize with the cleaved DNA probe on the electrode and to amplify the signal. The developed strategy offered a linear range from 5 aM to 5 fM with a detection limit of 1.2 aM. The biosensor was used to detect breast cancer-related biomarker in spiked serum with a good recovery [160].

Bartosik *et al.* developed a simple platform for the detection of the miRNA-522, which is known to induce the silencing of the AGR2 oncogene [161]. The strategy displayed in Fig. (**17**) was based on the use of the electroactivity of Os(VI)bipy complex which could specifically bind to 3'-end of ribose in an oligodeoxynucleotide [162]. The linear range was obtained from ~2 nM to 40 nM and the limit of detection was 2 nM [163].

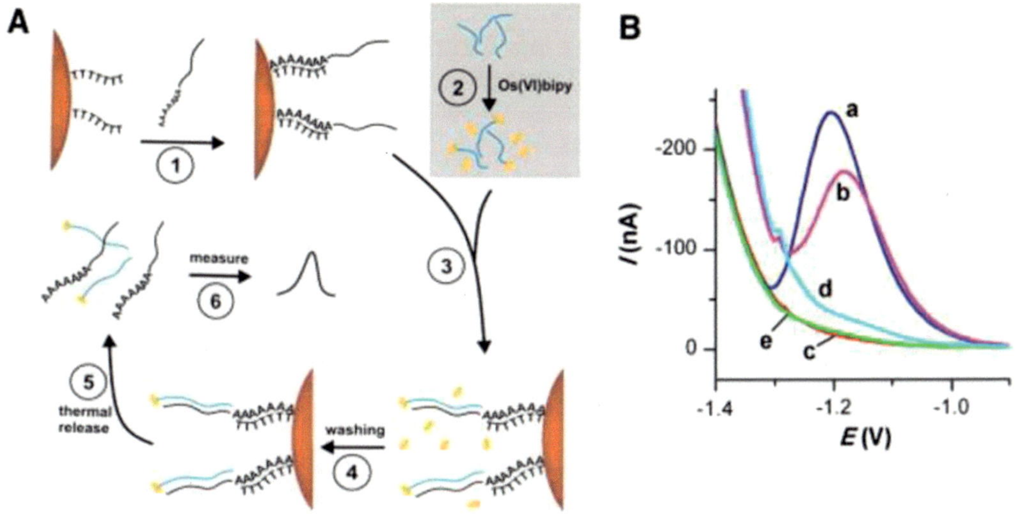

Fig. (17). Illustration of voltamperometric biosensors designed by Bartosiket al. for the detection of the miRNA-522 using [164] complex as a reporter.

A biosensor for the determination of miRNA-155 in plasma samples was designed by Azimzadeh *et al.* involving thiolated probes for the functionalization of gold nanorods which decorated the graphene oxide sheets on the glassy carbon electrode. The use of graphene sheets was justified by the improvement in the transport of electrons [165]. The intercalation of the label Oracet Blue and its reduction gave the electrochemical measured signal with a linear range from 2.0 fM to 8.0 pM and a detection limit of 0.6 fM. The designed platform was applied in the detection of the target in plasma of breast cancer patients [166].

Square Wave Voltammetry

The SWV technique is becoming more and more used by electrochemists. The current response to the potential excitation is sampled once with each forward pulse and once with each reverse pulse. Three current potential plots can be generated for forward current and reverse current *versus* potential as well as the difference between current and potential. The difference graph is usually used. The number of peaks appearing on the voltammogram corresponds to the number of electroactive species present and the height of the peak is proportional to the amount of these species in the bulk solution.

An SWV-based electrochemical biosensor for the determination of miR-21 was designed by Zhou *et al.* [167]. The amplification method in this work was based on the isothermal target recycling process and took advantage of DNA signal transducer and the kinetic and thermodynamic difference in DNA strand displacement reactions. The calibration plot was between 0.5 and 2000 pM with a detection limit of 0.056 pM. The platform was successfully applied to the determination of the target in total RNA from breast cancer cells (MCF-7).

Another breast cancer-biosensor was developed based on the detection of miR-21. The hybridization between the target, the thiolated capture probe, and the auxiliary probe induced the formation of a star trigon structure as illustrated in Fig. (**18**). The added endonuclease cleaved the capture probe releasing the capture probe's label and hence a decrease in the signal is noticed. Subsequent to this cleavage, the target and the auxiliary probe could form other star trigons with other capture probes. The linear range was obtained between 100 aM to 1 nM with a detection limit of 30 aM. A confirmation of the practical value of the developed strategy was achieved by the detection of the target miRNA in serum from both breast cancer patients and healthy donors. The overexpression of the miR-21 in cancer case is in good agreement with the results obtained using a commercial RT-qPCR [168].

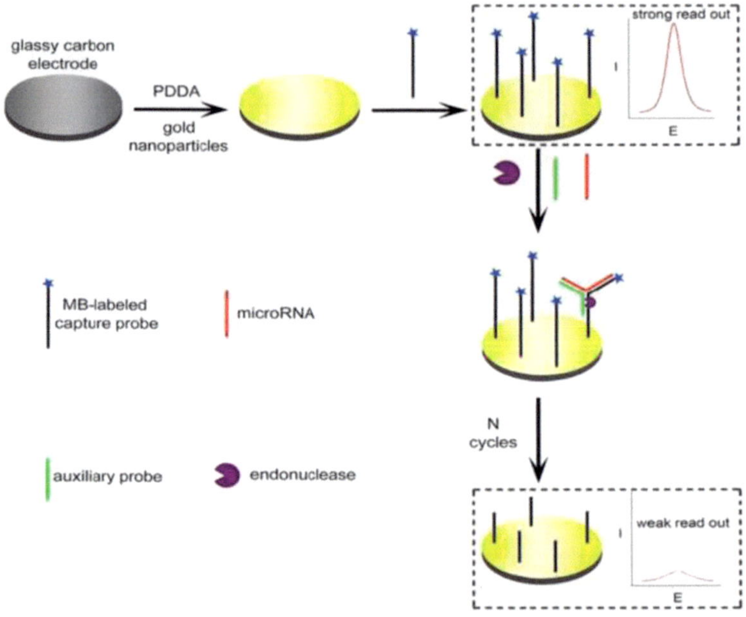

Fig. (18). Schematic illustration of the electrochemical microRNA biosensor. Printed with permission from [168].

Also, a biosensor that achieved the attomole levels of miR-21 detection was developed based on the use of large quantities of Cd^{2+} modified TiP as signal units. Complexes of molecules whose role has been demonstrated for electron transfer [150, 169] interact with DNA base-pairs and significantly enhanced the electrochemical signal. In addition, the strategy involved these molecules as an "electron bridge" for electron transport and signal enhancement. The hybridization between the immobilized thiolated capture DNA and half of the target miR-21 and the second one between the other half with the biotinylated detection DNA further conjugated with streptavidin-modified TiP−Cd^{2+} offered a sandwich structure. The obtained linear range was between 1.0 aM and 10.0 pM with 0.76 aM as a detection limit [170]. The developed biosensor was tested in the analysis of serum samples from leukemia, cervical, and breast cancer patients showing upregulation of the target micRNA-21 in cancer subjects compared to healthy donors. These results agreed to previously reported upregulation of this target in cancer cases patients [153, 171, 172].

Furthermore, the expression level of miR-21 was detected in serum collected from the breast, lung, and gastric cancer patients and was verified with long DNA concatamers-based strategy. This strategy, shown in Fig. (**19**), involved the use of an acridone derivative, DSA, which acted as a hybridization indicator through its intercalation into DNA duplexes. To improve the detection signal, the strategy relies on the use of a long DNA concatamers and p19-modified magnetic beads that bonded to the formed homoduplex for the specific enrichment. The calibration plot was from 20 to 100 aM with a detection limit of 6aM. An expected overexpression of the miRNA-21 was confirmed by this strategy [173].

A DNA circle capture probe with different target recognition domains was developed for simultaneous detection of miR-21 and miR-155. A tetrahedron DNA nanostructure (TDN) was immobilized on the Au/GCE electrode surface with at its top the DNA circle capture probe was initiated to recognize the two targets. This process was under the assistance of Helper strands, which could trigger mimetic proximity ligation assay to attach the beacons ferrocene and methylene blue. SWV responses of the biosensor achieved the limit of detection was 18.9 aMand 39.6 aM for miR-21 and miR-155 respectively. The developed strategy was applied for simultaneous detection of miR-21 in cervical cancer cells and miRNA-155 in human breast cancer giving consistent results [174].

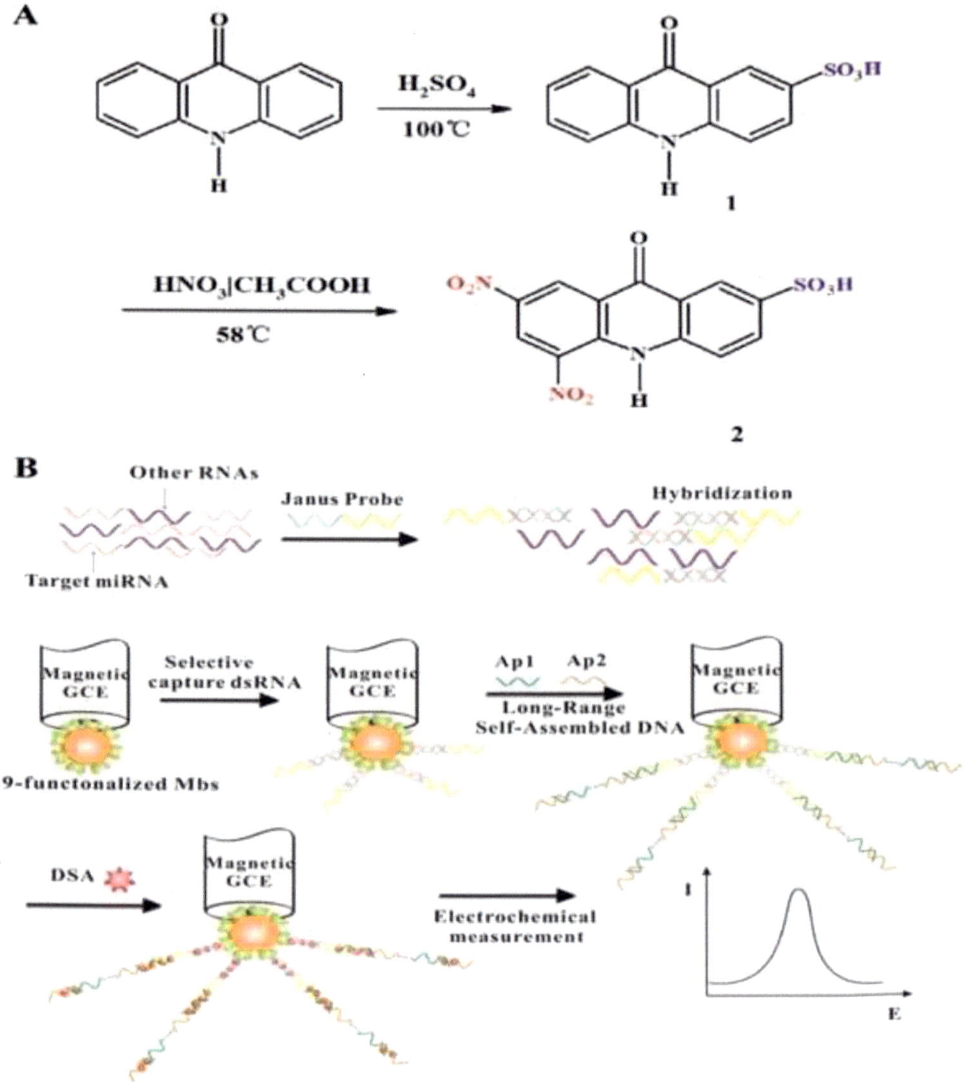

Fig. (19). Schematic illustration of the electrochemical microRNA biosensor. Printed with permission from [173].

Another multiplexed-based biosensor was developed for the simultaneous evaluation of miR-155 and miR-27b is illustrated in Fig. (**20**). Zhu *et al.* combined the high base-mismatch selectivity of a ligase chain reaction that ensured the high specificity of the analysis and the voltammetric signature of quantum dots barcodes in addition to their utility for the signal-amplification. Two reporters, PbQDs–Reporter1 and CdQDs–reporter2, conjugates, and two capture probes for each conjugate were used. The incubation of the targets was followed by T4 DNA ligase and the release of the disjoined QDs barcodes from the magnetic beads-conjugates. The developed biosensor offered a calibration plot of 50 fM–30 pM and 50 fM–1050 pM and limits of detection of 12 fM and 31 fM for miR-155 and miR-27b. This strategy was also verified in the recovery experiment in a biological matrix, respectively [175].

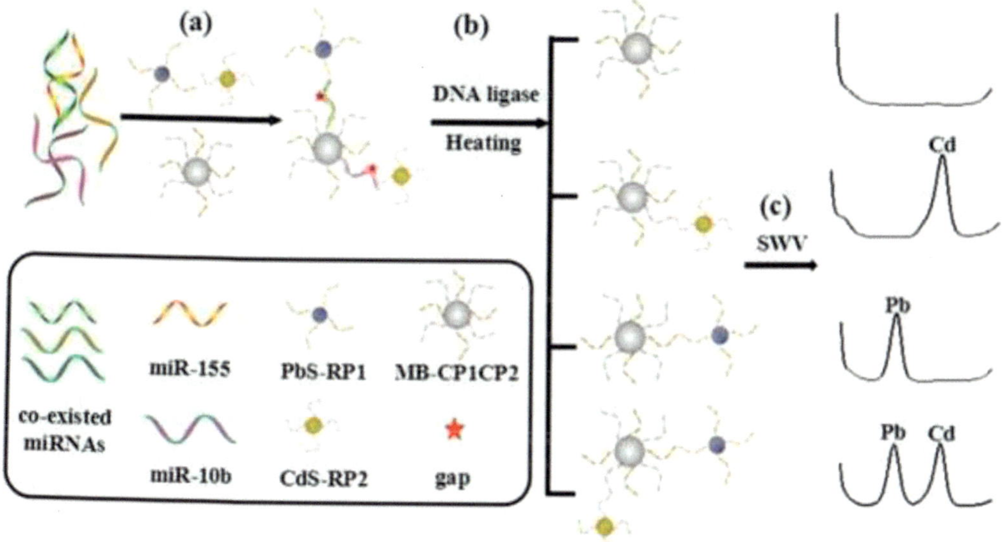

Fig. (20). Schematic illustration of the simultaneous electrochemical detection of multiple miRNA targets. Printed with permission from [175].

A three-mode sensor for the detection of three cancer biomarkers was developed by Labib et al. based on hybridization, p19 protein binding, and protein displacement. The immobilization of the thiolated probe on the gold electrode causing a modulation of the signal was the hybridization mode. The second model implied the addition of p-19 that recognized the formed hybrid and amplified the signal. Finally, the last mode was based on forcing the p19 to dissociate from the immobilized hybrid and to bind a newly formed hybrid non immobilized. This caused a shift back to the signal. The three developed modes could be accomplished on different electrodes or combined on one electrode. The combination of the three modalities offered a detection limit as low as 5 aM and a linear range between 10 aM and 1μM. The detection of miR-32, miR-122, and miR-21 in serum samples following the hybridization and the p-19 protein-based sensors were slightly higher than results from qPCR. This difference was ascribed to the nonspecific interactions with serum proteins, the added yeast RNA, and also p19 protein [176].

The same research group developed a CLL-biosensor by the determination of the biomarker microR-122. The strategy involved a four-way junction that consisted of a universal interfacial probe and two DNA adaptors, which could cooperatively hybridize with the probe and the target miRNA. A quadripartite complex with a four-way junction structure could be formed and could capture streptavidin molecules. Hence, increased the interfacial resistance of the sensor surface. The obtained calibration plot was from 10 aM to 1fM and a detection limit as low as 2 Am. The application of the developed biosensor in the detection of the miR-122 in serum from CLL patients and healthy donors revealed a higher expression of the target in cancer cases [177].

Electrochemical Impedance Spectroscopy

EIS is a technique that has enjoyed increasing use for over a century and this for applications such as the analysis of corrosion phenomena [178], the adsorption properties of molecules [179] or even for monitoring the operation of batteries and fuel cells [180]. As for impedimetric biosensors, they are used to track and measure changes in the surface of an electrode by measuring the resistance and capacitance of materials. Not requiring a label, this method is considered to be simple, based simply on the disturbance of a system at equilibrium by a sinusoidal excitation signal of low amplitude. Also, these easy methods and offering a wealth of information on surface conditions, are generally used to ensure that each step is carried out on the working electrodes [181]. However, these measurements may be limited by non-specific adsorptions, which considerably weaken the selectivity and sensitivity of this method. In order to overcome this disturbance, it is generally necessary to use blocking agents [182].

The most used redox probe in impedimetric-biosensors is $[Fe(CN)_6]^{4/3-}$. For instance, a hybridization-based biosensor was developed for the detection of the miRNA-199a in serum with application in Triple-Negative Breast Cancer. This strategy as illustrated in Fig. (**21**) involved the use of graphene oxide and gold nanorod-modified electrode and LNA probe. These probes contain methylene bridge between the 2′-O and 4-′C of ribose to "lock" it into a configuration more propitious for hybridization. This biosensor offered a linear range between 15 fM and 148 Pm and 4.5 fM as a detection limit. Tests in spiked serum samples gave a recovery between 93.3% to 104.6% [183].

A differential double-layer capacitance-based platform was based on Capaldo *et al.* The system was achieved at microfabricated gold electrodes, where an *in-situ* hybridization of a self-assembled monolayer of single-stranded occurred. the measure of the differential capacitance changes offered a medium detection limit of 1pM [184].

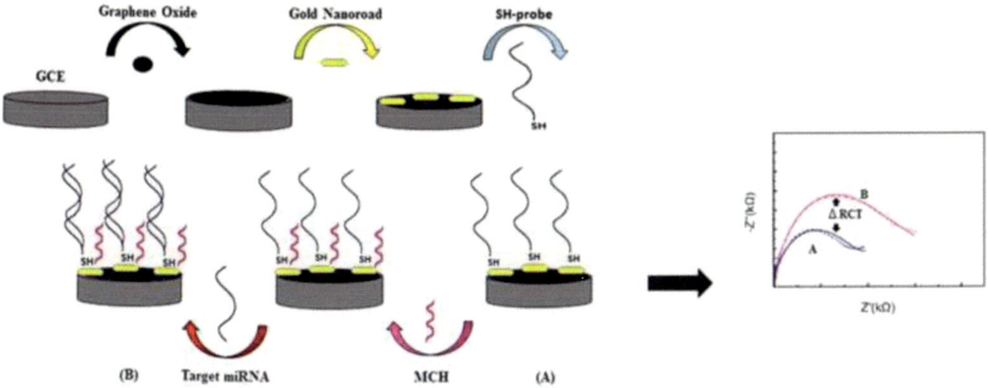

Fig. (21). Schematic illustration of the electrochemical detection of the miRNA-199a-5p. Printed with permission from [183].

Ren *et al.* developed a strategy that used a duplex-specific nuclease enzyme for the cleavage of the probe after the occurrence of the hybridization between the probe and the target. An isothermal amplification cycle was achieved due to the release of the target strands to the sample solution and their reapplication in other hybridizations. The obtained linear range was between 2.0 fM and 2.0 pM. Real sample tests allowed the detection of let-7b down to 1.0 fM. A direct profiling of miRNAs in serum samples and in total RNA extracted from cancer cells was reached [185].

An impedimetric biosensor based on the use of ZrO_2-RGO-modified electrode and catalyzed hairpin assembly process for a signal amplification was developed for the detection of microRNA-21. An application of the strategy in real samples including MCF-7 cells and human embryonic kidney cells (K293T) were achieved and showed overexpression of the target microRNA in MCF-7 cells [186] in good agreement with results from previous reports [187].

Wan *et al.* developed two amplification-based strategies illustrated in Fig. (**22**). The first one used a single DNAzyme and was based on the structure switch of the immobilized hairpin probe DNA to the DNAzyme triggered by the target. The second one used multiple-DNAzyme. It implied the implementation of the electrodes on DNAzyme-modified gold nanoparticles tags. The DNAzyme triggered the formation of an insulating film by the biocatalytic oxidation of 4-chloro-1-naphthol. This prompted a barrier against the electron transfer between the electrode and the redox probe in the electrolyte solution. The multiple-DNAzyme strategy offered a detection limit as low as 15 aM [188].

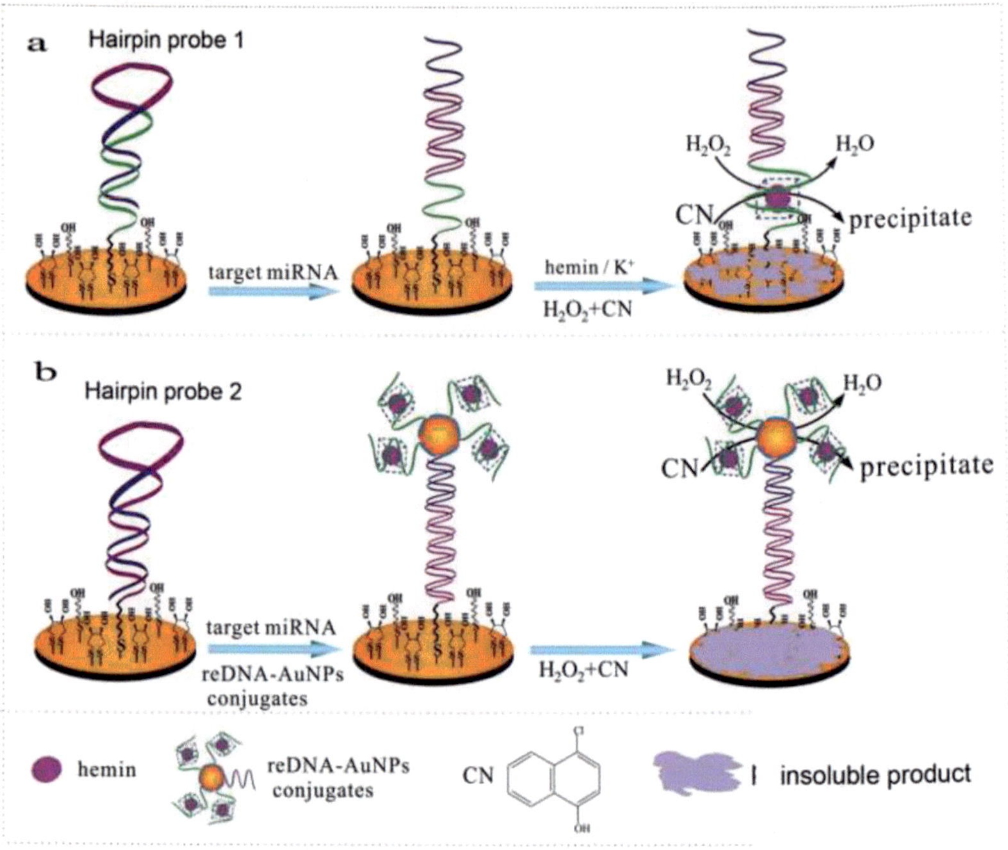

Fig. (22). Sensing of a target miRNA using electrochemical impedance spectroscopy by (a) single DNAzyme signal amplification strategy and (b) multiple-DNAzyme signal amplification strategy. Printed with permission from [188].

Nanomaterials-based amplification strategies have been also used with impedimetric techniques. Fig. (**23**) exemplifies a pencil graphite electrode-based strategy for the detection of cancer-biomarker, miR-125a. The working electrodes were modified with carbon black, multiwalled carbon nanotubes, and graphene oxide. The lowest detection limit (10 pM) was obtained with carbon black modification. The designed biosensor gave a linear range between 1 nM and 2 mM and was also investigated for the target detection in spiked serum with recoveries equal to 93% and 99% [189].

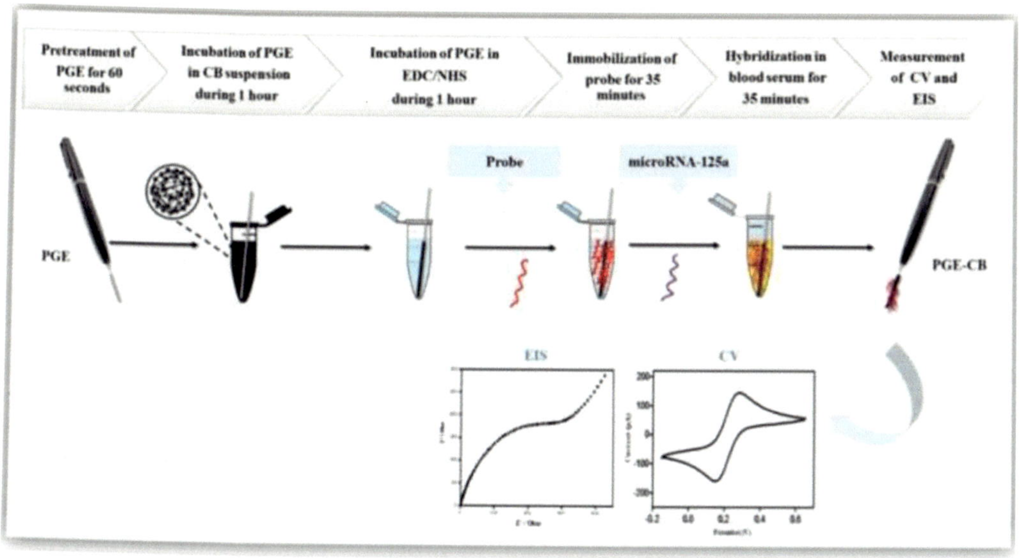

Fig. (23). Schematic illustration of the electrochemical detection of the miRNA-125a. Printed with permission from [189].

Another biosensor based on pencil graphite electrodes was developed by Eksin *et al.* for the detection of miR-660. The working electrodes were modified with chitosan-nitrogen doped reduced graphene oxide inducing an improvement of the conductivity and the electron transfer. The developed strategy showed a detection limit of 1.72 mg/mL and a linear range between 5 and 20 mg/mL in PBS *versus* 1.65 mg/mL as a detection limit with a calibration plot from 0 to 20 mg/mL in a mix of fetal bovine serum and PBS solution [190].

Another amplification strategy was developed by Voccia *et al.* for the detection miR-222, a lung tumors-related biomarker. This biosensor was based on the use of alkaline phosphatase-decorated liposomes and BCIP/NBT mixture. The strategy implied the immobilization of the thiolated DNA capture probes onto gold-nanostructured carbons surface and their hybridization with the target microRNA. Next, enzyme decorated liposomes were applied as labels of the biotinylated hybrids set up on the electrode surface through streptavidin assembly. The obtained limit of detection was as low as 0.400 pM and the linear range was from 1.70 to 900 pM with %RSD = 13. A recovery between 77% and 93% was demonstrated in spiked serum samples [191].

A dual-functional probe (biotin- molecular beacon-gold nanoparticles) biosensor was developed for the biorecognition and the signal generation in the of miR-21. The biotin-molecular beacon probe was activated by its hybridization with the target. Hence, the biotin previously protected biotin group became accessible for capture *via* supramolecular interaction. This occurred onto a neutravidin-modified electrode induced a decrease in the charge transfer resistance at the working electrode/electrolyte interface. The platform showed a linear range from 1 pM to 1000 pM, with a detection limit of 0.3 pM. An acceptable relative error was obtained in spiked serum samples [192].

A dual-mode sensor was developed for the determination of miR-141. The strategy was based on the use of synthesized CeO_2nanospherescodoped with Cu and Co (CuCo−CeO_2 NSs) in order to enhance the redox and electrocatalytic properties of CeO_2 toward H_2O_2 decomposition. This electrocatalysis of CuCo−CeO_2 nanospheres prompted the oxidation of DAB to form nonconductive insoluble precipitates, leading to an amplification of the electrochemical-impedimetric spectroscopy measured signal. DNAzyme was introduced by Mg^{2+} and could assist the microRNA recycling for more signal amplification. This dual strategy showed a linear range between 0.1 fM and 10 Nm with a detection limit as low as 33 aM. Tests were performed in prostate- cancer cells and cervical-cancer cells with consistent results [193].

OPTICAL DETECTION METHODS

Among the many types of biosensors, optical ones are the most attracting because of their low cost, rapid construction, small size, high performance, high sensitivity and selectivity, flexible geometry, and portability [194]. To date, optical based strategies are the most reported methods in literature for detecting miRNAs and are widely studied in the development of new biosensors [195]. Almost all optical techniques were adapted to detect cell-extracted or circulating miRNAs. In the following section, we discuss some of the most prominent optical miRNA biosensors. These studies mainly compromise four types: colorimetric, fluorescent, surface plasmon resonance and SERS.

FLUORESCENCE

Signal ON Biosensors

Fluorescence-based biosensors have an enhanced sensitivity and are appropriate for a wide range of practical applications. The strategies can be generally divided into two ways either by signal generation (signal ON) or signal quenching (signal OFF) following the hybridization process. To improve the sensitivity, researchers proposed several approaches. For instance, nanomaterials with unique properties were used to create new types of analytical tools in life science and biotechnology. Gold nanoparticles, silver nanoparticles, quantum dots, graphene oxide, and molybdenum disulfide nanosheets have been widely used in many biosensing applications [196]. CNPs demonstrate reversible and different binding affinities towards ssDNA/ssRNA probes *versus* dsDNA/dsRNA, which provides the applicability of CNPs into nucleic acid-based detection bioplatforms. For instance, Li *et al* [197]. reported a DNase I-aided cyclic enzymatic amplification method for miRNA determination based on the coupling use of nucleic acid probes with specific molecular recognition ability as well as CNPs. As illustrated in the Fig. (**24**), FAM-tagged ssDNA immobilized on the surface of the CNPs (a) causes fluorescence quenching. Subsequent addition of the target desorbs the heterohybrid RNA:DNA from the surface of particles (b). The addition of DNase I (c) that recognize the DNA strand in the heterohybrid (d). As a result, FAM-ssDNA is cleaved into small pieces and a strong fluorescence signal is generated (e). The designed strategy achieved satisfactory results for miRNA analysis in breast cancer cell lysate with a detection limit down to 3.2 pM.

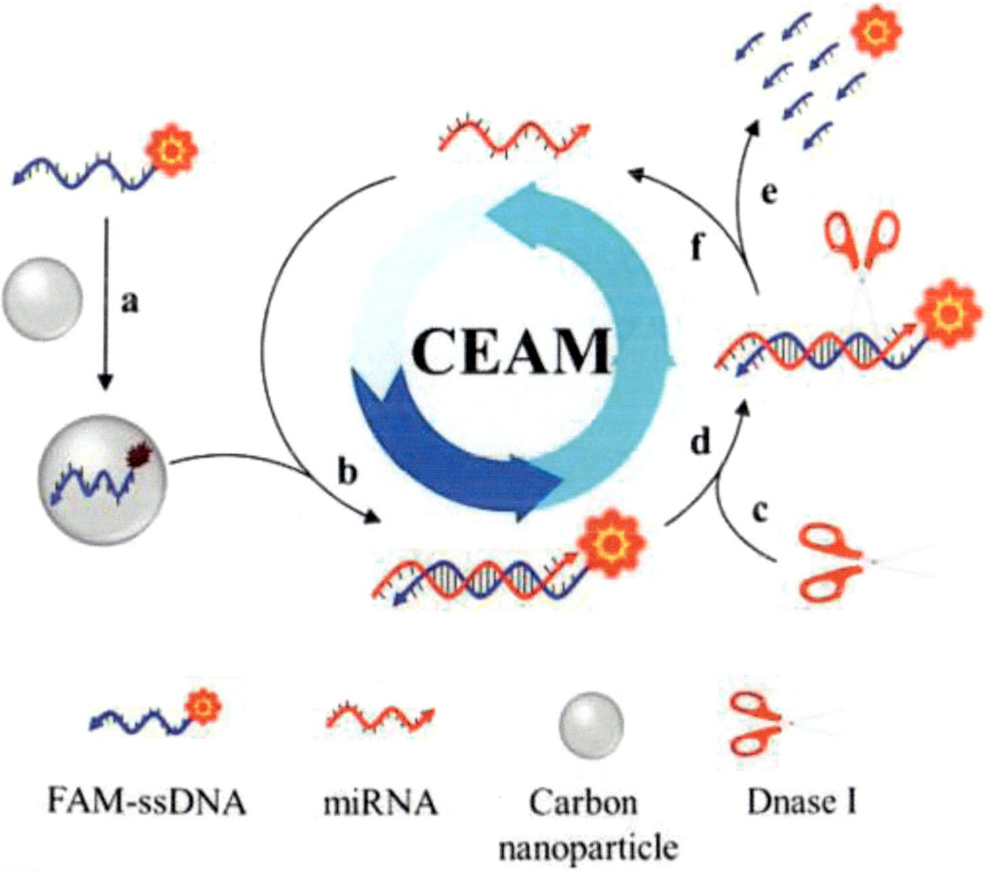

Fig. (24). Working principle of cyclic enzymatic amplification method (CEAM) for miRNA analysis. Reprinted with permission from [197].

In another study, Tang *et al.* [198] reported the design of a Janus nanosensor (Fig. **25**) for miRNA sensing in which the MPDA nanoparticle face consisting of a porous nanoquencher side and the gold side were functionalized with probes and signal amplifiers, respectively. The MPDA side generates the fluorescence recovery governed by target miRNA binding and heteroduplex release, while the gold side generates the amplification through the target recycling driven by the duplex cleavage *via* immobilized enzymes. The nanosensor was able to sensitively detect target miRNA with a low limit of 32 fM (in a linear range from 20 fM to 500 fM).

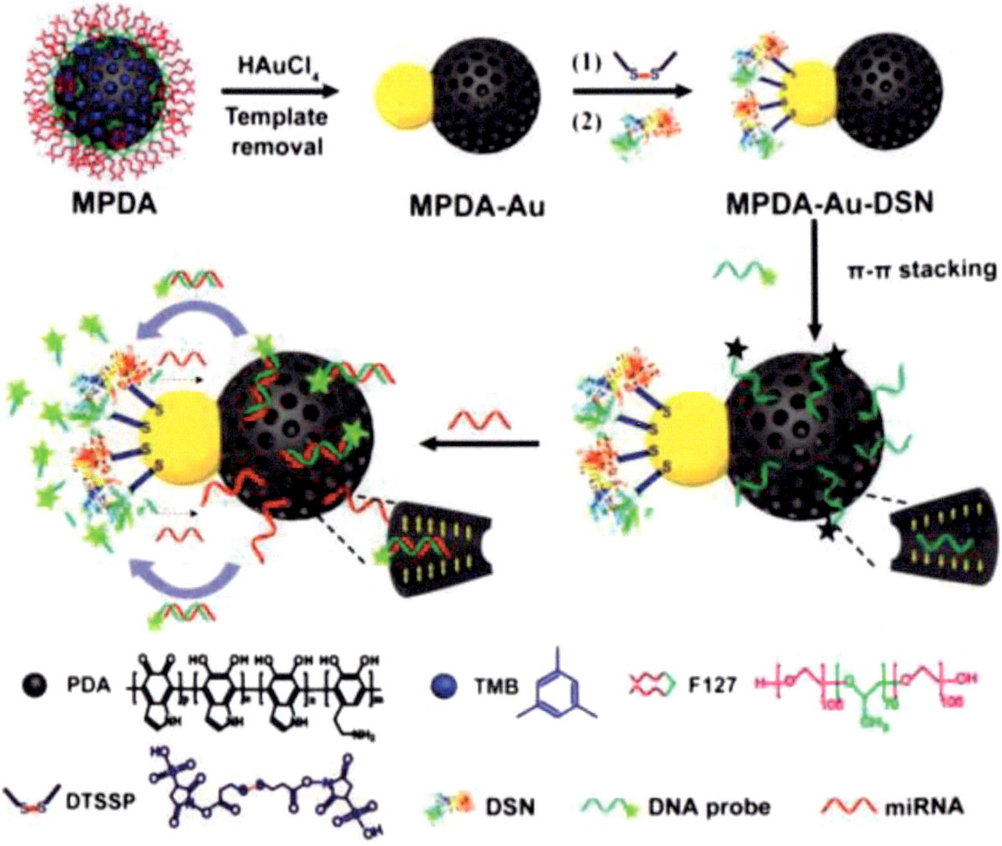

Fig. (25). Schematic illustration for the synthetic procedure and the miRNA detection application of Janus MPDA-Au nanoparticles that feature a mesoporous PDA moiety loaded with fluorescent DNA probes for miRNA recognition, and an asymmetric gold unit selectively immobilized with DSN/T7 for enzyme-assisted signal amplification. Reprinted with permission from [198].

Signal OFF Biosensors

MWCNT/AuNCs were also used as a novel fluorescence quenching platform. The quenching abilities of MWCNTs/AuNCs are much greater than conventionally used MWCNTs. In a recent study, Ma *et al.* [199] designed a sensitive biosensing platform for miR-155 detection using MWCNTs/AuNCs as a novel fluorescence quenching platform coupled with DSN-assisted recycling signal amplification. After the addition of target miR-155, DNA:RNA heteroduplexes were formed and released from MWCNTs/AuNCs to generate a strong fluorescence signal. In the presence of DSN, DNA/RNA heteroduplexes became a substrate for the enzymatic cleavage of DNA strands and initiated cyclic signal amplification (Fig. **26**). Moreover, by using DSN, the sensor showed excellent selectivity for miRNA-155 detection against other control miRNAs and a low detection limit of 33.4 fM was obtained.

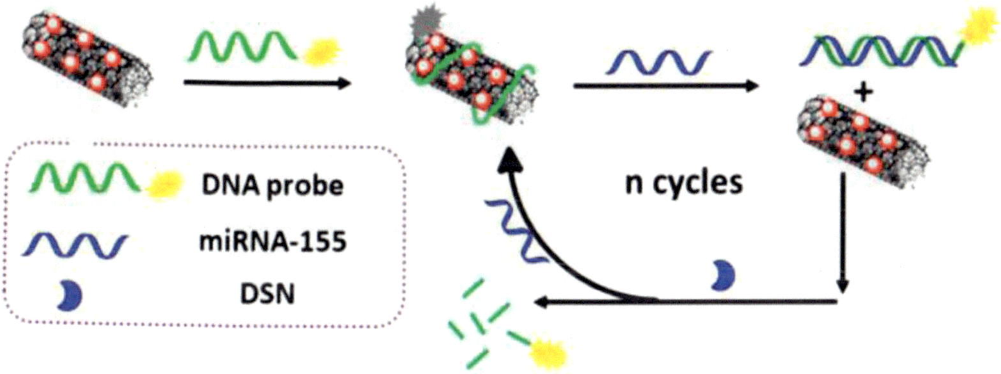

Fig. (26). Schematic illustration of the miRNA-155 assay using duplex-specific nuclease to release the fluorescent probe. Reprinted with permission from [199].

FRET Biosensors

FRET is a phenomenon that permits two emission intensities at different wavelengths simultaneously and is widely applied to detect miRNAs. This has been investigated by numerous researchers in recent years [200 - 204]. QDs are nanomaterials with absorption and emission characteristics that are dependent on size of QDs. With a suitable size, QDs can serve as ideal fluorescent markers for detection of multiple miRNA biomarkers with a high quantum yield and wide excitation range. The application of semiconductor QDs in FRET-based biosensing provides many advantages such as high sensitivity due to the brightness of QDs and homogeneous assay formats thanks to the biorecognition specific FRET signal [205, 206]. Currently, various DNA-QDs conjugates-based FRET strategies have been reported for miRNA detection. For instance, Ren *et al.* [207] reported a novel FRET strategy for miR-21 determination based on fluorescence-enhanced p19 proteins conjugated with a single quantum dot. The p19 protein molecule which can tightly bind only to the dsRNA formed in solution by hybridization of the specific anti-miR-21-Cy3 probe (receptor) to the single-stranded miR-21 (Fig. **27**). Fluorescence measurement showed that the probe can used to determine the content of miR-21 in breast cancer cell and a detection limit as low as 0.6 fM was achieved without employing any amplification techniques or purification steps.

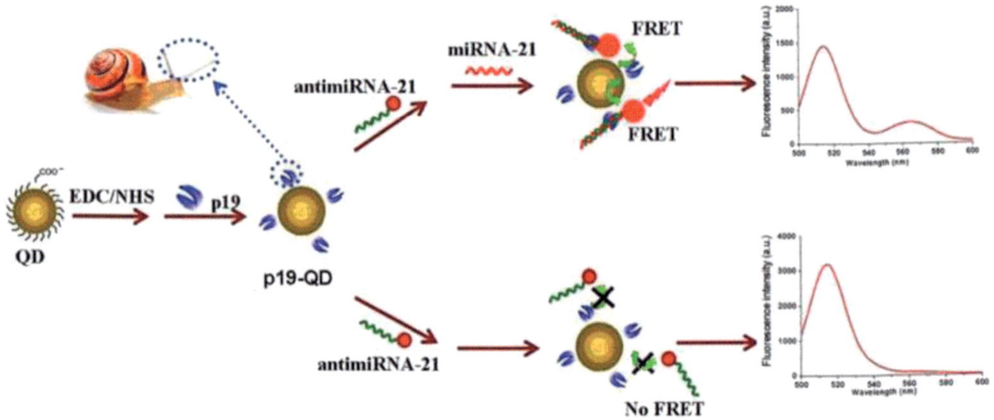

Fig. (27). Schematic of FRET strategy based on fluorescence-enhanced protein p19-conjugated single QD with multiplex antenna for one-step, specific and sensitive miRNAs detection. Reprinted with permission from [207].

A new methodology was described by Su and co-workers [203] for ultrahigh-sensitive and -selective miRNA "signal OFF" detection. The DNA-QDs conjugates have the advantages of the excellent optical properties of QDs and well-controlled recognition properties of DNA. With the addition of a target nucleic acid sequence, the fluorescence intensity of QDs was quenched by an organic quencher (BHQ2) *via* Förster resonance energy transfer. Furthermore, the nanosensor can detect as low as 10 fM miRNA also exhibited excellent selectivity. The fluorescence intensity of DNA-QDs have obviously decreased with the addition of a target miRNA because of energy transfer from QDs to BHQ2 and sandwiched heterohybrids were formed. In another interesting work employing FRET was designed to detect miR-155 in a new rapid, sensitive, and selective manner. The strategy uses a "sandwich-type" hybridization of oligonucleotides and FRET. A modified La(III)-based MOF and silver nanoparticles were employed as the energy donor–acceptor pair in fluorescence quenching through the FRET mechanism. This "turn OFF" bioplatform could sense and determine miR-155 biomarker low to 5.5 fM [200].

To achieve ultrahigh sensitive miRNA biosensors, signal amplification is a key point that should be considered. Nevertheless, many important miRNAs of interest are present at quite low abundance in biological samples. Thus, new sensitive and accurate miRNA amplification strategies, which are crucial for analysis of miRNAs are required. Liu *et al.* [208] designed a sensing system based on cooperative amplification combined with graphene oxide fluorescence switch-based circular exponential amplification and the labelling of multiple molecules with SYBR Green I. GO not only serves as a quencher to realize fluorescence quenching, but also serves as a protective agent to prevent miRNA adsorbed onto the surface of GO from being degraded by enzymes. In this assay, miRNA was hybridized with a portion of the hairpin probe and then acted as a primer to initiate a chain displacement reaction to form a complete double-stranded molecule. This strategy is able to induce significant fluorescence signal enhancement and further improve detection sensitivity. Another important biosensing device with highly sensitivity and excellent selectivity for rapid and facile detection of c-miRNAs has been developed by Fan *et al.* [209] using thioflavin T (ThT) as a fluorescent indicator. The sensing system consists of two unlabeled hairpin probes (HP1 and HP2) and a circular probe. Upon binding with the target miRNA, HP1 is opened, which serves as a toehold to hybridize with HP2. Since HP1-HP2 duplex is more stable than HP1-miRNA duplex, the target miRNA can be displaced from HP1, and again binds with a new HP1 to initiate another reaction cycle. Moreover, the formed HP1-HP2 duplex can be further used as a primer to initiate RCA with the circular probe, producing extremely long ssDNA molecules with repetitive sequence units, which can form into a large number of G-quadruplexes. These G-quadruplexes combined with ThT, resulting in a significantly enhanced fluorescent signal. This biosensor exhibits highly sensitivity toward target miRNA with a detection limit of 10 pM thanks to the double amplification and was successfully applied to detect miRNAs in cancer cells and tumor tissues.

Recently, another strategy reported by Zayani *et al.* [210]. The authors designed a dual-mode fluorescent/electrochemical strategy to detect femtomolar levels of miR-21 in blood serum samples (Fig. **28**). The nanosensor used a chemical amplification-based strategy for signal enhancement to achieve low levels of detection. 2,3-Diaminophenazine, as HRP enzymatic byproduct during the reduction of hydrogen peroxide and oxidation of o-PDA, is both fluorescent and redox-active. The competition of the target miRNA-21 and its biotinylated analog toward the same AuNPs-tagged probe induces a lower number of the biotinylated miRNA-21 on the surface of the nanoparticles when the level of the unlabeled target increases and consequently a lower number of SA/HRP labels and a lower fluorescent signal. The bioplatform has detection limits of 15fM and 19fM, and wide linear concentration ranges varying from 15fM (19 fM) to 100pM for the fluorescence and electrochemical bioassays, respectively.

The system was used to detect the levels of the target miRNA in blood serum samples from breast cancer patients and healthy donors to show that these levels are *ca.* 3 times higher in cancer patients in comparison with the healthy individuals, which is consistent with literature [211, 212].

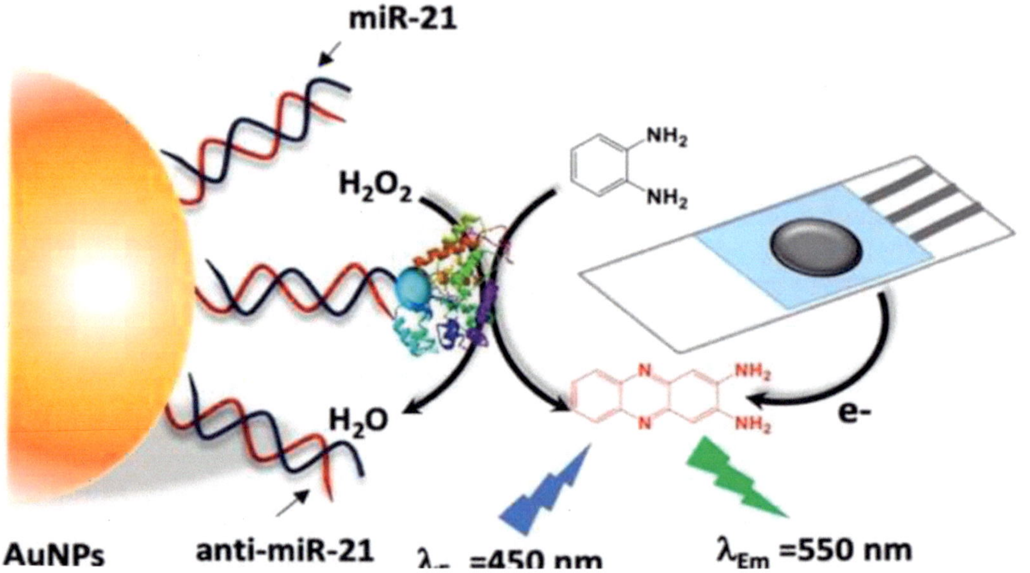

Fig. (28). Competition-based approach for fluorescent/electrochemical dual mode detection of miRNA-21 using HRP-based amplification producing fluorescent and redox-active species. Reprintedwith permission from [210].

Very recently, Peng *et al.* [213] combined CRISPR/Cas12a and CHA to design a high sensitive bioplatform for the detection of miRNAs. Indeed, miRNAs serve as a trigger for hairpin DNA assembly, which will be recognized by Cas12a/sgRNA ribonucleoprotein that induce trans-cleavage of a reporter probe. The combination of CHA/CRISPR system and SNP in DNA duplex formed by CHA allowed to improve the sensitivity more twelve times. The bioplatform was used to detect miR-21, miR-141 and miR-155 in different cancer cells (LO2, MCF-7 and A549) and in sera from healthy and cancer patients. The levels of expression determined by this method are very close to those determined by RT-qPCR.

UV-Visible

The colorimetric biosensors have the advantages of simplicity, rapidity and cost-effectiveness, and they enable the signal readout *via* color changes or even directly monitored with naked eyes. To this end, some smart materials like gold and magnetic nanoparticles, and quantum dots are decent choices. In particular, AuNPs are easy functionalization, have good optical performance, excellent biocompatibility, conductivity, catalytic properties, high density, high surface-t-

-volume ratio and can be fabricated in controlled manner, which make them ideal candidates for biosensing applications [214]. The functionalization can be made with different functional groups to tune the optical properties and the newly obtained particles will act as a signal provider in elegant detection platforms [215, 216]. For instance, based on the assembly of AuNPs into a core-satellite configuration, Park *et al.* [217] reported an on-chip colorimetric biosensor for miRNA detection. Core-AuNPs were first anchored on an APTES/OTMS-treated glass slide, then functionalized with two DNA probes to form the satellite-AuNPs. In presence of the target, it can partly hybridize with both probes to direct the assembly of core-AuNPs and satellite-AuNPs to form a core-satellite nanostructure, resulting in the color and spectrum changes. This biosensor can measure miRNA with a detection limit of 1 pM and a dynamic range of 10 orders of magnitude, and it exhibits good selectivity towards target miRNA.

Aggregation of oligonucleotide-modified AuNPs could be directly or indirectly triggered in the presence of target miRNA, leading to color change due to surface plasmon resonance [218]. For instance, RLS-based biosensor for miRNA was developed involving analyte-induced aggregation of gold nanoparticles for the selective determination of miR-21. The RLS sensor was fabricated by modifying AuNPs with two strands of cDNA sequence, which complement the sequence of target miRNA. When the target is introduced, the cDNAs hybridize with the target miRNAs to form a cDNA:miRNA heteroduplex. However, conventional colorimetric methods are not quite sensitive to sense low amount of miRNA. Consequently, several amplification strategies were applied to provide a low cost, rapid, and efficient alternative for miRNA sensing. Another simple, label-free, and enzyme-free colorimetric biosensor was developed [219] for the amplified detection of let-7a miRNA on the basis of dual signal amplification strategy. The sensing system mainly consists of four unlabeled hairpin probes termed H1, H2, H3, and H4. Upon sensing of the target miRNA, the forming H1–H2 duplex occurs and frees the target miRNA that can be recycled to trigger another reaction cycle (Fig. **29**). During this process, numerous split G-quadruplex structures are generated and further associate with cofactor hemin to form massive peroxidase-mimicking DNAzymes. The latter catalyzes the H_2O_2-mediated oxidation of colorless $ABTS^{2-}$ to the green-colored $ABTS^{\bullet-}$, inducing a remarkably amplified colorimetric signal. This newly developed sensing system exhibits high sensitivity toward miRNA with a detection limit of 7.4 fM and a large dynamic range of 6 orders of magnitude from 10 fM to 10 nM.

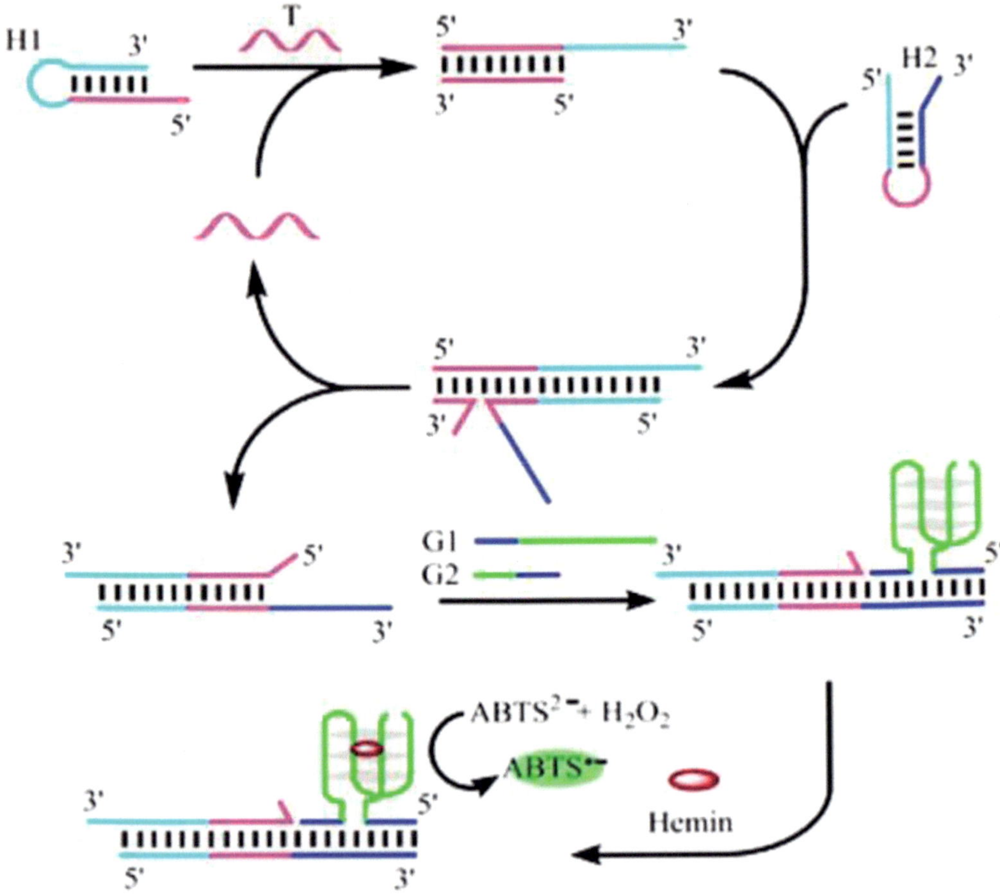

Fig. (29). Schematic illustration of typical catalyzed hairpin assembly strategy for detection of miRNA. Reprinted with permission from [219].

More recently, Ying *et al.* [220] described an enzyme assisted hybridization chain reaction (HCR) for colorimetric detection of miR-155. The sensing strategy is illustrated in Fig. (**30**). In this study, a biotinylated capture probe (b-CP) was first immobilized on streptavidin-coated plates. In the presence of target miRNA, the immobilized b-CP captures the miR-155. Subsequently, a second reporting sequence, containing half of the miR-155 and a toehold to initiate the hairpin H1 opening, triggers the HCR reaction producing a long dsDNA polymer with multiple FITC for signal amplification. Finally, multiple HRP molecules were immobilized onto the long-range DNA nanostructures through FITC/anti-FITC monoclonal antibody interactions on the microplate to oxidize TMB, which will produce a blue coloration. This approach enables the visual detection of miRNAs with a LOD of 31.8 fM and the detection of miRNA in serum samples.

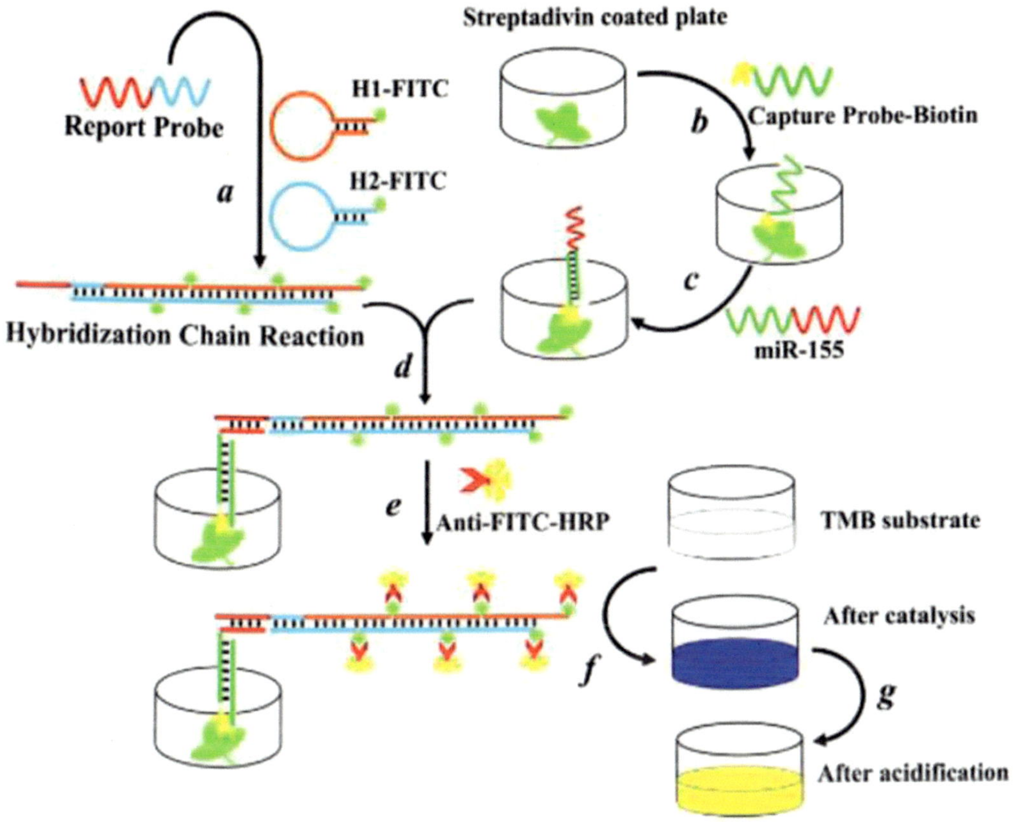

Fig. (30). Schematic representation of the sensing strategy for colorimetric detection of miR-155 based on enzyme assisted-HCR. Reprinted with permission from [220].

Additionally, Qiu *et al.* [221] built a platform that is able to detect miRNAs at low cost and high efficacy with a fM-level sensitivity and single-base specificity. This detection system contains isothermal amplification, detecting and reporting process based on RCA, CRISPR-dCas9, and split-HRP techniques. For the detection, miRNAs were isothermally amplified *via* RCA and used for *in vitro* dCas9 binding to several sites produced by the rolling circle amplification and split HRP which is joined when is located on two adjacent sites to enable restoring its enzymatic activity (Fig. **31**). A color change of the TMB substrate from light yellow to blue indicated the existence of specific miRNAs. The LOD of the designed assay was estimated to 35.4 aM.

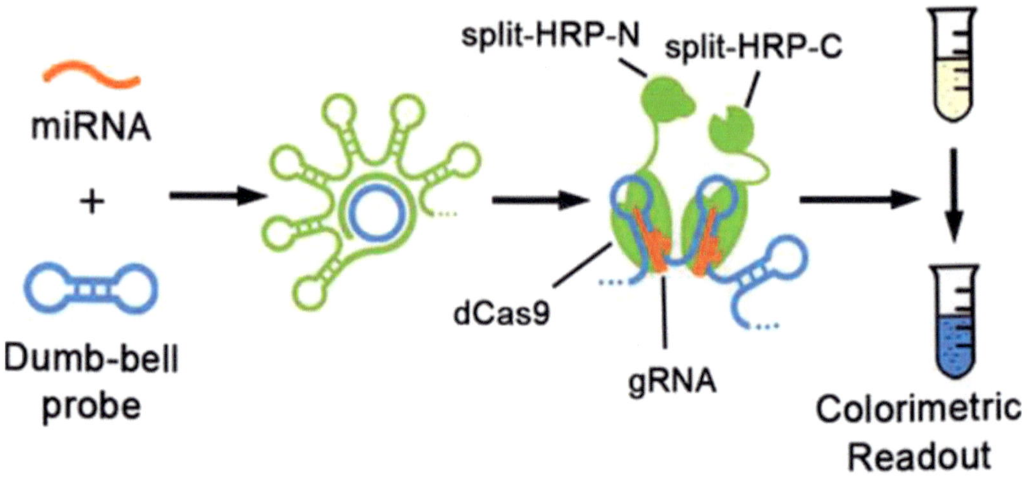

Fig. (31). Illustration of strategy for the colorimetric detection of miRNAs using CRISPR/dCas, rolling circle amplification and split HRP enzyme. Reprinted with permission from [221].

Alternatively, Persano *et al.* [222] developed a new method to detect miR-10a in biological samples. This technology was based on the isothermal nicking enzyme amplification reaction and subsequent hybridization of the amplification product with AuNPs and MBs (barcode system). Colorimetric detection and color changes can clearly be observed with naked eyes, due to target-induced capturing of the AuNP probes. This platform demonstrated an attomolar sensitivity at concentrations as low as 100 aM. Delkhahi and co-workers [223] used a novel, sensitive and specific miR-137 assay based on colorimetric detection of gold nanoparticles and hybridization chain reaction amplification (HCR). The strategy eliminates the need for enzymatic reactions, chemical changes, separation processes and sophisticated equipment. The detection process is visible with naked eyes and the detection limit for this method is 0.25nM, which is less than or at least comparable with the previous methods based on colorimetric of AuNPs.

In conclusion, colorimetric strategies offer an approach with low cost and easy equipment for detecting miRNAs, whereas further amplification techniques are also needed to accomplish notable efficiency.

Surface Plasmon Resonance

The optical properties of AuNPs are essentially linked to their Plasmon band, which is due to the collective oscillation of electrons on the surface of AuNPs occurring at a particular excitation wavelength. The Plasmon resonance band is strongly dependent on the size, shape and surface modification of the nanoparticles.

Meanwhile, AuNPs-based colorimetric assays are not sufficiently sensitive to detect very low concentrations of miRNAs. Furthermore, fluorescence techniques require fluorescent dyes or enzymes to produce them which can be expensive making label-free molecular-level quantification of miRNA is extremely challenging. SPR-based biosensors have significant enhanced sensitivity, appropriate for a wide range of practical applications. They are based on SPR, which is a label-free detection method that emerged during the last two decades as a suitable and reliable platform in clinical analysis for biomolecular interactions. The technique makes it possible to measure interactions in real-time with high sensitivity and without the need of labels [224]. These biosensors evaluate the change of refractivity of a material bound on a surface by measuring the resonance of free electrons in the metal films. Gold and silver NPs are the best options for use in SPR-based biosensors. Numerous nanomaterials were employed to improve the sensitivity of SPR signals. For example, gold, magnetic and silver nanoparticles were used to develop detection methods as a sandwich arrangement with a secondary-labeled molecule as an enhancer. For example, Sipova *et al.* [225] achieved rapid, label-free detection of miR-122 from mouse liver tissue at 0.2 nM, using a novel, high performance portable SPR sensor by performing an amplification step in which the captured miRNA is subsequently recognized by an antibody that exhibits affinity to the RNA:DNA heterohybrids. This approach allows the detection of target miRNA at low concentrations down to 2 pM. A similar strategy was reported by Nasheri *et al.* [226]. They directly detected synthetic miR-122 using a SPRi biosensor achieving a detection limit of 40 nM. After hybridization, the signal was amplified using the protein p19, which has affinity towards the hybrid RNA/RNA duplex. Although this strategy is interesting for demonstrating the utility of p19 for the recognition of miRNA-bound probes. Recently, Xue *et al.* [227] demonstrated the efficiency and ultra-sensitivity of the antimonene-based SPR sensor in the quantitative detection of cancer-associated miRNAs. Specifically, they applied the biosensor to detect miR-21 and miR-155, which are promising biomarkers for cancer diagnosis. This biosensor has a LOD of 10 aM, representing the highest sensitivity described thus far in miRNA detection based on direct detection and quantification of miRNA levels. A SPR biosensor for the detection of miRNA and cancer cell based on multiple signal amplification strategy proposed by Liu and his collogues [228]. Thiol-modified hairpin probe, including a sequence complementary to the target miRNA, was first immobilized on the Au film. In the presence of the target, the stem-loop structure of hairpin probe was unfolded, and then DNA-linked AuNPs were hybridized with the terminus of the unfolded hairpin probe. Subsequently, DNA-linked AuNPs initiated the formation of DNA super sandwich structure through the addition of two DNA reporters. Owing to the electronic coupling between localized plasmon of the AuNPs and the surface plasmon wave, as well as the enhancement of the refractive index of the medium over the Au film induced by DNA super sandwich structure (Fig. **32**). The overall SPR response was significantly enhanced. Next, numerous positively charged AgNPs were absorbed onto the long-range DNA super sandwich equably, resulting in a further increase of SPR response. Due to the enzyme free multiple signal amplification strategy, as low as *ca.* 0.6 fM miR-21 can be detected. In addition, this biosensor showed high selectivity toward single-base mismatch.

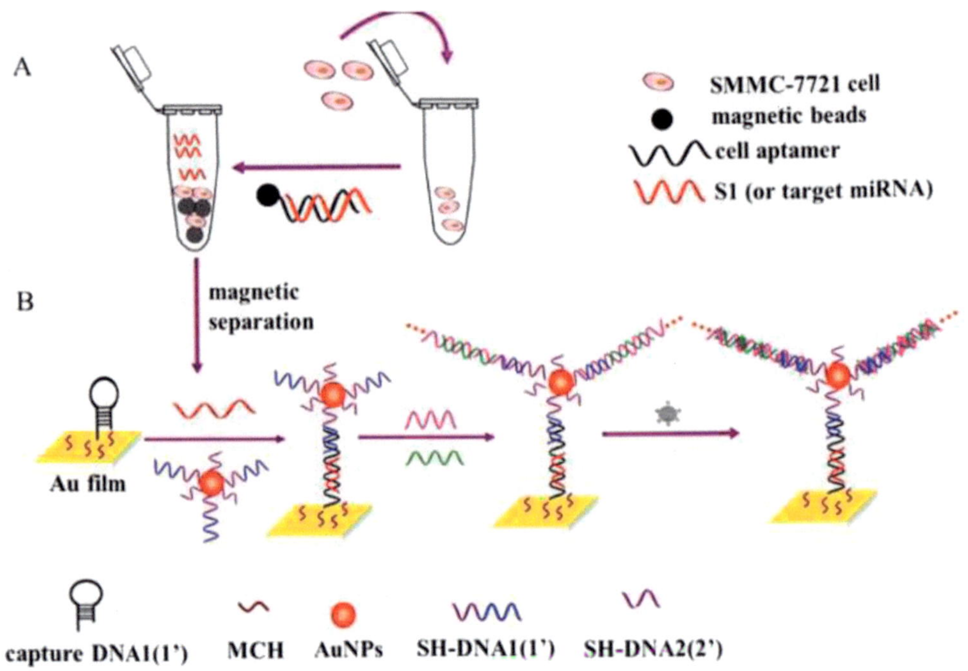

Fig. (32). Schematic representation of SPR biosensor based on multiple amplification strategy for miRNA and cancer cells detection. Reprinted with permission from [228].

More recently, a new biosensor based on two layers of GO/AuNPs composites for the detection of miR-141was reported [229]. As shown in the Fig. (**33**), by employing these two layers of GO/AuNPs composites, whereas one acted as a functionalized substrate on the sensor chip, provided a high specific surface area convenient for the immobilization of capture DNA molecules, while the other layer served as a signal-amplification element. The dual amplification strategy was achieved so that a measurement of miR-141 with a detection limit of 0.1 fM was obtained.

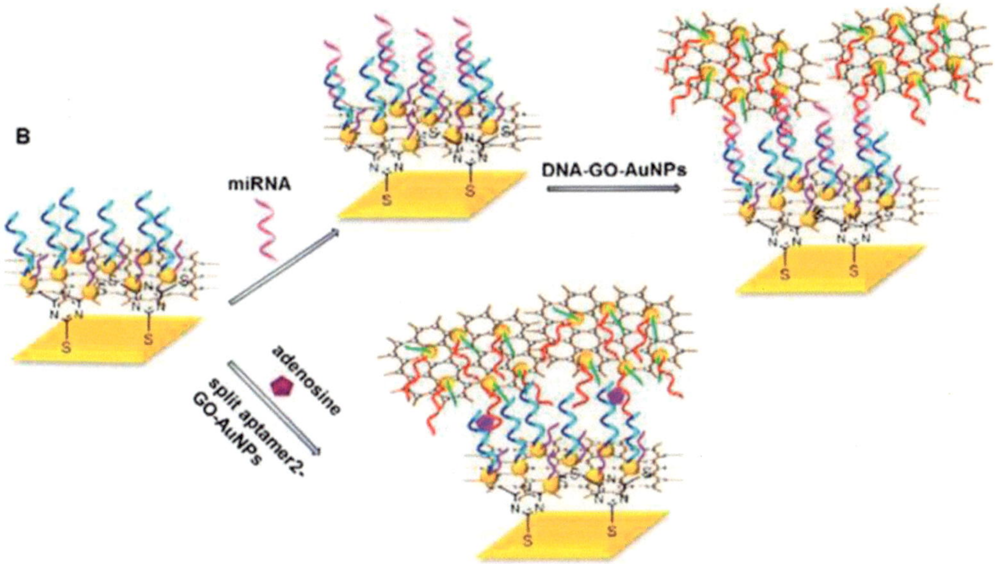

Fig. (33). Schematic illustration of the SPR biosensor based on the GO-AuNPs composites. Reprinted with permission from [229].

Various amplification techniques such as CHA and HCR were applied to SPR sensing platform. Hybridization chain reaction was widely used with SPR biosensing, where the hybridization between the target and its complementary strand immobilized on the electrode surface occurs and initiates the HCR process. For instance, Fan *et al.* [230] proposed an enzyme-based biosensor for let-7a miRNA quantitative analysis exploring the different affinity of ssDNA and dsDNA on GO. Helicase can initiate the HCR provoked by let-7a on the GO surface and the helicase-assisted HCR/GO sensor reduces the miRNA detection time from 4 h to 50 min. Furthermore, the sensitivity of this biosensor was two orders of magnitude higher than those in the absence of enzyme.Some strategies based on enzymatic reactions were also developed to improve SPR sensitivity. Wang *et al.* [231] developed an SPR biosensor the detection of miRNA using streptavidin as an enzyme for signal amplification. Streptavidin oligonucleotide complex was employed to increase the signal, to improve the detection sensitivity and to achieve a limit of detection to 1.7 fM of miR-122. Similarly, Another biosensor for miR-21 detection based on SPR imaging strategy based on the TMB instead of metal nanoparticles using poly(A) polymerase to induce an HRP-assisted oxidation of the TMB yielding a blue precipitate on the surface. This method significantly enhances the SPR signals. This is a simple, cost-effective, and feasible signal amplification methods [232].

Researchers also took advantage from enzyme-free methods for their signal amplification techniques. Recently, Li *et al.* [230] followed an interesting strategy for highly sensitive detection of miRNA by designing an isothermal amplification strategy, named multi-component nucleic acid enzyme-mediated mismatched catalyzed hairpin assembly. The H0 fragments could initiate the mismatched CHA cycles, resulting in the generation of massive hairpin H1–H2 complexes. As a result, the H1–H2 complexes and streptavidin were attached to the sensor surface, leading to a significantly amplified SPR signal readout. The established biosensor showed high sensitivity and selectivity with a wide dynamic range from 1 pM to 100 nM (Fig. **34**).

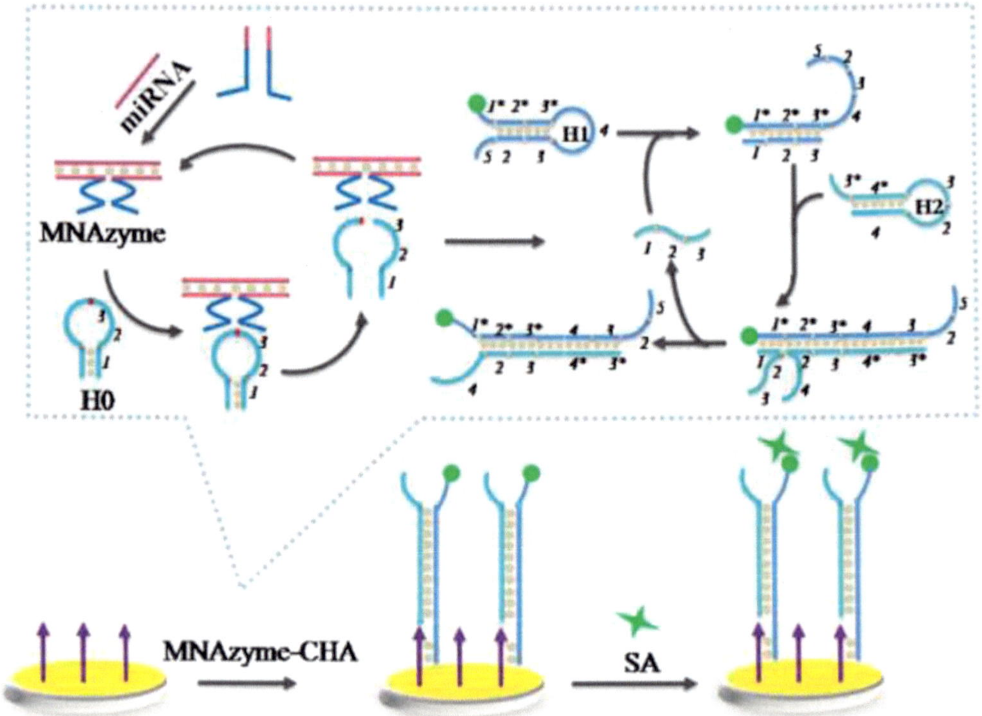

Fig. (34). Schematic representation of miRNA SPR biosensor. Reprinted with permission from [230].

An innovative approach was constructed by Li and co-workers [233] for a specific and highly sensitive detection of target miRNA employing the mismatched CHA amplification coupling with programmable streptavidin aptamer. The presence of target miRNA triggered the allosteric effect of CHA amplification, which brought about the recycling of the target miRNA and produced large amounts of CHA products and activated SA-aptamers. Meanwhile, the plentiful CHA products can hybridize with the capture probes on the sensor chip, and the massive activated SA-aptamers could capture the streptavidin to achieve enhancement and output of the detection signal. Benefiting from the outstanding performance of the enzyme-free CHA amplification and non-label SPR biosensor, the established biosensor exhibited simplified process, high sensitivity and good selectivity. Under the optimal conditions, this designed strategy could detect target miRNA down to 1 pM with a dynamic range from 5 pM to 100 nM and was successfully applied to the determination of target miRNA spiked into human total RNA samples. In a similar work, Wei *et al.* [234] used an enzyme-free SPRi biosensing method was developed for miRNA detection based on CHA and spherical nucleic acid. The hairpin H1 tethered on the sensor chip surface is unfolded by miRNA, and then the hybridized miRNA is released through the displacement of the hairpin H2 for the successive hybridization and assembly process (Fig. **35**). The emerging DNA fragments on the sensor chip surface after hairpins assembly are further used to hybridize with spherical nucleic acid, inducing a remarkably amplified SPR signal. This biosensing method is highly sensitive to miRNA with a detection limit of 53.7 fM and a linear range of 4 orders of magnitude.

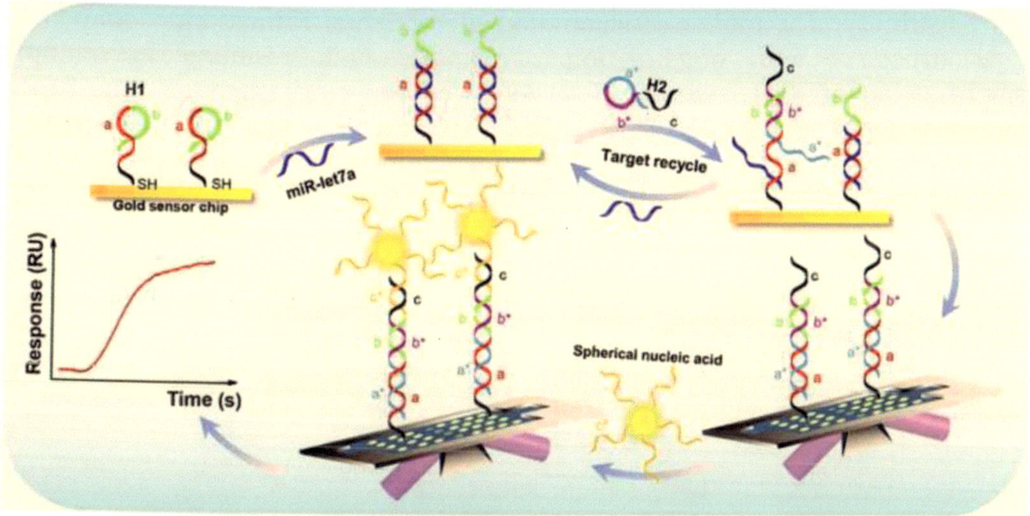

Fig. (35). Schematic illustration of the SPR biosensing method. Reprinted with permission from [234].

These biosensors provide powerful early detection and analysis that can be used to reduce the cost of patient care and therapy and prevents the extension of disease. Nevertheless, the SPR-based transduction cannot be used in studying small amounts of analyte with very low signal-to-noise ratios, because it measures the materials mass, binding to the sensor surface, thus, SPR-based biosensors are inappropriate for commercialization and are mostly to provide proof-of-concept for research purposes.

Surface-Enhanced Raman Scattering

SERS technology possesses a good deal of superiorities like high sensitivity, narrow spectral band and abundant fingerprint information, bringing a series of advantages for the detection of miRNAs. It facilitates the identification of samples at a molecular level. Furthermore, the sample preparation and operation are very easy and nondestructive, which is suitable for the detection of a wide variety of matrices. Therefore, it has been widely used to detect biomolecules at trace levels, such as nucleic acids, proteins and small molecules. To achieve ultra-trace detection of biomolecules, SERS signals should be further enhanced through either preparing efficient substrates or increasing the number of Raman signal molecules. A multiple signal amplification sandwich-type SERS biosensor for ultrasensitive detection of femtomolar miRNA was constructed by Shao *et al.* [235] involving a combination of AuNWs, silver stain and HCR. The capture unit, prepared by immobilizing the capture probe on the Fe_3O_4@AuNPs, can easily capture target miRNA and greatly simplify the separation step to improve reproducibility. The higher concentration of the target formed more sandwich-type structures with combination of capture unit, resulting in multiple amplification of SERS signals (Fig. **36**). The proposed sandwich-type SERS biosensor could detect miR-141 at the femtomolar level with a low detection limit of 0.03 fM.

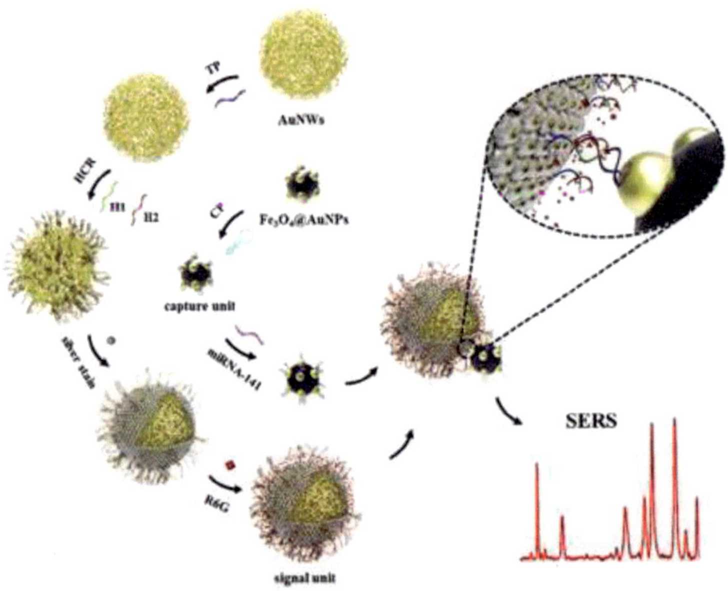

Fig. (36). Schematic diagram of the preparation procedure of the signal unit and the fabrication of the proposed multiple signal amplification sandwich-type SERS biosensor for miRNA detection. Reprinted with permission from [235].

Another intriguing sensitive SERS assay was reported by Zhang *et al.* [236] for multiplex detection of cancer-related miRNAs, namely miR-141, miR-429 and miR-200b, using three pairs of silica-coated, analyte-embedded Au nanoparticles (SA@GNPs) and Au-coated paramagnetic nanoparticles (Au@MNPs) conjugated with DNA probes specific for each miRNA target. The target detection was achieved by SERS excitation of magnetically concentrated SA@GNPs/target miRNA/Au@MNP complexes, which are formed by target-specific hybridization reactions. The detection limit of miRNAs in human blood serum was 120 fM. Wen *et al.* [237] also demonstrated a "signal OFF" SERS platform for ultrasensitive detection of miR-21 by integrating exonuclease-assisted target recycling amplification with a plasmon coupling enhancement effect. On this platform, Raman-labeled Au nanostar probes can be covalently linked with the thiolated aptamer on the Au-decorated silicon nanowire arrays (SiNWAs/Au) substrate, creating a coupled electromagnetic field between the substrate and the probes to enhance Raman signal. In the presence of miR-21, T7 exonuclease specifically hydrolyzed Aptamer on Apt/miRNA duplex to release miR-21. The regenerated element could then initiate another cycle of Apt/miRNA duplex formation and Aptamer cleavage. Due to the cascading integration between the target cycle process and the plasmon coupling effect, the present platform displayed a very low detection limit as little as 0.34 fM. Later, Pang *et al.* [238] developed a DSN-assisted dual-SERS biosensor for microR-10b in exosome and residual plasma of blood samples detection based on the Fe_3O_4 conjugates. In the presence of the target, it can hybridize with the complementary DNA probes. DSN enzyme was then added to selectively cleaves the DNA probe of the DNA/miRNA duplex, SERS tags can be released from the Fe_3O_4@Ag and SERS intensity quenching can be triggered, the released miRNA can enter the cycle to decluster other DNA and SERS tags. Due to the dual-SERS enhancement of the Fe_3O_4@Ag-SERS tag conjugates and the recycling signal amplification, a detection limit of 1 aM with single-base recognition can be performed by one step (Fig. **37**).

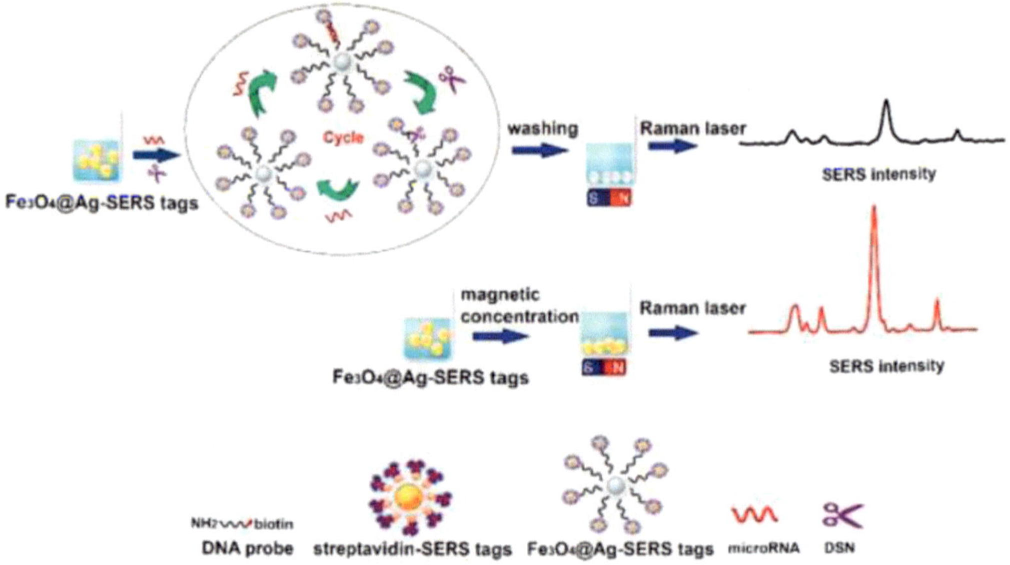

Fig. (37). DSN-assisted SERS detection of microRNA. Reprinted with permission from [238].

Another example was developed by Zhou *et al.* [239] for simultaneous detection of multiple liver cancer related miRNA biomarkers. The authors synthetized a novel nanogap-based SERS nanotags by modifying AuNPs with thiolated DNA and non-fluorescent small encoding molecules. Furthermore, they prepared hollow silver microspheres (Ag-HMSs) using bacteria as templates. Later, they used the DNA-conjugated SERS nanotags as SERS nanoprobes and the DNA-conjugated Ag-HMSs to capture the target with a detection limit of 10 fM. In a more recent work, Chen *et al.* [240, 241] designed an enzyme-free SERS platform to sensitively and reliably detect the target miR-21 using a corrective internal standard-based ratio-metric SERS probe coupled with mismatched CHA amplification. In this strategy, the target cyclically triggers the allosteric effects of mismatched CHA amplification and the 3′-R6G-labeled H1 is opened. Then, H2 hybridizes with H1 to form H1–H2 complex and the released miR-21 was free to participate in the next cycle of CHA reaction (Fig. **38**). Meanwhile, the H1–H2 complex can hybridize with the capture DNA on the SERS chip, making the Raman tag of R6G close to the surface of SERS substrate, and the SERS signal intensity arising from R6G labels increase while that from 4-ATP remain relatively unchanged. This platform exhibits sensitivity toward miR-21 with a limit of detection of 3.5 fM and a broad dynamic range from 10 fM to 100 nM.

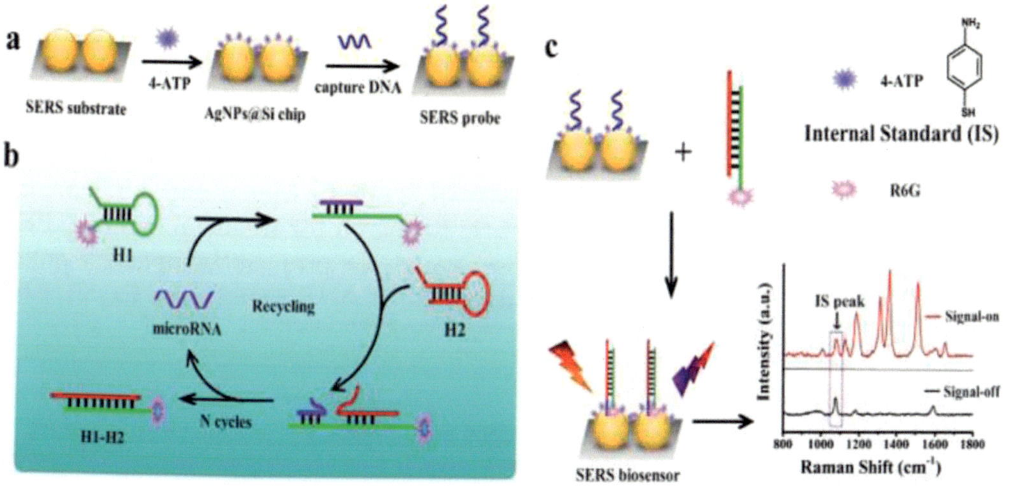

Fig. (38). Schematic of the ratiometric SERS platform based on mismatched CHA amplification for quantitative detection of miRNA-21. **(a)** Fabrication of the ISAgNPs@Si SERS probe. **(b)** The miRNA-induced mismatched CHA amplification process. **(c)** The principle of ratiometric SERS biosensor for miRNA-21 detection. Reprinted with permission from [240].

CONCLUDING REMARKS

The increasing number of research works evidencing the potential use of short non-coding RNAs and especially miRNAs as biomarkers for the diagnosis and prognosis of several diseases paved the way for the design of novel strategies to detect them using electrochemical and optical biosensors. Up to date, several interesting strategies have been devised, the most interesting ones are summarized in this chapter. Most of the biosensors reported in the literature are proofs-o--concept and need validation using cohorts of patients/control subjects to assess the results from the biosensing strategies to "gold" standard molecular biology techniques. Several other steps are necessary before some of these approaches find their way to the market to be used in hospitals and by health practitioners. Other non-coding RNAs, such as small-interacting RNAs (siRNAs), small nucleolar RNAs (snoRNAs), piwi-interacting RNAs (piRNAs), and circular RNAs (cirRNAs) and long non-coding RNAs (lncRNAs), are currently explored as new biomarkers for cancer diseases. Curiously, almost no literature references exist in their use as targets for biosensors, which could be an interesting area of research for beginners in this field.

CONSENT FOR PUBLICATION

Not applicable.

CONFLICT OF INTEREST

The authors declare no conflict of interest, financial or otherwise.

ACKNOWLEDGEMENTS

The authors gratefully thank the University of Tunis El Manar and the Tunisian Ministry of Higher Education and Scientific Research for financial support. PRF program is also acknowledged for funding through the projectsNanoFastResponse (ref.: PRF2017-D4P1), SmartBioSens (ref.: PRFCOV19-D2P2) and COVID-PP (ref.: PRFCOV19-D3P1).

ABBREVIATIONS

3-QD@DNA NC	triple-CdTe quantum dot labeled DNA nanocomposites;
Ag-HMSs	Hollow silver microspheres;
AgNPs	silver nanoparticles;
AuNWs	gold nanowires;
APTES	3-aminopropyltriethoxysilane;
Agol–4	Argonaute proteins 1-4 ;
AGO2	Argonaute-2;
BC	bladder cancer;
BCIP	5-bromo-4-chloro-3-indolyl phosphate;
BHQ2	organic quencher;
BRAF	B-Raf Proto-Oncogene;
BrC	breast cancer;
CA	carbohydrate antigen;
CC	cervical cancer;
CD44	cell-surface glycoprotein;
CEA	carcinoembryonic antigen;
CEAM	cyclic enzymatic amplification method;
CNPs	carbon nanoparticles;
CP	capture probe;
CRC	colorectal cancer;
CRISPR-Cas9	Clustered Regularly Interspaced Short Palindromic Repeats-associated protein 9;
CV	cyclic voltammetry;
DGCR8	DiGeorge Syndrome CriticalRegion-8;
dsRNA	double-strand RNA;
DSN	duplex-specific nuclease;

DPV	differential pulse voltammetry;
EC	esophageal cancer;
ECC	electrochemical–chemical–chemical;
EIS	electrochemical impedance spectroscopy;
EnC	endometrial cancer;
ELSIA	enzyme-linked immunoassay;
Fc-SH	6-ferrocenylhexanethiol;
FITC	fluorescein isothiocyanate;
FRET	Forster resonance energy transfer;
GC	gastric cancer;
GNPs	gold nanoplasmonic particles;
GO	graphene oxide;
HCC	hepatocellular cancer;
HER2	epidermal growth factor receptor 2;
HNSCC	head and neck squamous cell cancer;
HPLC	high performance liquid chromatography;
IARC	International Agency for Research on Cancer;
IUPAC	International Union of Pure and Applied Chemistry;
KRAS	Kirsten rat sarcoma 2 viral oncogene homolog;
LC	lung cancer;
LOD	Limit of detection;
miRs	microRNAs;
MNPs	magnetic nanoparticles;
MPDA	mesoporous polydopamine;
mRNAs	messenger RNAs;
MWCNT/AuNCs	multi-walled carbon nanotube-gold manocomposites;
MYC	Proto-Oncogene;
NBT	nitro blue tetrazolium;
NSCLC	non-small cell lung cancer;
OC	ovarian cancer;
OTMS	octadecyltrimethoxysilane;
PC	pancreatic cancer;
PCA	pyrenecarboxylic acid;
PIWI	P-element induced wimpy testis in Drosophila;
PDCD4	Programmed Cell Death 4;

PDMC	polymethylsiloxane;
PrC	prostate cancer;
pre-miRNAs	precursor miRNAs;
pri-miRNAs	primary miRNAs;
PSA	prostate specific antigen;
PTEN	Phosphatase and tensin homolog;
QDs	quantum dots;
RC	rolling circle amplification;
RCC	renal cell cancer;
RISC or miRISC	multiprotein RNA-induced silencing complex;
RLS	resource-limited settings;
SA	streptavidin;
SB	sulfobetaine-3-undecanethiol;
SC	skin cancer;
SensPEQ	electrocatalytic quadroprobe sensor ;
SERS	surface-enhanced Raman spectroscopy;
SiNW	silicon nanowire;
SPGE	Screen-Printed Gold Electrode;
SPR	surface resonance plasmon;
SPRY2	sprouty homolog 2;
ssDNA	single-stranded DNA;
TC	thyroid cancer;
ThT	Thioflavin T;
TiP	titanium phosphate nanoparticles;
TMB	3,3',5,5'-tétraméthylbenzidine;
TRBP	transactivation-responsive RNA-binding protein;
SWV	square-wave voltammetry;
UICC	Union for International Cancer Control;
UIP	universal interfacial probe.

REFERENCES

[1] WHO report on cancer: setting priorities, investing wisely and providing care for all. Geneva: World Health Organization 2020.

[2] Adams C, Torode J, Henshall S, Cazap E, Ryel AL, Grey N. The World Cancer Declaration: from resolution to action. Lancet Oncol 2011; 12(12): 1091-2. [http://dx.doi.org/10.1016/S1470-2045(11)70298-4] [PMID: 22041537]

[3] Mousa S, Mousa SA. Biosensors: the new wave in cancer diagnosis. Nanotechnol Sci Appl 2010; 4: 1-

10.
[http://dx.doi.org/10.2147/NSA.S13465] [PMID: 24198482]

[4] Peeling RW, Holmes KK, Mabey D, Ronald A. Rapid tests for sexually transmitted infections (STIs): the way forward. Sex Transm Infect 2006; 82 (Suppl. 5): v1-6.
[http://dx.doi.org/10.1136/sti.2006.024265] [PMID: 17151023]

[5] Turner APF. Biosensors: sense and sensibility. Chem Soc Rev 2013; 42(8): 3184-96.
[http://dx.doi.org/10.1039/c3cs35528d] [PMID: 23420144]

[6] Turner A, Karube I, Wilson GS. Biosensors: fundamentals and applications. Oxford university press 1987.

[7] Kimmel DW, LeBlanc G, Meschievitz ME, Cliffel DE. Electrochemical sensors and biosensors. Anal Chem 2012; 84(2): 685-707.
[http://dx.doi.org/10.1021/ac202878q] [PMID: 22044045]

[8] Grieshaber D, MacKenzie R, Vörös J, Reimhult E. Electrochemical biosensors-sensor principles and architectures. Sensors (Basel) 2008; 8(3): 1400-58.
[http://dx.doi.org/10.3390/s80314000] [PMID: 27879772]

[9] D'Orazio P. Biosensors in clinical chemistry. Clin Chim Acta 2003; 334(1-2): 41-69.
[http://dx.doi.org/10.1016/S0009-8981(03)00241-9] [PMID: 12867275]

[10] Gold P, Freedman SO. Specific carcinoembryonic antigens of the human digestive system. J Exp Med 1965; 122(3): 467-81.
[http://dx.doi.org/10.1084/jem.122.3.467] [PMID: 4953873]

[11] Koprowski H, Herlyn M, Steplewski Z, Sears HF. Specific antigen in serum of patients with colon carcinoma. Science 1981; 212(4490): 53-5.
[http://dx.doi.org/10.1126/science.6163212] [PMID: 6163212]

[12] Colomer R, Sole LA, Navarro M, Encabo G, Ruibal A, Salvador L. CA 15.3: early results of a new breast cancer marker. Anticancer Res 1986; 6(4): 683-4.
[PMID: 3463242]

[13] O'Brien TJ, Tanimoto H, Konishi I, Gee M. More than 15 years of CA 125: what is known about the antigen, its structure and its function. Int J Biol Markers 1998; 13(4): 188-95.
[http://dx.doi.org/10.1177/172460089801300403] [PMID: 10228899]

[14] Chatterjee SK, Zetter BR. Cancer biomarkers: knowing the present and predicting the future. Future Oncol 2005; 1(1): 37-50.
[http://dx.doi.org/10.1517/14796694.1.1.37] [PMID: 16555974]

[15] Barry MJ. Prostate-specificy-antigen testing for early diagnosis of prostate cancer. N Engl J Med 2001; 344(18): 1373-7.
[http://dx.doi.org/10.1056/NEJM200105033441806] [PMID: 11333995]

[16] Asif HM, Sultana S, Ahmed S, Akhtar N, Tariq M. HER-2 Positive Breast Cancer a Mini-Review Asian Pac J Cancer Prev 2016; 17(4): 1609-15.
[http://dx.doi.org/10.7314/APJCP.2016.17.4.1609] [PMID: 27221828]

[17] Romano G, Veneziano D, Acunzo M, Croce CM. Small non-coding RNA and cancer. Carcinogenesis 2017; 38(5): 485-91.
[http://dx.doi.org/10.1093/carcin/bgx026] [PMID: 28449079]

[18] Vo JN, Cieslik M, Zhang Y, *et al.* The Landscape of Circular RNA in Cancer. Cell 2019; 176(4): 869-881.e13.
[http://dx.doi.org/10.1016/j.cell.2018.12.021] [PMID: 30735636]

[19] Lee YS, Dutta A. MicroRNAs in Cancer. Annu Rev Pathol 2009; 4(1): 199-227.
[http://dx.doi.org/10.1146/annurev.pathol.4.110807.092222] [PMID: 18817506]

[20] Liu Y, Dou M, Song X, *et al.* The emerging role of the piRNA/piwi complex in cancer. Mol Cancer

2019; 18(1): 123.
[http://dx.doi.org/10.1186/s12943-019-1052-9] [PMID: 31399034]

[21] Ling H, Fabbri M, Calin GA. MicroRNAs and other non-coding RNAs as targets for anticancer drug development. Nat Rev Drug Discov 2013; 12(11): 847-65.
[http://dx.doi.org/10.1038/nrd4140] [PMID: 24172333]

[22] Kappel A, Keller A. miRNA assays in the clinical laboratory: workflow, detection technologies and automation aspects. Clinical Chemistry and Laboratory Medicine (CCLM) 2017; 55(5): 636-47.
[http://dx.doi.org/10.1515/cclm-2016-0467] [PMID: 27987355]

[23] Cai X, Hagedorn CH, Cullen BR. Human microRNAs are processed from capped, polyadenylated transcripts that can also function as mRNAs. RNA 2004; 10(12): 1957-66.

[24] Esteller M. Non-coding RNAs in human disease. Nat Rev Genet 2011; 12(12): 861-74.
[http://dx.doi.org/10.1038/nrg3074] [PMID: 22094949]

[25] Zhang X, Cozen AE, Liu Y, Chen Q, Lowe TM. Small RNA Modifications: Integral to Function and Disease. Trends Mol Med 2016; 22(12): 1025-34.
[http://dx.doi.org/10.1016/j.molmed.2016.10.009] [PMID: 27840066]

[26] Stefani G, Slack FJ. Small non-coding RNAs in animal development. Nat Rev Mol Cell Biol 2008; 9(3): 219-30.
[http://dx.doi.org/10.1038/nrm2347] [PMID: 18270516]

[27] Akkilic N, Geschwindner S, Höök F. Single-molecule biosensors: Recent advances and applications. Biosens Bioelectron 2020; 151: 111944.
[http://dx.doi.org/10.1016/j.bios.2019.111944] [PMID: 31999573]

[28] Krützfeldt J, Rajewsky N, Braich R, *et al.* Silencing of microRNAs in vivo with 'antagomirs'. Nature 2005; 438(7068): 685-9.
[http://dx.doi.org/10.1038/nature04303] [PMID: 16258535]

[29] Esquela-Kerscher A, Slack FJ. Oncomirs — microRNAs with a role in cancer. Nat Rev Cancer 2006; 6(4): 259-69.
[http://dx.doi.org/10.1038/nrc1840] [PMID: 16557279]

[30] Osada H, Takahashi T. MicroRNAs in biological processes and carcinogenesis. Carcinogenesis 2007; 28(1): 2-12.
[http://dx.doi.org/10.1093/carcin/bgl185] [PMID: 17028302]

[31] Wienholds E, Plasterk RHA. MicroRNA function in animal development. FEBS Lett 2005; 579(26): 5911-22.
[http://dx.doi.org/10.1016/j.febslet.2005.07.070] [PMID: 16111679]

[32] Lu J, Getz G, Miska EA, *et al.* MicroRNA expression profiles classify human cancers. Nature 2005; 435(7043): 834-8.
[http://dx.doi.org/10.1038/nature03702] [PMID: 15944708]

[33] Ebert MS, Sharp PA. Roles for microRNAs in conferring robustness to biological processes. Cell 2012; 149(3): 515-24.
[http://dx.doi.org/10.1016/j.cell.2012.04.005] [PMID: 22541426]

[34] Sharma PC, Gupta A. MicroRNAs: potential biomarkers for diagnosis and prognosis of different cancers. Transl Cancer Res 2020; 9(9): 5798-818.
[http://dx.doi.org/10.21037/tcr-20-1294] [PMID: 35117940]

[35] Kozomara A, Birgaoanu M, Griffiths-Jones S. miRBase: from microRNA sequences to function. Nucleic Acids Res 2019; 47(D1): D155-62.
[http://dx.doi.org/10.1093/nar/gky1141] [PMID: 30423142]

[36] Grundhoff A, Sullivan CS. Virus-encoded microRNAs. Virology 2011; 411(2): 325-43.
[http://dx.doi.org/10.1016/j.virol.2011.01.002] [PMID: 21277611]

[37] Nair V, Zavolan M. Virus-encoded microRNAs: novel regulators of gene expression. Trends Microbiol 2006; 14(4): 169-75.
[http://dx.doi.org/10.1016/j.tim.2006.02.007] [PMID: 16531046]

[38] Cai X, Hagedorn CH, Cullen BR. Human microRNAs are processed from capped, polyadenylated transcripts that can also function as mRNAs. RNA 2004; 10(12): 1957-66.
[http://dx.doi.org/10.1261/rna.7135204] [PMID: 15525708]

[39] Han J, Lee Y, Yeom KH, *et al.* Molecular basis for the recognition of primary microRNAs by the Drosha-DGCR8 complex. Cell 2006; 125(5): 887-901.
[http://dx.doi.org/10.1016/j.cell.2006.03.043] [PMID: 16751099]

[40] Yi R, Qin Y, Macara IG, Cullen BR. Exportin-5 mediates the nuclear export of pre-microRNAs and short hairpin RNAs. Genes Dev 2003; 17(24): 3011-6.
[http://dx.doi.org/10.1101/gad.1158803] [PMID: 14681208]

[41] Winter J, Jung S, Keller S, Gregory RI, Diederichs S. Many roads to maturity: microRNA biogenesis pathways and their regulation. Nat Cell Biol 2009; 11(3): 228-34.
[http://dx.doi.org/10.1038/ncb0309-228] [PMID: 19255566]

[42] Ha M, Kim VN. Regulation of microRNA biogenesis. Nat Rev Mol Cell Biol 2014; 15(8): 509-24.
[http://dx.doi.org/10.1038/nrm3838] [PMID: 25027649]

[43] Kai K, Dittmar RL, Sen S. Secretory microRNAs as biomarkers of cancer. Semin Cell Dev Biol 2018; 78: 22-36.
[http://dx.doi.org/10.1016/j.semcdb.2017.12.011] [PMID: 29258963]

[44] Condrat CE, Thompson DC, Barbu MG, *et al.* miRNAs as Biomarkers in Disease: Latest Findings Regarding Their Role in Diagnosis and Prognosis. Cells 2020; 9(2): 276.
[http://dx.doi.org/10.3390/cells9020276] [PMID: 31979244]

[45] Helwak A, Kudla G, Dudnakova T, Tollervey D. Mapping the human miRNA interactome by CLASH reveals frequent noncanonical binding. Cell 2013; 153(3): 654-65.
[http://dx.doi.org/10.1016/j.cell.2013.03.043] [PMID: 23622248]

[46] Krek A, Grün D, Poy MN, *et al.* Combinatorial microRNA target predictions. Nat Genet 2005; 37(5): 495-500.
[http://dx.doi.org/10.1038/ng1536] [PMID: 15806104]

[47] Chevillet J, Lee I, Briggs H, He Y, Wang K. Issues and prospects of microRNA-based biomarkers in blood and other body fluids. Molecules 2014; 19(5): 6080-105.
[http://dx.doi.org/10.3390/molecules19056080] [PMID: 24830712]

[48] Peplow PV, Martinez B. MicroRNAs as biomarkers of diabetic retinopathy and disease progression. Neural Regen Res 2019; 14(11): 1858-69.
[http://dx.doi.org/10.4103/1673-5374.259602] [PMID: 31290435]

[49] Zhang J, Zhao H, Gao Y, Zhang W. Secretory miRNAs as novel cancer biomarkers. Biochim Biophys Acta Rev Cancer 2012; 1826(1): 32-43.
[http://dx.doi.org/10.1016/j.bbcan.2012.03.001] [PMID: 22440944]

[50] Di Leva G, Garofalo M, Croce CM. MicroRNAs in Cancer. In: Abbas AK, Galli SJ, Howley PM, editors Annual Review of Pathology: Mechanisms of Disease, Vol 9 Annual Review of Pathology-Mechanisms of Disease. 2014; p. 287-314..
[http://dx.doi.org/10.1146/annurev-pathol-012513-104715]

[51] Rottiers V, Näär AM. MicroRNAs in metabolism and metabolic disorders. Nat Rev Mol Cell Biol 2012; 13(4): 239-50.
[http://dx.doi.org/10.1038/nrm3313] [PMID: 22436747]

[52] Bottani M, Banfi G, Lombardi G. Circulating miRNAs as Diagnostic and Prognostic Biomarkers in Common Solid Tumors: Focus on Lung, Breast, Prostate Cancers, and Osteosarcoma. J Clin Med

2019; 8(10): 1661.
[http://dx.doi.org/10.3390/jcm8101661] [PMID: 31614612]

[53] Weber JA, Baxter DH, Zhang S, *et al.* The microRNA spectrum in 12 body fluids. Clin Chem 2010; 56(11): 1733-41.
[http://dx.doi.org/10.1373/clinchem.2010.147405] [PMID: 20847327]

[54] Ludwig N, Leidinger P, Becker K, *et al.* Distribution of miRNA expression across human tissues. Nucleic Acids Res 2016; 44(8): 3865-77.
[http://dx.doi.org/10.1093/nar/gkw116] [PMID: 26921406]

[55] Pogribny IP. MicroRNAs as biomarkers for clinical studies. Exp Biol Med (Maywood) 2018; 243(3): 283-90.
[http://dx.doi.org/10.1177/1535370217731291] [PMID: 28914096]

[56] Fu Q, Yang F, Xiang T, *et al.* A novel microRNA signature predicts survival in liver hepatocellular carcinoma after hepatectomy. Sci Rep 2018; 8(1): 7933.
[http://dx.doi.org/10.1038/s41598-018-26374-9] [PMID: 29785036]

[57] Francavilla A, Turoczi S, Tarallo S, Vodicka P, Pardini B, Naccarati A. Exosomal microRNAs and other non-coding RNAs as colorectal cancer biomarkers: a review. Mutagenesis 2020; 35(3): 243-60.
[http://dx.doi.org/10.1093/mutage/gez038] [PMID: 31784760]

[58] Kluiver J, Poppema S, de Jong D, *et al.* BIC and miR-155 are highly expressed in Hodgkin, primary mediastinal and diffuse large B cell lymphomas. J Pathol 2005; 207(2): 243-9.
[http://dx.doi.org/10.1002/path.1825] [PMID: 16041695]

[59] Ryu JK, Hong SM, Karikari CA, Hruban RH, Goggins MG, Maitra A. Aberrant MicroRNA-155 expression is an early event in the multistep progression of pancreatic adenocarcinoma. Pancreatology 2010; 10(1): 66-73.
[http://dx.doi.org/10.1159/000231984] [PMID: 20332664]

[60] Liu B-Y, Nie H, Wang M, *et al.* microRNA-155 is downregulated in gastric cancer cells and involved in cell metastasis. Oncol Rep 2012; 27(6): 1960-6.
[http://dx.doi.org/10.3892/or.2012.1719] [PMID: 22426647]

[61] Qin W, Ren Q, Liu T, Huang Y, Wang J. MicroRNA-155 is a novel suppressor of ovarian cancer-initiating cells that targets CLDN1. FEBS Lett 2013; 587(9): 1434-9.
[http://dx.doi.org/10.1016/j.febslet.2013.03.023] [PMID: 23523916]

[62] Calin GA, Sevignani C, Dumitru CD, *et al.* Human microRNA genes are frequently located at fragile sites and genomic regions involved in cancers. Proc Natl Acad Sci USA 2004; 101(9): 2999-3004.
[http://dx.doi.org/10.1073/pnas.0307323101] [PMID: 14973191]

[63] Deng S, Calin GA, Croce CM, Coukos G, Zhang L. Mechanisms of microRNA deregulation in human cancer. Cell Cycle 2008; 7(17): 2643-6.
[http://dx.doi.org/10.4161/cc.7.17.6597] [PMID: 18719391]

[64] Cozar JM, Robles-Fernandez I, Rodriguez-Martinez A, *et al.* The role of miRNAs as biomarkers in prostate cancer. Mutat Res Rev Mutat Res 2019; 781: 165-74.
[http://dx.doi.org/10.1016/j.mrrev.2019.05.005] [PMID: 31416574]

[65] Chen B, Xia Z, Deng YN, *et al.* Emerging microRNA biomarkers for colorectal cancer diagnosis and prognosis. Open Biol 2019; 9(1): 180212.
[http://dx.doi.org/10.1098/rsob.180212] [PMID: 30958116]

[66] Bhat SA, Majid S, Rehman MU. Scenario and future prospects of microRNAs in gastric cancer: A review. Iran J Basic Med Sci 2019; 22(4): 345-52.
[http://dx.doi.org/10.22038/ijbms.2019.32399.7765] [PMID: 31168337]

[67] Yeh CH, Moles R, Nicot C. Clinical significance of microRNAs in chronic and acute human leukemia. Mol Cancer 2016; 15(1): 37.
[http://dx.doi.org/10.1186/s12943-016-0518-2] [PMID: 27179712]

[68] Yete S, Saranath D. MicroRNAs in oral cancer: Biomarkers with clinical potential. Oral Oncol 2020; 110: 105002.
[http://dx.doi.org/10.1016/j.oraloncology.2020.105002] [PMID: 32949853]

[69] Aggarwal V, Priyanka K, Tuli HS. Emergence of Circulating MicroRNAs in Breast Cancer as Diagnostic and Therapeutic Efficacy Biomarkers. Mol Diagn Ther 2020; 24(2): 153-73.
[http://dx.doi.org/10.1007/s40291-020-00447-w] [PMID: 32067191]

[70] Hayes C, Chayama K. MicroRNAs as Biomarkers for Liver Disease and Hepatocellular Carcinoma. Int J Mol Sci 2016; 17(3): 280.
[http://dx.doi.org/10.3390/ijms17030280] [PMID: 26927063]

[71] Wang C, Ding M, Xia M, *et al.* A Five-miRNA Panel Identified From a Multicentric Case–control Study Serves as a Novel Diagnostic Tool for Ethnically Diverse Non-small-cell Lung Cancer Patients. EBioMedicine 2015; 2(10): 1377-85.
[http://dx.doi.org/10.1016/j.ebiom.2015.07.034] [PMID: 26629532]

[72] Hu Y, Wang H, Chen E, Xu Z, Chen B, Lu G. Candidate microRNAs as biomarkers of thyroid carcinoma: a systematic review, meta-analysis, and experimental validation. Cancer Med 2016; 5(9): 2602-14.
[http://dx.doi.org/10.1002/cam4.811] [PMID: 27465286]

[73] Stojanovic J, Tognetto A, Tiziano DF, *et al.* MicroRNAs expression profiles as diagnostic biomarkers of gastric cancer: a systematic literature review. Biomarkers 2019; 24(2): 110-9.
[http://dx.doi.org/10.1080/1354750X.2018.1539765] [PMID: 30387681]

[74] Babashah S, Sadeghizadeh M, Tavirani MR, Farivar S, Soleimani M. Aberrant microRNA expression and its implications in the pathogenesis of leukemias. Cell Oncol (Dordr) 2012; 35(5): 317-34.
[http://dx.doi.org/10.1007/s13402-012-0095-3] [PMID: 22956261]

[75] Momen-Heravi F, Bala S. Emerging role of non-coding RNA in oral cancer. Cell Signal 2018; 42: 134-43.
[http://dx.doi.org/10.1016/j.cellsig.2017.10.009] [PMID: 29056500]

[76] Hamam R, Hamam D, Alsaleh KA, *et al.* Circulating microRNAs in breast cancer: novel diagnostic and prognostic biomarkers Cell Death Dis 2017; 8(9):e3045.
[http://dx.doi.org/10.1038/cddis.2017.440]

[77] Wang C, Ding M, Xia M, *et al.* A five-miRNA panel identified from a multicentric case–control study serves as a novel diagnostic tool for ethnically diverse non-small-cell lung cancer patients. EBioMedicine 2015; 2(10): 1377-85.
[http://dx.doi.org/10.1016/j.ebiom.2015.07.034] [PMID: 26629532]

[78] Hu Y, Wang H, Chen E, Xu Z, Chen B, Lu G. Candidate microRNAs as biomarkers of thyroid carcinoma: a systematic review, meta-analysis, and experimental validation. Cancer Med 2016; 5(9): 2602-14.
[http://dx.doi.org/10.1002/cam4.811] [PMID: 27465286]

[79] Filella X, Foj L. miRNAs as novel biomarkers in the management of prostate cancer. Clinical Chemistry and Laboratory Medicine (CCLM) 2017; 55(5): 715-36.
[http://dx.doi.org/10.1515/cclm-2015-1073] [PMID: 26751899]

[80] de Carvalho INSR, de Freitas RM, Vargas FR. Translating microRNAs into biomarkers: What is new for pediatric cancer? Med Oncol 2016; 33(5): 49.
[http://dx.doi.org/10.1007/s12032-016-0766-4] [PMID: 27085875]

[81] Letelier P, Riquelme I, Hernández A, Guzmán N, Farías J, Roa J. Circulating MicroRNAs as Biomarkers in Biliary Tract Cancers. Int J Mol Sci 2016; 17(5): 791.
[http://dx.doi.org/10.3390/ijms17050791] [PMID: 27223281]

[82] Resnick KE, Alder H, Hagan JP, Richardson DL, Croce CM, Cohn DE. The detection of differentially expressed microRNAs from the serum of ovarian cancer patients using a novel real-time PCR

platform. Gynecol Oncol 2009; 112(1): 55-9.
[http://dx.doi.org/10.1016/j.ygyno.2008.08.036] [PMID: 18954897]

[83] Fadaka AO, Pretorius A, Klein A. Biomarkers for Stratification in Colorectal Cancer: MicroRNAs. Cancer Contr 2019; 26: 1.
[http://dx.doi.org/10.1177/1073274819862784] [PMID: 31431043]

[84] Lai X, Wang M, McElyea SD, Sherman S, House M, Korc M. A microRNA signature in circulating exosomes is superior to exosomal glypican-1 levels for diagnosing pancreatic cancer. Cancer Lett 2017; 393: 86-93.
[http://dx.doi.org/10.1016/j.canlet.2017.02.019] [PMID: 28232049]

[85] Fang Z, Tang J, Bai Y, *et al.* Plasma levels of microRNA-24, microRNA-320a, and microRNA-423-5p are potential biomarkers for colorectal carcinoma. J Exp Clin Cancer Res 2015; 34(1): 86.
[http://dx.doi.org/10.1186/s13046-015-0198-6] [PMID: 26297223]

[86] Lin XJ, Chong Y, Guo ZW, *et al.* A serum microRNA classifier for early detection of hepatocellular carcinoma: a multicentre, retrospective, longitudinal biomarker identification study with a nested case-control study. Lancet Oncol 2015; 16(7): 804-15.
[http://dx.doi.org/10.1016/S1470-2045(15)00048-0] [PMID: 26088272]

[87] Pan C, Yan X, Li H, *et al.* Systematic literature review and clinical validation of circulating microRNAs as diagnostic biomarkers for colorectal cancer. Oncotarget 2017; 8(40): 68317-28.
[http://dx.doi.org/10.18632/oncotarget.19344] [PMID: 28978119]

[88] Guo S, Zhang J, Wang B, *et al.* A 5-serum miRNA panel for the early detection of colorectal cancer. OncoTargets Ther 2018; 11: 2603-14.
[http://dx.doi.org/10.2147/OTT.S153535] [PMID: 29780253]

[89] Ye J, Xu M, Tian X, Cai S, Zeng S. Research advances in the detection of miRNA. J Pharm Anal 2019; 9(4): 217-26.
[http://dx.doi.org/10.1016/j.jpha.2019.05.004] [PMID: 31452959]

[90] Androvic P, Valihrach L, Elling J, Sjoback R, Kubista M. Two-tailed RT-qPCR: a novel method for highly accurate miRNA quantification. Nucleic Acids Res 2017; 45(15): e144.
[http://dx.doi.org/10.1093/nar/gkx588] [PMID: 28911110]

[91] Su WZ, Ren LF. MiRNA-199 inhibits malignant progression of lung cancer through mediating RGS17. Eur Rev Med Pharmacol Sci 2019; 23(8): 3390-400.
[PMID: 31081094]

[92] Xiao G, Jia W-Z, Yu T, *et al.* MicroRNA-190 regulates FOXP2 genes in human gastric cancer. OncoTargets Ther 2016; 9: 3643-51.
[http://dx.doi.org/10.2147/OTT.S103682] [PMID: 27382302]

[93] Liu J, Jiang Y, Wan Y, Zhou S, Thapa S, Cheng W. MicroRNA□665 suppresses the growth and migration of ovarian cancer cells by targeting HOXA10. Mol Med Rep 2018; 18(3): 2661-8.
[http://dx.doi.org/10.3892/mmr.2018.9252] [PMID: 30015865]

[94] Cheng Y, Dong L, Zhang J, Zhao Y, Li Z. Recent advances in microRNA detection. Analyst (Lond) 2018; 143(8): 1758-74.
[http://dx.doi.org/10.1039/C7AN02001E] [PMID: 29560992]

[95] Li C, Li Z, Jia H, Yan J. One-step ultrasensitive detection of microRNAs with loop-mediated isothermal amplification (LAMP). Chem Commun (Camb) 2011; 47(9): 2595-7.
[http://dx.doi.org/10.1039/C0CC03957H] [PMID: 21173961]

[96] Mukama O, Nie C, Habimana JD, *et al.* Synergetic performance of isothermal amplification techniques and lateral flow approach for nucleic acid diagnostics. Anal Biochem 2020; 600: 113762.
[http://dx.doi.org/10.1016/j.ab.2020.113762] [PMID: 32387190]

[97] Sun Y, Tian H, Liu C, Sun Y, Li Z. One-step detection of microRNA with high sensitivity and specificity via target-triggered loop-mediated isothermal amplification (TT-LAMP). Chem Commun

(Camb) 2017; 53(80): 11040-3.
[http://dx.doi.org/10.1039/C7CC06140D] [PMID: 28937697]

[98] Tian W, Li P, He W, Liu C, Li Z. Rolling circle extension-actuated loop-mediated isothermal amplification (RCA-LAMP) for ultrasensitive detection of microRNAs. Biosens Bioelectron 2019; 128: 17-22.
[http://dx.doi.org/10.1016/j.bios.2018.12.041] [PMID: 30616213]

[99] Yin P, Choi HMT, Calvert CR, Pierce NA. Programming biomolecular self-assembly pathways. Nature 2008; 451(7176): 318-22.
[http://dx.doi.org/10.1038/nature06451] [PMID: 18202654]

[100] Liu J, Zhang Y, Xie H, Zhao L, Zheng L, Ye H. Applications of Catalytic Hairpin Assembly Reaction in Biosensing. Small 2019; 15(42): 1902989.
[http://dx.doi.org/10.1002/smll.201902989] [PMID: 31523917]

[101] He C, Wang M, Sun X, *et al.* Integrating PDA microtube waveguide system with heterogeneous CHA amplification strategy towards superior sensitive detection of miRNA. Biosens Bioelectron 2019; 129: 50-7.
[http://dx.doi.org/10.1016/j.bios.2019.01.003] [PMID: 30682689]

[102] Dai W, Zhang J, Meng X, *et al.* Catalytic hairpin assembly gel assay for multiple and sensitive microRNA detection. Theranostics 2018; 8(10): 2646-56.
[http://dx.doi.org/10.7150/thno.24480] [PMID: 29774065]

[103] Ali MM, Li F, Zhang Z, *et al.* Rolling circle amplification: a versatile tool for chemical biology, materials science and medicine. Chem Soc Rev 2014; 43(10): 3324-41.
[http://dx.doi.org/10.1039/c3cs60439j] [PMID: 24643375]

[104] Gu L, Yan W, Liu L, Wang S, Zhang X, Lyu M. Research progress on rolling circle amplification (RCA)-based biomedical sensing. Pharmaceuticals (Basel) 2018; 11(2): 35.
[http://dx.doi.org/10.3390/ph11020035] [PMID: 29690513]

[105] Li J, Lin L, Yu J, Zhai S, Liu G, Tian L. Fabrication and biomedical applications of "polymer-like" nucleic acids enzymatically produced by rolling circle amplification. ACS Appl Bio Mater 2019; 2(10): 4106-20.
[http://dx.doi.org/10.1021/acsabm.9b00622] [PMID: 35021425]

[106] Garbarino F, Minero GAS, Rizzi G, Fock J, Hansen MF. Integration of rolling circle amplification and optomagnetic detection on a polymer chip. Biosens Bioelectron 2019; 142: 111485.
[http://dx.doi.org/10.1016/j.bios.2019.111485] [PMID: 31301578]

[107] Ciftci S, Cánovas R, Neumann F, *et al.* The sweet detection of rolling circle amplification: Glucose-based electrochemical genosensor for the detection of viral nucleic acid. Biosens Bioelectron 2020; 151: 112002.
[http://dx.doi.org/10.1016/j.bios.2019.112002] [PMID: 31999596]

[108] Dirks RM, Pierce NA. Triggered amplification by hybridization chain reaction. Proc Natl Acad Sci USA 2004; 101(43): 15275-8.
[http://dx.doi.org/10.1073/pnas.0407024101] [PMID: 15492210]

[109] Bi S, Yue S, Zhang S. Hybridization chain reaction: a versatile molecular tool for biosensing, bioimaging, and biomedicine. Chem Soc Rev 2017; 46(14): 4281-98.
[http://dx.doi.org/10.1039/C7CS00055C] [PMID: 28573275]

[110] Yang L, Liu C, Ren W, Li Z. Graphene surface-anchored fluorescence sensor for sensitive detection of microRNA coupled with enzyme-free signal amplification of hybridization chain reaction. ACS Appl Mater Interfaces 2012; 4(12): 6450-3.
[http://dx.doi.org/10.1021/am302268t] [PMID: 23182299]

[111] Guo Q, Yu Y, Zhang H, Cai C, Shen Q. Electrochemical sensing of exosomal microRNA based on hybridization chain reaction signal amplification with reduced false-positive signals. Anal Chem 2020;

92(7): 5302-10.
[http://dx.doi.org/10.1021/acs.analchem.9b05849] [PMID: 32148013]

[112] Shoemark A, Frost E, Dixon M, *et al.* Accuracy of Immunofluorescence in the Diagnosis of Primary Ciliary Dyskinesia. Am J Respir Crit Care Med 2017; 196(1): 94-101.
[http://dx.doi.org/10.1164/rccm.201607-1351OC] [PMID: 28199173]

[113] Kim B. Western blot techniques Molecular Profiling. Springer 2017; pp. 133-9.

[114] L K, L Z, M MR Miniaturized Electrochemical Sensors to Facilitate Liquid Biopsy for Detection of Circulating Tumor Markers In: M T, editor Applications of Microfluidic Systems in Biology and Medicine Bioanalysis (Advanced Materials, Methods, and Devices) Singapore: Springer. 2019.
[http://dx.doi.org/10.1007/978-981-13-6229-3_4]

[115] Johnson BN, Mutharasan R. Biosensor-based microRNA detection: techniques, design, performance, and challenges. Analyst (Lond) 2014; 139(7): 1576-88.
[http://dx.doi.org/10.1039/c3an01677c] [PMID: 24501736]

[116] Thévenot DR, Toth K, Durst RA, Wilson GS. Electrochemical biosensors: recommended definitions and classification. Biosens Bioelectron 2001; 16(1-2): 121-31.
[PMID: 11261847]

[117] Zouari M, Campuzano S, Pingarrón JM, Raouafi N. Competitive RNA-RNA hybridization-based integrated nanostructured-disposable electrode for highly sensitive determination of miRNAs in cancer cells. Biosens Bioelectron 2017; 91: 40-5.
[http://dx.doi.org/10.1016/j.bios.2016.12.033] [PMID: 27987409]

[118] Yan LX, Huang XF, Shao Q, *et al.* MicroRNA miR-21 overexpression in human breast cancer is associated with advanced clinical stage, lymph node metastasis and patient poor prognosis. RNA 2008; 14(11): 2348-60.
[http://dx.doi.org/10.1261/rna.1034808] [PMID: 18812439]

[119] Campuzano S, Torrente-Rodríguez RM, López-Hernández E, *et al.* Magnetobiosensors based on viral protein p19 for microRNA determination in cancer cells and tissues. Angew Chem Int Ed 2014; 53(24): 6168-71.
[http://dx.doi.org/10.1002/anie.201403270] [PMID: 24789269]

[120] Zhou Y, Wang M, Meng X, Yin H, Ai S. Amplified electrochemical microRNA biosensor using a hemin-G-quadruplex complex as the sensing element. RSC Advances 2012; 2(18): 7140-5.
[http://dx.doi.org/10.1039/c2ra20487h]

[121] Zhou Y, Zhang Z, Xu Z, Yin H, Ai S. MicroRNA-21 detection based on molecular switching by amperometry. New J Chem 2012; 36(10): 1985-91.
[http://dx.doi.org/10.1039/c2nj40253j]

[122] Zeng D, Wang Z, Meng Z, *et al.* DNA tetrahedral nanostructure-based electrochemical miRNA biosensor for simultaneous detection of multiple miRNAs in pancreatic carcinoma. ACS Appl Mater Interfaces 2017; 9(28): 24118-25.
[http://dx.doi.org/10.1021/acsami.7b05981] [PMID: 28660759]

[123] Wang J, Chen J, Chang P, *et al.* MicroRNAs in plasma of pancreatic ductal adenocarcinoma patients as novel blood-based biomarkers of disease. Cancer Prev Res (Phila) 2009; 2(9): 807-13.
[http://dx.doi.org/10.1158/1940-6207.CAPR-09-0094] [PMID: 19723895]

[124] Huang YL, Mo S, Gao ZF, *et al.* Amperometric biosensor for microRNA based on the use of tetrahedral DNA nanostructure probes and guanine nanowire amplification. Mikrochim Acta 2017; 184(8): 2597-604.
[http://dx.doi.org/10.1007/s00604-017-2246-8]

[125] Gao ZF, Huang YL, Ren W, Luo HQ, Li NB. Guanine nanowire based amplification strategy: Enzyme-free biosensing of nucleic acids and proteins. Biosens Bioelectron 2016; 78: 351-7.
[http://dx.doi.org/10.1016/j.bios.2015.11.070] [PMID: 26649493]

[126] Liu YQ, Zhang M, Yin BC, Ye BC. Attomolar ultrasensitive microRNA detection by DNA-scaffolded silver-nanocluster probe based on isothermal amplification. Anal Chem 2012; 84(12): 5165-9. [http://dx.doi.org/10.1021/ac300483f] [PMID: 22655700]

[127] Cheng FF, Jiang N, Li X, *et al.* Target-triggered triple isothermal cascade amplification strategy for ultrasensitive microRNA-21 detection at sub-attomole level. Biosens Bioelectron 2016; 85: 891-6. [http://dx.doi.org/10.1016/j.bios.2016.06.008] [PMID: 27311114]

[128] Pei X, Zhang B, Tang J, Liu B, Lai W, Tang D. Sandwich-type immunosensors and immunoassays exploiting nanostructure labels: A review. Anal Chim Acta 2013; 758: 1-18. [http://dx.doi.org/10.1016/j.aca.2012.10.060] [PMID: 23245891]

[129] Shu J, Tang D. Current advances in quantum-dots-based photoelectrochemical immunoassays. Chem Asian J 2017; 12(21): 2780-9. [http://dx.doi.org/10.1002/asia.201701229] [PMID: 28880459]

[130] Zhou Q, Tang D. Catalytic hairpin assembly-mediated surface charge density on the electrode for sensitive potentiometric detection of microRNA-21 in IgA-nephropathy. Biochem Eng J 2018; 140: 9-16. [http://dx.doi.org/10.1016/j.bej.2018.09.004]

[131] Goda T, Masuno K, Nishida J, *et al.* A label-free electrical detection of exosomal microRNAs using microelectrode array. Chem Commun (Camb) 2012; 48(98): 11942-4. [http://dx.doi.org/10.1039/c2cc36111f] [PMID: 23073155]

[132] Wadhera T, Kakkar D, Wadhwa G, Raj B. Recent advances and progress in development of the field effect transistor biosensor: A review. J Electron Mater 2019; 48(12): 7635-46. [http://dx.doi.org/10.1007/s11664-019-07705-6]

[133] Cai B, Huang L, Zhang H, Sun Z, Zhang Z, Zhang GJ. Gold nanoparticles-decorated graphene field-effect transistor biosensor for femtomolar MicroRNA detection. Biosens Bioelectron 2015; 74: 329-34. [http://dx.doi.org/10.1016/j.bios.2015.06.068] [PMID: 26159152]

[134] Gao A, Lu N, Dai P, Li T, Wang Y. Label-free and ultrasensitive detection of microrna biomarkers in lung cancer cells based on silicon nanowire FET biosensors IEEE. p. 2439-42. [http://dx.doi.org/10.1109/Transducers.2013.6627299]

[135] Hwang MT, Heiranian M, Kim Y, *et al.* Ultrasensitive detection of nucleic acids using deformed graphene channel field effect biosensors. Nat Commun 2020; 11(1): 1543. [http://dx.doi.org/10.1038/s41467-020-15330-9] [PMID: 32210235]

[136] Gao A, Yang X, Tong J, *et al.* Multiplexed detection of lung cancer biomarkers in patients serum with CMOS-compatible silicon nanowire arrays. Biosens Bioelectron 2017; 91: 482-8. [http://dx.doi.org/10.1016/j.bios.2016.12.072] [PMID: 28073028]

[137] Seenivasan R, Maddodi N, Setaluri V, Gunasekaran S. An electrochemical immunosensing method for detecting melanoma cells. Biosens Bioelectron 2015; 68: 508-15. [http://dx.doi.org/10.1016/j.bios.2015.01.022] [PMID: 25636023]

[138] Wang J, Li J, Baca AJ, *et al.* Amplified voltammetric detection of DNA hybridization *via* oxidation of ferrocene caps on gold nanoparticle/streptavidin conjugates. Anal Chem 2003; 75(15): 3941-5. [http://dx.doi.org/10.1021/ac0344079] [PMID: 14572067]

[139] Wang J, Yi X, Tang H, Han H, Wu M, Zhou F. Direct quantification of microRNA at low picomolar level in sera of glioma patients using a competitive hybridization followed by amplified voltammetric detection. Anal Chem 2012; 84(15): 6400-6. [http://dx.doi.org/10.1021/ac203368h] [PMID: 22788545]

[140] Meng L, Jin J, Yang G, Lu T, Zhang H, Cai C. Nonenzymatic electrochemical detection of glucose based on palladium-single-walled carbon nanotube hybrid nanostructures. Anal Chem 2009; 81(17): 7271-80.

[http://dx.doi.org/10.1021/ac901005p] [PMID: 19715358]

[141] Cardoso AR, Moreira FTC, Fernandes R, Sales MGF. Novel and simple electrochemical biosensor monitoring attomolar levels of miRNA-155 in breast cancer. Biosens Bioelectron 2016; 80: 621-30. [http://dx.doi.org/10.1016/j.bios.2016.02.035] [PMID: 26901459]

[142] Labib M, Khan N, Berezovski MV. Protein electrocatalysis for direct sensing of circulating microRNAs. Anal Chem 2015; 87(2): 1395-403. [http://dx.doi.org/10.1021/ac504331c] [PMID: 25495265]

[143] Selvaraju T, Das J, Han SW, Yang H. Ultrasensitive electrochemical immunosensing using magnetic beads and gold nanocatalysts. Biosens Bioelectron 2008; 23(7): 932-8. [http://dx.doi.org/10.1016/j.bios.2007.09.010] [PMID: 17977708]

[144] Karunakaran C, Bhargava K, Benjamin R. Biosensors and bioelectronics. Elsevier 2015.

[145] Zouari M, Campuzano S, Pingarrón JM, Raouafi N. Femtomolar direct voltammetric determination of circulating miRNAs in sera of cancer patients using an enzymeless biosensor. Anal Chim Acta 2020; 1104: 188-98. [http://dx.doi.org/10.1016/j.aca.2020.01.016] [PMID: 32106951]

[146] Liu L, Xu Q, Hao S, Chen Y. A quasi-direct LC-MS/MS-based targeted proteomics approach for miRNA quantification *via* a covalently immobilized DNA-peptide probe. Sci Rep 2017; 7(1): 5669. [http://dx.doi.org/10.1038/s41598-017-05495-7] [PMID: 28720752]

[147] Zouari M, Campuzano S, Pingarrón JM, Raouafi N. Determination of miRNAs in serum of cancer patients with a label- and enzyme-free voltammetric biosensor in a single 30-min step. Mikrochim Acta 2020; 187(8): 444. [http://dx.doi.org/10.1007/s00604-020-04400-w] [PMID: 32661767]

[148] Mohammadniaei M, Go A, Chavan SG, *et al.* Relay-race RNA/barcode gold nanoflower hybrid for wide and sensitive detection of microRNA in total patient serum. Biosens Bioelectron 2019; 141: 111468. [http://dx.doi.org/10.1016/j.bios.2019.111468] [PMID: 31279178]

[149] Shuai HL, Huang KJ, Chen YX, Fang LX, Jia MP. Au nanoparticles/hollow molybdenum disulfide microcubes based biosensor for microRNA-21 detection coupled with duplex-specific nuclease and enzyme signal amplification. Biosens Bioelectron 2017; 89(Pt 2): 989-97. [http://dx.doi.org/10.1016/j.bios.2016.10.051] [PMID: 27825521]

[150] Zhou C, Huang R, Zhou X, Xing D. Sensitive and specific microRNA detection by RNA dependent DNA ligation and rolling circle optical signal amplification. Talanta 2020; 216: 120954. [http://dx.doi.org/10.1016/j.talanta.2020.120954] [PMID: 32456939]

[151] Lu Z, Tang H, Wu D, *et al.* Amplified voltammetric detection of miRNA from serum samples of glioma patients *via* combination of conducting magnetic microbeads and ferrocene-capped gold nanoparticle/streptavidin conjugates. Biosens Bioelectron 2016; 86: 502-7. [http://dx.doi.org/10.1016/j.bios.2016.07.010] [PMID: 27442080]

[152] Wang F, Zheng Z, Guo J, Ding X. Correlation and quantitation of microRNA aberrant expression in tissues and sera from patients with breast tumor. Gynecol Oncol 2010; 119(3): 586-93. [http://dx.doi.org/10.1016/j.ygyno.2010.07.021] [PMID: 20801493]

[153] Hong CY, Chen X, Liu T, *et al.* Ultrasensitive electrochemical detection of cancer-associated circulating microRNA in serum samples based on DNA concatamers. Biosens Bioelectron 2013; 50: 132-6. [http://dx.doi.org/10.1016/j.bios.2013.06.040] [PMID: 23850778]

[154] Liu W, Zhong H, Wang R, Seeman NC. Crystalline two-dimensional DNA-origami arrays. Angew Chem Int Ed 2011; 50(1): 264-7. [http://dx.doi.org/10.1002/anie.201005911] [PMID: 21053236]

[155] Dietz H, Douglas SM, Shih WM. Folding DNA into twisted and curved nanoscale shapes. Science

2009; 325(5941): 725-30.
[http://dx.doi.org/10.1126/science.1174251] [PMID: 19661424]

[156] Li Y, Chang Y, Yuan R, Chai Y. Highly efficient target recycling-based netlike Y-DNA for regulation of electrocatalysis toward methylene blue for sensitive DNA detection. ACS Appl Mater Interfaces 2018; 10(30): 25213-8.
[http://dx.doi.org/10.1021/acsami.8b08545] [PMID: 29979026]

[157] Silvestrini M, Fruk L, Moretto LM, Ugo P. Detection of DNA hybridization by methylene blue electrochemistry at activated nanoelectrode ensembles. J Nanosci Nanotechnol 2015; 15(5): 3437-42.
[http://dx.doi.org/10.1166/jnn.2015.10214] [PMID: 26504963]

[158] Han S, Liu W, Yang S, Wang R. Facile and Label-Free Electrochemical Biosensors for MicroRNA Detection Based on DNA Origami Nanostructures. ACS Omega 2019; 4(6): 11025-31.
[http://dx.doi.org/10.1021/acsomega.9b01166] [PMID: 31460200]

[159] Li B, Liu F, Peng Y, *et al.* Two-stage cyclic enzymatic amplification method for ultrasensitive electrochemical assay of microRNA-21 in the blood serum of gastric cancer patients. Biosens Bioelectron 2016; 79: 307-12.
[http://dx.doi.org/10.1016/j.bios.2015.12.051] [PMID: 26720919]

[160] Yang B, Zhang S, Fang X, Kong J. Double signal amplification strategy for ultrasensitive electrochemical biosensor based on nuclease and quantum dot-DNA nanocomposites in the detection of breast cancer 1 gene mutation. Biosens Bioelectron 2019; 142: 111544.
[http://dx.doi.org/10.1016/j.bios.2019.111544] [PMID: 31376717]

[161] Hrstka R, Nenutil R, Fourtouna A, *et al.* The pro-metastatic protein anterior gradient-2 predicts poor prognosis in tamoxifen-treated breast cancers. Oncogene 2010; 29(34): 4838-47.
[http://dx.doi.org/10.1038/onc.2010.228] [PMID: 20531310]

[162] Trefulka M, Bartošík M, Paleček E. Facile end-labeling of RNA with electroactive Os(VI) complexes. Electrochem Commun 2010; 12(12): 1760-3.
[http://dx.doi.org/10.1016/j.elecom.2010.10.016]

[163] Bartosik M, Trefulka M, Hrstka R, Vojtesek B, Palecek E. Os(VI)bipy-based electrochemical assay for detection of specific microRNAs as potential cancer biomarkers. Electrochem Commun 2013; 33: 55-8.
[http://dx.doi.org/10.1016/j.elecom.2013.04.009]

[164] O'Dea JJ, Osteryoung J, Osteryoung RA. Theory of square wave voltammetry for kinetic systems. Anal Chem 1981; 53(4): 695-701.
[http://dx.doi.org/10.1021/ac00227a028]

[165] Pumera M. Electrochemistry of graphene: new horizons for sensing and energy storage. Chem Rec 2009; 9(4): 211-23.
[http://dx.doi.org/10.1002/tcr.200900008] [PMID: 19739147]

[166] Azimzadeh M, Rahaie M, Nasirizadeh N, Ashtari K, Naderi Manesh H. An electrochemical nanobiosensor for plasma miRNA-155, based on graphene oxide and gold nanorod, for early detection of breast cancer. Biosens Bioelectron 2016; 77: 99-106.
[http://dx.doi.org/10.1016/j.bios.2015.09.020] [PMID: 26397420]

[167] Zhou L, Wang J, Chen Z, *et al.* A universal electrochemical biosensor for the highly sensitive determination of microRNAs based on isothermal target recycling amplification and a DNA signal transducer triggered reaction. Mikrochim Acta 2017; 184(5): 1305-13.
[http://dx.doi.org/10.1007/s00604-017-2129-z]

[168] Miao P, Wang B, Yu Z, Zhao J, Tang Y. Ultrasensitive electrochemical detection of microRNA with star trigon structure and endonuclease mediated signal amplification. Biosens Bioelectron 2015; 63: 365-70.
[http://dx.doi.org/10.1016/j.bios.2014.07.075] [PMID: 25127470]

[169] Abi A, Ferapontova EE. Unmediated by DNA electron transfer in redox-labeled DNA duplexes end-tethered to gold electrodes. J Am Chem Soc 2012; 134(35): 14499-507. [http://dx.doi.org/10.1021/ja304864w] [PMID: 22876831]

[170] Cheng FF, He TT, Miao HT, Shi JJ, Jiang LP, Zhu JJ. Electron transfer mediated electrochemical biosensor for microRNAs detection based on metal ion functionalized titanium phosphate nanospheres at attomole level. ACS Appl Mater Interfaces 2015; 7(4): 2979-85. [http://dx.doi.org/10.1021/am508690x] [PMID: 25588109]

[171] Zhang X, Wu D, Liu Z, *et al.* An ultrasensitive label-free electrochemical biosensor for microRNA-21 detection based on a 2′-O-methyl modified DNAzyme and duplex-specific nuclease assisted target recycling. Chem Commun (Camb) 2014; 50(82): 12375-7. [http://dx.doi.org/10.1039/C4CC05541A] [PMID: 25187259]

[172] Zhuang J, Tang D, Lai W, Chen G, Yang H. Immobilization-free programmable hairpin probe for ultrasensitive electronic monitoring of nucleic acid based on a biphasic reaction mode. Anal Chem 2014; 86(16): 8400-7. [http://dx.doi.org/10.1021/ac501986k] [PMID: 25084479]

[173] Li C, Liu Z, Cai S, *et al.* An electrochemical microRNA biosensor based on protein p19 combining an acridone derivate as indicator and DNA concatamers for signal amplification. Electrochem Commun 2015; 60: 185-9. [http://dx.doi.org/10.1016/j.elecom.2015.09.012]

[174] Xu S, Chang Y, Wu Z, Li Y, Yuan R, Chai Y. One DNA circle capture probe with multiple target recognition domains for simultaneous electrochemical detection of miRNA-21 and miRNA-155. Biosens Bioelectron 2020; 149: 111848. [http://dx.doi.org/10.1016/j.bios.2019.111848] [PMID: 31726271]

[175] Zhu W, Su X, Gao X, Dai Z, Zou X. A label-free and PCR-free electrochemical assay for multiplexed microRNA profiles by ligase chain reaction coupling with quantum dots barcodes. Biosens Bioelectron 2014; 53: 414-9. [http://dx.doi.org/10.1016/j.bios.2013.10.023] [PMID: 24201005]

[176] Labib M, Khan N, Ghobadloo SM, Cheng J, Pezacki JP, Berezovski MV. Three-mode electrochemical sensing of ultralow microRNA levels. J Am Chem Soc 2013; 135(8): 3027-38. [http://dx.doi.org/10.1021/ja308216z] [PMID: 23362834]

[177] Labib M, Ghobadloo SM, Khan N, Kolpashchikov DM, Berezovski MV. Four-way junction formation promoting ultrasensitive electrochemical detection of microRNA. Anal Chem 2013; 85(20): 9422-7. [http://dx.doi.org/10.1021/ac402416z] [PMID: 24047131]

[178] Nishikata A, Ichihara Y, Tsuru T. An application of electrochemical impedance spectroscopy to atmospheric corrosion study. Corros Sci 1995; 37(6): 897-911. [http://dx.doi.org/10.1016/0010-938X(95)00002-2]

[179] Strašák L, Dvořák J, Hasoň S, Vetterl V. Electrochemical impedance spectroscopy of polynucleotide adsorption. Bioelectrochemistry 2002; 56(1-2): 37-41. [http://dx.doi.org/10.1016/S1567-5394(02)00019-1] [PMID: 12009440]

[180] Gomadam PM, Weidner JW. Analysis of electrochemical impedance spectroscopy in proton exchange membrane fuel cells. Int J Energy Res 2005; 29(12): 1133-51. [http://dx.doi.org/10.1002/er.1144]

[181] Katz E, Willner I. Probing biomolecular interactions at conductive and semiconductive surfaces by impedance spectroscopy: routes to impedimetric immunosensors, DNA-sensors, and enzyme biosensors. Electroanalysis. Electroanalysis 2003; 15(11): 913-47. [http://dx.doi.org/10.1002/elan.200390114]

[182] Rickert J, Göpel W, Beck W, Jung G, Heiduschka P. A 'mixed' self-assembled monolayer for an impedimetric immunosensor. Biosens Bioelectron 1996; 11(8): 757-68.

[http://dx.doi.org/10.1016/0956-5663(96)85927-6] [PMID: 8639283]

[183] Ebrahimi A, Nikokar I, Zokaei M, Bozorgzadeh E. Design, development and evaluation of microRNA-199a-5p detecting electrochemical nanobiosensor with diagnostic application in Triple Negative Breast Cancer. Talanta 2018; 189: 592-8.
[http://dx.doi.org/10.1016/j.talanta.2018.07.016] [PMID: 30086965]

[184] Capaldo P, Alfarano SR, Ianeselli L, *et al.* Circulating Disease Biomarker Detection in Complex Matrices: Real-Time, *In Situ* Measurements of DNA/miRNA Hybridization *via* Electrochemical Impedance Spectroscopy. ACS Sens 2016; 1(8): 1003-10.
[http://dx.doi.org/10.1021/acssensors.6b00262]

[185] Ren Y, Deng H, Shen W, Gao Z. A highly sensitive and selective electrochemical biosensor for direct detection of microRNAs in serum. Anal Chem 2013; 85(9): 4784-9.
[http://dx.doi.org/10.1021/ac400583e] [PMID: 23594156]

[186] Zhang K, Zhang N, Zhang L, Wang H, Shi H, Liu Q. Label-free impedimetric sensing platform for microRNA-21 based on ZrO_2 -reduced graphene oxide nanohybrids coupled with catalytic hairpin assembly amplification. RSC Advances 2018; 8(29): 16146-51.
[http://dx.doi.org/10.1039/C8RA02453G] [PMID: 35542230]

[187] Li S, Xu L, Ma W, *et al.* Dual-Mode Ultrasensitive Quantification of MicroRNA in Living Cells by Chiroplasmonic Nanopyramids Self-Assembled from Gold and Upconversion Nanoparticles. J Am Chem Soc 2016; 138(1): 306-12.
[http://dx.doi.org/10.1021/jacs.5b10309] [PMID: 26691742]

[188] Wan J, Liu X, Zhang Y, Gao Q, Qi H, Zhang C. Sensitive impedimetric detection of microRNAs using a hairpin probe based on DNAzyme-functionalized gold nanoparticle tag-initiated deposition of an insulating film on gold electrode. Sens Actuators B Chem 2015; 213: 409-16.
[http://dx.doi.org/10.1016/j.snb.2015.02.123]

[189] Yammouri G, Mandli J, Mohammadi H, Amine A. Development of an electrochemical label-free biosensor for microRNA-125a detection using pencil graphite electrode modified with different carbon nanomaterials. J Electroanal Chem (Lausanne) 2017; 806: 75-81.
[http://dx.doi.org/10.1016/j.jelechem.2017.10.012]

[190] Eksin E, Bikkarolla SK, Erdem A, Papakonstantinou P. Chitosan/nitrogen doped reduced graphene oxide modified biosensor for impedimetric detection of microRNA. Electroanalysis 2018; 30(3): 551-60.
[http://dx.doi.org/10.1002/elan.201700663]

[191] Voccia D, Bettazzi F, Fratini E, Berti D, Palchetti I. Improving impedimetric nucleic acid detection by using enzyme-decorated liposomes and nanostructured screen-printed electrodes. Anal Bioanal Chem 2016; 408(26): 7271-81.
[http://dx.doi.org/10.1007/s00216-016-9593-x] [PMID: 27178553]

[192] Azzouzi S, Mak WC, Kor K, Turner APF, Ali MB, Beni V. An integrated dual functional recognition/amplification bio-label for the one-step impedimetric detection of Micro-RNA-21. Biosens Bioelectron 2017; 92: 154-61.
[http://dx.doi.org/10.1016/j.bios.2017.02.014] [PMID: 28213328]

[193] Xue S, Li Q, Wang L, You W, Zhang J, Che R. Copper- and Cobalt-Codoped CeO_2 Nanospheres with Abundant Oxygen Vacancies as Highly Efficient Electrocatalysts for Dual-Mode Electrochemical Sensing of MicroRNA. Anal Chem 2019; 91(4): 2659-66.
[http://dx.doi.org/10.1021/acs.analchem.8b03778] [PMID: 30652475]

[194] Damborský P, Švitel J, Katrlík J. Optical biosensors. Essays Biochem 2016; 60(1): 91-100.
[http://dx.doi.org/10.1042/EBC20150010] [PMID: 27365039]

[195] Kilic T, Erdem A, Ozsoz M, Carrara S. microRNA biosensors: Opportunities and challenges among conventional and commercially available techniques. Biosens Bioelectron 2018; 99: 525-46.
[http://dx.doi.org/10.1016/j.bios.2017.08.007] [PMID: 28823978]

[196] Huang J, Ye L, Gao X, Li H, Xu J, Li Z. Molybdenum disulfide-based amplified fluorescence DNA detection using hybridization chain reactions. J Mater Chem B Mater Biol Med 2015; 3(11): 2395-401. [http://dx.doi.org/10.1039/C4TB01986E] [PMID: 32262070]

[197] Li H, Li Y, Li W, Cui L, Huang G, Huang J. A carbon nanoparticle and DNase I-Assisted amplified fluorescent biosensor for miRNA analysis. Talanta 2020; 213: 120816. [http://dx.doi.org/10.1016/j.talanta.2020.120816] [PMID: 32200921]

[198] Tang J, Xing Y, Wang Z, Yang M, Zhang J, Cai K. Janus nanoparticles with asymmetrically subcompartmentalized sensing and amplification modules toward fluorescence detection of microRNA. Sens Actuators B Chem 2020; 320: 128438. [http://dx.doi.org/10.1016/j.snb.2020.128438]

[199] Ma H, Xue N, Li Z, Xing K, Miao X. Ultrasensitive detection of miRNA-155 using multi-walled carbon nanotube-gold nanocomposites as a novel fluorescence quenching platform. Sens Actuators B Chem 2018; 266: 221-7. [http://dx.doi.org/10.1016/j.snb.2018.03.071]

[200] Afzalinia A, Mirzaee M. Ultrasensitive Fluorescent miRNA Biosensor Based on a "Sandwich" Oligonucleotide Hybridization and Fluorescence Resonance Energy Transfer Process Using an Ln(III)-MOF and Ag Nanoparticles for Early Cancer Diagnosis: Application of Central Composite Design. ACS Appl Mater Interfaces 2020; 12(14): 16076-87. [http://dx.doi.org/10.1021/acsami.0c00891] [PMID: 32207913]

[201] Mahani M, Mousapour Z, Divsar F, Nomani A, Ju H. A carbon dot and molecular beacon based fluorometric sensor for the cancer marker microRNA-21. Mikrochim Acta 2019; 186(3): 132. [http://dx.doi.org/10.1007/s00604-019-3233-z] [PMID: 30707293]

[202] Borghei YS, Hosseini M, Ganjali MR. Fluorometric determination of microRNA *via* FRET between silver nanoclusters and CdTe quantum dots. Mikrochim Acta 2017; 184(12): 4713-21. [http://dx.doi.org/10.1007/s00604-017-2512-9]

[203] Su S, Fan J, Xue B, *et al.* DNA-conjugated quantum dot nanoprobe for high-sensitivity fluorescent detection of DNA and micro-RNA. ACS Appl Mater Interfaces 2014; 6(2): 1152-7. [http://dx.doi.org/10.1021/am404811j] [PMID: 24380365]

[204] Jou AF, Lu CH, Ou YC, *et al.* Diagnosing the miR-141 prostate cancer biomarker using nucleic acid-functionalized CdSe/ZnS QDs and telomerase. Chem Sci (Camb) 2015; 6(1): 659-65. [http://dx.doi.org/10.1039/C4SC02104E] [PMID: 28706633]

[205] Freeman R, Willner I. Optical molecular sensing with semiconductor quantum dots (QDs). Chem Soc Rev 2012; 41(10): 4067-85. [http://dx.doi.org/10.1039/c2cs15357b] [PMID: 22481608]

[206] Resch-Genger U, Grabolle M, Cavaliere-Jaricot S, Nitschke R, Nann T. Quantum dots *versus* organic dyes as fluorescent labels. Nat Methods 2008; 5(9): 763-75. [http://dx.doi.org/10.1038/nmeth.1248] [PMID: 18756197]

[207] Ren X, Xue Q, Wen L, Li X, Wang H. Fluorescence-enhanced p19 proteins-conjugated single quantum dot with multiplex antenna for one-step, specific and sensitive miRNAs detection. Anal Chim Acta 2019; 1053: 114-21. [http://dx.doi.org/10.1016/j.aca.2018.11.060] [PMID: 30712556]

[208] Liu H, Li L, Wang Q, Duan L, Tang B. Graphene fluorescence switch-based cooperative amplification: a sensitive and accurate method to detection microRNA. Anal Chem 2014; 86(11): 5487-93. [http://dx.doi.org/10.1021/ac500752t] [PMID: 24823448]

[209] Fan T, Mao Y, Liu F, Zhang W, Yin J, Jiang Y. Dual signal amplification strategy for specific detection of Circulating microRNAs based on Thioflavin T. Sens Actuators B Chem 2017; 249: 1-7. [http://dx.doi.org/10.1016/j.snb.2017.04.079]

[210] Zayani R, Rabti A, Ben Aoun S, Raouafi N. Fluorescent and electrochemical bimodal bioplatform for femtomolar detection of microRNAs in blood sera. Sens Actuators B Chem 2021; 327: 128950. [http://dx.doi.org/10.1016/j.snb.2020.128950]

[211] Drakaki A, Hatziapostolou M, Polytarchou C, *et al.* Functional microRNA high throughput screening reveals miR-9 as a central regulator of liver oncogenesis by affecting the PPARA-CDH1 pathway. BMC Cancer 2015; 15(1): 542. [http://dx.doi.org/10.1186/s12885-015-1562-9] [PMID: 26206264]

[212] Yu Y, Yao Y, Yan H, *et al.* A Tumor-specific MicroRNA Recognition System Facilitates the Accurate Targeting to Tumor Cells by Magnetic Nanoparticles. Mol Ther Nucleic Acids 2016; 5: e318. [http://dx.doi.org/10.1038/mtna.2016.28] [PMID: 27138178]

[213] Peng S, Tan Z, Chen S, Lei C, Nie Z. Integrating CRISPR-Cas12a with a DNA circuit as a generic sensing platform for amplified detection of microRNA. Chem Sci (Camb) 2020; 11(28): 7362-8. [http://dx.doi.org/10.1039/D0SC03084H] [PMID: 33133487]

[214] Li C, Wang Z, Wang L, Zhang C. Biosensors for epigenetic biomarkers detection: A review. Biosens Bioelectron 2019; 144: 111695. [http://dx.doi.org/10.1016/j.bios.2019.111695] [PMID: 31526982]

[215] Li J, Liu Q, Xi H, Wei X, Chen Z. Y-shaped DNA duplex structure-triggered gold nanoparticle dimers for ultrasensitive colorimetric detection of nucleic acid with the dark-field microscope. Anal Chem 2017; 89(23): 12850-6. [http://dx.doi.org/10.1021/acs.analchem.7b03391] [PMID: 29120162]

[216] Gharatape A, Yari Khosroushahi A. Optical Biomarker-based Biosensors for Cancer/Infectious Disease Medical Diagnoses. Appl Immunohistochem Mol Morphol 2019; 27(4): 278-86. [http://dx.doi.org/10.1097/PAI.0000000000000586] [PMID: 28968262]

[217] Park J, Yeo JS. Colorimetric detection of microRNA miR-21 based on nanoplasmonic core–satellite assembly. Chem Commun (Camb) 2014; 50(11): 1366-8. [http://dx.doi.org/10.1039/C3CC48154A] [PMID: 24346179]

[218] Zhao H, Qu Y, Yuan F, Quan X. A visible and label-free colorimetric sensor for miRNA-21 detection based on peroxidase-like activity of graphene/gold-nanoparticle hybrids. Anal Methods 2016; 8(9): 2005-12. [http://dx.doi.org/10.1039/C5AY03296B]

[219] Wu H, Liu Y, Wang H, Wu J, Zhu F, Zou P. Label-free and enzyme-free colorimetric detection of microRNA by catalyzed hairpin assembly coupled with hybridization chain reaction. Biosens Bioelectron 2016; 81: 303-8. [http://dx.doi.org/10.1016/j.bios.2016.03.013] [PMID: 26985582]

[220] Ying N, Sun T, Chen Z, *et al.* Colorimetric detection of microRNA based hybridization chain reaction for signal amplification and enzyme for visualization. Anal Biochem 2017; 528: 7-12. [http://dx.doi.org/10.1016/j.ab.2017.04.007] [PMID: 28434989]

[221] Qiu XY, Zhu LY, Zhu CS, *et al.* Highly effective and low-cost microRNA detection with CRISPR-Cas9. ACS Synth Biol 2018; 7(3): 807-13. [http://dx.doi.org/10.1021/acssynbio.7b00446] [PMID: 29486117]

[222] Persano S, Guevara ML, Wolfram J, *et al.* Label-free isothermal amplification assay for specific and highly sensitive colorimetric miRNA detection. ACS Omega 2016; 1(3): 448-55. [http://dx.doi.org/10.1021/acsomega.6b00109] [PMID: 27713932]

[223] Delkhahi S, Rahaie M, Rahimi F. Design and fabrication a gold nanoparticle-DNA based nanobiosensor for detection of microRNA involved in Alzheimer's disease. J Fluoresc 2017; 27(2): 603-10. [http://dx.doi.org/10.1007/s10895-016-1988-8] [PMID: 27909844]

[224] Nguyen H, Park J, Kang S, Kim M. Surface plasmon resonance: a versatile technique for biosensor

applications. Sensors (Basel) 2015; 15(5): 10481-510.
[http://dx.doi.org/10.3390/s150510481] [PMID: 25951336]

[225] Šípová H, Zhang S, Dudley AM, Galas D, Wang K, Homola J. Surface plasmon resonance biosensor for rapid label-free detection of microribonucleic acid at subfemtomole level. Anal Chem 2010; 82(24): 10110-5.
[http://dx.doi.org/10.1021/ac102131s] [PMID: 21090631]

[226] Nasheri N, Cheng J, Singaravelu R, Wu P, McDermott MT, Pezacki JP. An enzyme-linked assay for the rapid quantification of microRNAs based on the viral suppressor of RNA silencing protein p19. Anal Biochem 2011; 412(2): 165-72.
[http://dx.doi.org/10.1016/j.ab.2011.01.030] [PMID: 21284927]

[227] Salahandish R, Ghaffarinejad A, Omidinia E, *et al.* Label-free ultrasensitive detection of breast cancer miRNA-21 biomarker employing electrochemical nano-genosensor based on sandwiched AgNPs in PANI and N-doped graphene. Biosens Bioelectron 2018; 120: 129-36.
[http://dx.doi.org/10.1016/j.bios.2018.08.025] [PMID: 30172235]

[228] Liu R, Wang Q, Li Q, Yang X, Wang K, Nie W. Surface plasmon resonance biosensor for sensitive detection of microRNA and cancer cell using multiple signal amplification strategy. Biosens Bioelectron 2017; 87: 433-8.
[http://dx.doi.org/10.1016/j.bios.2016.08.090] [PMID: 27589408]

[229] Li Q, Wang Q, Yang X, Wang K, Zhang H, Nie W. High sensitivity surface plasmon resonance biosensor for detection of microRNA and small molecule based on graphene oxide-gold nanoparticles composites. Talanta 2017; 174: 521-6.
[http://dx.doi.org/10.1016/j.talanta.2017.06.048] [PMID: 28738618]

[230] Li X, Cheng W, Li D, *et al.* A novel surface plasmon resonance biosensor for enzyme-free and highly sensitive detection of microRNA based on multi component nucleic acid enzyme (MNAzyme)-mediated catalyzed hairpin assembly. Biosens Bioelectron 2016; 80: 98-104.
[http://dx.doi.org/10.1016/j.bios.2016.01.048] [PMID: 26807523]

[231] Yang Y, Wang Q, Guo D. A novel strategy for analyzing RNA-protein interactions by surface plasmon resonance biosensor. Mol Biotechnol 2008; 40(1): 87-93.
[http://dx.doi.org/10.1007/s12033-008-9066-3] [PMID: 18465270]

[232] Aoki H, Corn RM, Matthews B. MicroRNA detection on microsensor arrays by SPR imaging measurements with enzymatic signal enhancement. Biosens Bioelectron 2019; 142: 111565.
[http://dx.doi.org/10.1016/j.bios.2019.111565] [PMID: 31404878]

[233] Li J, Lei P, Ding S, *et al.* An enzyme-free surface plasmon resonance biosensor for real-time detecting microRNA based on allosteric effect of mismatched catalytic hairpin assembly. Biosens Bioelectron 2016; 77: 435-41.
[http://dx.doi.org/10.1016/j.bios.2015.09.069] [PMID: 26453904]

[234] Wei X, Liu D, Zhao M, *et al.* An enzyme-free surface plasmon resonance imaging biosensing method for highly sensitive detection of microRNA based on catalytic hairpin assembly and spherical nucleic acid. Anal Chim Acta 2020; 1108: 21-7.
[http://dx.doi.org/10.1016/j.aca.2020.02.055] [PMID: 32222240]

[235] Shao H, Lin H, Guo Z, *et al.* A multiple signal amplification sandwich-type SERS biosensor for femtomolar detection of miRNA. Biosens Bioelectron 2019; 143: 111616.
[http://dx.doi.org/10.1016/j.bios.2019.111616] [PMID: 31472412]

[236] Zhang H, Fu C, Wu S, *et al.* Magnetic-capture-based SERS detection of multiple serum microRNA biomarkers for cancer diagnosis. Anal Methods 2019; 11(6): 783-93.
[http://dx.doi.org/10.1039/C8AY02423E]

[237] Wen S, Su Y, Dai C, *et al.* Plasmon Coupling-Enhanced Raman Sensing Platform Integrated with Exonuclease-Assisted Target Recycling Amplification for Ultrasensitive and Selective Detection of microRNA-21. Anal Chem 2019; 91(19): 12298-306.

[http://dx.doi.org/10.1021/acs.analchem.9b02476] [PMID: 31486639]

[238] Pang Y, Wang C, Lu L, Wang C, Sun Z, Xiao R. Dual-SERS biosensor for one-step detection of microRNAs in exosome and residual plasma of blood samples for diagnosing pancreatic cancer. Biosens Bioelectron 2019; 130: 204-13.
[http://dx.doi.org/10.1016/j.bios.2019.01.039] [PMID: 30745282]

[239] Zhou W, Tian YF, Yin BC, Ye BC. Simultaneous surface-enhanced Raman spectroscopy detection of multiplexed microRNA biomarkers. Anal Chem 2017; 89(11): 6120-8.
[http://dx.doi.org/10.1021/acs.analchem.7b00902] [PMID: 28488851]

[240] Chen J, Wu Y, Fu C, *et al.* Ratiometric SERS biosensor for sensitive and reproducible detection of microRNA based on mismatched catalytic hairpin assembly. Biosens Bioelectron 2019; 143: 111619.
[http://dx.doi.org/10.1016/j.bios.2019.111619] [PMID: 31454694]

[241] Chen Z, Lin Y, Ma X, *et al.* Multicolor biosensor for fish freshness assessment with the naked eye. Sens Actuators B Chem 2017; 252: 201-8.
[http://dx.doi.org/10.1016/j.snb.2017.06.007]

CHAPTER 14

Electrochemical Biosensor for Cancer Biomarkers Detection

Md Arifuzzaman[1], **Mostafa Kamal Masud**[2,3], **Asif Ahmed**[4], **Md Morsaline Billah**[4] and **Md Nazmul Islam**[5,6,*]

[1] *Institute of Tissue Banking and Biomaterial Research, Atomic Energy Research Establishment, Savar, Dhaka-1349 Bangladesh*

[2] *Australian Institute for Bioengineering and Nanotechnology (AIBN), The University of Queensland, Brisbane, QLD, 4072 Australia*

[3] *International Center for Materials Nanoarchitectonics (WPI-MANA), National Institute for Materials Science, Tsukuba, Ibaraki, 305-0044 Japan*

[4] *Biotechnology and Genetic Engineering Discipline, Khulna University, Khulna 9208, Bangladesh*

[5] *School of Health & Life Sciences, Teesside University, Middlesbrough TS1 3BA, United Kingdom*

[6] *National Horizons Centre, Teesside University, Darlington DH1 1HG, United Kingdom*

Abstract: Biosensors are common analytical devices, capable of sensing a myriad of biological analytes, including cancer biomarkers. Although biosensors have different transducer types, electrochemical biosensors provide fast analysis time, high sensitivity, and the ability to perform complex measurements such as multiplexed analysis or screening tests for early diagnosis and prognosis of cancer. This chapter describes the background and theory of electrochemical sensors and introduces the main readout techniques. Innovative electrochemical biosensing strategies for analysis and quantification of important early cancer biomarkers, which include circulating nucleic acids (*e.g.*, circulating tumour DNA, gene mutations, and microRNA) proteins, circulating tumour cells, and extracellular vesicles are discussed with the recent developments to provide an overview of the possible academic and clinical approaches.

Keywords: Biosensor, Early Detection, Electrochemistry, Voltammetry, Impedance, Biomarker, Exosomes, microRNA.

[*] **Corresponding author Md Nazmul Islam:** School of Health & Life Sciences, Teesside University, Middlesbrough TS1 3BA, United Kingdom and National Horizons Centre, Teesside University, Darlington DH1 1HG, United Kingdom; E-mail: mdnazmul.islam@tees.ac.uk

Farhadul Islam (Ed.)

INTRODUCTION

Cancer is one of the leading causes of death and an important barrier to increasing life expectancy across the globe [1]. A failure to improve the survival from cancer is largely a consequence of the failure of the diagnostic system due to late diagnosis. Early detection of cancer holds the greatest promise for reducing the economic and health burden associated with cancer [2]. Despite the recent rapid development of early diagnostic methods and precision medicine, current practices are expensive and laboratory-based methods such as imaging (CT, MRI, X-Ray), and serological tests. However, these diagnostic approaches are considered unreliable due to non-specific and often intermittent symptoms. These also lead to over-investigation and put a significant burden on hospital resources, with the possibility of exposing patients to ionising radiation as well as the risks and discomfort associated with invasive approaches. Therefore, the development of new low-cost diagnostic tools which can facilitate early detection of cancer with high precision, has become a priority [3].

The choice of an accurate biomarker panel is important for early cancer diagnosis and cancer surveillance. An ideal tumour marker should be specific, sensitive, and readily available in biological fluids such as blood and urine. In addition to their correlation with therapeutic monitoring, biomarkers should have a suitable baseline level to lower risk stratification and prognostic evaluation of patients with cancer [3]. Cancer biomarkers are comprised of a variety of molecular entities of cellular, sub-cellular or supramolecular origin, such as nucleic acids (*e.g.*, mutation, altered RNA profiling, epigenetic alteration, *etc.*), proteins and their functional subgroups (*e.g.*, enzymes, glycoproteins, tumour antigens and receptors), cells (*e.g.*, circulating tumour cells (CTCs) and extracellular vesicles (*e.g.*, tumour derived exosomes).

In recent years, circulating biomarkers, such as CTCs, extracellular vesicles, cell-free DNA (cfDNA), circulating tumour DNA (ctDNA) and microRNA have become increasingly popular as suitable candidates for liquid biopsies [4, 5]. The detection approaches for these biomarkers are generally limited to several molecular biology-based methods such as polymerase chain reaction (PCR) and next-generation sequencing (NGS) [5]. Despite their analytical reliability, the scope of these approaches at point of care, as well as resource-limited settings, is much limited.

To address these limitations, there is an increasing interest in the advancement of biosensor-based technologies for the detection of early cancer. Biosensors are analytical instruments capable of calculating the concentration of an analyte of interest in a biological or chemical reaction and can produce signals. Output single may be quantitative or qualitative depending on functionality and/or biomedical need [6, 7]. Portable electrochemical biosensors represent an inexpensive solution to provide a rapid measurement of biomarkers with clinically relevant sensitivity and specificity [8]. Electrochemical biosensors based on amplification-free direct detection assays are suitable for decentralized laboratory and point-of-care settings. Several electrochemical sensors do not require enzymatic amplification steps, which can provide a faster response and require a simpler workflow [9].

In this chapter, we presented a brief overview of the biosensor with a specific focus on the principle and mechanism of electrochemical biosensors and how they can be utilized for sensing cancer biomarkers.

SOME KEY TERMS IN BIOSENSOR-BASED ASSAYS

Biomarkers and Analytes. Cancer biomarkers could either be a biological molecule or biological processes induced by the tumour itself or by other noncancerous tissues. Tumour biomarkers can be diagnostic (determine the presence and types of cancer), prognostic (give information on the patient's overall cancer outcomes with or without standard treatment), or predictive (to understand which treatment the patient is most likely to respond to or benefit from) [3]. Certain biomarkers can be diagnostic, prognostic, and predictive at the same time. Depending on their localization in the body (*e.g.*, in biological fluids such as blood, urine, or saliva; in tissues; or in cells), the biomarkers can be noninvasive, minimally invasive or invasive. In biosensor-based assays, the target biomarker is known as an 'analyte' [10].

Matrix. Every molecule of a sample except the target analyte is known as a matrix. Detailed knowledge of the matrix is important as the analytical performance of an assay can be significantly influenced by interference of non-specific molecules of the matrix. Matrix interference could arise from the signals caused by non-target molecules or fouling of the sensor due to the adsorption of non-specific molecules on the sensor surface [10].

Transducer. The component of a biosensor that can convert the bio-recognition event into a quantifiable signal is known as a transducer [10]. The extent of target analyte–bioreceptor interactions or biorecognition events is related (usually proportionate) to the signals produced by transducers.

Sensitivity and Specificity. Sensitivity refers to the quantitative ability of a biosensor to detect a true portion of a target analyte within a given sample comprising the total target analyte. In other words, sensitivity reflects a true positive rate of an analyte in a given sample. Specificity can be defined as the ratio of true positives to total outcomes, which also include false positives. It is essential for a biosensor to detect cancer biomarkers to ensure the required level of sensitivity and specificity as the biomarkers remain in trace and varying amounts in a complex biological mixture [11].

Limit of Detection (LOD). Limit of detection (LOD) refers to the smallest amount of analyte for a biosensor to detect. Generally, LOD is the concentration that produces a signal greater than three times of the standard deviation of a blank sample. This can be calculated from the calibration curve because the concentration is equivalent to three times of the standard deviation at the ordinal intercept. LOD should not be limited to a specific concentration, and the presence of the target analyte can only be concluded with a given probability, that is, the noise from the sensor is very minimal [11].

Selectivity. Selectivity refers to the ability of the biosensor to respond only to the target analyte. In the complex mixture of the biological matrix, ensuring selectivity is very challenging [10].

Reproducibility. Reproducibility can be defined as the capacity of a biosensor to produce an identical response in a similar type of experiment. Both the precision and accuracy of the biosensor are characteristics of repeatability. Precision refers to the ability of a biosensor to produce consistent results every time the experiment is conducted, while accuracy denotes the ability of a biosensor to produce values close to the true values in multiple measurements [10, 11].

Stability. Stability is also regarded as one of the important characteristics to be considered for biosensor fabrication. Environmental factors, such as temperature, light and moisture, influence the stability of a biosensor and the biorecognition events. The physical properties and redox characteristics of the bioreceptors onto the transduction surface are also considered important factors for the design of a biosensor [10].

TYPES OF BIOSENSORS

"Biosensors, as classically defined, incorporate biological or biologically derived sensing elements that harness the exquisite specificity and sensitivity of living systems in conjunction with electronic transducers and processors, to either provide data or to directly actuate an appropriate response". Biosensors usually consist of three main components: (1) a recognition element (receptor) that interacts directly with a target analyte (*e.g.*, aptamer, DNA, antigen, antibody, *etc.*); (2) a signal transducer capable of converting an analyte-bioreceptor recognition event into a detectable signal; and (3) associated electronics and a readout device that interpret the transmitted signal and produce a quantifiable response [7]. Biosensors can be classified into different types depending on the transducers and readout methods, such as electrochemical biosensors, optical biosensors, magnetic biosensors, piezoelectric biosensors, gravimetric biosensors, and mechanical biosensors. However, electrochemical and optical biosensors are most widely employed in the detection of cancer biomarkers.

Electrochemical Biosensors. An electrochemical biosensor transduces the biorecognition events, such as enzyme-target (substrate) and antigen-antibody interaction, and adsorbed molecules to electrical signals in the form of current, voltage, impedance, *etc*. Since the discovery of glucose biosensors, various types of biosensors have been introduced and commercialised for diverse applications [12, 13]. It generally comprises a three-electrode system (working electrode, reference electrode and a counter electrode). Electrochemical transducers possess a wide range of readout methods, including i) amperometry, which measures the redox (oxidation or reduction) current of electroactive species; ii) conductometry, which relies on the conductometric of enzyme reactions and biological membranes; iii) potentiometry, which measures the potential difference of working electrode and a reference electrode without any current flows between them; and iv) impedimetry, which relies on the measurement of current flow hindrance induced by biorecognition events taking place on biosensor surface. Electrochemical biosensors are robust, easy to miniaturize, and have a wide range of detection limits, even when a trace amount of analyte is present. In addition, it can provide rapid response generated from molecular recognition, electrocatalytic activity and signal enhancement for ultrasensitive detection [14 - 16].

Optical Biosensors. Optical biosensors contain an optical transduction system obtained from the optical signal. The signal strength is proportional to analyte concentration [17, 18]. Fluorescence, luminescence, internal reflection, surface plasmon resonance, absorption, and light scattering spectroscopy are some examples of different forms of the optical transducer. Optical sensors have the capacity to remove external disturbances and are small and cost-effective. A variety of biomolecules such as enzymes, antibodies, antigens, receptors, nucleic acids, entire cells, and tissues can serve as biorecognition elements. Both label-free (signal is created directly by the bio-recognition events taking place onto transducer surface) and label-based (a label is used to generate colorimetric, fluorescent, or luminescent signals) detection can be conducted on optical biosensing platforms [17, 19].

Magnetic Biosensors. Magnetic biosensors contain magnetic (*e.g*., paramagnetic or super-paramagnetic) particles, or composites to detect biological interactions or biorecognition events of analytes. It can monitor the differences in magnetic characteristics or magnetically induced effects such as changes in coil inductance, resistance, or magneto-optical properties [20]. They have many advantages, such as limited background noise effects; the sensor can be controlled by an external magnetic field, allowing magnetic field-induced enhancement of signals generated from biorecognition events [20].

ELECTROCHEMICAL READOUT METHODS

Electrochemical sensing platforms have evolved from the concept of centralized laboratory to point-of-care testing. A variety of strategies for analyte recognition and signal transduction have allowed the development of different types of electrochemical assays (Fig. **1**) [9]. The most commonly used electrochemical sensing methods for detecting cancer biomarkers are discussed below:

Cyclic Voltammetry (CV). CV determines the redox potential and electrochemical reaction rate of a target analyte in solution. It is the most basic and fundamental technique to investigate the redox behavior of an electrolyte solution or response of a modified electrode in each electrode system. In addition, it can provide information about sensor fabrication steps for the detection of cancer biomarkers. In the CV process, the voltage is swept between two potential values at a fixed rate, however, when the voltage reaches the final potential (V_f), the scan is reversed, and the voltage is swept back to the initial potential (V_i). The current is measured between the working electrode and the counter electrode, whereas the voltage is recorded between the reference electrode and the working electrode. CV is represented as current *versus* voltage (known as a voltammogram) in a plot.

Differential Pulse Voltammetry (DPV). DPV is a differential technique that is the first derivative of a linear voltammogram. It is one of the most widely utilized techniques. For each redox reaction, a single peak is observed, which provides the characteristic potential and current. A series of pulses are overlaid on the cyclic voltammetry staircase waveform in pulsed voltammetry. The pulse voltammogram has a wave-like form, with a peak produced from the first derivative. The half-wave potential ($E^{1/2}$), which corresponds to the potential at half the wave height, provides qualitative information about an analyte in linear sweep voltammetry (LSV). Likewise, the peak potential, Ep, in DPV can be roughly identified with $E^{1/2}$. As a result, the DPV can depict the discrepancies in measured currents and applied potentials. DPV is more sensitive than linear sweep approaches because of its potential to produce less capacitive current. Furthermore, when it comes to biosensor fabrication, DPV provides a significant advantage over CV. CV is typically used for exploratory purposes and gives important information such as process reversibility and the types of redox processes present in a study (matrix, analyte, and electrode), whereas DPV is utilized for quantitative determinations. For instance, several RNA biosensors based on DPV technique have been reported, where adsorption of analytes on the electrode surfaces substantially reduced the DPV signals which were proportional to the amount of target analytes [21, 22].

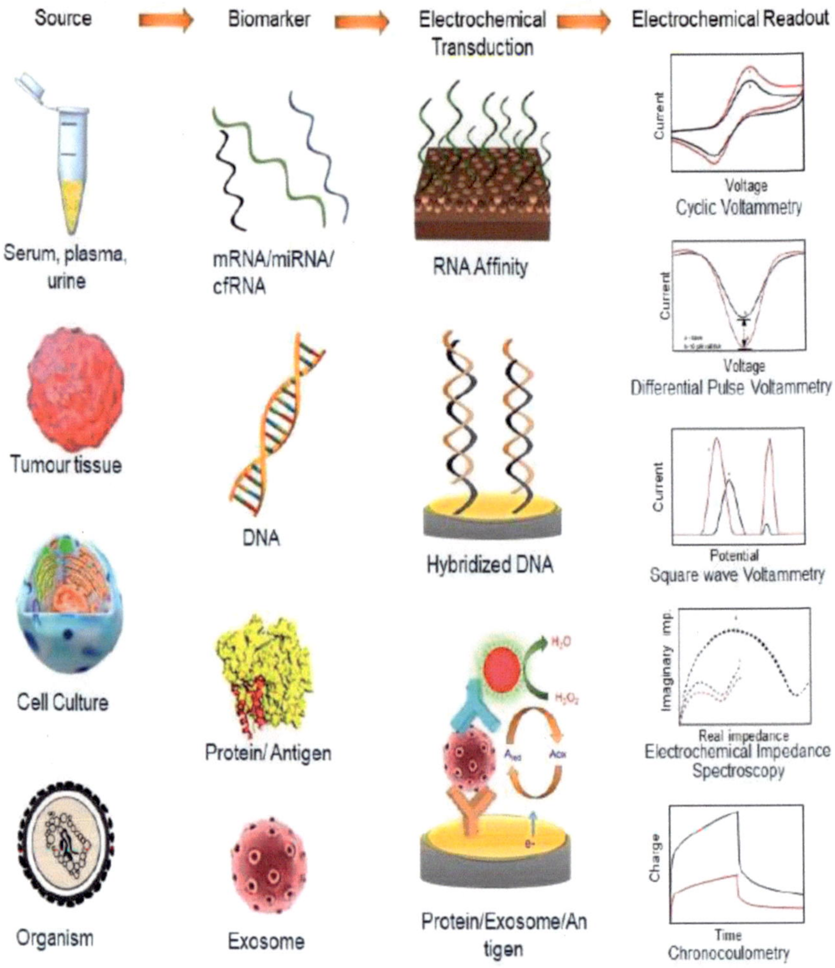

Fig. (1). A schematic representation of sample source, biomarkers, molecular recognition event and various electrochemical readout strategies for cancer biomarker detection.

Square-wave Voltammetry (SWV). In the SWV technique, the signal-to-noise ratio changes by the square root of the scan rate. The improvement in the signal is proportional to the time between the application of the pulse and the measurement of current. The timing of SWV is frequency dependent, which indicates with the frequency rises, the time constant falls and the measured faradaic current rises, giving the voltammogram sharper peaks. By evaluating the kinetics and mechanism of the electrode process, it is possible to analyse the distinctive properties of electrode materials in SWV [23]. In SWV, the current–potential curves show well-defined profiles and are often symmetrical. This is because the current is measured alone at the end of each semiperiod, and variations in height and width of the potential pulse are always constant within a given range of potentials [24].

Chronoamperometry. Chronoamperometry is an amperometric technique that involves the application of a square-wave potential to a working electrode and measuring the steady state current as a function of time. Diffusion layer at the electrode surface increases or decreases, causing changes in the current. At the electrode surface, analyte concentration declines to zero, and diffusion regulates the transport of analyte from bulk solution in an increasing concentration to the electrode [14]. As a result, the concentration gradient develops away from the electrode surface. This technique is closely related to the Cottrell equation that defines the current-time dependence for linear diffusion control at a planar electrode [25].

Electrochemical Impedance Spectroscopy (EIS). EIS is a very useful technique that can generate quantifiable signal changes in response to small changes in analyte concentration. In EIS, an alternating potential is applied to the working electrode at a range of frequencies. This results in an alternating current from the redox reaction (charge transfer) of the electrochemical species present at the working electrode surface [14]. EIS can investigate any inherent material characteristics that can influence the conductivity, resistivity, or capacitivity of an electrochemical system. EIS can be used to analyze and characterize electrode materials and different layers of a biosensor, such as studying polymer deterioration. Impedance approaches can be used to monitor changes in electrical characteristics caused by biorecognition events at the surface of modified electrodes, which is important for electrochemical sensing.

ELECTROCHEMICAL SENSOR FOR NUCLEIC ACID BIOMARKERS

Detection of nucleic acid biomarkers is generally confined to several classic molecular biology-based methods, such as polymerase chain reaction (PCR) and next-generation sequencing (NGS). Despite their reliability, the scope of these methods is limited outside of centralized laboratories. Conversely, electrochemical sensors for nucleic acid biomarkers are suitable for analysis either in decentralized laboratory facilities or at the point of care settings [9]. Due to their high sensitivity, many electrochemical sensors can detect endogenous concentrations of nucleic acids without the need for amplification steps [5].

Electrochemical DNA Sensors

CfDNA and CtDNA. The terms circulating cell-free DNA (cfDNA) and circulating tumour DNA (ctDNA) are often used as synonyms, causing general confusion. cfDNA is short (~130-180 base pairs) double-stranded DNA in body fluids, and an increased level of cfDNA is related with tumour progression [26]. ctDNA denotes a fraction of the cfDNA that originates from tumours and may carry the same genetic signatures of a primary tumour. While the overall level of cfDNA is quantified to aid diagnostics and prognosis, ctDNA analysis involves specific detection of its surrogate markers such as its epigenetic and molecular aberrations. Despite huge potentials in precision medicine, routine use of cfDNA and ctDNA as biomarkers in clinical setup is yet to be demonstrated. Existing methodologies are limited by biological (*e.g.*, high fragmentation, low stability, and rare abundance of cfDNA), technical (*e.g.*, ineffective extraction procedures) and clinical (*e.g.*, requirement of big set of control samples, patient heterogeneity, *etc.*) challenges.

Recently, microfabricated devices based on electrochemical readout of ctDNA have gained considerable attention as they can address some of the above challenges and are amenable to multiplexing [26, 27]. Kelley group has reported some of the important developments relating to chip-based electrochemical ctDNA sensors [27, 28]. For example, DPV readout was used to analyse mutated ctDNA in cancer samples. In this method, DNA samples were heat-denatured to produce single-stranded DNA (ssDNA) followed by an incubation with single-stranded clutch probes (Fig. **2I**, **A**). The pair of clutch probes prevents the reassociation of ssDNAs with complementary strands. Peptide nucleic acid (PNA) complementary to the wildtype strands of target DNA was further added, which allowed specific hybridization of PNA with perfectly matched wildtypes, while keeping the target of interest (*i.e.*, mutated ctDNA strands) unhybridized. The sample was then placed on a nanostructured microelectrode which was pre-functionalized with another set of PNA probes complementary to the mutant target ctDNA strand (Fig. **2I**, **B**). Therefore, only the target mutant ctDNA was hybridized to an immobilized PNA probe on the sensor surface. Note that, non-targets were already hybridized in the previous step, and eventually were washed way, thereby prevented from binding on the sensor. Following target hybridization, in the presence of an electrocatalytic reporter system comprising Ruthenium hexaammine(III) chloride ($[Ru(NH3)_6]^{3+}$) and ferricyanide ($[Fe(CN)_6]^{3-}$), DPV was used to obtain an electrochemical signal. On the electrode surface, positively charged $[Ru(NH3)_6]^{3+}$ is electrostatically attracted to the negatively charged phosphate backbone of the mutant ctDNA-PNA duplex. Upon providing a reduction potential to the electrode, target bound $[Ru(NH3)_6]^{3+}$ is reduced to $[Ru(NH3)_6]^{3+}$. When the system was further coupled with $[Fe(CN)_6]^{3-}$, there was a sharp amplification in the current. This is because, being a stronger oxidant than $[Ru(NH3)_6]^{2+}$, $[Fe(CN)_6]^{3-}$ in the diffusion layer oxidizes $[Ru(NH3)_6]^{2+}$to regenerate $[Ru(NH3)_6]^{3+}$ to initiate multiple turnovers of $Ru(NH_3)_6^{3+}$ thereby generating a high electrocatalytic current. The electrochemical signal is directly related to the increased concentration of anionic phosphates of target ctDNA at the electrode surface and can be calculated as the direct function of the amounts of target of interest present in the sample. This assay can detect as low as 1 fg/μL of a target mutation in the presence of 100 pg/μL of wild-type DNA. Due to the high potential of ctDNA-based biosensors in precision medicine, it has been studied extensively in several reviews [26, 29, 30].

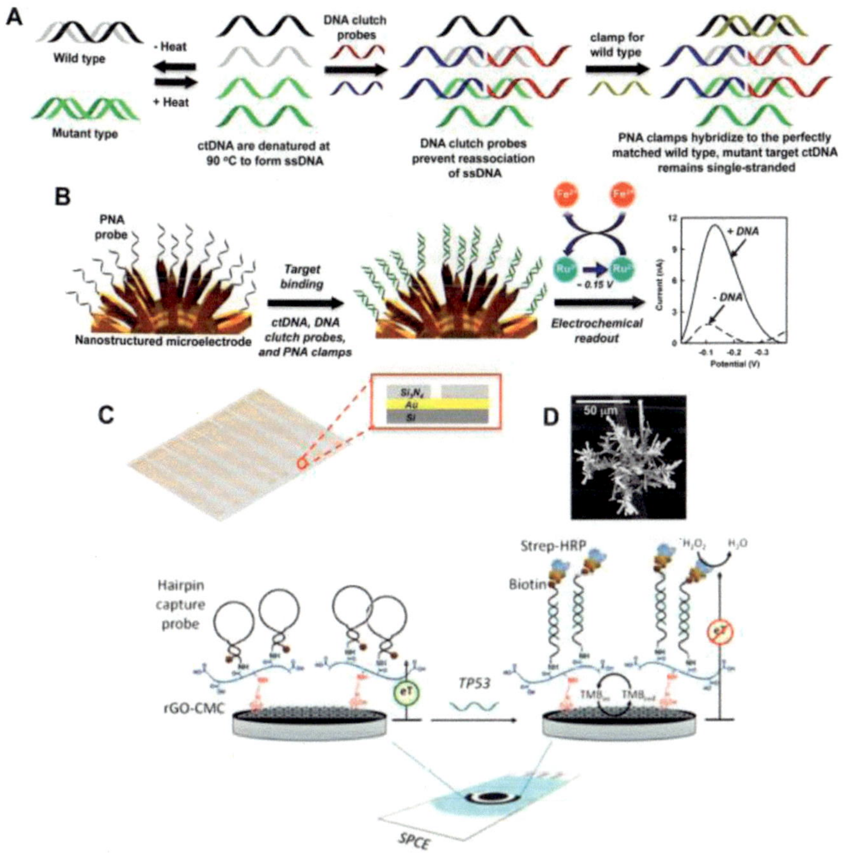

Fig. (2). Electrochemical sensors for detecting mutations in **(I)** ctDNA and **(II)** TP53 gene. I) Adapted with permission from Das *et al.* (27), copyright: 2016 American Chemical Society. II) Reprinted with permission from de Ávila *et al.* (31), copyright: 2015 American Chemical Society.

Mutation. The analysis of gene mutations (*e.g.*, mismatched base pairs, genomic sequence variations such single nucleotide polymorphisms, SNPs) plays a crucial role in early cancer diagnostics. Avila *et al.* illustrated an electrochemical sensor for the detection of SNP on p53 tumour suppressor (TP53) gene [31]. In this assay, a single base mismatch sequence of TP53 genotype (containing hot-spot mutation of G → A at codon 175 of exon 5) was chosen as a target which has a predominant role in altering cell cycle regulation during cancer progression. Screen-printed carbon electrodes (SPCEs) were fabricated with reduced graphene oxide– carboxymethylcellulose (rGO-CMC) hybrid nanomaterial. The 5′-end of the DNA hairpin capture probe was modified with biotin while an amino-C--modifier was tagged at its 3′-end. The probe was then covalently immobilized on the functionalized SPCE surface using carbodiimide chemistry (*i.e.*, EDC-NHS coupling). Next, using the strong affinity between biotin and streptavidin, streptavidin-coated horse radish peroxidase (strep-HRP) was attached on 5′-end of the capture probe. The electrochemical readout was performed *via* amperometric responses measured upon the addition of 3,3′,5,5′- tetramethylbenzidine (TMB) as a redox mediator in the presence of H_2O_2. TMB is considered an excellent electrochemical substrate for a trace amount of HRP. Thus, the amount of the complex oxidative product (diimine) generated in TMB oxidation measured by amperometry is directly related to the available amount of HRP, which in turn represents the extent of target hybridisation. Being specific, when target TP53 is present in the sample, it hybridizes with the HRP-tagged probe and the hairpin structures open up, thereby allowing HRP to oxidize TMB, resulting in a sharp increase in the current. When a single base mismatch target is hybridized, a significantly higher current than that of the no-target is observed. The current resulting from the mutant TP53 hybridization was found to be lower than that of the wildtype TP53, which was clearly distinguishable. Note that, in this sensor, the fabrication of functional hybrid nanomaterials on the electrode has considerably improved the assay performance towards a single base mismatch detection. This is because, the rGO-CMC hybrid offered an enormous surface area allowing a larger number of immobilized probes on the surface with enough spacing for optimal hybridization and amplified electrochemical signal. Barton group reported some of the early and phenomenal works on the development of electrochemical sensors for mutation based on DNA charge transport mechanism [13, 32, 33].

DNA Methylation. DNA methylation is an epigenetic phenomenon involving the addition of a methyl group to cytosine nucleotides (5 methylcytosine, 5mC) where the original DNA sequence remains unchanged. Both global DNA hypomethylation (*i.e.*, loss of the 5mC across the entire genome) and gene-specific hypermethylation (*i.e.*, an increase in locus-specific 5mC at regulatory regions) are crucial signatures for the early diagnosis of cancer. Bisulfite conversion of DNA is the most common step for the analysis of DNA methylation. To further quantify the level of methylation, bisulfite-treated DNA is read *via* other amplification or quantification approaches such as methylation-specific polymerase chain reaction (MS-PCR). However, the uncertainty of complete bisulfite conversion, inability to detect 5-methylcytosine oxidation products, DNA degradation, mispriming and amplification error (*i.e.,* PCR bias) are some of the associated issues.

There have been efforts to develop bisulfite treatment-free methods to analyse DNA methylation. One of the most straightforward strategies reported was the direct electrochemical oxidation of 5mC [15]. However, direct electrochemical oxidation of 5mC has been considered difficult because of the instability of unmodified metal electrodes at the extreme positive oxidation potential of 5mC. Moreover, the oxidative peak potentials of cytosine (C), thymine (T) and 5mC are in close range. This makes the discrimination of 5mC from the C and T bases from their oxidation peak very challenging. To address these issues, innovative inert electrode materials with wider potential windows and higher electrode activity have been developed [15]. Kato *et al.* used electron cyclotron resonance (ECR) to deposit sp^2 and sp^3 carbon mixture on a sputtered nanocarbon film electrode to produce a highly stable electrode which gave a significant potential difference (130–150 mV) between 5mC and C (Fig. **3I**) [34]. Polypyrrole functionalized graphene nanowall-modified electrodes showed strong enhancement in the potential resolution (184 mV) between 5mC and C oxidation [35].

Exploiting the physicochemical property of DNA, an electrochemical methylation assay was recently developed [36]. The assay demonstrated that a differential level of DNA methylation resulted in fundamental differences in DNA solvation properties and DNA-gold affinity between cancerous and normal genomes (Fig. **3II**). This feature can work as a universal signature for cancer. Purified DNA samples were directly added to a disposable Au electrode and allowed to physically adsorb. A $[Fe(CN)6]^{3-/4-}$ redox system was used to quantify the amount of adsorbed DNA *via* DPV, whereby adsorbed negatively charged DNA prevents $[Fe(CN)6]^{3-/4-}$ from reaching the electrode surface resulting in a significant current reduction. The DPV current change (% i_r) obtained was proportional to the adsorption level of DNA on gold electrodes, which in turn provided information on the 5mC landscape of a given genomic DNA, present in the genome.

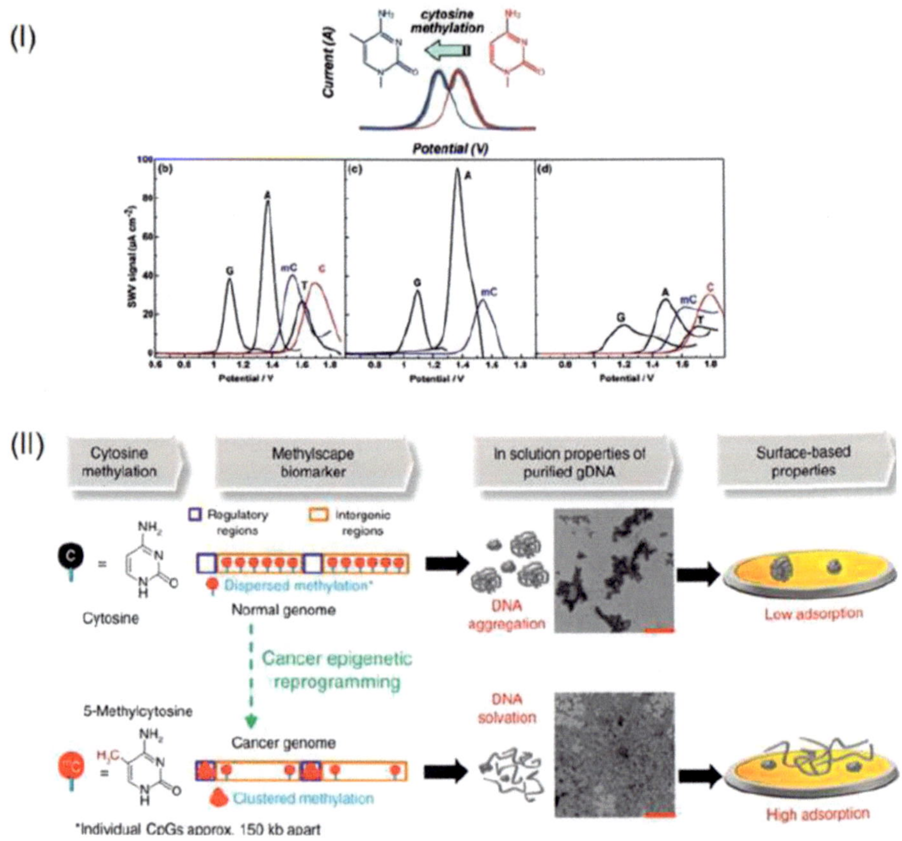

Fig. 3 (I). Direct electrochemical oxidation-based detection of 5-methylcytosine (5mC). **(II)** Electrochemical detection of global DNA methylation using physicochemical properties of methylated and unmethylated cytosine. (I) Reproduced with permission from D. Kato *et al.* (34) Copyright (2008) American Chemical Society. (II) Reproduced from A.A.I. Sina *et al.*(36) Copyright (2018) http://creativecommons.org/licenses/by/4.0/.

Electrochemical RNA Sensors

Non-coding transcripts such as microRNA (miRNA), and long non-coding RNA (lncRNA) have shown improved diagnostic, prognostics, and therapeutic potentiality for cancer management. miRNA, a short molecule consisting of 20-22 nucleotides, has become a crucial biomarker for early diagnostics of cancer due to their key regulatory roles, including translational repression and mRNA degradation [5]. Circulating miRNAs in body fluids are an important candidate for developing liquid biopsies. Since the discovery of miRNA, a great number of electrochemical biosensors have been developed [5, 16]. Most of these sensors rely on an isolation and purification step, followed by the hybridization of target

RNA sequences with capture probes and resultant readout. miRNA sensing, however, is inherently challenging, and there are two important considerations. First, the requirement of highly specific strategies (to avoid interference from other non-target miRNAs with sequence similarity and size homology and intermediates of miRNA biogenesis). Second, the requirement of ultrasensitive assay due to its low abundance in biological samples. To meet the sensitivity requirement, many electrochemical assays have been reported, which involve the incorporation of multiple signal amplification steps [25, 37, 38]. Signal amplification can be attained using electrocatalytic electrode materials, multifunctional nanomaterials modified electrodes, enzymatic and electrocatalytic reactions [16].

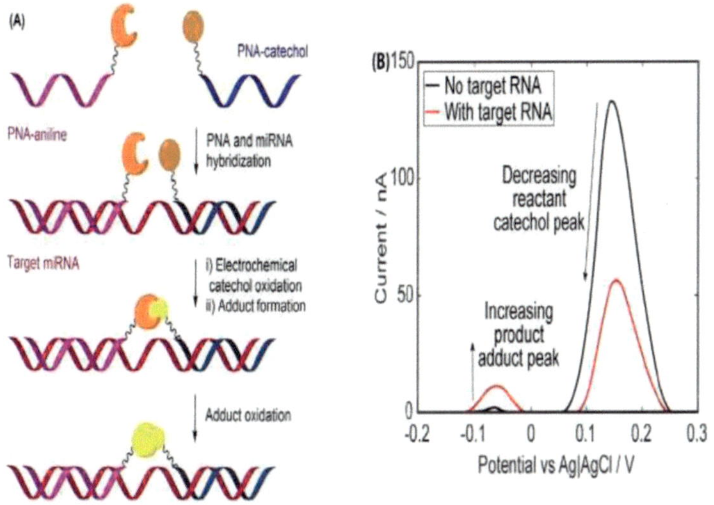

Fig. (4). Electrochemical quantification of miRNA using PNA probes **(A)** Schematic representation electrochemical oligonucleotide templated (EOTR) miRNA assay. **(B)** Differential Pulse Voltametric (DPV) response in the presence (red line) and absence (black line) of target miRNA. Reproduced with permission from Gillespie *et al.* (39) copyright: 2020 Elsevier.

To increase the assay specificity, dynabead and new magnetic functional nanomaterials involving multiple binding and washing steps were used [20]. Recently, Gillespie *et al.* reported a highly specific electrochemical miRNA assay *via* demonstrating the first example of electrochemical oligonucleotide-templated reaction (EOTR) (Fig. **4**) [39]. Two peptide nucleic acid (PNA) probes were synthesised and functionalized with a 4-methyl-cathecol and aniline molecules at their N- and C-terminus, respectively. These two probe heads were designed to allow simultaneous hybridisation to the same miRNA target to bring the probe heads in close proximity to each other, enabling the formation of an electroactive adduct. Both the reduction of the quinone peak and the adduct peak were recorded by DPV in the absence (Fig. **4B**, black line) or presence (Fig. **4B**, red line) of the target miRNA. Upon addition of a template, a significant increase in adduct formation between the first and second scan was observed along with a consumption of the quinone probe, whereas adduct formation was significantly reduced in the absence of a target. Electrochemical detection of this biorthogonal reaction showed a direct correlation between the amount of adduct formed and target miR-141 concentration. For more information on electrochemical miRNA sensors, please refer to the following reviews [5, 16, 40].

ELECTROCHEMICAL SENSORS FOR PROTEIN BIOMARKERS

There are a large range of protein-based tumour biomarkers such as carcinoembryonic antigen (CEA), squamous cell carcinoma antigen (SCCA), vascular endothelial growth factor (VEGF), epidermal growth factor receptor (EGFR), human epidermal growth factor receptor 2 (HER2), mucin 1 (MUC 1), breast cancer type 1 and 2 susceptibility proteins (BRCA1 and BRCA2) and DNA methyltransferase (DNA-MTase) [9]. There are some intrinsic challenges to the development of protein biosensors. These include (i) unlike nucleic acids, protein cannot be amplified; (ii) optimal ambient environment (temperature, pH) is needed to maintain its structural stability; (iii) large nonspecific interference from plenty of other proteins present in crude biological samples. Over the years, great progress has been made in addressing these obstacles to the development of electrochemical sensors [9]. For example, a proof-of-concept impedimetric sensor was developed to detect early breast cancer biomarker VEGF [41]. In this sensor, the recognition layer of the gold electrode was made up of a self-assembled monolayer of 3-Mercaptopropionic acid (3-MPA) linked to VEGF receptor-1. EIS was used to derive the charge transfer resistance (R_{ct}), which showed that the assay can quantify VEGF in the linear range between 10 pg/mL and 70 pg/mL. In another aptamer-based protein sensor, MUC1 was detected using DPV. The aptamer specific for MUC1 was modified with a thiol moiety at one end and a biotin label at the other end, which was further functionalised on HRP labelled gold nanoparticles (AuNPs) *via* a gold-thiol bond. The fabricated AuNPs were then immobilised on a glassy carbon electrode (GCE) which was pre-functionalised with streptavidin-modified multiwall carbon nanotubes (MWCNTs). The assay demonstrated an LOD of 268.6 µg/ L.

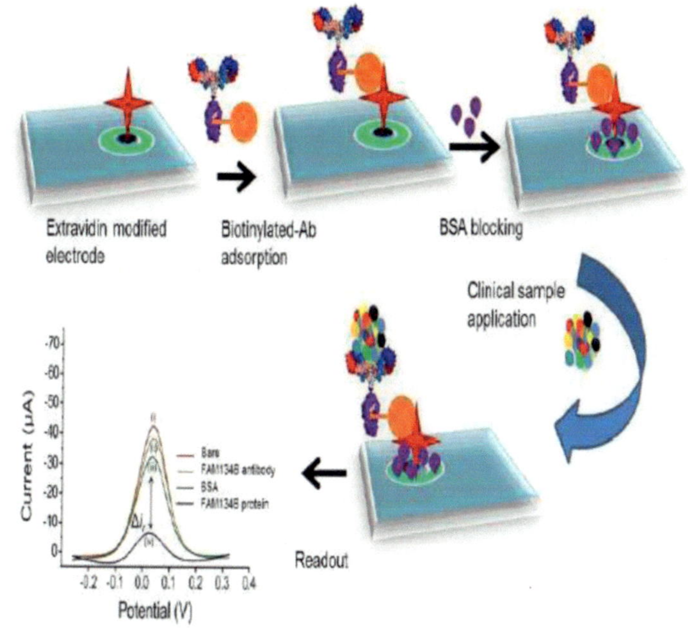

Fig. (5). Detection of FAM134B protein in colon cancer. Schematic shows the steps involved in the fabrication of electrochemical assay for the detection of FAM134B protein.

Islam *et al.* developed a rapid and sensitive electrochemical protein sensor for the detection of FAM134B protein biomarker in serum samples derived from colon cancer patients (Fig. **5**) [42]. In this biosensor, an ExtrAvidin®-modified screen-printed carbon electrode was modified with an anti-FAM134B antibody. The sensor surface was blocked with bovine serum albumin (BSA) to minimise the non-specific binding of sample. $[Fe(CN)_6]^{3-/4-}$ was used as the redox system where surface attached antibody- target conjugate hindered the interfacial electron transfer reaction of $[Fe(CN)_6]^{3-/4-}$. This resulted in a decrease in DPV current, allowing the quantification of the FAM134B protein biomarker with a LOD of 10 pg μL^{-1}.

ELECTROCHEMICAL SENSORS FOR CIRCULATING TUMOUR CELLS

Quantification of circulating tumour cells (CTCs), which account for 1 to 10 cells in 10^5-10^6 peripheral blood, can be crucial in cancer diagnostics and patient prognosis. A major challenge of the FDA□approved Cell Search-based CTC analysis is the 'biological noise' associated with low sensitivity, and specificity. Recent progress in microfabrication techniques has also enabled the development of several integrated electrochemical sensor (*e.g.*, microfluidic devices with electrochemical sensor) for CTC capture and detection. Generally, CTCs can be enriched by commercial kits based on immunoaffinity or biophysical property. Electrochemical methods can then be employed to quantify the cells.

Feng *et al.* designed an EIS-based CTC sensor. In this sensor, the gold working electrode was modified with epithelial cell adhesion molecule (EpCAM), which could bind over-expressed MCF-7 cells [44]. Due to the binding of CTCs, electron transfer at the electrode-reporter molecule interface was hindered, resulting in changes in impedance. This biosensor obtained a low detection limit of 10 cells mL^{-1}. In another study, an array nanochannel–ion channel hybrid coupled with an electrochemical sensor was demonstrated for CTC capture and detection [45]. The ion channel surface of the sensor was fabricated with aptamer probes which can selectively bind surface protein markers of CTCs. Based on altered mass-transfer properties, the captured CTCs were quantified using the electrochemical linear sweep voltammetry (LSV) technique. The method was reported to capture and detect as low as 100 cells mL^{-1} of leukemia CCRF-CEM CTCs. Fig. (**6**) shows the schematic representation of an electrochemical CTC sensor that uniquely employed multiple signal amplification steps. First, the CTCs were isolated and enriched by magnetic manipulation of EpCAM-tagged nanomaterials. Then, CTCs were linked with an aptamer–primer DNA sequence. To amplify the detection signal, rolling circle amplification (RCA) was performed for an increase in DNA loading onto the electrode. The reaction of the DNA molecules with molybdate generated an electrochemical current that is proportional to the number of CTCs. There are two useful articles that comprehensively reviewed CTC biosensing and identified challenges in CTC analysis [46, 47].

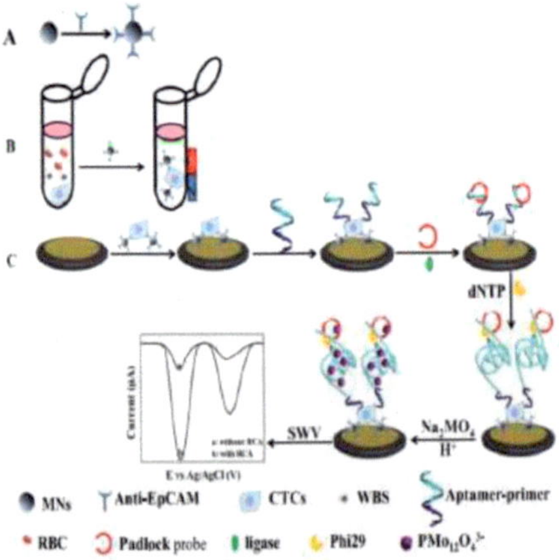

Fig. (6). Illustration of electrochemical measurement of circulating tumour cells (CTC) *via* rolling circle signal amplification: **(A)** Formation of Anti-EpCAM-MNs; **(B)** Recognition and Isolation of CTCs by Anti-EpCAM-MNs; **(C)** Electrochemical Detection of CTCs. (EpCAM: epithelial cell adhesion molecule; MNs: magnetic nanospheres). Reproduced with permission from [43]. Copyright: 2019 American Chemical Society.

ELECTROCHEMICAL SENSORS FOR EXTRACELLULAR VESICLES

Circulating tumour-derived exosomes in accessible bodily fluids such as blood, urine, saliva, and plasma have emerged as promising biomarkers for a range of cancers. Exosomes are nanoscale (≈30–150 nm) extracellular vesicles that regulate immune system function, particularly in tumorigenesis, as well as condition future metastatic sites for the attachment and growth of tumour tissue [48]. It has several advantages over traditional "soluble" biomarkers. These advantages include: their stability *in vivo* and in storage; their utility as a non-invasive biopsy; and that mechanical methods can be used to separate exosomes from "in-solution" signalling moieties that confound many traditional proteomic approaches used for biomarker identification.

Yadav *et al.* developed an electrochemical sensor to detect breast cancer-specific exosomes [49]. Here, an extravidin-modified screen-printed electrode functionalized with biotinylated anti-CD9 antibody was employed to capture generic exosomes from cell culture media. This is followed by the capture of breast-cancer-specific exosomes sandwiching between surface-bound CD9 and breast cancer-specific anti-human epidermal growth factor receptor 2 (HER-2) antibodies. The tumour-specific exosomes were then quantified with DPV, in the presence of $[Fe(CN)_6]^{3-/4-}$ redox system. Engineered superparamagnetic gold-coated nanomaterials based magnetic collection, purification and enrichment of exosome biomarkers were incorporated in a recently reported electrochemical platform [50]. This approach uniquely avoided commercial or laboratory-based pre-processing of exosomes. Jeong *et al.* developed an exosome sensor termed 'iMEX', which shows high potential for point-of-care testing [51]. The sensor is composed of eight channels, each containing a potentiostat. Eight magnets were placed under the potentiostat to allow immunomagnetic separation of exosomes. On the sensor, magnetic beads labelled with generic antibody (anti-CD63), were used to isolate bulk exosomes. HRP labelled tumour-specific antibody was then used to capture the cancer-specific exosomes selectively. After several magnetic washing and purification steps, the exosome biomarker was quantified *via* amperometry. iMEX is relatively rapid (assay time <1.0 h) and can detect as low as $<10^5$ vesicles in biological samples. A review by Boriachek *et al.* comprehensively covered a different aspect of exosome biosensors [48].

CONCLUSION

Current cancer diagnostics and therapeutics can be considered as "one size fits all" which is largely ineffective and expensive. In addition to causing overtreatment to many patients, it also results in the undertreatment of aggressive cancer. To overcome this, precision medicine-based cancer management is needed where electrochemical sensor-based personalized diagnostics can play a crucial role. An electrochemical biosensor is preferred for point-of-care (POC) examination due to its quick analytical response, downsizing potential, and ease of operation.

However, several issues must be addressed before they are implemented in routine clinical applications. Careful consideration should be taken for biosensor fabrication so that the biosensor surface becomes resistant to biofouling and the molecular detection events minimise off-target effects that can lead to false negatives and false positives. Significant research efforts are needed to develop innovative sampling approaches to simplify the downstream operations of electrochemical diagnostics. Multiplexed electrochemical biosensors that can analyze multiple biomarkers and continuously monitor biomarkers in real-time would reduce the need for frequent sampling. This would also help to avoid inaccurate results associated with tumor heterogeneity. Integration of electrochemical biosensors into fully automated systems is also required for point-of-care management of cancer. Full automation will facilitate the generation of accurate results even in the absence of trained personnel. Nevertheless, new advances in materials science, molecular biology, nanotechnology, and artificial intelligence are increasingly providing insights into electrochemical sensor platforms. This, in the future, will result in the development of new state-of-t-e-art electrochemical biosensors which can meet the demand for precision medicine-based cancer management

CONSENT FOR PUBLICATION

Not applicable.

CONFLICT OF INTEREST

The authors declare no conflict of interest, financial or otherwise.

ACKNOWLEDGEMENT

This work was supported by the Royal Society of Chemistry Research Fund Grant (R20-6411 to Md Nazmul Islam).

REFERENCES

[1] Sung H, Ferlay J, Siegel RL, *et al.* Global Cancer Statistics 2020: GLOBOCAN Estimates of Incidence and Mortality Worldwide for 36 Cancers in 185 Countries. CA Cancer J Clin 2021; 71(3): 209-49.
[http://dx.doi.org/10.3322/caac.21660] [PMID: 33538338]

[2] Loomans-Kropp HA, Umar A. Cancer prevention and screening: the next step in the era of precision

medicine. npj Precision Oncology 2019; 3(1):3.

[3] Chang JYH, Ladame S. Diagnostic, prognostic, and predictive biomarkers for cancer. In: Ladame S, Chang JYH, Eds. Bioengineering Innovative Solutions for Cancer 2020; 3-21. [http://dx.doi.org/10.1016/B978-0-12-813886-1.00001-2]

[4] Perakis S, Speicher MR. Emerging concepts in liquid biopsies. BMC Med 2017; 15(1): 75. [http://dx.doi.org/10.1186/s12916-017-0840-6] [PMID: 28381299]

[5] Islam MN, Masud MK, Haque MH, *et al.* RNA biomarkers: diagnostic and prognostic potentials and recent developments of electrochemical biosensors. Small Methods 2017; 1(7)1700131 [http://dx.doi.org/10.1002/smtd.201700131]

[6] Jayanthi VSPKSA, Das AB, Saxena U. Recent advances in biosensor development for the detection of cancer biomarkers. Biosens Bioelectron 2017; 91 (Suppl. C): 15-23. [http://dx.doi.org/10.1016/j.bios.2016.12.014] [PMID: 27984706]

[7] Vigneshvar S, Sudhakumari CC, Senthilkumaran B, Prakash H. Recent Advances in Biosensor Technology for Potential Applications – An Overview. Front Bioeng Biotechnol 2016; 4(11): 11. [http://dx.doi.org/10.3389/fbioe.2016.00011] [PMID: 26909346]

[8] Labib M, Sargent EH, Kelley SO. Electrochemical Methods for the Analysis of Clinically Relevant Biomolecules. Chem Rev 2016; 116(16): 9001-90. [http://dx.doi.org/10.1021/acs.chemrev.6b00220] [PMID: 27428515]

[9] Sage AT, Besant JD, Lam B, Sargent EH, Kelley SO. Ultrasensitive electrochemical biomolecular detection using nanostructured microelectrodes. Acc Chem Res 2014; 47(8): 2417-25. [http://dx.doi.org/10.1021/ar500130m] [PMID: 24961296]

[10] Bhalla N, Jolly P, Formisano N, Estrela P. Introduction to biosensors. Essays Biochem 2016; 60(1): 1-8. [http://dx.doi.org/10.1042/EBC20150001] [PMID: 27365030]

[11] O'Hare D. Biosensors and Sensor Systems. In: Yang G-Z, Ed. Body Sensor Networks 2014; 55-115. [http://dx.doi.org/10.1007/978-1-4471-6374-9_2]

[12] Clark LC Jr, Lyons C. Electrode systems for continuous monitoring in cardiovascular surgery. Ann N Y Acad Sci 1962; 102(1): 29-45. [http://dx.doi.org/10.1111/j.1749-6632.1962.tb13623.x] [PMID: 14021529]

[13] Drummond TG, Hill MG, Barton JK. Electrochemical DNA sensors. Nat Biotechnol 2003; 21(10): 1192-9. [http://dx.doi.org/10.1038/nbt873] [PMID: 14520405]

[14] Islam MN, Channon RB. Electrochemical sensors. In: Ladame S, Chang JYH, Eds. Bioengineering Innovative Solutions for Cancer 2020; 47-71. [http://dx.doi.org/10.1016/B978-0-12-813886-1.00004-8]

[15] Hossain T, Mahmudunnabi G, Masud MK, *et al.* Electrochemical biosensing strategies for DNA methylation analysis. Biosens Bioelectron 2017; 94: 63-73. [http://dx.doi.org/10.1016/j.bios.2017.02.026] [PMID: 28259051]

[16] Masud MK, Umer M, Hossain MSA, Yamauchi Y, Nguyen NT, Shiddiky MJA. Nanoarchitecture Frameworks for Electrochemical miRNA Detection. Trends Biochem Sci 2019; 44(5): 433-52. [http://dx.doi.org/10.1016/j.tibs.2018.11.012] [PMID: 30686572]

[17] Damborský P, Švitel J, Katrlík J. Optical biosensors. Essays Biochem 2016; 60(1): 91-100. [http://dx.doi.org/10.1042/EBC20150010] [PMID: 27365039]

[18] Mancuso V, Stramba-Badiale C, Cavedoni S, Cipresso P. Biosensors and biofeedback in clinical psychology reference module in neuroscience and biobehavioral psychology Reference Module in Neuroscience and Biobehavioral Psychology: Elsevier 2020.

[19] Nazmul Islam M, Yadav S, Hakimul Haque M, *et al.* Optical biosensing strategies for DNA

methylation analysis. Biosens Bioelectron 2017; 92: 668-78.
[http://dx.doi.org/10.1016/j.bios.2016.10.034] [PMID: 27836605]

[20] Masud MK, Na J, Younus M, *et al.* Superparamagnetic nanoarchitectures for disease-specific biomarker detection. Chem Soc Rev 2019; 48(24): 5717-51.
[http://dx.doi.org/10.1039/C9CS00174C] [PMID: 31720618]

[21] Islam MN, Gopalan V, Haque MH, *et al.* A PCR-free electrochemical method for messenger RNA detection in cancer tissue samples. Biosens Bioelectron 2017; 98: 227-33.
[http://dx.doi.org/10.1016/j.bios.2017.06.051] [PMID: 28688308]

[22] Haque MH, Gopalan V, Islam MN, *et al.* Quantification of gene-specific DNA methylation in oesophageal cancer *via* electrochemistry. Anal Chim Acta 2017; 976 (Suppl. C): 84-93.
[http://dx.doi.org/10.1016/j.aca.2017.04.034] [PMID: 28576321]

[23] Simões FR, Xavier MG. Simões FR, Xavier MG. 6 - Electrochemical Sensors. In: Da Róz AL, Ferreira M, de Lima Leite F, Oliveira ON, editors. Nanoscience and its Applications: William Andrew Publishing 2017; 155-78.

[24] Osteryoung JG, Osteryoung RA. Square wave voltammetry. Anal Chem 1985; 57(1): 101-10.
[http://dx.doi.org/10.1021/ac00279a004]

[25] Kamal Masud M, Islam MN, Haque MH, *et al.* Gold-loaded nanoporous superparamagnetic nanocubes for catalytic signal amplification in detecting miRNA. Chem Commun (Camb) 2017; 53(58): 8231-4.
[http://dx.doi.org/10.1039/C7CC04789D] [PMID: 28681881]

[26] Gorgannezhad L, Umer M, Islam MN, Nguyen NT, Shiddiky MJA. Circulating tumor DNA and liquid biopsy: opportunities, challenges, and recent advances in detection technologies. Lab Chip 2018; 18(8): 1174-96.
[http://dx.doi.org/10.1039/C8LC00100F] [PMID: 29569666]

[27] Das J, Ivanov I, Sargent EH, Kelley SO. DNA Clutch Probes for Circulating Tumor DNA Analysis. J Am Chem Soc 2016; 138(34): 11009-16.
[http://dx.doi.org/10.1021/jacs.6b05679] [PMID: 27513828]

[28] Das J, Ivanov I, Montermini L, Rak J, Sargent EH, Kelley SO. An electrochemical clamp assay for direct, rapid analysis of circulating nucleic acids in serum. Nat Chem 2015; 7(7): 569-75.
[http://dx.doi.org/10.1038/nchem.2270] [PMID: 26100805]

[29] Li X, Ye M, Zhang W, *et al.* Liquid biopsy of circulating tumor DNA and biosensor applications. Biosens Bioelectron 2019; 126: 596-607.
[http://dx.doi.org/10.1016/j.bios.2018.11.037] [PMID: 30502682]

[30] Campuzano S, Serafín V, Gamella M, Pedrero M, Yáñez-Sedeño P, Pingarrón JM. Opportunities, Challenges, and Prospects in Electrochemical Biosensing of Circulating Tumor DNA and its Specific Features. Sensors (Basel) 2019; 19(17): 3762.
[http://dx.doi.org/10.3390/s19173762] [PMID: 31480367]

[31] Esteban-Fernández de Ávila B, Araque E, Campuzano S, *et al.* Dual functional graphene derivative-based electrochemical platforms for detection of the TP53 gene with single nucleotide polymorphism selectivity in biological samples. Anal Chem 2015; 87(4): 2290-8.
[http://dx.doi.org/10.1021/ac504032d] [PMID: 25597471]

[32] Boon EM, Ceres DM, Drummond TG, Hill MG, Barton JK. Mutation detection by electrocatalysis at DNA-modified electrodes. Nat Biotechnol 2000; 18(10): 1096-100.
[http://dx.doi.org/10.1038/80301] [PMID: 11017050]

[33] Kelley S, Boon EM, Barton JK, Jackson NM, Hill MG. Single-base mismatch detection based on charge transduction through DNA. Nucleic Acids Res 1999; 27(24): 4830-7.
[http://dx.doi.org/10.1093/nar/27.24.4830] [PMID: 10572185]

[34] Kato D, Sekioka N, Ueda A, *et al.* A nanocarbon film electrode as a platform for exploring DNA methylation. J Am Chem Soc 2008; 130(12): 3716-7.

[http://dx.doi.org/10.1021/ja710536p] [PMID: 18314986]

[35] Wang P, Han P, Dong L, Miao X. Direct potential resolution and simultaneous detection of cytosine and 5-methylcytosine based on the construction of polypyrrole functionalized graphene nanowall interface. Electrochem Commun 2015; 61: 36-9.
[http://dx.doi.org/10.1016/j.elecom.2015.09.025]

[36] Sina AAI, Carrascosa LG, Liang Z, *et al.* Epigenetically reprogrammed methylation landscape drives the DNA self-assembly and serves as a universal cancer biomarker. Nat Commun 2018; 9(1): 4915.
[http://dx.doi.org/10.1038/s41467-018-07214-w] [PMID: 30514834]

[37] Islam MN, Masud MK, Nguyen NT, *et al.* Gold-loaded nanoporous ferric oxide nanocubes for electrocatalytic detection of microRNA at attomolar level. Biosens Bioelectron 2018; 101 (Suppl. C): 275-81.
[http://dx.doi.org/10.1016/j.bios.2017.09.027] [PMID: 29096366]

[38] Islam MN, Gorgannezhad L, Masud MK, *et al.* Graphene-Oxide-Loaded Superparamagnetic Iron Oxide Nanoparticles for Ultrasensitive Electrocatalytic Detection of MicroRNA. ChemElectroChem 2018; 5(17): 2488-95.
[http://dx.doi.org/10.1002/celc.201800339]

[39] Gillespie P, Channon RB, Meng X, Islam MN, Ladame S, O'Hare D. Nucleic acid sensing *via* electrochemical oligonucleotide-templated reactions. Biosens Bioelectron 2021; 176112891.
[http://dx.doi.org/10.1016/j.bios.2020.112891] [PMID: 33397596]

[40] Gillespie P, Ladame S, O'Hare D. Molecular methods in electrochemical microRNA detection. Analyst (Lond) 2019; 144(1): 114-29.
[http://dx.doi.org/10.1039/C8AN01572D] [PMID: 30375585]

[41] Sezgintürk MK. A new impedimetric biosensor utilizing VEGF receptor-1 (Flt-1): Early diagnosis of vascular endothelial growth factor in breast cancer. Biosens Bioelectron 2011; 26(10): 4032-9.
[http://dx.doi.org/10.1016/j.bios.2011.03.025] [PMID: 21515041]

[42] Islam F, Haque MH, Yadav S, *et al.* An electrochemical method for sensitive and rapid detection of FAM134B protein in colon cancer samples. Sci Rep 2017; 7(1): 133.
[http://dx.doi.org/10.1038/s41598-017-00206-8] [PMID: 28273937]

[43] Shen C, Liu S, Li X, Yang M. Electrochemical Detection of Circulating Tumor Cells Based on DNA Generated Electrochemical Current and Rolling Circle Amplification. Anal Chem 2019; 91(18): 11614-9.
[http://dx.doi.org/10.1021/acs.analchem.9b01897] [PMID: 31452368]

[44] Shen H, Yang J, Chen Z, *et al.* A novel label-free and reusable electrochemical cytosensor for highly sensitive detection and specific collection of CTCs. Biosens Bioelectron 2016; 81: 495-502.
[http://dx.doi.org/10.1016/j.bios.2016.03.048] [PMID: 27016910]

[45] Cao J, Zhao XP, Younis MR, Li ZQ, Xia XH, Wang C. Ultrasensitive Capture, Detection, and Release of Circulating Tumor Cells Using a Nanochannel–Ion Channel Hybrid Coupled with Electrochemical Detection Technique. Anal Chem 2017; 89(20): 10957-64.
[http://dx.doi.org/10.1021/acs.analchem.7b02765] [PMID: 28929739]

[46] Costa C, Abal M, López-López R, Muinelo-Romay L. Biosensors for the detection of circulating tumour cells. Sensors (Basel) 2014; 14(3): 4856-75.
[http://dx.doi.org/10.3390/s140304856] [PMID: 24618729]

[47] den Toonder J. Circulating tumor cells: the Grand Challenge. Lab Chip 2011; 11(3): 375-7.
[http://dx.doi.org/10.1039/c0lc90100h] [PMID: 21206959]

[48] Boriachek K, Islam MN, Möller A, *et al.* Biological Functions and Current Advances in Isolation and Detection Strategies for Exosome Nanovesicles. Small 2018; 14(6)1702153.
[http://dx.doi.org/10.1002/smll.201702153] [PMID: 29282861]

[49] Yadav S, Boriachek K, Islam MN, *et al.* An Electrochemical Method for the Detection of Disease-

Specific Exosomes. ChemElectroChem 2017; 4(4): 967-71.
[http://dx.doi.org/10.1002/celc.201600391]

[50] Boriachek K, Masud MK, Palma C, *et al.* Avoiding Pre-Isolation Step in Exosome Analysis: Direct Isolation and Sensitive Detection of Exosomes Using Gold-Loaded Nanoporous Ferric Oxide Nanozymes. Anal Chem 2019; 91(6): 3827-34.
[http://dx.doi.org/10.1021/acs.analchem.8b03619] [PMID: 30735354]

[51] Jeong S, Park J, Pathania D, Castro CM, Weissleder R, Lee H. Integrated Magneto–Electrochemical Sensor for Exosome Analysis. ACS Nano 2016; 10(2): 1802-9.
[http://dx.doi.org/10.1021/acsnano.5b07584] [PMID: 26808216]

SUBJECT INDEX

A

B

Farhadul Islam (Ed.)

D

E

F

G

H

O

P

Q

R

S

T

U

V

Made in the USA
Las Vegas, NV
03 November 2026

57423614R00238